Introduction to
Human Nutrition

The Nutrition Society Textbook Series

Introduction to Human Nutrition

Introduction to Human Nutrition: a global perspective on food and nutrition
Body composition
Energy metabolism
Nutrition and metabolism of proteins and amino acids
Digestion and metabolism of carbohydrates
Nutrition and metabolism of lipids
Dietary reference standards
The vitamins
Minerals and trace elements
Measuring food intake
Food composition
Food and nutrition: policy and regulatory issues
Nutrition research methodology
Food safety: a public health issue of growing importance
Food and nutrition-related diseases: the global challenge

Nutrition and Metabolism

Core concepts of nutrition
Molecular nutrition
The regulation of food intake
Integration of metabolism 1: Energy
Integration of metabolism 2: Carbohydrates and lipids
Integration of metabolism 3: Protein and amino acids
Phytochemicals
Pregnancy and lactation
Growth and aging
Gastrointestinal tract
Cardiovascular system
The skeletal system
The immune and inflammatory systems
The sensory systems
Physical activity
Overnutrition
Undernutrition
The brain

Public Health Nutrition

An overview of public health nutrition
Nutrition epidemiology
Food choice
Assessment of nutritional status at individual and population level
Assessment of physical activity
Overnutrition
Undernutrition
Eating disorders, dieting and food fads
PHN strategies for nutrition: intervention at the level of individuals
PHN strategies for nutrition: intervention at the ecological level
Food and nutrition guidelines
Fetal programming
Cardiovascular disease
Cancer
Osteoporosis
Diabetes
Vitamin A deficiency
Iodine deficiency
Iron deficiency
Maternal and child health
Breast feeding
Adverse outcomes in pregnancy

Clinical Nutrition

General principles of clinical nutrition
Metabolic and nutritional assessment
Overnutrition
Undernutrition
Metabolic disorders
Eating disorders
Adverse reactions to foods
Nutritional support
Ethical and legal issues
Gastrointestinal tract
The liver
The pancreas
The kidney
Blood and bone marrow
The lung
Immune and inflammatory systems
Heart and blood vessels
The skeleton
Traumatic diseases
Infectious diseases
Malignant diseases
Pediatric nutrition
Cystic fibrosis
Clinical cases
Water and electrolytes

Introduction to Human Nutrition

Second Edition

Edited on behalf of The Nutrition Society by

Michael J Gibney

Susan A Lanham-New

Aedin Cassidy

Hester H Vorster

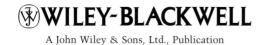

A John Wiley & Sons, Ltd., Publication

This edition first published 2009
First edition published 2002
© 2009, 2002 by The Nutrition Society

Blackwell Publishing was acquired by John Wiley & Sons in February 2007. Blackwell's publishing programme has been merged with Wiley's global Scientific, Technical, and Medical business to form Wiley-Blackwell.

Registered office
John Wiley & Sons Ltd, The Atrium, Southern Gate, Chichester, West Sussex, PO19 8SQ, United Kingdom

Editorial offices
9600 Garsington Road, Oxford, OX4 2DQ, United Kingdom
2121 State Avenue, Ames, Iowa 50014-8300, USA

For details of our global editorial offices, for customer services and for information about how to apply for permission to reuse the copyright material in this book please see our website at www.wiley.com/wiley-blackwell.

Library of Congress Cataloging-in-Publication Data

Introduction to human nutrition / edited on behalf of the Nutrition Society by Michael J. Gibney . . . [et al.]. – 2nd ed.
    p. ; cm. – (The human nutrition textbook series)
  Includes bibliographical references and index.
  ISBN 978-1-4051-6807-6 (pbk. : alk. paper)   1. Nutrition.   I. Gibney, Michael J.   II. Nutrition Society
(Great Britain)   III. Series.
  [DNLM: 1. Nutrition Physiology   2. Food. QU 145 I623 2009]

  QP141.I665 2009
  612.3–dc22

                          2008035123

A catalogue record for this book is available from the British Library.

Set in 10 on 12 pt Minion by SNP Best-set Typesetter Ltd., Hong Kong
Printed in Singapore by Fabulous Printers Pte Ltd

Contents

Contributors   vii

Series Foreword   ix

Preface   xi

Acknowledgments   xii

1. **Introduction to Human Nutrition: A Global Perspective on Food and Nutrition**   1
   HH Vorster

2. **Body Composition**   12
   P Deurenberg

3. **Energy Metabolism**   31
   A Astrup and A Tremblay

4. **Nutrition and Metabolism of Proteins and Amino Acids**   49
   NK Fukagawa and Y-M Yu

5. **Digestion and Metabolism of Carbohydrates**   74
   J Mathers and TMS Wolever

6. **Nutrition and Metabolism of Lipids**   86
   BA Griffin and SC Cunnane

7. **Dietary Reference Standards**   122
   KM Younger

8. **The Vitamins**   132
   DA Bender

9. **Minerals and Trace Elements**   188
   JJ Strain and KD Cashman

10. **Measuring Food Intake**   238
    UE MacIntyre

11. **Food Composition**   276
    HC Schönfeldt and JM Holden

12. **Food and Nutrition: Policy and Regulatory Issues**   293
    MJ Gibney and A McKevitt

13. **Nutrition Research Methodology**   305
    JA Martínez and MA Martínez-González

14. **Food Safety: A Public Health Issue of Growing Importance**   324
    A Reilly, C Tlustos, J O'Connor, and L O'Connor

15. **Food and Nutrition-Related Diseases: The Global Challenge**   350
    HH Vorster and MJ Gibney

Index   361

Contributors

Professor Arne Astrup
Head, Department of Human Nutrition,
Faculty of Life Sciences,
University of Copenhagen,
Copenhagen, Denmark

Dr David A Bender
Sub-Dean (Education),
University College London Medical School,
London, UK

Professor Kevin D Cashman
Department of Food and Nutritional Sciences,
University College Cork,
Ireland

Dr Stephen C Cunnane
Departments of Medicine, Physiology and
  Biophysics and Research Center on Aging,
Université de Sherbrooke
Canada

Professor Paul Deurenberg
Associate Professor in Nutrition,
Department of Human Nutrition,
Wageningen University,
The Netherlands
Visiting Professor,
University Tor Vergata, Rome, Italy
Nutrition Consultant, Singapore

Professor Naomi K Fukagawa
Department of Medicine,
University of Vermont,
Burlington, Vermont, USA

Professor Michael J Gibney
Department of Clinical Medicine,
Trinity College, Dublin,
Ireland

Dr Bruce A Griffin
Reader in Nutritional Metabolism,
Nutritional Sciences Division,
Faculty of Health and Medical Sciences,
University of Surrey,
Guildford, UK

Joanne M Holden
Nutrient Data Laboratory,
Beltsville,
Maryland, USA

Una E MacIntyre
Institute for Human Nutrition,
University of Limpopo,
Medunsa,
South Africa

Dr Aideen McKevitt
School of Biomedical Sciences,
University of Ulster,
Northern Ireland

Professor J Alfredo Martínez
Intitute of Nutrition and Food Sciences,
University of Navarra,
Spain

Professor Miguel A Martínez-González
Department of Preventive Medicine and Public
  Health,
University of Navarra,
Spain

Professor John Mathers
Human Nutrition Research Centre,
Institute for Ageing and Health
University of Newcastle, UK

Dr Judith O'Connor
Food Safety Authority of Ireland,
Dublin, Ireland

Dr Lisa O'Connor
Food Safety Authority of Ireland,
Dublin, Ireland

Alan Reilly
Food Safety Authority of Ireland,
Dublin, Ireland

Professor Hettie C Schönfeldt
School of Agricultural and Food Science
University of Pretoria,
South Africa

Professor JJ (Sean) Strain
Professor of Human Nutrition,
Northern Ireland Centre for Food and Health,
University of Ulster,
Coleraine, Northern Ireland

Christina Tlustos
Food Safety Authority of Ireland,
Dublin, Ireland

Angelo Tremblay
Preventive and Social Medicine,
Laval University,
Ste-Foy, Québec,
Canada

Professor Hester H Vorster
Director of the Centre of Excellence for Nutrition
Faculty of Health Sciences,
North-West University
Potchefstroom, South Africa

Dr Thomas MS Wolever
Department of Nutritional Sciences,
Faculty of Medicine,
University of Toronto,
Canada

Dr Kate M Younger
Lecturer in Human Nutrition,
School of Biological Sciences,
Dublin Institute of Technology,
Ireland

Dr Yong-Ming Yu
Department of Surgery,
Massachusetts General Hospital and Shriners Burns
    Hospital,
Harvard Medical School,
Boston, Massachusetts, USA

Series Foreword

The early decades of the twentieth century were a period of intense research on constituents of food essential for normal growth and development, and saw the discovery of most of the vitamins, minerals, amino acids and essential fatty acids. In 1941, a group of leading physiologists, biochemists and medical scientists recognized that the emerging discipline of nutrition needed its own learned society and the Nutrition Society was established. Our mission was, and remains, "*to advance the scientific study of nutrition and its application to the maintenance of human and animal health*". The Nutrition Society is the largest learned society for nutrition in Europe and we have over 2000 members worldwide. You can find out more about the Society and how to become a member by visiting our website at www.nutsoc.org.uk

The ongoing revolution in biology initiated by large-scale genome mapping and facilitated by the development of reliable, simple-to-use molecular biological tools makes this a very exciting time to be working in nutrition. We now have the opportunity to obtain a much better understanding of how specific genes interact with nutritional intake and other lifestyle factors to influence gene expression in individual cells and tissues and, ultimately, affect our health. Knowledge of the polymorphisms in key genes carried by a patient will allow the prescription of more effective, and safe, dietary treatments. At the population level, molecular epidemiology is opening up much more incisive approaches to understanding the role of particular dietary patterns in disease causation. This excitement is reflected in the several scientific meetings that the Nutrition Society, often in collaboration with sister learned societies in Europe, organizes each year. We provide travel grants and other assistance to encourage students and young researchers to attend and participate in these meetings.

Throughout its history a primary objective of the Society has been to encourage nutrition research and to disseminate the results of such research. Our first journal, *The Proceedings of the Nutrition Society*, recorded, as it still does, the scientific presentations made to the Society. Shortly afterwards, *The British Journal of Nutrition* was established to provide a medium for the publication of primary research on all aspects of human and animal nutrition by scientists from around the world. Recognizing the needs of students and their teachers for authoritative reviews on topical issues in nutrition, the Society began publishing *Nutrition Research Reviews* in 1988. In 1997, we launched *Public Health Nutrition*, the first international journal dedicated to this important and growing area. All of these journals are available in electronic, as well as in the conventional paper form and we are exploring new opportunities to exploit the web to make the outcomes of nutritional research more quickly and more readily accessible.

To protect the public and to enhance the career prospects of nutritionists, the Nutrition Society is committed to ensuring that those who practice as nutritionists are properly trained and qualified. This is recognized by placing the names of suitably qualified individuals on our professional registers and by the award of the qualifications Registered Public Health Nutritionist (RPHNutr) and Registered Nutritionist (RNutr). Graduates with appropriate degrees but who do not yet have sufficient postgraduate experience can join our Associate Nutritionist registers. We undertake accreditation of university degree programs in public health nutrition and are developing accreditation processes for other nutrition degree programs.

Just as in research, having the best possible tools is an enormous advantage in teaching and learning. This is the reasoning behind the initiative to launch this series of human nutrition textbooks designed for use worldwide. This was achieved by successfully launching the first series in multiple languages including Spanish, Portuguese and Greek. The Society is deeply indebted to Professor Mike Gibney and his team of editors for their tireless work in the last 10 years to bring the first edition of this series of textbooks to its successful fruition worldwide. We look forward to this new edition under the stewardship of Dr Susan Lanham-New in equal measure. Read, learn and enjoy.

Professor Ian Macdonald
President of the Nutrition Society

Preface

The Nutrition Society Textbook Series started ten years ago as an ambitious project to provide undergraduate and graduate students with a comprehensive suite of textbooks to meet their needs in terms of reference material for their studies. By all accounts the project has been successful and the Nutrition Society Textbook Series have been adapted by all of the best academic nutrition units across the globe. The series has been translated into Spanish and Portuguese.

This second edition of *Introduction to Human Nutrition* is an update of the very basic foundations for the study of human nutrition. Although little has changed, all authors have made whatever updates are necessary and we have made some re-arrangements of some chapters. The study of human nutrition at universities across the globe is rapidly expanding as the role of diet in health becomes more evident. Indeed, the sequencing of the human genome has highlighted the narrower range of genes controlling human biology, emphasising the critically important role of the environment including diet in human health. Moreover, we now recognize the important role that diet plays in interacting with our genome both *in utero* and in the immediate period of post natal development.

The study of human nutrition needs a solid base in the physiology and biochemistry of human metabolism and that is the basis of the textbook *Nutrition and Metabolism*. The present textbook is designed to serve two needs. Firstly, many will use this book as an introduction to human nutrition and go no further. Students in pharmacy, food science, agriculture and the like may take introductory modules to human nutrition and leave the subject there but be well informed in the area. Those who will go on to study human nutrition will find within this textbook an introduction to the many areas of diet and health that they will go on to study in greater depths using the remaining textbooks in the Nutrition Society series. Besides the basic biology, students will be introduced to the concept of food policy and to the dual challenges to the global food supply, both over and under nutrition.

As I write, I am handing over the leadership of the Nutrition Society Textbook Series to Dr Susan Lanham-New at the University of Surrey who has agreed to take on this important task for the Society. I would like to thank all those with whom I have worked with on this project and to wish Sue and her new team all the very best.

Michael J Gibney

The Nutrition Society Textbook Series Editors

Outgoing Editor-in-Chief
Professor Michael J Gibney
University College Dublin, Ireland

Assistant Editor
Julie Dowsett
University College Dublin, Ireland

Incoming Editor-in-Chief
Susan A Lanham-New
University of Surrey, UK

Assistant Editor
Jennifer Norton
The Nutrition Society, UK

Acknowledgments

With grateful appreciation to all those who have served on the International Scientific Committee and the Textbook Editors, without whom this task would be insurmountable and to all the authors who gave time to make this edition possible. Very special thanks must go to Mike Gibney and Julie Dowsett, for their effort and dedication in seeing this textbook of the second edition through to publication.

1
Introduction to Human Nutrition: A Global Perspective on Food and Nutrition

Hester H Vorster

Key messages

- Human nutrition is a complex, multifaceted scientific domain indicating how substances in foods provide essential nourishment for the maintenance of life.
- To understand, study, research, and practice nutrition, a holistic integrated approach from molecular to societal level is needed.
- Optimal, balanced nutrition is a major determinant of health. It can be used to promote health and well-being, to prevent ill-health and to treat disease.
- The study of the structure, chemical and physical characteristics, and physiological and biochemical effects of the more than 50 nutrients found in foods underpins the understanding of nutrition.

- The hundreds of millions of food- and nutrition-insecure people globally, the coexistence of undernutrition and overnutrition, and inappropriate nutritional behaviors are challenges that face the nutritionist of today.
- Nutrition practice has a firm and well-developed research and knowledge base. There are, however, many areas where more information is needed to solve global, regional, communal and individual nutrition problems.
- The development of ethical norms, standards, and values in nutrition research and practice is needed.

1.1 Orientation to human nutrition

The major purpose of this series of four textbooks on nutrition is to guide the nutrition student through the exciting journey of discovery of nutrition as a science. As apprentices in nutrition science and practice students will learn how to collect, systemize, and classify knowledge by reading, experimentation, observation, and reasoning. The road for this journey was mapped out millennia ago. The knowledge that nutrition – what we choose to eat and drink – influences our health, well-being, and quality of life is as old as human history. For millions of years the quest for food has helped to shape human development, the organization of society and history itself. It has influenced wars, population growth, urban expansion, economic and political theory, religion, science, medicine, and technological development.

It was only in the second half of the eighteenth century that nutrition started to experience its first renaissance with the observation by scientists that intakes of certain foods, later called nutrients, and eventually other substances not yet classified as nutrients, influence the function of the body, protect against disease, restore health, and determine people's response to changes in the environment. During this period, nutrition was studied from a medical model or paradigm by defining the chemical structures and characteristics of nutrients found in foods, their physiological functions, biochemical reactions and human requirements to prevent, first, deficiency diseases and, later, also chronic noncommunicable diseases.

Since the late 1980s nutrition has experienced a second renaissance with the growing perception that the knowledge gained did not equip mankind to solve the global problems of food insecurity and malnutrition. The emphasis shifted from the medical or pathological paradigm to a more psychosocial, behavioral one in which nutrition is defined as a basic human right, not only essential for human development but also as an outcome of development.

In this first, introductory text, the focus is on principles and essentials of human nutrition, with the main purpose of helping the nutrition student to develop a holistic and integrated understanding of this complex, multifaceted scientific domain.

1.2 An integrated approach

Human nutrition describes the processes whereby cellular organelles, cells, tissues, organs, systems, and the body as a whole obtain and use necessary substances obtained from foods (nutrients) to maintain structural and functional integrity. For an understanding of how humans obtain and utilize foods and nutrients from a molecular to a societal level, and of the factors determining and influencing these processes, the study and practice of human nutrition involve a spectrum of other basic and applied scientific disciplines. These include molecular biology, genetics, biochemistry, chemistry, physics, food science, microbiology, physiology, pathology, immunology, psychology, sociology, political science, anthropology, agriculture, pharmacology, communications, and economics. Nutrition departments are, therefore, often found in Medical (Health) or Social Science, or Pharmacy, or Agriculture Faculties at tertiary training institutions. The multidisciplinary nature of the science of nutrition, lying in both the natural (biological) and social scientific fields, demands that students of nutrition should have a basic understanding of many branches of science and that they should be able to integrate different concepts from these different disciplines. It implies that students should choose their accompanying subjects (electives) carefully and that they should read widely in these different areas.

1.3 A conceptional framework for the study of nutrition

In the journey of discovery into nutrition science it will often be necessary to put new knowledge, or new applications of old knowledge, into the perspective of the holistic picture. For this, a conceptual framework of the multidisciplinary nature of nutrition science and practice may be of value. Such a concep-

tual framework, illustrating the complex interactions between internal or constitutional factors and external environmental factors which determine nutritional status and health, is given in Figure 1.1.

On a genetic level it is now accepted that nutrients dictate phenotypic expression of an individual's genotype by influencing the processes of transcription, translation, or post-translational reactions. In other words, nutrients can directly influence genetic (DNA) expression, determining the type of RNA formed (transcription) and also the proteins synthesized (translation). For example, glucose, a carbohydrate macronutrient, increases transcription for the synthesis of glucokinase, the micronutrient iron increases translation for the synthesis of ferritin, while vitamin K increases post-translational carboxylation of glutamic acid residues for the synthesis of prothrombin. Nutrients, therefore, influence the synthesis of structural and functional proteins, by influencing gene expression within cells.

Nutrients also act as substrates and cofactors in all of the metabolic reactions in cells necessary for the growth and maintenance of structure and function. Cells take up nutrients (through complex mechanisms across cell membranes) from their immediate environment, also known as the body's internal environment. The composition of this environment is carefully regulated to ensure optimal function and survival of cells, a process known as homeostasis, which gave birth to a systems approach in the study of nutrition.

Nutrients and oxygen are provided to the internal environment by the circulating blood, which also removes metabolic end-products and harmful substances from this environment for excretion through the skin, the kidneys, and the large bowel.

The concerted function of different organs and systems of the body ensures that nutrients and oxygen are extracted or taken up from the external environment and transferred to the blood for transport and delivery to the internal environment and cells. The digestive system, for example, is responsible for the ingestion of food and beverages, the breakdown (digestion and fermentation) of these for extraction of nutrients, and the absorption of the nutrients into the circulation, while the respiratory system extracts oxygen from the air. These functions are coordinated and regulated by the endocrine and central nervous

Levels of human function (factors)	Accompanying scientific disciplines of study

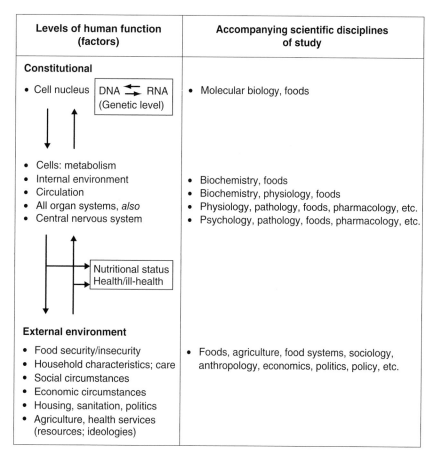

Figure 1.1 Conceptual framework for a holistic, integrated understanding of human nutrition.

systems in response to the chemical and physical composition of the blood and internal environment, and to cellular needs.

The health or disease state of the different organs and systems will determine the nutrient requirements of the body as a whole.

The central nervous system is also the site or "headquarters" of the higher, mental functions related to conscious or cognitive, spiritual, religious, and cultural behaviors, which will determine, in response to the internal and external environments, what and how much will be eaten. What and how much is eaten will further depend on what is available, influenced by a host of factors determining food security. All of these factors, on an individual, household, community, national, or international level, shape the external environment.

During the first renaissance of nutrition, emphasis was placed on the study of nutrients and their func-

tions. A medical, natural science or biological model underpinned the study of the relationships between nutrition and health or ill-health. During the second renaissance, these aspects are not neglected, but expanded to include the study of all other external environmental factors that determine what and how much food and nutrients are available on a global level. These studies are underpinned by social, behavioral, economic, agricultural, and political sciences. The study of human nutrition therefore seeks to understand the complexities of both social and biological factors on how individuals and populations maintain optimal function and health, how the quality, quantity and balance of the food supply are influenced, what happens to food after it is eaten, and the way that diet affects health and well-being. This integrated approach has led to a better understanding of the causes and consequences of malnutrition, and of the relationship between nutrition and health.

1.4 Relationship between nutrition and health

Figure 1.2 shows that individuals can be broadly categorized into having optimal nutritional status or being undernourished, overnourished, or malnourished. The major causes and consequences of these nutritional states are indicated. It is important to realize that many other lifestyle and environmental factors, in addition to nutrition, influence health and well-being, but nutrition is a major, modifiable, and powerful factor in promoting health, preventing and treating disease, and improving quality of life.

1.5 Nutrients: the basics

People eat food, not nutrients; however, it is the combination and amounts of nutrients in consumed foods that determine health. To read one must know the letters of the alphabet; to do sums one must be able to count, add, subtract, multiply, and divide. To understand nutrition, one must know about nutrients. The study of nutrients, the ABC and numeric calculations of nutrition, will form a major part of the student's nutrition journey, and should include:

- the chemical and physical structure and characteristics of the nutrient
- the food sources of the nutrient, including food composition, the way in which foods are grown, harvested, stored, processed and prepared, and the effects of these on nutrient composition and nutritional value
- the digestion, absorption, circulatory transport, and cellular uptake of the nutrient, as well as regulation of all these processes
- the metabolism of the nutrient, its functions, storage, and excretion
- physiological needs (demands or requirements) for the nutrient in health and disease, and during special circumstances (pregnancy, lactation, sport events), as well as individual variability
- interactions with other nutrients, nonnutrients (phytochemicals), antinutrients, and drugs

Nutritional situation		Health consequences, outcomes
Optimum nutrition Food-secure individuals with adequate, balanced and prudent diets	→	Health, well-being, normal development, high quality of life
Undernutrition: hunger Food-insecure individuals living in poverty, ignorance, politically unstable environments, disrupted societies, war	→	• Decreased physical and mental development • Compromised immune systems • Increased infectious diseases • Vicious circle of undernutrition, underdevelopment, poverty
Overnutrition Overconsumption of food, especially macronutrients, plus: • low physical activity • smoking, stress, alcohol abuse	→	Obesity, metabolic syndrome, cardiovascular disease, type 2 diabetes mellitus, certain cancers: chronic NCDs, often characterized by overnutrition of macronutrients and undernutrition of micronutrients
Malnutrition Nutrition transition: Individuals and communities previously food insecure → confronted with abundance of palatable foods → some undernourished, others too many macronutrients and too few micronutrients	→	Double burden of infectious diseases plus NCDs, often characterized by overnutrition of macronutrients and undernutrition of micronutrients

Figure 1.2 Relationship between nutrition and health. NCD, noncommunicable disease.

- the consequences of underconsumption and over-consumption of nutrients
- the therapeutic uses of the nutrient
- factors influencing food and nutrition security and food safety.

There are more than 50 known nutrients (including amino acids and fatty acids) and many more chemicals in food thought to influence human function and health (Box 1.1). Nutrients do not exist in isolation, except for water and others in some pharmaceutical preparations. In foods, in the gut during digestion, fermentation and absorption, in the blood during transport, and in cells during metabolism, nutrients interact with each other. Therefore, a particular nutrient should not be studied in isolation, but integrated with other nutrients and seen in the context of total body function. The study of nutrition also includes how to determine nutrient requirements to make recommendations for intakes and how nutritional status is monitored by measuring intakes, anthropometry, body composition, biochemical markers reflecting nutritional status, and the clinical signs of malnutrition.

This knowledge of nutrients and their functions will enable the nutritionist to advise individuals what and how much to eat. However, this knowledge is not sufficient to understand and address the global problem of malnutrition facing mankind today. This perception has resulted in the cultivation of social science disciplines to support knowledge from the biological sciences to address global malnutrition.

1.6 Global malnutrition

It is a major tragedy that millions of people currently live with hunger, and fear starvation. This is despite the fact that food security or "access for all at all times, to a sustainable supply of nutritionally adequate and safe food for normal physical and mental development and healthy, productive lives" is a basic human right embedded in the constitution of most developing countries. It is also despite the fact that sufficient food is produced on a global level (see Box 1.2). Food

---

Box 1.2

Food insecurity: when people live with hunger, and fear starvation.
Food security: access for all, at all times, to a sustainable, affordable supply of nutritionally adequate and safe food for normal physical and mental development and healthy, productive lives.

Box 1.1 Classes of nutrients for human nutrition

Class/category	Subclass/category	Nutrient examples
Carbohydrates (macronutrients)	Monosaccharides Disaccharides Polysaccharides	Glucose, fructose, galactose Sucrose, maltose, lactose Starch and dietary fiber
Proteins (macronutrients)	Plant and animal source proteins	Amino acids ($n = 20$): aliphatic, aromatic, sulfur-containing, acidic, basic
Fats and oils (lipids) (macronutrients)	Saturated fatty acids Monounsaturated fatty acids Polyunsaturated fatty acids (n-3, n-6, n-9)	Palmitic and stearic acid Oleic (*cis*) and elaidic (*trans*) fatty acids Linoleic, α-linolenic, arachidonic, eicosapentaenoic, docosahexaenoic acid
Minerals (micronutrients)	Minerals and electrolytes Trace elements	Calcium, sodium, phosphate, potassium, iron, zinc, selenium, copper, manganese, molybdenum, fluoride, chromium
Vitamins (micronutrients)	Fat soluble	Retinol (A), calciferols (D), tocopherols (E), vitamin K
	Water soluble	Ascorbic acid (C), thiamine (B_1), riboflavin (B_2), niacin (B_3), pyridoxine (B_6), folate, cobalamin (B_{12})
Water	Water	Water

insecurity is an obstacle to human rights, quality of life, and human dignity. It was estimated that, during the last decade of the twentieth century, 826 million people were undernourished: 792 million in developing countries and 34 million in developed countries. In developing countries, more than 199 million children under the age of 5 years suffer from acute or chronic protein and energy deficiencies. An estimated 3.5–5 billion people are iron deficient, 2.2 billion iodine deficient, and 140–250 million vitamin A deficient. This has led to several global initiatives and commitments, spearheaded by a number of United Nations organizations, to reduce global undernutrition, food insecurity, hunger, starvation, and micronutrient deficiencies. Some progress has been made in reducing these numbers, but the problems are far from solved. Some of the initiatives are:

- the 1990 United Nations Children's (Emergency) Fund (UNICEF)-supported World Summit for Children, with a call to reduce severe and moderate malnutrition among children under 5 years of age by half the 1990 rate by the year 2000, including goals for the elimination of micronutrient malnutrition
- the 1992 World Health Organization/Food and Agriculture Organization (WHO/FAO) International Conference on Nutrition that reinforced earlier goals and extended them to the elimination of death from famine
- the 1996 FAO-supported World Food Summit during which 186 heads of state and governments pledged their political will and commitment to a plan of action to reduce the number of undernourished people to half their 1996 number by 2015
- the establishment in 1997 of the Food Insecurity and Vulnerability Information and Mapping System (FIVIMS) and their Interagency Working Group (IAWG), which consists of 26 international organizations and agencies with a shared commitment to reduce food insecurity and vulnerability and its multidimensional causes rooted in poverty; information about these initiatives can be accessed at: http://www.fao.org/
- Millennium Development Goals: the United Nations articulated eight goals, ranging from halving extreme poverty and hunger, halting the spread of the human immunodeficiency virus (HIV)/acquired immunodeficiency syndrome (AIDS) and providing universal primary education, to be reached by the target

date of 2015; the blueprint of these goals was agreed to by all the world's countries and leading development institutions.

A 2001 report from the FAO indicated that in 1997–1999 there were 815 million undernourished people in the world, of whom 777 million were in developing countries, 27 million in transitional countries and 11 million in the industrialized countries. The annual decrease in undernourished people from the 1990–1992 period was 6 million. To reach the World Food Summit's goal of halving the number of undernourished in developing countries by 2015, it is estimated that the annual decrease required is 22 million.

Clearly, this is a huge challenge for food and nutrition scientists and practitioners. It would need a holistic approach and understanding of the complex, interacting factors that contribute to malnutrition on different levels. These include immediate, intermediate, underlying, and basic causes:

- individual level or immediate causes: food and nutrient intake, physical activity, health status, social structures, care, taboos, growth, personal choice
- household level or intermediate causes: family size and composition, gender equity, rules of distribution of food within the household, income, availability of food, access to food
- national level or underlying causes: health, education, sanitation, agriculture and food security, war, political instability, urbanization, population growth, distribution and conflicts, war, natural disasters, decreased resources
- international level or basic causes: social, economic and political structures, trade agreements, population size, population growth distribution, environmental degradation.

To address these causes of undernutrition food-insecure and hungry communities and individuals must be empowered to be their own agents of food security and livelihood development. Complicating the task of fighting food insecurity and hunger are natural disasters such as droughts, floods, cyclones and extreme temperatures, ongoing wars and regional conflicts, as well as the devastating impact of HIV and AIDS, especially in sub-Saharan Africa.

In many developing countries, indigenous people have changed their diets and physical activity patterns to those followed in industrialized countries. Supplementary feeding programs in these countries have often been associated with increasing trends towards obesity, insulin resistance, and the emergence of chronic diseases of lifestyle in some segments of these populations, while other segments are still undernourished.

The coexistence of undernutrition and overnutrition, leading to a double burden of infectious and chronic, noncommunicable diseases, and the multifactorial causes of malnutrition, call for innovative approaches to tackle both undernutrition and overnutrition in integrated nutrition and health-promoting programs, focusing on optimal nutrition for all.

1.7 Relationship between nutrition science and practice

The journey through the scientific domain of nutrition will, at a specialized stage, fork into different roads. These roads will lead to the different scopes or branches of nutrition science that are covered in the second, third, and fourth texts of this series. These different branches of nutrition science could lead to the training of nutrition specialists for specific practice areas.

The main aim of nutrition professionals is to apply nutrition principles to promote health and wellbeing, to prevent disease, and/or to restore health (treat disease) in individuals, families, communities and the population. To help individuals or groups of people to eat a balanced diet, in which food supply meets nutrient needs, involves application of nutrition principles from a very broad field to almost every facet of human life. It is therefore not surprising that these different branches or specialties of nutrition have evolved and are developing. They include clinical nutrition, community nutrition, public health, and public nutrition. It can be expected that there will be overlap in the practice areas of these specialties.

- The clinical nutritionist will counsel individuals from a biomedical–disease–behavioral paradigm to promote health, prevent disease, or treat disease. The clinical nutritionist will mostly work within the health service (facility-based settings such as hospitals, clinics, private practice).
- The community nutritionist, with additional skills from the psychosocial behavioral sciences, should

be aware of the dynamics within particular communities responsible for nutritional problems. These would include household food security, socioeconomic background, education levels, childcare practices, sanitation, water, energy sources, healthcare services, and other quality-of-life indicators. The community nutritionist will design, implement, and monitor appropriate, community-participatory programs to address these problems.
- The public health or public nutritionist covers the health and care practice areas but will also be concerned with food security (agricultural) and environmental issues on a public level. The public health or public nutritionist will, for example, be responsible for nutrition surveillance, and the design, implementation, and monitoring of dietary guidelines that address relevant public health problems. A background knowledge in economics, agriculture, political science, and policy design is essential for the formulation and application of nutrition policy in a country.

Many developing countries will not have the capacity or the financial resources to train and employ professionals for different specialties. However, future specialized training and employment of different professionals could result in a capacity to address nutritional problems more effectively.

1.8 Nutrition milestones: the development of nutrition as a science

Ancient beliefs

Throughout human existence people have attributed special powers to certain foods and developed beliefs and taboos regarding foods. These were often based on climatic, economic, political, or religious circumstances and principles, but also on observations regarding the relationship between the consumption of certain foods and health.

Recorded examples are ancient Chinese and Indian philosophers who advised on the use of warming and cooling foods and spices for certain conditions and for "uplifting the soul," the Mosaic laws documented in the Old Testament which distinguished between clean and unclean foods, the fasting and halal practices of Islam, and the Benedictine monks from Salerno who preached the use of hot and moist versus cold and dry foods for various purposes. Hippocrates, the father of modern medicine, who lived from 460 to about 377 BC, and later Moses Maimonides, who lived in the twelfth century, urged people to practice abstemiousness and a prudent lifestyle. They, and others, advised that, for a long and healthy life, one should avoid too much fat in the diet, eat more fruit, get ample sleep, and be physically active – advice that is still incorporated in the modern, science-based dietary guidelines of the twenty-first century!

Cultural beliefs

The perception that food represents more than its constituent parts is still true. Eating together is an accepted form of social interaction. It is a way in which cultural habits and customs, social status, kinship, love, respect, sharing, and hospitality are expressed. Scientists and nutrition professionals realize that, when formulating dietary guidelines for traditional living people, cultural beliefs and taboos should be taken into account and incorporated. There are numerous examples of traditional food habits and diets, often based on what was available. Today, with the world becoming a global village, cultures have learned from each other, and dietary patterns associated with good health, such as the Mediterranean diet, are becoming popular among many cultures.

The first renaissance: development of an evidence base

The knowledge of the specific health effects of particular diets, foods, and nutrients is now firmly based on the results of rigid scientific experimentation. Nutrition developed gradually as a science, but advanced with rapid strides during the twentieth century. There are numerous meticulously recorded examples of how initial (often ancient and primitive) observations about diet and health relationships led to the discovery, elucidation of function, isolation, and synthesis of the different nutrients. Perhaps the most often quoted example is James Lind's description in 1772 of how citrus fruit could cure and prevent scurvy in seamen on long voyages. The anti-scurvy factor (ascorbic acid or vitamin C) was only isolated in 1921, characterized in 1932, and chemically synthesized in 1933. Other examples of nutritional milestones are the induction of beriberi in domestic fowl by Eijkman in 1897, the observation of Takaki in 1906

that beriberi in Japanese sailors could be prevented by supplementing their polished rice diets with wheat bread, and, eventually, the isolation of the responsible factor, thiamine or vitamin B_1, by Funk in 1911. Others are the Nobel Prize-winning discovery by Minot and Murphy in 1926 that pernicious anemia is a nutritional disorder due to a lack of vitamin B_{12} in the diet, the description of kwashiorkor as a protein-deficiency state by Cecily Williams in 1935, and the discovery of resistant starch and importance of colonic fermentation for humans by nutritionists of the Dunn Clinical Nutrition Centre in the 1980s.

The history of modern nutrition as practiced today is an exciting one to read, and students are encouraged to spend some time on it. It is often characterized by heartbreaking courage and surprising insights. An example of the former is the carefully documented clinical, metabolic, and pathological consequences of hunger and starvation by a group of Jewish doctors in 1940 in the Warsaw ghetto: doctors who themselves were dying of hunger. An example of the latter is the studies by Price, an American dentist, who tried to identify the dietary factors responsible for good dental and overall health in people living traditional lifestyles. He unwittingly used a fortigenic paradigm in his research, examining the strengths and factors that keep people healthy, long before the term was defined or its value recognized.

At present, thousands of nutrition scientists examine many aspects of nutrition in laboratories and field studies all over the world and publish in more than 100 international scientific nutrition journals. This means that nutrition science generates new knowledge based on well-established research methodologies. The many types of experiments, varying from molecular experimentation in the laboratory, through placebo-controlled, double-blinded clinical interventions, to observational epidemiological surveys, and experiments based on a health (fortigenic) or a disease (pathogenic) paradigm, will be addressed in this volume (Chapter 13). The peer-review process of published results has helped in the development of guidelines to judge how possible, probable, convincing, and applicable results from these studies are. New knowledge of nutrients, foods, and diet relationships with health and disease is, therefore, generated through a process in which many scientists examine different pieces of the puzzle all over the world in controlled scientific experiments. Therefore, nutrition practice today has a firm research base that enables nutritional professionals to practice evidence-based nutrition.

The second renaissance: solving global malnutrition

There is little doubt that improved nutrition has contributed to the improved health and survival times experienced by modern humans. However, global figures on the prevalence of both undernutrition and overnutrition show that millions of people do not have enough to eat, while the millions who eat too much suffer from the consequences of obesity. It is tempting to equate this situation to the gap between the poor and the rich or between developing and developed countries, but the situation is much more complex. Obesity, a consequence of overnutrition, is now a public health problem not only in rich, developed, food-secure countries but also in developing, food-insecure countries, especially among women. Undernutrition, the major impediment to national development, is the biggest single contributor to childhood death rates, and to impaired physical growth and mental development of children in both developing and developed countries. Moreover, a combination of undernutrition and overnutrition in the same communities, in single households, and even in the same individual is often reported. Examples are obese mothers with undernourished children and obese women with certain micronutrient deficiencies. The perception that these global problems of malnutrition will be solved only in innovative, multidisciplinary, and multisectoral ways has led to the second, very recent renaissance in nutrition research and practice.

1.9 Future challenges for nutrition research and practice

Basic, molecular nutrition

The tremendous development in recent years of molecular biology and the availability of sophisticated new techniques are opening up a field in which nutrient–gene interactions and dietary manipulation of genetic expression will receive increasing attention (see Chapter 15). The effects of more than 12 000

different substances in plant foods, not yet classified as nutrients, will also be examined. These substances are produced by plants for hormonal, attractant, and chemoprotective purposes, and there is evidence that many of them offer protection against a wide range of human conditions. It is possible that new functions of known nutrients, and even new nutrients, may be discovered, described, and applied in the future.

Clinical and community nutrition

Today, the focus has moved from simple experiments with clear-cut answers to studies in which sophisticated statistics have to be used to dissect out the role of specific nutrients, foods, and diets in multifactorial diseases. Nutrition epidemiology is now established as the discipline in which these questions can be addressed. A number of pressing problems will have to be researched and the results applied, for example:

- the biological and sociological causes of childhood obesity, which is emerging as a global public health problem
- the nutrient requirements of the elderly: in the year 2000, more than 800 million of the Earth's inhabitants were older than 60 years; to ensure a high-quality life in the growing elderly population, much more needs to be known about their nutrient requirements
- the relationships between nutrition and immune function and how improved nutrition can help to defend against invading microorganisms; in the light of the increasing HIV/AIDS pandemic, more information in this area is urgently needed
- dietary recommendations: despite sufficient, convincing evidence about the effects of nutrients and foods on health, nutritionists have generally not been very successful in motivating the public to change their diets to more healthy ones. We need to know more about why people make certain food choices in order to design culturally sensitive and practical dietary guidelines that will impact positively on dietary choices. The food-based dietary guidelines that are now being developed in many countries are a first step in this direction.

Public health nutrition

The single most important challenge facing mankind in the future is probably to provide adequate safe food and clean water for all in an environmentally safe way that will not compromise the ability of future generations to meet their needs. In addition to the hundreds of millions not eating enough food to meet their needs for a healthy, active life, an additional 80 million people have to be fed each year. The challenge to feed mankind in the future calls for improved agriculture in drought-stricken areas such as sub-Saharan Africa, the application of biotechnology in a responsible way, interdisciplinary and intersectorial cooperation of all involved, and a better distribution of the food supply so that affordable food is accessible by all. The need for sustained economic growth in poor countries is evident.

Nutritionists have an important part to play in ensuring food security for all, a basic human right, in the future. One of their main functions would be to educate and inform populations not to rely too heavily on animal products in their diet, the production of which places a much heavier burden on the environment than plant foods. A major challenge would be to convince political leaders and governments that addressing undernutrition (the major obstacle in national development) in sustainable programs should be the top priority in developing and poor communities. Another challenge is to develop models based on the dynamics within communities and, using a human rights approach, to alleviate undernutrition without creating a problem of overnutrition. There are examples where such models, incorporated into community development programs, have been very successful (e.g., in Thailand).

Functional foods: a new development

Functional foods are new or novel foods, developed to have specific health benefits, in addition to their usual functions. Examples are spreads with added phytosterols, to lower serum low-density lipoprotein cholesterol and the risk of coronary heart disease, and the development of starchy products with resistant starch and lower glycemic indices, to help control blood glucose levels. The development and testing of functional foods is an exciting new area. These foods may help to improve or restore nutritional status in many people. However, much more should be known about suitable biomarkers to test their efficacy, variability in human response to specific food products, safety, consumer understanding, and how their health messages must be formulated, labeled, and communicated.

Food safety

The continued provision of safe food, free from microorganisms, toxins, and other hazardous substances that cause disease, remains a huge challenge. Recent experiences with animals suffering from bovine spongiform encephalopathy (BSE or mad cow disease) or from foot-and-mouth disease, or birds infected with the influenza A virus (bird flu), have shown how quickly a national problem can become an international one because of global marketing of products. The list of possible hazardous substances in foods emphasizes the need for continuous monitoring of the food supply by health officials (Figure 1.3).

Microbial contamination Bacteria and mold (fungi) producing toxins and aflatoxins Toxins cause "food poisoning" and aflatoxins are carcinogenic	
Natural toxins Such as cyanide in cassava, solanine in potatoes; can be produced by abnormal circumstances, could be enzyme inhibitors or antivitamins	**Agricultural residues** Pesticides such as DDT or hormones used to promote growth such as bovine somatotrophin
Environmental contamination Heavy metals and minerals Criminal adulteration, industrial pollution Substances from packaging materials Changes during cooking and processing of foods	**Intentional additives** Artificial sweeteners Preservatives Phytochemicals Modified carbohydrates (for functional foods)

Figure 1.3 Potential hazardous substances in food. DDT, dichloro-diphenyl-trichloroethane.

1.10 Perspectives on the future

Nutrition research and practice, although it has been around for many years, is in its infancy as a basic and applied scientific discipline. The present and future nutrition student will take part in this very exciting second renaissance of nutrition and see its maturation. However, to influence effectively the nutrition and health of individuals and populations, the nutritionist will have to forge links and partnerships with other health professionals and policy-makers, and will have to develop lateral thinking processes. The magnitude and complexity of nutritional problems facing mankind today demand concerted multidisciplinary and multisectorial efforts from all involved to solve them. Therefore, the principal message to take on a nutrition science journey is that teamwork is essential: one cannot travel this road on one's own; partners from different disciplines are needed. Another essential need is the continuous development of leadership in nutrition. Leaders on every level of research and practice are necessary to respond to the existing challenges of global malnutrition and to face future challenges.

The modern advances in molecular biology and biotechnology on the one hand, and the persistence of global malnutrition on the other, increasingly demand a re-evaluation of ethical norms, standards, and values for nutrition science and practice. Direction from responsible leaders is needed (Box 1.3). There is an urgent need for ethical guidelines and a code of conduct for partnerships between food industries, UN agencies, governments, and academics. These partnerships are necessary for addressing global malnutrition in sustainable programs.

Box 1.3 Future challenges that require exceptional leadership

- Basic molecular nutrition
  - Nutrient–gene interactions
  - Role of phytochemicals in health
  - New nutrients? New functions?
- Community and public health nutrition
  - Childhood obesity
  - Requirements of the elderly
  - Dietary recommendations
  - Nutrition of patients with human immunodeficiency virus/acquired immunodeficiency syndrome
- Public nutrition
  - To feed mankind
  - Food security
- Functional foods
  - To ensure that novel foods are effective and safe
- Food safety
  - Continuous monitoring
- Partnerships with other disciplines
- Leadership

The student in nutrition, at the beginning of this journey of discovery of nutrition as a science, must make use of the many opportunities to develop leadership qualities. May this be a happy, fruitful, and lifelong journey with many lessons that can be applied in the research and practice of nutrition to make a difference in the life of all.

Further reading

Websites

http://whq.libdoc.who.int/trs/who_trs_916
http://www.who.int/nutrition/en
http://www.ifpri.org
http://fao.org/ag/agn/nutrition/profiles_en.stm

2
Body Composition

Paul Deurenberg

Key messages

- Body composition data are used to evaluate nutritional status, growth and development, water homeostasis, and specific disease states.
- Human body composition is studied at atomic, molecular, cellular, tissue, and whole body levels. The levels are interrelated.
- A "normal weight" human body consists of approximately 98% oxygen, carbon, hydrogen, nitrogen, and calcium; of 60–70% water, 10–35% fat (depending on gender), 10–15% protein, and 3–5% minerals.
- The variation in body composition between individuals is large, mainly because of variations in fat mass. Variations in fat-free mass are smaller.
- Several direct, indirect, and doubly indirect techniques are available to measure body composition, each with its own distinct advantages and disadvantages.
- The choice of method will be influenced by the availability of instrumentation, invasiveness, and radiation danger to subjects, price, accuracy required, and application objectives.
- Interpretation and application of data from body composition measurements should be carried out with care and should take into account the limitations of the method used, age, gender, and ethnic group.

2.1 Introduction

Mankind has long been fascinated with the composition of the human body. Centuries ago, the Greeks dissected human cadavers to obtain an insight into the structure and build of the human body, and drawings from the Middle Ages of gross muscle structures grace the walls of many famous art galleries. They are prized not only for their artistic merit, but also for what they reveal of the work of the dissectionists of that era. With progress in the development of analytical chemical methods in the twentieth century, these studies of body composition were applied to body tissues, fetuses, and cadavers of newborns. Scientists such as Mitchell, Widdowson, and Forbes performed the most important work of chemical analyses in adult cadavers during the 1940s and 1950s. Today, neutron activation analysis allows the chemical composition of the human body to be studied *in vivo*. These early chemical analyses of the body gave insights into the changes occurring during growth and development. They also form the basis for a number of methods now widely used to assess body composition *in vivo*.

Today, it is known that many diseases and disorders are related to abnormal body composition or to changes in body composition. The most common of these conditions is obesity, in which the amount of body fat is excessively high, leading to abnormalities in lipid and carbohydrate metabolism, high blood pressure, and adult-onset diabetes. At the other end of the nutritional spectrum, energy and protein malnutrition results in a decrease in the amount of fat and protein stores in the body, and many diseases are related to abnormalities in total body water or to the distribution of body water across the intracellular and extracellular spaces.

Because of the high variability between subjects in chemical body composition, mainly due to the high variation in body fat stores, the concept of fat-free mass (FFM) was introduced at the end of the nineteenth century. If body composition data are expressed as a proportion of the FFM, data become much more consistent between individuals. For example, the fraction of water in the FFM (0.73 ± 0.02) is very consistent across individuals, whereas the between-subject variation is two to three times higher if expressed per kilogram of body weight. This high variability in body components led to the definition of a "reference man," an imaginary person with a given body composition.

In this chapter a (global) description of the composition of the healthy human body is given and discussed at the following levels:

- atomic
- molecular
- cellular
- tissue
- whole body.

Of the many methods available to measure body composition, a few are highlighted and a short description of each is given. For more detailed information, the books by Forbes (1987) and Heymsfield *et al.* (2005) on human body composition are recommended for further reading.

2.2 Five levels of body composition

Human body composition can be studied at the atomic, molecular, cellular, tissue, and whole body level. These five levels are related to each other. For example, information at the atomic level can be used, subject to certain assumptions, to provide information at the whole body level.

Atomic level

Many chemical elements (atoms) are found in the human body, but the six elements oxygen, carbon, hydrogen, nitrogen, calcium, and phosphorus are the most abundant and together account for more than 98% of body weight (Table 2.1). Indeed, the 11 most common elements account for 99.5% of the atomic body composition. This information was initially based on chemical analysis of carcasses, but today the information can also be obtained by *in vivo* neutron activation analysis (IVNAA). The classical chemical cadaver analysis, as carried out mainly in the 1940s,

Table 2.1 Body composition at the atomic level of a 70 kg reference man

Atomic element	Amount (kg)	Amount (% body weight)
Oxygen	43	61
Carbon	16	23
Hydrogen	7	10
Nitrogen	1.8	2.6
Calcium	1.0	1.4
Phosphorus	0.6	0.8
Total	69.4	98.8

Box 2.1

The water content in the body varies with age. In a fetus, the water content slowly decreases from more than 90% after conception to about 80% before delivery at about 7 months of gestation. A newborn has about 70% body water, which is about 82% of the fat-free mass. This value slowly decreases further to 72% of the fat-free mass until the body is chemically mature at age 15–18 years. In general, males have more body water (related to body weight) than females, as their body fat content is lower.

still forms the basis for many *in vivo* techniques that are used to assess body composition.

Molecular level

The chemical elements in the human body are bound in molecules and, in very global terms, the main compartments are water, lipids, proteins, minerals, and carbohydrates. The total amount of water in the body is high and, depending on the body fat content, can be as high as 60–70% of total body weight. Total body water can be divided into intracellular water and extracellular water, and the ratio of the two is an important health parameter that is disturbed in many diseases (Box 2.1).

Lipids appear in the human body in different forms. Essential structural lipids such as the phospholipids (cell membranes) and sphingomyelin (nervous system) form only a minor part of the total lipids in the body. The nonessential lipids, mostly triglycerides or triacylglycerol (fat), are the most abundant. They are the energy store of the adult human body, insulate against cold, protect vital organs such as the kidneys against mechanical damage, and, to a certain extent, enhance the body's appearance. In a "normal weight" healthy adult, the amount of body fat varies between 10% and 25% in men and between 15% and 35% in

Table 2.2 Body composition at the molecular level of a 70 kg reference man

Component	Amount (kg)	Amount (% body weight)
Water		
Extracellular	18	26
Intracellular	24	34
Lipid		
Essential	1.5	2.1
Nonessential	12	17
Protein	10.1	14.4
Mineral	3.7	5.3
Carbohydrate	0.5	0.6
Total	69.8	99.4

Table 2.3 Body composition at the tissue level of a 70 kg reference man

Tissue/organ	Amount (kg)	Amount (% body weight)
Muscle	28	40
Adipose tissue	15	21.4
Blood	5.5	7.9
Bone	5	7.1
Skin	2.6	3.7
Liver	1.8	2.6
Total	57.9	82.7

women. In severe obesity body fat can be as high as 60–70% of body weight.

Body protein varies between 10% and 15%. It is higher in males than in females, as males generally have more muscles. There is no protein storage in the body and, generally speaking, loss of protein coincides with a loss of functionality given the high protein content and high protein turnover rates in vital organs.

The amount of minerals in the body varies between 3% and 5%, again dependent on body fat. Calcium and phosphorus are the two main minerals. They are found mainly in bones. Carbohydrates are found in the body as glucose (blood sugar) and glycogen, a polysaccharide in muscle and liver cells that serves as a short-term energy store. The amount of carbohydrates in the body rarely exceeds 500 g. Table 2.2 gives the body composition of the reference man at a molecular level.

Cellular level

At the cellular level, body composition can be described in terms of body cell mass, extracellular fluids, and extracellular solids. The body cell mass includes the cells with all their contents, such as water, proteins, and minerals. Extracellular fluid contains about 95% water, which is plasma in the intravascular space and interstitial fluid in the extravascular space. Extracellular solids are mainly proteins (e.g., collagen) and minerals (bone minerals and soluble minerals in the extracellular fluid). Body composition at the cellular level is not easy to measure, owing to its complex nature. As will be discussed later, the ^{40}K method can be used to assess body cell mass and some dilution techniques, for example bromide dilution, can be used to assess extracellular water.

Tissue level

Cells with equal functions form tissues, including muscular, connective, epithelial, and nervous tissue. Bones are connective tissue and consist mainly of hydroxyapatite, $[Ca_3(PO_4)_2]_3Ca(OH)_2$, bedded in a protein matrix. A rather simple body composition model at the tissue level would be:

$$Body\ weight = adipose\ tissue + skeletal\ muscle + bone + organs + rest$$

Several of these components can now be measured with, for example, computed tomography (CT) or magnetic resonance imaging (MRI) for adipose tissue; creatinine excretion or N-methyl-histidine excretion in 24 h urine for skeletal muscle; dual-energy X-ray absorptiometry (DXA) for bones; and MRI or ultrasound for organs. Body composition at the tissue level is given in Table 2.3.

Whole body level

Body composition measurements at the whole body level use simple body parameters to give an insight into body composition. Formulae, based on statistical relationships that have been established in earlier studies between body parameters (e.g., skinfold thickness) and information on body composition (e.g., body fat by density), also enable the assessment of body composition. Another example is the assessment of body water based on weight, height, age, and gender.

2.3 Relationships between different levels of body composition

The five levels of body composition are interrelated. This means that information at one level can be trans-

Box 2.2

Adipose tissue is made of adipocytes, which are cells that store triglycerides in the form of small fat droplets. Adipose tissue contains about 80% triglycerides and some 1–2% protein (enzymes), and the remaining part is water plus electrolytes. During weight loss adipose tissue decreases: the actual fat loss will be about 80% of the actual weight loss.

Table 2.4 Methods used to determine body composition

Direct	Indirect	Doubly indirect
Carcass analyses	Densitometry	Weight/height indices
IVNAA	Deuterium oxide dilution	Skinfolds/ultrasound
	^{40}K counting	Circumferences/diameters
	More-compartment models	Impedance
	DXA	Infrared interactance
	CT/MRI scans	Creatinine excretion

IVNAA, *in vivo* neutron activation analysis; DXA, dual-energy X-ray absorptiometry; CT, computed tomography; MRI, magnetic resonance imaging.

lated to another level. This is important as it forms the basis of many techniques used to determine body composition. In the context of this chapter, only a few examples are given. After determining the amount of calcium in the body by, for example, IVNAA (atomic level), the amount of bone can be calculated assuming that a certain amount of total body calcium is in the skeletal tissue. Determination of total body potassium (by ^{40}K or IVNAA) enables the assessment of the body cell mass, as most of the body potassium is known to be intracellular. Skinfold thickness measurements (total body level) enable the assessment of body fat (molecular level). Formulae used for these calculations are component based, property based, or sometimes a combination. Component-based formulae are based on fixed relationships between components. An example is the calculation of total body water from measured hydrogen: the chemical formula of water determines the factor. Property-based formulae are based on established statistical relationships between variables. An example is the prediction of body fat percentage (body composition parameter) from skinfold thickness (property) (Box 2.2). Property-based formulae tend to be population specific, which limits the widespread application.

Most body composition techniques that are in use today are based on assumptions, often derived from carcass analyses or experimentally derived from observational studies. Violation of these assumptions leads to biased results, and some methods are more prone to bias than others. In the following short description of different methodologies, the most important assumptions are highlighted.

2.4 Body composition techniques

Body composition techniques can be described in terms of direct, indirect, and doubly indirect methods.

- In direct methods, the body component of interest is determined directly without or with only minor assumptions. Examples are chemical carcass analyses and IVNAA for the atomic components.
- In indirect techniques, the body component of interest is determined indirectly. Examples are the determination of body protein from body nitrogen, assuming a constant conversion factor of 6.25 from nitrogen to protein, and the determination of body cell mass using ^{40}K. In both examples, assumptions are used. These assumptions may not be valid in the given situation or for the subject(s) under study and hence could lead to biased results.
- Doubly indirect methods rely on a statistical relationship between easily measurable body parameter(s) and the body component of interest. Examples are the assessment of skeletal muscle mass by creatinine excretion and the assessment of body fat from skin-fold thickness. Table 2.4 gives an overview of the most common methods.

2.5 Direct methods

Carcass analysis

The (chemical) analysis of carcasses is a time-consuming exercise and requires very precise approaches to the task. The carcass has to be carefully dissected into the different tissues that are then exactly weighed, after which the chemical analyses have to be performed. To avoid errors it is important that no unaccounted water losses occur during the analytical work. As early as the nineteenth century, it was recognized that the variation in chemical body composition was reduced when results were expressed as a fraction of the fat-free body. The data on the chemical composition of only a few human cadavers form the basis for the assumptions that are normally used in indirect methods. These chemical analyses were performed in five men and one woman. It was concluded that, on the basis of FFM, the mean amounts of water, protein, and minerals in the body are 72.6%, 20.5%, and 6.9%, respectively. The variability in these figures is about 13% for protein and minerals and 4% for water. Although one can question the quality of these data as a basis for other methods (low number, high variation in age, variation in gender, some carcasses were not analyzed immediately after death), they form the basis for many indirect and doubly indirect body composition methods. Chemical carcass analysis also revealed that the amount of potassium in the FFM is fairly constant. This fact is used as the basis for the calculation of the amount of FFM or for body cell mass from total body potassium, determined by ^{40}K scanning.

In the 1980s, cadaver studies were performed again in the "Brussels study." Unfortunately, only information at a tissue level and not at atomic or molecular level was collected. However, the need for cadaver studies has greatly diminished given that the same information can now be obtained *in vivo* by IVNAA.

In vivo *neutron activation analysis*

IVNAA is a relatively new body composition technique that allows the determination of specific chemical elements in the body. The body is bombarded with fast neutrons of known energy level. The neutrons can be captured by chemical elements (as part of molecules) in the body, resulting in a transition state of higher energy for that element – energy that is finally emitted as gamma rays. For example, capture of neutrons by nitrogen results in the formation of the isotope ^{15}N, which will emit the excess energy as gamma rays:

$$^{14}N + {}^{1}n \rightarrow {}^{15}N^* + \text{gamma rays}$$

where ^{14}N is nitrogen with atomic mass 14, ^{15}N is nitrogen with atomic mass 15, and ^{1}n is a neutron.

With IVNAA, many elements in the body can be determined, including calcium, phosphorus, nitrogen, oxygen, potassium, and chlorine.

The information obtained at the atomic level can be converted to more useful information. For example, from total body nitrogen total body protein can be calculated as 6.25 times the total nitrogen, assuming that body protein consists of 16% nitrogen. The advantage of the method is that the chemical body composition can be determined *in vivo* and can be compared with other, indirect, techniques. For fundamental studies and for validation of existing techniques in special groups of subjects, for example in different ethnic groups, elderly subjects, obese subjects, or in the diseased state, the methodology can be of great importance. The disadvantage of IVNAA is not only the price. The subject is irradiated, with the radiation dose used depending on the number and kind of elements to be determined. It is relatively low for nitrogen (0.26 mSv) but high for calcium (2.5 mSv).

2.6 Indirect methods

Densitometry

The densitometric method assumes that the body consists of two components, a fat mass, in which all "chemical" fat is located, and the FFM, which consists of (fat-free) bones, muscles, water, and organs. Chemically, the FFM consists of water, minerals, protein, and a small amount of carbohydrate, the last often being neglected. The density of the fat mass is 0.900 kg/l and, from carcass analysis data, the density of the FFM can be calculated as 1.100 kg/l, depending on the relative amount of minerals, protein, and water in the FFM (Box 2.3).

The density of the total body depends on the ratio of fat mass to FFM. Once the density of the body has been determined, the percentage of fat in the body (BF%) can be calculated by Siri's formula (Box 2.4):

$$BF\% = (495/\text{body density}) - 450$$

Body density can be determined by several techniques, the oldest and perhaps most accurate being underwater weighing. Behnke first used the technique, showing that excess body weight in American football players was not the result of excess fat but of enlarged muscle mass.

In underwater weighing, the weight of the subject is first measured in air and then while totally immersed in water. The difference between weight in air and weight under water is the upwards force, which equals the weight of the displaced water (Archimedes' law),

Box 2.3

The density of the fat-free mass (FFM) can be calculated if its composition is known.

In the calculation example below it is assumed that the FFM consists of 73.5% water, 19.6% protein, and 6.9% minerals with densities (at 37°C) of 0.993, 1.340, and 3.038 kg/l, respectively. In addition, it is assumed that the volumes of the separate compartments can be added up to the total volume of the FFM (in fact, the compartments do not "mix"). Thus, the volume of the FFM equals the sum of the other compartments:

$$FFM_{volume} = Water_{volume} + Mineral_{volume} + Protein_{volume}$$

As volume is weight/density, the equation can be written as:

$$100/Density_{FFM} = 73.5/0.993 + 6.9/3.038 + 19.6/1.340$$

From this, the density of the FFM can be calculated as 1.0999 kg/l.

It is obvious that differences in composition of the FFM will result in a different density.

Box 2.4

Siri's formula can be derived assuming that the body consists of fat mass (FM) and fat-free mass (FFM). If body weight is assumed to be 100% and body fat is x%, then FFM is $100 - x$%. It is assumed that the volumes of these two compartments can be added up to total body volume. Then:

$$Body_{volume} = FM_{volume} + FFM_{volume}$$

As volume is weight/density, the equation can be written as:

$$100/body\ density = x/0.9 + (100 - x)/1.1$$

From this, body fat percentage (BF%) can be calculated as:

$$BF\% = 495/density - 450$$

The general formula to calculate BF% from body density (D_b) is:

$$BF\% = \frac{1}{D_b} \times \left(\frac{D_{FFM} \times D_{FM}}{D_{FFM} - D_{FM}} \right) - \left(\frac{D_{FM}}{D_{FFM} - D_{FM}} \right)$$

In general, a lower density of the FFM than 1.1 kg/l will result in an overestimation of BF% if Siri's formula is used. It is likely that the density of the FFM is lower in elderly people, owing to bone mineral loss (osteoporosis).

Densitometry (using Siri's equation) overestimates body fat compared with a four-compartment model (see Figure 2.7).

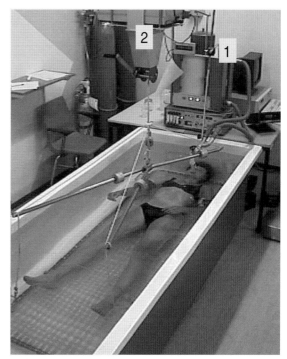

Figure 2.1 Underwater weighing. The subject is submerged completely and breathes via a respirometer (1) for simultaneous residual lung volume measurement. Weight (*W*) (2) under water (uw) is recorded and density (*D*) is calculated as $D_{body} = W_{air}/(W_{air} - W_{uw})$. Corrections are made for water temperature and lung volume: percentage of fat in the body = $495/D_{body} - 450$.

from which, after correction for the water temperature (density), the displaced water volume (and thus the body volume) can be calculated. Corrections must be made for residual lung volume and air in the gut. Figure 2.1 shows an underwater weighing. The technique gives very reproducible results within about 1% of BF%. The absolute error in determined body fat is assumed to be maximal 3% of BF%. This error is mainly due to violation of the assumption that the density of the FFM equals 1.100 kg/l in the subject under study. It can be argued that in certain subjects or groups of subjects this assumption may be violated, as for example in young children and in pregnant women. Use of Siri's formula will then lead to biased conclusions. Some laboratories have attempted to use water displacement instead of underwater weighing, but the technique failed, mainly because of the difficulty in accurately reading the water level in the tank.

An air-displacement method has been commercially available since 1995. This method measures body volume after placing the subject in a small, airtight chamber and increasing the pressure by adding a known amount of air into the chamber. Boyle Gay-Lussac's law enables the calculation of body volume. Corrections are made for temperature and humidity changes, and lung volume is assessed simultaneously.

Research to date has generally shown good agreement between underwater weighing and air displacement. Air displacement is better accepted by the volunteers, but some experience difficulties because of the breathing pattern to be followed or because of claustrophobia.

Dilution techniques

Carcass analyses revealed that the amount of water in the FFM is relatively constant at about 73%. Total body water (TBW) can be determined by dilution techniques. Dilution techniques are generally based on the equation:

$$C_1 \times V_1 = C_2 \times V_2 = \text{Constant}$$

where C is the tracer (deuterium oxide, tritium, or ^{18}O water) concentration and V is the volume.

When a subject is given a known amount of a tracer ($C_1 \times V_1$), which is known to be diluted in a given body compartment, the volume of that body compartment can be calculated from the dose given and the concentration of the tracer in that compartment after equilibrium has been reached. Suitable tracers for the determination of TBW are deuterium oxide, tritium oxide, and ^{18}O-labeled water. Other tracers can also be used, such as alcohol and urea, but they are less suitable because they are partly metabolized (alcohol) or because they are actively excreted from the body (urea) during the dilution period. After giving a subject the tracer and allowing around 3–5 hours for equal distribution throughout the body, determination of the concentration of deuterium in blood, saliva, or urine allows the calculation of TBW (Box 2.5).

Alternatively, other tracers can be used, such as tritium oxide and ^{18}O-labeled water, and the tracer can be given intravenously, which is advantageous when the subject has gastrointestinal disorders. The reproducibility of the method is 1–3%, depending on the tracer used and the analytical method chosen. From TBW, the FFM, and hence fat mass, can be calculated, assuming that 73% of the FFM is water:

$$BF\% = 100 \times (\text{Weight} - \text{TBW}/0.73)/\text{Weight}$$

The precision for estimations of body fat is about 3–4% of body weight. As with the densitometric method, this error is due to violations of the assumption used (i.e., that the relative amount of water in the FFM is constant and equals 73% of the FFM). In sub-

---

Box 2.5

A person with a body weight of 75 kg is given an exactly weighed dose of 15 g deuterium oxide. This deuterium oxide is allowed to be equally distributed in the body water compartment for about 3–5 hours. Then, blood is taken and the deuterium concentration in the sample is determined. Assuming the plasma level to be 370 mg/kg, the "deuterium space" can be calculated as 15 000/370 = 40.5 kg. As deuterium exchanges in the body with hydroxyl groups from other molecules, the deuterium space has to be corrected for this nonaqueous dilution (4–5%). Thus, total body water is 0.95 × 15 000/370 = 38.5 kg. Assuming a hydration of the fat-free mass of 73%, the body fat percentage of this 75 kg weight subject would be: 100 × [75 − (38.5/0.73)/75] = 29.7%.

Box 2.6

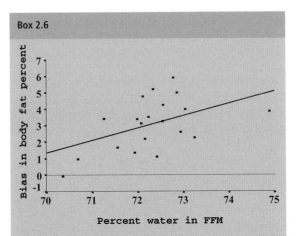

For the computation of body composition from dual-energy X-ray absorptiometry, especially body fat and lean tissue, several assumptions are made, one of which is a constant hydration of the fat-free mass (FFM). The figure shows that the bias in calculated body fat percentage depends on the hydration of the FFM. Reference is a four-compartment model.

---

jects with a larger than 73% water content in the FFM (pregnant women, morbid obese subjects, and patients with edema), the factor 0.73 will result in an overestimation of the FFM. A three-compartment model of the body that contains fat mass, water, and dry FFM has a lower bias than a two-compartment model. An overestimation of body fat by densitometry, for example because of a relatively high amount of water in the FFM, will be counteracted by an underestimation using the dilution method (see also Box 2.6).

The use of tracers that do not cross the cell membrane enables the determination of extracellular water (ECW). Commonly used tracers in this respect are bromide salts or sodium-24. Intracellular water (ICW) cannot be determined directly and is calculated as the difference between TBW and ECW.

Total body potassium

Chemical carcass analysis has revealed that the amount of potassium in the fat-free body is relatively constant, although the amount of potassium in different tissues varies widely. The determination of total body potassium (TBK) is relatively easy, owing to the natural occurrence of three potassium isotopes (^{39}K, ^{40}K, and ^{41}K), in constant relative amounts, of which ^{40}K is radioactive (gamma emission). Counting the emission of the gamma rays from the body reveals the amount of radioactive potassium, from which TBK and hence FFM can be calculated. The chamber in which the subject is scanned has to be carefully shielded to avoid any background radiation (cosmic radiation). The scanning of the body for potassium lasts for 20–30 min and the reproducibility is 2–3%.

Several authors have shown that the amount of potassium in the FFM is different between males and females, is lower in obese subjects, and is probably also age dependent. Thus, TBK is much more useful as a measure of body cell mass (BCM) than as a measure of FFM. However, this discrepancy can be used to calculate the "quality" of FFM, defined as the ratio of cellular to extracellular components of FFM, or operationally as BCM/FFM. Thus, when TBK is used to assess BCM, and another method such as hydrodensitometry or DXA is used to assess FFM independently, it can be shown that the quality of FFM declines with age, along with the quantity (Figure 2.2). When potassium values are used to calculate intracellular water, BCM, or FFM, assuming constant amounts of potassium in these body components, the same errors can occur as with densitometry and dilution techniques.

Although the technique is easy to apply in patients, the high cost of the scanning instrumentation limits its use other than in research settings.

Dual-energy X-ray absorptiometry

During DXA (also known as DEXA), the body or part of the body is scanned with X-rays of two distinct levels of energy. The attenuation of the tissues for the two different levels of radiation depends on its chemical composition and is detected by photocells. The

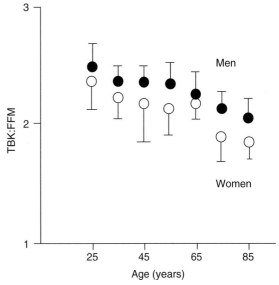

Figure 2.2 Difference in total body potassium (TBK) content of the fat-free mass (FFM) between men and women and the relationship with age.

instrument's software generates a two-dimensional picture of the body or the body compartment under study. The software can calculate several body components: bone mineral content and bone mineral density, lean mass, and adipose tissue fat mass. These calculations are possible for each of the body parts, e.g., for legs, trunk, spine, femur, and arms. However, the method cannot distinguish between subcutaneous adipose tissue and discrete adipose tissue sites such as perirenal adipose tissue. The reproducibility of DXA is very high, varying from about 0.5% for bone mineral density to about 2% for total body composition. The reproducibility for regional body composition is less. The method is quick and easy to perform and places very few demands on the subject. The radiation dose (0.02 mSv) is only a fraction of the radiation dose of a normal chest radiograph, and hardly higher than the normal background. Apart from repeated scanning, the radiation dose should not be a limiting factor in terms of volunteers being exposed to hazardous levels of radiation. A disadvantage of the method is that the attenuation of the X-rays depends on the thickness of the tissue. Therefore, correction for the body size has to be made. Compared with traditional methods, DXA scanning is easy and widely available which, in turn, leads to prediction equations for body composition based on DXA. However, as with other methods, DXA relies on certain assumptions (Box 2.6) and there are many publications showing that the error in body composition measurements using DXA can be considerable (Figure 2.3). Moreover, identical machines, even using the same software versions, can give different results in scanning the same person.

Multicompartment models

Two-compartment models, consisting of fat mass and FFM, lack validity in many situations where the composition of the body is "abnormal." Examples already mentioned are pregnancy, morbid obesity, and the elderly. A combination of techniques often results in more valid estimates, as is the case when, for example, body density and body water are combined. In this particular case, the body is divided into three compartments:

$$\text{Body weight} = \text{Fat mass} + \text{Body water} + \text{Dry fat-free mass}$$

In this three-compartment model the variation of the water content in the FFM is accounted for. There are fewer assumptions in this model, leading to more valid results. Modern techniques such as DXA enable the valid and precise measurement of bone mineral, from which total body mineral can be estimated. When the mineral content of the body is combined with body density and body water, a four-compartment model of the body is generated:

$$\text{Body weight} = \text{Fat mass} + \text{Water} + \text{Minerals} + \text{Protein}$$

In this model, most of the variation in the amounts of the chemical components is accounted for, resulting in a very reliable body composition measure (Box 2.7). Four-compartment models can also be obtained using other techniques. For example, the measurement of calcium, phosphorus, and nitrogen with IVNAA in combination with TBW provides information for a model consisting of fat, minerals, protein, and water. In the literature, models based on six compartments are also described. However, they do not provide much additional information and the increased technical error negates the methodological advantage.

More-compartment models enable the best possible estimate of body composition for populations as

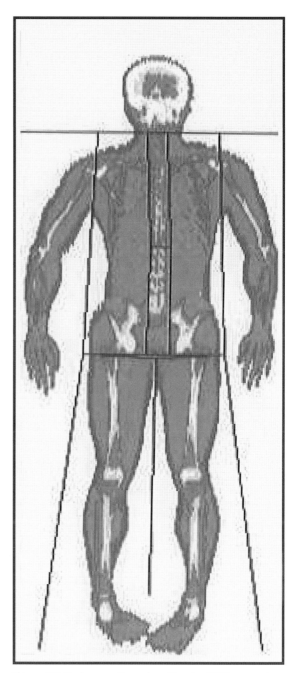

Figure 2.3 Dual-energy X-ray absorptiometer (DXA) scan using a HOLOGIC whole-body DXA (QDR-4500). Subcutaneous body fat, bone, and muscle are distinguished by different colors.

Box 2.7

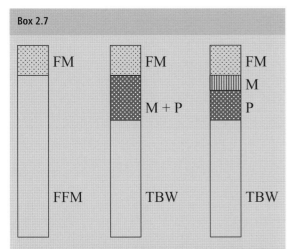

The first bar represents a two-compartment model of body composition, in which the body is divided into fat mass and fat-free mass (FFM). In the second bar, the FFM is divided into water and a "dry" FFM, consisting of protein and mineral. The third bar shows a four-compartment model in which the body is divided into water, protein, mineral, and fat. The four-compartment model shown has only minor assumptions and provides body composition data that are very accurate.

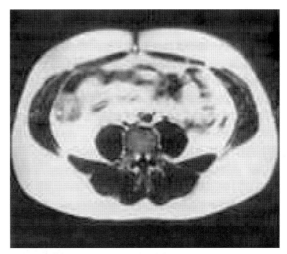

Figure 2.4 Magnetic resonance imaging scan at the L4 level in an obese subject. The white areas in the image are adipose tissue. Subcutaneous adipose tissue and intra-abdominal adipose tissue are separated by the abdominal muscles.

well as for individuals. Although some studies comparing body composition from four-compartment models show that mean values generally agree with simpler approaches, there are also studies showing directional bias of two-compartment body composition models. For this reason, more-compartment models should ideally be used as a reference (gold standard). However, only a limited number of laboratories can perform all of the necessary measurements for the calculation of maximum compartment models. Moreover, the data are expensive to collect, and measurements are time-consuming and not very practical in clinical situations.

Imaging techniques

CT scanning enables the visualization of tissues in cross-sectional slices of the body. The thickness of those slices can vary, but is normally about 1 cm. During CT scanning a source of X-rays rotates perpendicularly around the body or a body segment, while photodetectors, opposite to the source, register the attenuation of the X-rays after they have passed through the body in the various directions. The information received by the photodetectors is used to generate images. Software enables the calculation of the amounts of tissues with different attenuation, for example adipose tissue against nonadipose tissue. The CT technique was introduced for body composition assessments in the 1980s and is now widely used, predominantly for measurements of body fat distribution. Figure 2.4 shows a scan of the abdomen at the level of the umbilicus, made by MRI, a technique that gives comparable information. The precision of the calculation of a tissue area or tissue volume from the same scan(s) is very accurate, with an error of about 1%. Partial volume effects (pixels that contain tissue with different attenuation) may influence the accuracy and reproducibility of the method.

A single CT scan provides only relative data, for example in a scan of the abdomen the relative amount of visceral adipose tissue to subcutaneous adipose tissue. Multiple CT scanning allows the calculation of tissue volumes. From adipose tissue volumes (tissue level) and an assumed density and composition of the adipose tissue, the amount of fat mass (molecular level) can be calculated. Multiplying tissue volumes with specific densities of these tissues (determined *in vitro*) allows a recalculation of the body weight, a necessary but not sufficient exercise for validation of a whole body technique. Research in this area has shown that the CT technique allows the determination of total body composition, with an error of estimate for fat mass of 3–3.5 kg (compared with densitometry).

CT scanning is expensive and, because of the relatively high level of radiation, the method is limited to subjects for whom scanning is indicated on clinical grounds. An alternative method to CT scanning is MRI, which has the advantage that no ionizing radiation is involved.

During MRI, the signals emitted when the body is placed in a strong magnetic field are collected and, as with CT scanning, the data are used to generate a visual cross-sectional slice of the body in a certain region. The determination of adipose tissue versus nonadipose tissue is based on the shorter relaxation time of adipose tissue than of other tissues that contain more protons or differ in resonance frequency. MRI has the advantage over CT scanning that the subject is not exposed to ionizing radiation. However, the time necessary to make an MRI image is relatively long (minutes versus seconds using CT), which has implications for the quality of the image. Any movement of the subject, even the movements of the intestinal tract when making images in the abdominal region, will decrease the quality of the image.

As with CT scanning, images can be combined to obtain information on total body composition. Information about organ size can be obtained with a high accuracy. For example, MRI is used to study the contribution of various organs to the resting metabolic rate of the total body.

Both CT scanning and MRI are expensive, and therefore their use will remain limited to a few laboratories and for very specific situations.

2.7 Doubly indirect methods

Anthropometry

Weight/height indices

A weight/height index aims to correct body weight for height. As a measure of body composition, for example body fat, a weight/height index should have a high correlation with body fat, but also a low correlation with body height, otherwise in short people body fat would be systematically overestimated or underestimated.

In the literature, a number of weight/height indices have been proposed. Examples are the Quetelet index or body mass index (BMI: weight/height^2), the Broca index [weight/(height − 100)], and the Benn index (weight/height^p, in which the exponent p is popula-

Table 2.5 Classification of weight in adults according to body mass index

Classification	Body mass index (kg/m^2)	Risk of comorbidities
Underweight	<18.5	Low
Normal range	18.5–24.9	Average
Overweight	>25.0	
Preobese	25.0–29.9	Increased
Obese class I	30.0–34.9	Moderate
Obese class II	35.0–39.9	Severe
Obese class III	>40	Very severe

Reproduced with permission of the World Health Organization.

tion specific). The Quetelet index or BMI is the most widely used index today. Its correlation with body fat is high (depending on the age group $r = 0.6–0.8$) and the correlation with body height is generally low. The World Health Organization (WHO) promotes the BMI as a crude indicator for weight judgment. In Table 2.5 the cut-off points for underweight, normal weight, overweight, and obesity according to the WHO are given. These cut-off values are based on the relation of BMI with mortality and with risk factors for disease as found in Caucasian populations. For non-Caucasian populations other cut-off values may apply (WHO, 2004).

The cut-off values for BMI as in Table 2.5 cannot be used in children. In younger children, weight compared with height is relatively low, and so is the BMI. During growth, the increase in weight is larger than the increase in height and, consequently, the BMI increases with age during the pubertal phase of life. There are age-related BMI cut-off values for obesity for children.

The BMI can also be used as a predictor for the percentage of body fat. Several studies have been published in which a good relationship between the BMI and the amount of body fat (either as fat mass or as body fat percentage) was demonstrated. The relationship between BMI and body fat percentage is age and gender dependent and is different among certain ethnic groups (Box 2.8). When using such age- and gender-specific prediction equations, body fat percentage can be predicted with an error of 3–5%. This error is similar to the prediction error of other doubly indirect methods, for example skinfold thickness or total body bioelectrical impedance measurements. The disadvantage of these prediction formulae is that they obviously cannot be used in certain subjects or

Box 2.8

Recent studies have shown that the relationship between body mass index (BMI) and body fat percentage differs among ethnic groups. For example, compared with Caucasian populations some Asian populations have 3–5% more body fat for the same BMI, age, and gender. These differences can be explained by differences in body build or frame size, subjects with a smaller frame having more body fat at the same BMI.

These differences can have important consequences for the definition of obesity (based on BMI cut-off values) and the prevalence of obesity in a population. In Indonesia, obesity has recently been redefined as BMI ≥ 27 kg/m^2. At this BMI, Indonesians have a similar body fat to Caucasians with a BMI of 30 kg/m^2. The lowering of the cut-off point for obesity from 30 to 27 kg/m^2 increased the prevalence of obesity from less than 5% to over 10%.

Recently an Expert Consultation of the World Health Organization (WHO) resulted in new guidelines to redefine "action points" in non-Caucasian populations. For this not only was the different relationship between BMI and body fat percentage important, but also the high levels of cardiovascular risk factors at low BMI values (WHO, 2004).

Box 2.9

From Table 2.6 it can be seen that for the same amount of subcutaneous fat (identical skinfold thickness) women have more body fat than men. This is because of the higher internal (organ) fat content in women. It can also be seen (in both females and males) that at equal skinfold thickness older people have more body fat: with age the amount of internal fat increases.

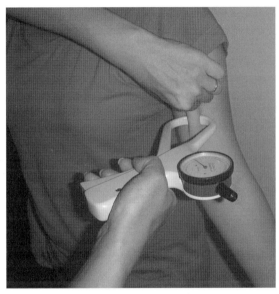

Figure 2.5 Measurement of the biceps skinfold.

groups of subjects such as pregnant women or body-builders. However, other predictive methods also have their limitations in these subjects.

TBW can also be predicted from weight and height, and numerous prediction formulae have been published. The standard error of estimate of these equations is, however, considerable.

Skinfold thickness measurements

Body fat is located both internally and subcutaneously. If one assumes a constant relationship between subcutaneous fat and total body fat, then total body fat can be estimated by measuring the amount of the subcutaneous adipose tissue. The amount of subcutaneous tissue can be estimated by measuring the thickness of the subcutaneous fat layer at different sites of the body using a skinfold caliper, infrared interactance, or ultrasound measurements. In a given age group, the relation between subcutaneous fat and total fat is indeed relatively constant. However, the relationship is different between males and females, females having relatively more internal fat (Box 2.9). Thus, it is possible by using age- and gender-specific prediction equations to assess the total amount of body fat by measuring skinfolds at different sites of the body.

Skinfolds can be measured all over the body. The most often measured skinfolds for the assessment of

total body fat are skinfolds on the upper arm biceps (Figure 2.5) and triceps, under the scapula (subscapular) and above the iliac crest (suprailiac). The sum of more skinfolds is normally used to reduce the error in measurement and to correct for possible differences in subcutaneous body fat distribution between subjects within the same age and gender group. Various prediction formulae for body fat from skinfold thickness have been published. For children, in whom the relationship between skinfold thickness and body fat depends on biological age, separate formulae must be used.

Measuring skinfolds adequately requires a trained and experienced observer, otherwise excessively large errors in the assessment of the body fat can occur. A disadvantage of the method is that the subject has to be partly undressed. This hampers the use of the method in epidemiological studies. In bed-ridden or seriously ill patients the measurement of the trunk

Table 2.6 Body fat percentage from the sum of four skinfolds (biceps, triceps, subscapular, suprailiac) in males and females of different ages[a]

Skinfolds (mm)	Age (Males)					Age (Females)				
	17–29	30–39	40–49	≥50	60–87	17–29	30–39	40–49	≥50	60–87
20	8	12	12	13	24	14	17	20	22	34
30	13	16	18	19	27	20	22	25	27	37
40	16	19	21	23	29	23	26	28	30	39
50	19	22	25	27	31	27	28	31	33	41
60	21	24	27	29	32	29	31	33	36	42
70	23	25	29	32	33	31	33	35	38	43
80	25	27	31	34	34	33	34	37	40	44
90	26	28	33	36	35	35	36	38	41	45
100	28	29	34	37	36	36	37	40	43	46
110	29	30	36	39	37	38	39	41	44	47
120	30	31	37	40	37	39	40	42	45	48
130	31	32	38	42	38	40	41	43	46	48
140	32	33	39	43	38	41	42	44	47	49
150	33	34	40	44	39	42	43	45	48	49

[a]Based on data from Durnin and Womersley (1974) for the age groups 17 to ≥50 and on Visser *et al.* (1994) for the elderly.

skinfold thicknesses can be difficult. This can be overcome by measuring only the skinfold thickness at the upper arm, for example the triceps. However, the error can be large because the triceps does not necessarily represent the total amount of subcutaneous fat. With advancing age, the triceps skinfold becomes less representative of total body fat.

In elderly subjects, the correlation between skinfold thickness and total body fat as measured by densitometry is generally lower than in young and middle-aged adults. This is due to an increased amount of internal fat in the elderly. Obese subjects are difficult to measure and the error is large even when measured by trained observers. This is also the case in subjects with edema, in whom the thickness of the subcutaneous adipose tissue is easily overestimated. In patients with human immunodeficiency virus (HIV) lipodystrophy, peripheral subcutaneous fat may be almost absent, while abdominal fat is increased. In this situation, skinfolds can be very misleading as indicators of total body fat, and should be used only to assess regional fat.

The calculation of the body fat percentage once the skinfolds have been measured is very simple. For a given skinfold thickness, the amount of body fat can be read from a table (Table 2.6).

The prediction error in body fat percentage is 3–5% compared with densitometry, depending on age,

gender, and level of body fatness. Given the possible error in densitometry (3%), this means that in extreme cases body fat from skinfolds can be as much as 10–15% off.

Other anthropometric variables

Measurements of widths of skeletal diameters provide an indication of the amount of skeletal mass. There are formulae that allow the calculation of the skeletal mass from body height, wrist diameter, and knee diameter. The current reference data for ideal weight in the USA use the elbow diameter to classify people into three types of body build.

In elderly subjects, the measurement of stature can be difficult owing to kyphosis and/or shrinkage of the spinal vertebrae. Knee height can then be used to predict the maximal stature during lifetime. Arm span is also used for that purpose. However, one has to realize that the current prediction formulae are developed in younger populations, in which the relationship between stature and surrogate measurements may be different. In addition, the prediction error (3–5 cm) is relatively high. Knee height can also be used by itself (without predicting total stature), when comparing stature-adjusted body composition between young and old people.

Circumferences of the extremities or the trunk are used to obtain information on body composition.

From the mid-arm circumference, in combination with the triceps skinfold thickness, information on muscle mass and fat mass of the upper arm can be obtained. Circumferences of the trunk at waist, hip, and upper thigh level are used as indicators of body fat distribution. The WHO suggests an upper limit waist-to-hip circumference ratio above 0.85 for females and 1.00 for males for abdominal fat distribution. Diameters can also be used to gain insights into body fat distribution. A high sagittal diameter compared with transverse diameter of the abdomen is indicative of an enlarged amount of visceral fat. However, it has to be kept in mind that the relationship between these anthropometric parameters of body fat distribution and the intra-abdominal fat determined by CT or MRI scan is generally low. Changes in internal fat detected by MRI are only weakly associated with changes in these anthropometric parameters of fat distribution.

Infrared interactance

The principle of infrared interactance is based on differences in absorbance and reflection of infrared light in different tissues. When the absorbance of near-infrared light (700–1100 nm) is measured at well-defined sites of the body, information on the thickness of the subcutaneous adipose tissue layer can be obtained. In the prediction formulae used, many other parameters are included, such as weight, height, age, and gender, and it has been argued that the prediction of body fat depends more on these parameters than on the measured infrared interaction.

Ultrasound measurements

Ultrasound measurements can also be used to study several aspects of body composition. With ultrasound measurements, the thickness of the subcutaneous fat layer can be determined and total body fat can be calculated. A good reflection signal depends heavily on the absence of connective tissue between adipose tissue and muscle. The main difficulty in ultrasound measurements is the exact application of the ultrasound transducer perpendicular to the tissue without any pressure. In the literature, several studies report a good correlation between skinfold thicknesses measured by calipers and those measured by ultrasound. The correlation of skinfolds with total body fat was higher than when using ultrasound, suggesting that

skinfold thickness measurements have a better predictive value.

Internal abdominal body fat can also be assessed with ultrasound. Studies have shown that ultrasound measurements provide a better method than anthropometry to assess internal abdominal fat depots.

Bioelectrical impedance

In bioelectrical impedance, a small alternating current is applied to the body. It is assumed that the body consists of different components, of which water and dissolved electrolytes are able to conduct the current. Hence, body impedance is a measure of body water. The electrical resistance or impedance of an electrolyte solution depends on several factors, of which the most important are the amount of electrolytes (pure water does not conduct the current), the kind of electrolytes, and the temperature of the solution. If currents of low frequency (<5 kHz) are used, body impedance is a measure of ECW, as a low-frequency current cannot penetrate the cell membrane, which acts, with its layers of protein, lipids, and proteins, as an electrical capacitor. With increasing frequencies the capacitor features of the cell membrane diminish and gradually ICW also participates in the conductance of the current, resulting in lower impedance values at higher frequencies. Hence, at higher frequencies, TBW is measured. TBW and ECW can be predicted from impedance at high and low frequency, respectively, using empirically derived prediction formulae. Other parameters are often taken into consideration, such as body weight, age, and gender.

Most prediction equations are based on statistical relationships between empirically measured impedance index values (height²/impedance) and body water values obtained by dilution techniques such as deuterium oxide dilution (for TBW) and bromide dilution (for ECW). As body water in healthy subjects is an assumed fixed part (73%) of the FFM, bioelectrical impedance measurements can also be used for the prediction of the FFM and hence body fat percentage. For those prediction equations, the impedance index was related to measures of FFM, normally obtained by densitometry or by DXA.

Body impedance depends on the frequency of the current used and on body water distribution between the extracellular and intracellular space and between the different geometrical body compartments (legs, trunk, and arms). This calls for extreme caution in the

Box 2.10

The relative validity of impedance prediction formulae can be demonstrated by a simple calculation example. A man, aged 35 years, of height 170 cm, weight 75 kg, and measured impedance (from foot to hand) 400 Ω, has a predicted fat-free mass (FFM) of 64.7 kg according to Lukaski et al. (1986) and a predicted FFM of 60.5 kg according to Segal et al. (1988). Both prediction formulae were developed in US populations and were cross-validated. The instrument used was the same and the method of reference in both studies was underwater weighing.

interpretation of calculated body composition values in situations where body water distribution can be disturbed, as is the case, for example, in dialysis patients and in ascites. In general, prediction formulae based on impedance values are strongly population specific, and age and gender are important contributors. Differences between populations and individuals are partly caused by differences in body build (e.g., relatively long legs), which is not surprising, as the legs contribute most to total body impedance relative to other parts of the body (Box 2.10).

Currently available impedance analyzers vary in their electrical features and in their principles. Many companies have developed impedance analyzers for personal use, anticipating considerable interest among the public in determining their body fat percentage. There are instruments that measure impedance from foot to foot while standing on a weighing scale and provide not only body weight but also body fat percentage. Other instruments measure impedance from hand to hand and allow the reading of body fat percentage, using a built-in software program in which weight, height, age, and gender have to be entered. Combinations of foot-to-foot and hand-to-hand impedance analyzers are also marketed.

As for all other impedance analyzers, the incorporated formulae are population specific and have a prediction error of 4–5%. This means that, apart from a systematic error (prediction formula is not valid), the value can be as much as 10% off in extreme cases. This kind of error is similar to the possible error in skinfold thickness measurements, and hence impedance is no better than skinfold thickness measurements. The advantage of impedance analyzers is that there is no need to undress and measurements are less prone to observer bias.

Total body electrical conductivity

Total body electrical conductivity (TOBEC) was developed in the 1970s. The principle of the method is that conductive material (body water and dissolved electrolytes) that is placed in an electromagnetic field will cause an inductive current, which is related to the amount of conductive material. In practice, the subject lies on a stretcher, which enters the inner space of an electric wire coil, through which a high-frequency current (2.5–5 MHz) passes. The measurement is very quick (it takes only seconds), painless, and without any risk to the subject. The reproducibility of a measurement is within 2% and the error in the predicted FFM was found to be about 3 kg in a group of adult subjects, which is similar to, for example, skinfold thickness measurements or impedance measurements. The TOBEC method is especially suitable for measurements in infants and young children, in whom bioelectrical impedance measurements are difficult or impossible to perform, owing to movement. The main disadvantage of the method is the high price.

Creatinine excretion and N-methyl-histidine excretion

In the muscle cell, creatine phosphate, necessary for the energy metabolism of the cell, degenerates to creatinine at a constant daily rate of about 2%. It is assumed that 1 g of excreted creatinine is equivalent to 18–22 kg of muscle mass. As the cell cannot recycle creatinine, the kidneys excrete it. Since metabolized creatine phosphate is not the only source of urinary creatinine (e.g., creatinine in ingested meat is also excreted immediately), the validity of the method is dubious. A day-to-day coefficient of variation in the excretion of creatinine of almost 20% is reported, when the subject is "free living" and the urine is sampled over constant periods of 24 hours. The high variation is due to the ingestion of creatinine with nonvegetarian meals, differences in physical activity levels, and variation in creatinine excretion within the phase of the menstrual cycle. After careful standardization, which includes a controlled diet, the day-to-day variability in excretion can be decreased to about 5%. To obtain a reliable assessment of the creatinine excretion, sampling of urine over multiple 24 hour periods is necessary.

The excretion of 3-methylhistidine has also been proposed as a measure for muscle mass. FFM determined by densitometry correlates well with excreted 3-methylhistidine. The chemical determination of 3-methylhistidine is, however, more complicated than that of creatinine. A unique feature of 3-methylhistidine is that it gives a measure of muscle protein breakdown. Given the greater expense of measuring 3-methylhistidine and the limited benefit for muscle mass estimates, it is probably best to use it primarily for turnover studies.

The main disadvantages of creatinine and 3-methylhistidine excretion as measures for body composition are the large variability in excretion, the necessity to follow a controlled (meat-free) diet for several days before and during the urine collections, and the difficulties associated with collecting 24 hour urine samples.

Use and misuse of body composition data

Information on the body composition of groups of subjects or individuals is important, as body composition is an indicator of nutritional status and also provides information about acute water homeostasis. Depending on what information is needed, several methods are available. However, all have their advantages and limitations. The price of the method (both the instrument and the required personnel), the eventual stress and danger (e.g., radiation) for the subject, and the time necessary to obtain the information determine the choice of the method, as well as

the required accuracy. The use in epidemiological studies is different than that in clinical situations or in physiological research. Table 2.7 provides a "buyer's guide" to the several methods discussed in this chapter. It is difficult to generalize as to which method should be used in a given study. Apart from the factors mentioned in Table 2.7, availability plays an important role. Some situations are discussed below.

For the description of body fatness of a large general population group, the calculation of the body fat percentage from the BMI may be as good as or even better than the more expensive information obtained from bioelectrical impedance or the laborious measurement of skinfold thicknesses. Whichever method is to be used for the prediction of body fat percentage in the population, it is important to remember that the formulae used should have been validated in the population under study. The fact that a formula is cross-validated by the authors who published the formula does not mean that the formula is valid in another population. The use of the Durnin and Womersley (1974) equations for estimating body fat from the sum of four skinfolds may be correct if the population is adult but younger than about 60 years. In older subjects, the amount of body fat is likely to be underestimated with these formulae. Therefore, their use and thoughtless interpretation in the elderly would lead to completely wrong conclusions about

Table 2.7 Buyer's guide to different methods used to determine body composition

Method	Accuracy	Expenses	Radiation	Time	Convenience for subject
Carcass analysis	+ + +	− −			
Neutron activation	+ + +	− −	− −	+ +	+ +
Densitometry	+ +	+		+ +	+/−
Dilution method	+ +	+/−	(−)	+	+
^{40}K method	+ +	−		+ +	+ +
DXA	+ + +	+/−	−	+ +	+ +
More-compartment models	+ + +	−	−	−	+
CT scanning	+ +	−	− −	+ +	+ +
MRI scanning	+ +	−		+ +	+
Anthropometry	+	+ + +		+ +	+
Infrared interactance	+	+ +		+ +	+ +
Bioelectrical impedance	+	+		+ + +	+ + + +
TOBEC	+	−		+ +	+ +
Creatinine/N-methylhistidine excretion	+	+		−	−

DXA, dual-energy X-ray absorptiometry; CT, computed tomography; MRI, magnetic resonance imaging; TOBEC, total body electrical conductivity.
+ + +, excellent; + +, very good; +, good; +/−, reasonable; −, bad; − −, very bad.

body composition in the elderly and changes in body composition with age. For the same reason, the BMI as an indicator of body fatness is only suitable when corrections for age and gender are made; for example, a BMI of 25 kg/m^2 at the age of 20 years reflects a much lower percentage of body fat than at the age of 70 years. Body fat in females is always higher than body fat in males with the same BMI and age. Recent studies have shown that the relationship between BMI and body fat percentage also differs among ethnic groups. Figure 2.6 gives a good insight on how misleading a low BMI can be. The biodata also show the differences in body build, which is at least part of the reason for the paradox. Prediction equations based on impedance are dependent on body build,

among other factors, and there are no universally valid prediction equations based on impedance. Choice of method to assess body composition in a population would also take into consideration within- and between-observer variability. Thus, impedance may be better than skinfold thickness measurements in a study of 1000 people, where variability between technicians is important. One may argue that, for population studies, a slight overestimation or under-estimation of body fat is not important. However, if, for example, obesity is defined as a certain amount of body fat that is achieved at a certain distinct level of BMI, even minor differences in body fat percentage or in BMI will result in large differences in the preva-lence of obesity.

	Dutch	Asian
Age (years)	21	22
Height (cm)	175.6	158.0
Weight (kg)	77.2	43.9
Relative sitting height	0.53	0.55
Wrist (cm)	5.6	4.4
Knee (cm)	9.1	8.4
Arm span (cm)	177.0	157.5
Waist (cm)	82.0	62.2
Hip (cm)	104.0	87.0
BMI	25.0	17.6
BF (%)	31.1	29.6

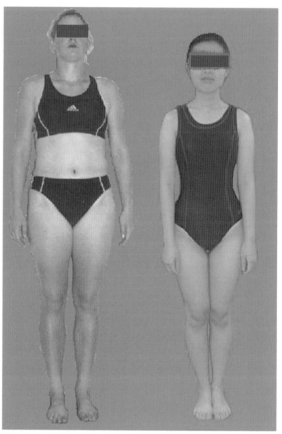

Figure 2.6 The difference in the relationship between BMI and body fat percentage across populations is best demonstrated in this figure and the given biodata. Note that the two young women are the same age and their percentage body fat as determined by a chemical four-compartment model (bias free!) is the same. The Asian woman has relatively shorter legs and a more slender body build (determined as height/(sum of knee and wrist diameter). Relative leg length and "slenderness" are main determining factors in the BMI/percentage body fat relationship in addition to physical activity level.

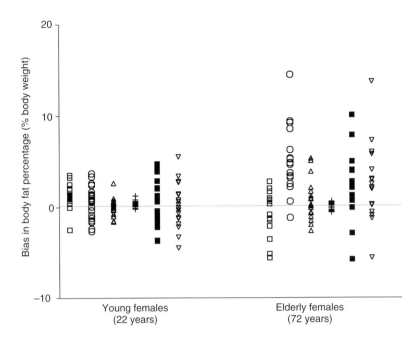

Figure 2.7 Individual differences in measured body fat percentage compared with a chemical four-compartment model in 20 young and 20 elderly females using various techniques. *y*-axis, BF% from four-compartment model minus: □, densitometry (Siri); ○, deuterium dilution; △, DXA; +, three-compartment model (Siri); ■, skinfold thickness; ∇, bioelectrical impedance.

In physiological studies where, for example, energy metabolism has to be corrected for body composition, a systematic bias in body composition results may lead to completely wrong conclusions. When a body composition formula or method systematically overestimates the FFM in obese subjects, a "normal" resting metabolic rate in obese subjects would be underestimated after "correction" for differences in body composition (expressed as kJ/kg FFM). This may lead to the conclusion that obese subjects have lower metabolic rates, which might have caused their excess adipose tissue stores. This argument does not even imply whether the FFM can be treated as one entity in different populations instead of different components such as the heart, liver, or muscles (Gallagher *et al.*, 1998). These considerations are important for comparative studies between groups (e.g., obese versus nonobese, elderly versus young or middle-aged), but also for longitudinal studies (e.g., weight-loss studies).

The use of bioelectrical impedance to predict changes in FFM, TBW, or body fat during weight loss is questionable. The difference in body water distribution (anatomically as well as intracellular/extracellular) before and after weight loss may be considerable, leading to a different and systematic bias of the prediction equation. In such a study it may be better to report changes in impedance values instead of changes in predicted body composition. Another example is the very low change in impedance after water removal in patients with ascites. Despite the fact that a considerable amount of water is removed from the body, the change in total body impedance is low as the trunk hardly contributes to total body impedance.

All methods have their limitations, doubly indirect more than indirect methods. Figure 2.7 shows the individual errors in body fat percentage from densitometry, DXA, deuterium dilution, a chemical three-compartment model, skinfold thicknesses, and bioelectrical impedance in young and elderly women compared with body fat percentage obtained from a four-compartment model. It is obvious that errors can be considerable, both at a group level and especially at an individual level in the elderly. Many of these errors can be explained by the violation of assumptions. This clearly shows that information on body composition must be used with an awareness of the limitations of the techniques.

2.8 Perspectives on the future

Given the importance of body composition to evaluate nutritional status and to gain information on certain disease processes, it can be expected that more easy-to-use methods and instrumentation will be developed and become available in the future. Application and interpretation of data from these methods should be used with an awareness of possible limitations, as mentioned above. There is a growing perception that, because of differences in body build, frame size, and possibly also other variables, there are differences in the relationship between BMI and body fat percentage among ethnic groups. Some Aboriginal and Asian people have a higher fat percentage and therefore greater risk for several chronic diseases at a given BMI than Caucasian populations. Conversely, Africans often have higher bone density than Caucasians. Much more research is needed to define the optimal BMI values that will correlate with optimal health and the lowest risk of disease for different populations.

Acknowledgment

This chapter has been revised and updated by Paul Deurenberg based on the original chapter by Paul Deurenberg and Ronenn Roubenoff. For more information on this topic visit www.nutritiontexts.com

References

Durnin JVGA, Womersley J. Body fat assessed from total body density and its estimation from skinfold thickness: measure-ments on 481 men and women aged from 17 to 72 years. *Br J Nutr* 1974; **32**: 77–97.

Forbes GB. *Human Body Composition*. Springer, New York, 1987.

Gallagher D, Belmonte D, Deurenberg P, Wang Z-M, Krasnow N, Pi-Sunyer FX, Heymsfield SB. Organ-tissue mass measurement by MRI allows accurate in vivo modeling of REE and metabolic active tissue mass. *Am J Physiol* 1998: **275**: E249–258.

Heymsfield SB, Lohman TG, Wang ZW, Going SB. *Human Body Composition*, 2nd edn. Human Kinetics, Champaign, IL, 2005.

Lukaski HC, Bolonchuk WW, Hall CB, Siders WA. Validity of tetrapolar bioelectrical impedance method to assess human body composition. *J Appl Physiol* 1986; **60**: 1327–1332.

Segal KR, Van Loan M, Fitzgerald PI, Hodgdon JA, Van Itallie TB. Lean body mass estimation by bio-electrical impedance analysis: a four site cross-validation study. *Am J Clin Nutr* 1988; **47**: 7–14.

Visser M, Heuvel van den E, Deurenberg P. Prediction equations for the estimation of body composition in the elderly using anthropometric data. *Br J Nutr* 1994; **71**: 823–833.

WHO Expert Consultation. Appropriate body-mass index for Asian populations and its implications for policy and intervention strategies. *Lancet* 2004; **363**: 157–163.

Further reading

Siri WE. Body composition from fluid spaces and density: analysis of methods. In: Brozek J, Henschel A, eds. *Techniques for Measuring Body Composition*. National Academy of Sciences, Washington, DC, 1961: 223–244.

Snijder WS, Cook MJ, Nasset ES, *et al. Report of the Task Group on Reference Man*. Pergamon Press, Oxford, 1984.

Wang Z-M, Pierson RN, Heymsfield SB. The five-level model; a new approach to organise body composition rsearch. *Am J Clin Nutr* 1992; **56**: 19–28.

World Health Organization. *Obesity: Preventing and Managing the Global Epidemic*. WHO, Geneva, 1998.

3
Energy Metabolism

Arne Astrup and Angelo Tremblay

Key messages

- Energy balance in the body is the balance between how much energy is consumed and how much is expended. Positive balance is when intake exceeds expenditure and is associated with increases in body energy stores (weight gain). During negative balance, as in periods of starvation, body energy stores are depleted.
- Energy intake corresponds to the energy content of macronutrients in foods. Carbohydrate provides 16.8 kJ/g, protein also 16.8 kJ/g, and fat 37.8 kJ/g. In addition, alcohol provides 29.4 kJ/g.
- Total energy expenditure constitutes approximately two-thirds of the energy expended by the body to maintain basic physiological functions plus the thermic effect of a meal and energy expended during physical movement. The basic physiological functions include heart beat, muscle function, and respiration (resting or basal metabolic rate). The thermic effect of a meal is about 10% of the caloric value of the meal needed to digest, metabolize, and store ingested macronutrients. The energy expended during physical activity is energy expended when skeletal muscles are used for any type of physical movement. In infants and children, the cost of growth is added.
- Energy requirement is the amount of food energy needed to balance energy expenditure in order to maintain body size, body composition, and level of physical activity, consistent with long-term good health. This includes the energy needs for optimal growth and development in children, and the needs of pregnancy and lactation (deposition of tissue and secretion of milk).
- Body mass index (BMI) classifies weight relative to height squared and is the most accepted and widely used crude index of obesity. A BMI of 18–24.9 kg/m^2 is regarded as normal for adults, between 25 and 29.9 kg/m^2 as overweight, and >30 kg/m^2 as obese.
- Energy expenditure can be measured by direct methods (calorimetry) or indirect methods, in which oxygen consumption and carbon dioxide production are used to calculate energy expenditure. However, the modern gold standard is measurement by doubly labeled water, which is a noninvasive method used to measure total energy expenditure over periods of 7–14 days while subjects are living in their usual environments.
- Hunger is the physiological need to eat and results in actions to attempt to obtain food for consumption. Appetite is a psychological desire to eat and is related to the pleasant sensations that are often associated with food. Thus, hunger is more of an intrinsic instinct, whereas appetite is often a learned response.

3.1 Introduction

Definition and conceptualization of energy balance

The average adult human consumes close to 1 000 000 calories (4000 MJ) per year. Despite this huge energy intake, most healthy individuals are able to strike a remarkable balance between how much energy is consumed and how much energy is expended, thus resulting in a state of energy balance in the body. This accurate balance between energy intake and energy expenditure is an example of homeostatic control and results in maintenance of body weight and body energy stores. This regulation of energy balance is achieved over the long term despite large fluctuations in both energy intake and energy expenditure within and between days. The accuracy and precision by which the body maintains energy balance is highlighted by the fact that even a small error in the system can have detrimental consequences over time. If energy intake chronically exceeds energy expenditure by as little as 105 kJ/day, then, over time, a person will become substantially obese. The achievement of energy balance is driven by the first law of thermodynamics, which states that energy can be neither destroyed nor created. This principle necessitates that when energy intake equals energy expenditure, body energy stores must remain constant. This chapter explains how the body is able to achieve this state of energy balance through control of energy intake and energy expenditure. In addition, the various ways that body energy stores can be measured and some examples of conditions in which energy balance may be disrupted are summarized. Particular emphasis is placed on obesity, which is the end-result of a positive energy balance and is now considered one of the major nutritional disorders.

Components of energy balance

Energy intake
Energy intake is defined as the caloric or energy content of food as provided by the major sources of dietary energy: carbohydrate (16.8 kJ/g), protein (16.8 kJ/g), fat (37.8 kJ/g), and alcohol (29.4 kJ/g).

Energy storage
The energy that is consumed in the form of food or drinks can either be stored in the body in the form of fat (the major energy store), glycogen (short-term energy/carbohydrate reserves), or protein (rarely used by the body for energy except in severe cases of starvation and other wasting conditions, as discussed later in the chapter), or be used by the body to fuel energy-requiring events.

Energy expenditure
The energy that is consumed in the form of food is required by the body for metabolic, cellular, and mechanical work such as breathing, heart beat, and muscular work, all of which require energy and result in heat production. The body requires energy for a variety of functions. The largest use of energy is needed to fuel the basal metabolic rate (BMR), which is the energy expended by the body to maintain basic physiological functions (e.g., heart beat, muscle contraction and function, respiration). BMR is the minimum level of energy expended by the body to sustain life in the awake state. It can be measured after a 12 hour fast while the subject is resting physically and mentally, and maintained in a thermoneutral, quiet environment. The BMR is slightly elevated above the metabolic rate during sleep, because energy expenditure increases above basal levels owing to the energy cost of arousal. Because of the difficulty in achieving BMR under most measurement situations, resting metabolic rate (RMR) is frequently measured using the same measurement conditions stated for BMR. Thus, the major difference between BMR and RMR is the slightly higher energy expended during RMR (~ 3%) owing to less subject arousal and non-fasting conditions. Because of this small difference, the terms basal and resting metabolic rate are often used interchangeably. RMR occurs in a continual process throughout the 24 hours of a day and remains relatively constant within individuals over time. In the average adult human, RMR is approximately 4.2 kJ/min. Thus, basal or resting metabolic rate is the largest component of energy expenditure and makes up about two-thirds of total energy expenditure.

In addition to RMR, there is an increase in energy expenditure in response to food intake. This increase in metabolic rate after food consumption is often referred to as the thermic effect of a meal (or meal-induced thermogenesis) and is mainly the energy that is expended to digest, metabolize, convert, and store ingested macronutrients, named obligatory thermogenesis. The measured thermic effect of a meal is usually higher than the theoretical cost owing to a facultative component caused by an activation of the sympathoadrenal system, which increases energy expenditure through peripheral β-adrenoceptors. The energy cost associated with meal ingestion is primarily influenced by the composition of the food that is consumed, and also is relatively stable within individuals over time. The thermic effect of a meal usually constitutes approximately 10% of the caloric content of the meal that is consumed. The third source of energy expenditure in the body is the increase in metabolic rate that occurs during physical activity, which includes exercise as well as all forms of physical activity. Thus, physical activity energy expenditure (or the thermic effect of exercise) is the term frequently used to describe the increase in metabolic rate that is caused by use of skeletal muscles for any type of physical movement. Physical activity energy expenditure is the most variable component of daily energy expenditure and can vary greatly within and between individuals owing to the volitional and variable nature of physical activity patterns.

In addition to the three major components of energy expenditure, there may be a requirement for energy for three other minor needs.

- The energy cost of growth occurs in growing individuals, but is negligible except within the first few months of life.
- Adaptive thermogenesis is heat production during exposure to reduced temperatures, and occurs in humans, e.g., during the initial months of life and during fever and other pathological conditions, but also as a contributor to daily energy expenditure.
- Thermogenesis is increased by a number of agents in the environment, including in foods and beverages. Nicotine in tobacco is the most important one, and heavy smokers may have a 10% higher energy expenditure than nonsmokers of similar body size and composition and physical activity. Caffeine and derivatives in coffee, tea, and chocolate, capsaicin in hot chilies, and other substances in foods and drinks may possess minor thermogenic effects that affect energy expenditure.

Energy balance

Energy balance occurs when the energy content of food is matched by the total amount of energy that is expended by the body. An example of energy balance would be the scenario cited at the outset of this chapter in which, over a year, the average adult consumes and expends 1 000 000 calories, resulting in no net change in the energy content of the body. When energy intake exceeds energy expenditure, a state of positive energy balance occurs. Thus, positive energy balance occurs when excessive overfeeding relative to energy needs occurs, and the body increases its overall energy stores. Examples of positive energy balance include periods around major festivals when overeating and inactivity generally prevail, and during pregnancy and lactation when the body purposefully increases its stores of energy. When energy intake is lower than energy expenditure, a state of negative energy balance occurs, for example during periods of starvation. In this regard, evidence suggests that, under conditions of substantial energy imbalance, be it positive or negative, energy expenditure may reach a level that is beyond what could be predicted by body weight changes. This so-called "adaptive thermogenesis" might contribute to the occurrence of resistance to lose fat in the context of obesity treatment or the achievement of a new body weight plateau following overfeeding. It is important to note that energy balance can occur regardless of the levels of energy intake and expenditure; thus, energy balance can occur in very inactive individuals as well as in highly active individuals provided that adequate energy sources are available. It is also important to think of energy balance in terms of the major sources of energy, i.e., carbohydrate, protein, and fat. For example, carbohydrate balance occurs when the body balances the amount of carbohydrate ingested with that expended for energy.

3.2 Energy intake

Sources of dietary energy

As mentioned above, the sources of energy in the food we eat include the major macronutrients: protein, carbohydrate, and fat, as well as alcohol. Carbohydrate and protein provide 16.8 kJ of energy for each gram; alcohol provides 29.4 kJ/g, whereas fat is the most energy dense, providing 37.8 kJ/g. Note that 4.2 kJ is defined as the amount of heat that is required to raise the temperature of 1 liter of water by 1°C. The energy content of food can be measured by bomb calorimetry, which involves combusting a known weight of food inside a sealed chamber and measuring the amount of heat that is released during this process. Thus, 1 g of pure fat would release 37.8 kJ during its complete combustion, whereas 1 g of pure carbohydrate would release 16.8 kJ. Thus, if the gram quantities of any type of food are known, the energy content can easily be calculated. For example, if a protein-rich nutrition snack contains 21 g of carbohydrate, 6 g of fat, and 14 g of protein, then the total energy content is $(21 \times 16.8) + (6 \times 37.8) + (14 \times 16.8) = 814.8$ kJ. The macronutrient composition of food is typically assessed in the percentage contribution of each macronutrient to the total number of calories. If a food has a carbohydrate content of 21 g, which is 352.8 kJ, and the total energy content is 820 kJ the proportion of energy derived from carbohydrate is 43%; the fat content is 6 g, or 226.8 kJ, equivalent to 28% of the energy; and the protein contributes 14 g, 235.2 kJ and 29% of the energy.

Regulation of food intake

Appetite, hunger, and satiety

The quality and quantity of food that is consumed are closely regulated by the body. Food intake is regulated by a number of factors involving complex interactions among various hormones, neuroendocrine factors, the central nervous system, and organ systems (e.g., brain and liver), and environmental and external factors.

Appetite is usually defined as a psychological desire to eat and is related to the pleasant sensations that are often associated with specific foods. Scientifically, appetite is used as a general term of overall sensations related to food intake.

Hunger is usually defined as the subjective feeling that determines when food consumption is initiated and can be described as a nagging, irritating feeling that signifies food deprivation to a degree that the next eating episode should take place.

Satiety is considered as the state of inhibition over eating that leads to the termination of a meal, and is related to the time interval until the next eating episode. Thus, hunger and satiety are more intrinsic instincts, whereas appetite is often a learned response.

The internal factors that regulate the overall feeling of hunger and satiety include the central nervous system (primarily the hypothalamus and the vagus nerve), the major digestive organs such as the stomach and liver, and various hormones. In addition, environmental factors (e.g., meal pattern and composition, food availability, smell and sight of foods, climate), emotional factors (e.g., stress), and some diseased states (e.g., anorexia, trauma, infection) may influence the feelings of both hunger and appetite. The factors that influence appetite include factors external to the individual (e.g., climate, weather), specific appetite cravings, specific learned dislikes or avoidance (e.g., alcohol), intrinsic properties of food (e.g., taste, palatability, texture), cultural practices or preferences, specific effects of some drugs and diseases, and metabolic factors such as hormones and neurotransmitters. Some of these factors are described in further detail below.

The classic way to describe the complex appetite-regulating system is the satiety cascade put forth by John Blundell. The satiety cascade describes four distinctly different but overlapping categories of mechanisms involved in acute within-meal feeling of satiety (referred to as satiation) and the inbetween-meal satiety (Figure 3.1).

Factors influencing food intake

Digestive factors

Several factors in the digestive system exert a short-term influence over food intake. The presence of food

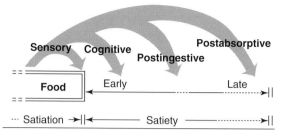

Figure 3.1 The satiety cascade by John Blundell (1987). The four categories of mechanisms are sensory, cognitive, postingestive, and postabsorptive. The sensoric phase includes stimuli mediated via sensory fibers in the cranial nerves and relates to the palatability of the ingested meal including smell, taste, temperature, and texture. The cognitive phase of the satiety cascade represents learned, known, and assumed properties of the ingested food. In the postingestive phase the gastrointestinal tract is involved in a number of satiety signals both via chemo- and mechanoreceptors and appetite-regulating peptides from the gut and pancreas either entering circulation and acting directly in the CNS or signaling via the vagus nerve. Important satiety signals in the postabsorptive phase include circulating nutrients, signals derived from differences in energy turnover, substrate oxidation, and neurohormonal factors. Reprinted from Blundell *et al.* (1987), copyright 1987 with permission of Elsevier.

and drink in the stomach and intestine and the resultant pressure that they exert may regulate food intake. This effect is known as gastrointestinal distension. In addition, the stomach produces a hormone called cholecystokinin (CCK) in response to food intake, which may, in turn, regulate food intake. Furthermore, when subjects have fat or carbohydrate infused directly into the small intestine, they report feelings of satiety. This suggests that factors in the intestine regulate food intake. Indeed, receptors in the intestine have been identified that recognize the presence of specific macronutrients; these receptors are linked to the brain and therefore can communicate directly with the central nervous system, resulting in regulation of energy balance. In addition, other gastrointestinal hormones, such as glucagon-like peptide-1 and -2 (GLPs), CCK, and glucose-dependent insulinotropic polypeptide (GIP) are likely to play a role in the mediation of gut events and brain perception of hunger and satiety.

Central nervous system factors

The main contributory factor regulating food intake in the central nervous system is the hypothalamus. The hypothalamus is linked to specific parts of the brain that are known to modify feeding behavior, specifically the paraventricular nuclei and the nigro-striatal tract. These areas of the brain respond to various neurotransmitters as well as sympathetic nervous system activity. In general, food intake will decrease as sympathetic nervous system activity increases, and vice versa.

Circulating factors

After consumption of a meal, food is broken down into its basic components (i.e., carbohydrate is broken down to glucose, protein to amino acids, and fats or triglycerides to glycerol and fatty acids) and the circulating levels of some of these breakdown products increase in the blood. Consequently, glucose, amino acids, glycerol, and fatty acids are further metabolized, primarily in the liver, or used for immediate energy (e.g., in muscle or brain). There is evidence to suggest that this resultant metabolism, especially in the liver, may in turn regulate food intake. After meal consumption, the circulating levels of nutrients fall (within minutes for glucose, several hours for triglycerides) and the feelings of hunger return. The link from nutrient metabolism to central control of food intake occurs through signals from the liver to the brain via the vagus nerve. Thus, circulating factors provide a link between the digestive system and the central nervous system, which provides another system for regulating food intake.

Signals from the periphery

Leptin is a hormone that is produced by fat cells and communicates with the central nervous system through leptin receptors in the hypothalamus. Reduced production of leptin, or lack of sensitivity of the hypothalamus to leptin, may regulate food intake and play a key role in the etiology of rare forms of obesity in humans. Leptin and the other peripheral hormones with a central effect on appetite are divided into two broad categories: (1) the so-called adiposity signals, which are tonically active providing information on body fat stores to the CNS and (2) the satiety signals which are released in response to food intake and are thought to be involved in short-term regulation of energy intake. Currently known adiposity signals are insulin, leptin, and adiponectin, which are considered as long-acting signals reducing energy intake. Among the satiety signals are the hunger hormone ghrelin, which is secreted in the stomach, and the short-acting

gut- and pancreas-derived satiety signals CCK, peptide YY (PYY), GLP-1, oxyntomodulin (OXM), and pancreatic polypeptide (PP). Many of the peripheral satiety signals have receptors in the arcuate nucleus (ARC) of the hypothalamus, which plays an important role in appetite regulation. The ARC contains neuropeptide Y (NPY)- and agouti-related peptide (AgRP)-expressing neurons acting to stimulate food intake along with the adjacent pro-opiomelanocortin (POMC) and cocaine- and amphetamine-regulated transcript (CART)-expressing neurons which inhibit feeding. Besides the ARC, the nucleus of the solitary tract (NTS) and the area postrema (AP) receive appetite-regulating inputs from vagal afferents and circulating factors and are connected to the hypothalamic nuclei controlling food intake.

External factors

Various nonphysiological or external factors are also known to modify food intake, and these effects may be mediated through the intrinsic factors described above. Psychological factors such as depression may lead to either increased or decreased food intake, or changes in the consumption of specific types of foods. Environmental factors are also important, the most obvious being food availability. Even when food is available, some of the specific properties of foods make them more or less appealing, thereby modifying food intake. Important physical characteristics of food include taste, texture, color, temperature, and presentation. Other cultural influences in the environment, such as time of day, social factors, peer influence, and cultural preferences, can also play a role in influencing food intake.

3.3 Energy expenditure

Concept of energy expenditure

The process of energy expenditure and the oxidation or combustion of food for energy in the body is analogous to a woodstove that burns wood to release heat in a controlled fashion. In this analogy, large chunks of wood are fed to the stove and the wood is gradually combusted in the presence of oxygen to release carbon dioxide, water vapor, and heat. Similarly, in the body, the food consumed is oxidized or combusted in the presence of oxygen to release carbon dioxide, water, and heat. When ingested food is used for energy, however, the release and transfer of energy occur through a series of tightly regulated metabolic pathways in which the potential energy from food is released slowly and gradually over time. This process ensures that the body is provided with a gradual and constant energy store, rather than relying on a sudden release of energy from an immediate combustion of ingested food. As a simple example of how the body uses food for energy, consider the combustion of a simple glucose molecule:

$$C_6H_{12}O_6 + 6O_2 \rightarrow 6H_2O + 6CO_2 + Heat$$

Similar chemical reactions can be described for the combustion of other sources of energy, such as fat and other types of carbohydrates. These types of reaction occur continuously in the body and constitute energy expenditure. As discussed previously, the three major sources of energy expenditure in the body are to fuel RMR, the thermic effect of meals, and physical activity. As discussed in more detail below, energy expenditure can be measured by assessment of total heat production in the body (direct calorimetry) or by assessment of oxygen consumption and carbon dioxide production (indirect calorimetry).

Historical aspects of energy expenditure

The burning or combustion of food in the body was originally described in the classic experiments of Lavoisier, who worked in France in the late eighteenth century. Lavoisier discovered that a candle would burn only in the presence of oxygen. In addition, he was the first to describe how living organisms produced heat in a similar way, as they required oxygen for life and combusted food as they released heat. His experiments were the first to document the heat production of living organisms. Working before the invention of electricity, he built the first calorimeter in which a small animal was placed in a sealed chamber. Lavoisier packed ice into a sealed pocket around the chamber (he could only perform these studies in the winter when ice was collected from the ground), and then placed the chamber and ice layer inside an insulated chamber. Lavoisier then collected and measured the volume of melting water. Since the ice layer was insulated from the outside world, the only way that the ice could melt was by the increase in heat produced by the living animal. Lavoisier therefore measured the volume of melted ice water, and, by so doing, was able to calculate accurately the amount of heat that had to be produced by the animal to melt the measured amount of ice.

Measurement of energy expenditure

Lavoisier's device was the first calorimeter that was used to measure heat production. This approach is termed direct calorimetry because heat production is measured directly. Direct calorimeters have been designed for measuring heat production in humans, but this approach is technically demanding, especially in human studies, and is now infrequently used. Indirect calorimetry measures energy production via respiratory gas analysis. This approach is based on oxygen consumption and carbon dioxide production that occurs during the combustion (or oxidation) of protein, carbohydrate, fat, and alcohol, as shown in the example of glucose combustion. Respiratory gas analysis can easily be achieved in humans either over short measurement periods at rest or during exercise using a face mask, mouthpiece, or canopy system for gas collection, and over longer periods of 24 hours (and longer) with subjects living in a metabolic chamber. BMR is typically measured by indirect calorimetry under fasted conditions while subjects lie quietly at rest in the early morning for 30–40 min. The thermic effect of a meal is typically measured by monitoring the changes in metabolic rate by indirect calorimetry for 3–6 hours following consumption of a test meal of known caloric content. The energy expended in physical activity can be measured under laboratory conditions, also using indirect calorimetry during standard activities. In addition, free-living physical activity-related energy expenditure over extended periods of up to 2 weeks can be measured by the combination of doubly labeled water (DLW) to measure total energy expenditure (see below), and indirect calorimetry to measure resting energy expenditure and the thermic effect of a meal. Indirect calorimetry has an added advantage in that the ratio of carbon dioxide production to oxygen consumption (the respiratory quotient, or RQ) is indicative of the type of substrate (i.e., fat versus carbohydrate) being oxidized, for example carbohydrate oxidation has a RQ of 1.0 and fat oxidation has a RQ close to 0.7.

Energy expenditure can be assessed from indirect calorimetry in a simple, less accurate way by ignoring the contribution of protein oxidation or by collecting urine during the measurement to analyze the excreted nitrogen. The latter approach is preferable because it gives a more accurate estimate of energy expenditure and RQ.

Step 1

First, the contribution of protein oxidation to oxygen consumption ($\dot{V}O_2$) and carbon dioxide production ($\dot{V}CO_2$) is estimated based on the knowledge that the nitrogen content of protein is 1/6.25:

$$\dot{V}O_{2(prot)} = n \times 6.25 \times 0.97$$
$$\dot{V}CO_{2(prot)} = n \times 6.25 \times 0.77$$

where V is volume, 0.97 and 0.77 are liters of O_2 consumed and CO_2 produced by the biological oxidation of 1 g of protein, respectively, and prot is protein.

Step 2

Next, nonprotein $\dot{V}O_2$ ($\dot{V}O_{2(nonprot)}$) and nonprotein $\dot{V}CO_2$ ($\dot{V}CO_{2(nonprot)}$) are calculated:

$$\dot{V}O_{2(nonprot)} = \dot{V}O_2 - \dot{V}O_{2(prot)}$$
$$\dot{V}CO_{2(nonprot)} = \dot{V}CO_2 - \dot{V}CO_{2(prot)}$$
$$\dot{V}O_{2(nonprot)} = C \times 0.828 + F \times 2.03$$
$$\dot{V}CO_{2(nonprot)} = C \times 0.828 + F \times 1.43$$

where C and F are grams of oxidized carbohydrate and fat, respectively, and can be found by solving the two equations with two unknowns; O_2 and CO_2 produced by the combustion of 1 g of carbohydrate is 0.828 liters, whereas the combustion of 1 g triglyceride consumes 2.03 liters O_2 and produces 1.43 liters CO_2. The protein oxidation (P) is $n \times 6.25$ g.

Step 3

The RQ is defined as:

$$\dot{V}CO_2/\dot{V}O_2$$

Nonprotein RQ ($RQ_{(nonprot)}$) is calculated by the equation:

$$RQ_{(nonprot)} = \dot{V}CO_{2(nonprot)}/\dot{V}O_{2(nonprot)}$$

Step 4

Next, energy expenditure can be calculated:

$$\text{Energy expenditure (kJ/min)}$$
$$= [19.63 + 4.59 (RQ_{(nonprot)} - 0.707]$$
$$\times \dot{V}O_{2(nonprot)} + 18.78 \times \dot{V}O_{2(nonprot)}$$

or

$$\text{Energy expenditure (kJ/min)} =$$
$$17 \times P + 17.5 \times C + 38.9 \times F$$

where 17, 17.5, and 38.9 are the heat produced (kJ) by the combustion of 1 g of protein, glycogen, and triglyceride, respectively.

The equations are produced by the insertion of the heat equivalent for carbohydrate and fat, and are valid even though there is a quantitative conversion of carbohydrate to lipid (*de novo* lipogenesis) or glyconeogenesis.

The caloric equivalent for O_2 is similar to the three main substrates: 21 kJ/l O_2 for carbohydrate, 19 kJ/l O_2 for fat, and 17.8 kJ/l O_2 for protein (which contributes only modestly to energy expenditure). Energy expenditure can therefore be calculated with reasonable accuracy by the equation:

$$\text{Energy expenditure (kJ/min)} = 20 \text{ kJ/l} \times \dot{V}O_2 \text{ (l/min)}$$

With pure fat oxidation the RQ is 0.707, with pure carbohydrate oxidation it is 1.0, and with pure protein oxidation it is approximately 0.8.

Step 5

Oxidation of protein (P), carbohydrate (C), and fat (F) can be calculated by the following equations, where n is the unit g/min:

$$P \text{ (g/min)} = 6.25 \times n$$
$$C \text{ (g/min)} = 4.55 \times \dot{V}CO_2 - 3.21 \times \dot{V}O_2 - 2.87$$
$$F \text{ (g/min)} = 1.67 \times \dot{V}O_2 - 1.67 \times \dot{V}CO_2 - 1.92 \times n$$

3.4 Factors that influence energy expenditure

Resting metabolic rate

Each of the components of energy expenditure is determined by various factors. RMR is highly variable between individuals (±25%), but is very consistent within individuals (<5%). Since RMR occurs predominantly in muscle and the major organs of the body, the main source of individual variability in RMR is an individual's amount of organ and muscle mass. Thus, fat-free mass (FFM; the total mass of the body that is not fat, i.e., predominantly organs and muscle) explains 60–80% of the variation in RMR between individuals. This concept can be explained using the woodstove analogy; the larger the woodstove (or FFM), the larger the amount of heat production (or the larger the RMR). Since FFM is a heterogeneous mixture of all nonfat body components, the metabolic rate associated with each kilogram of

FFM is dependent on the quality of the FFM, in terms of hydration and relative contribution of the different organs that make up the FFM. For example, skeletal muscle constitutes approximately 43% of total mass in an adult, but contributes only 22–36% of the RMR, whereas the brain, which constitutes approximately only 2% of mass, contributes 20–24% of the RMR. In addition, the metabolic cost of each kilogram of FFM decreases with developmental progression, probably owing to developmental increases in the muscle mass to organ mass ratio within FFM. Thus, the relationship between RMR and FFM is not linear across all ages and is estimated to be 331.8 kJ/kg between the ages of 0 and 2.5 years, 151.2 kJ/kg in children aged 4–7 years, 88.2 kJ/kg during adolescence, and 151.2 kJ/kg in adulthood.

Although fat mass is generally thought to be metabolically inert, it significantly contributes to variations in RMR. This is likely explained, at least in part, by neurobiological effects (e.g., changes in sympathetic nervous system activity) resulting from variations in fat mass which affect the metabolism of other tissues. RMR is also influenced by fat mass, even though fat mass is generally thought to be metabolically inert. Fat mass contributes in the order of 42.0–54.6 kJ/kg to RMR. This difference is independent of the gender difference in FFM; in other words, if one studied a group of males and females of identical FFM and similar age, RMR would be higher in males than in females by around 210.0 kJ/day. This gender difference is consistent across the lifespan, and the source of the difference is not well understood (Table 3.1). More active people tend to have a higher RMR than inactive individuals. This difference may be explained in part by the residual effects of chronic exercise on metabolic rate. In other words, RMR appears to be elevated because of the long-lasting effects of the thermic effect of exercise. However, other factors are also involved, since the higher RMR in more active individuals persists long after the last bout of exercise has been completed. Collectively, FFM, fat mass, age, gender, and physical activity explain 80–90% of the variance in RMR. In addition, a portion of the unique variance in RMR across individuals has been ascribed to genetic factors, although the specific source of this genetic variation has not yet been identified. Other factors that have been shown to influence metabolic rate include thyroid hormones (higher levels increase

Table 3.1 Variation in total energy expenditure (TEE) as a function of resting metabolic rate (RMR) among various populations

Study group	Average TEE/RMR (range)
5-year-old children in Arizona, USA	1.37 (1.15–1.70)
Obese women in the UK	1.39 (1.20–1.77)
Elderly women in Vermont, USA	1.42 (1.25–1.82)
5-year-old children in Vermont, USA	1.44 (1.11–1.77)
Elderly men in Vermont, USA	1.50 (1.30–2.11)
Obese Pima Indians	1.56 (1.03–1.99)
Adolescents in the UK	1.56
Dutch adults	1.64
Obese women in New York, USA	1.68
Young men in Boston, USA	1.70 (1.38–2.32)
Obese women in New York, USA	1.73
Elderly men in Boston, USA	1.74
Young men in the UK	1.88 (1.44–2.57)
Young men in Boston, USA	1.98 (1.57–2.60)
Mount Everest climbers	2.0
Tour de France cyclists	5.3
Burns patients	1.3

Range of TEE/RMR is given in parentheses for studies in which the individual data were reported.

metabolic rate) and sympathetic nervous system activity.

Several prediction equations have been developed to estimate RMR from other simple measures. These equations are often useful for making estimates in clinical situations when measurement of RMR cannot be achieved, or for estimating energy needs for other individuals. The classic equations of Harris and Benedict are frequently used for this purpose. These equations were developed from limited measures performed in the early 1900s, and predict RMR from age, height, and weight, and may be of limited accuracy. More recent equations have been developed in larger groups of subjects and can predict RMR from body weight (Table 3.2). These new equations have been shown to be more accurate.

Thermic effect of feeding

The thermic effect of meal ingestion is primarily influenced by the quantity and macronutrient quality of the ingested calories. The thermic effect of food has also been termed meal-induced thermogenesis, or the specific dynamic action of food. The increase in metabolic rate that occurs after meal ingestion occurs over an extended period of at least 5 hours; the cumulative energy cost is equivalent to around 10% of the energy ingested. In other words, if one consumed a mixed meal of 2.1 MJ, the body would require 210.0 kJ to

Table 3.2 Simple equations for estimating resting metabolic rate (RMR) from body weight according to gender and age

Age (years)	RMR (kJ/day)	
	Equation for males	Equation for females
0–3	$(60.9 \times wt) - 54$	$(61.0 \times wt) - 51$
3–10	$(22.7 \times wt) + 495$	$(22.5 \times wt) + 499$
10–18	$(17.5 \times wt) + 651$	$(12.2 \times wt) + 746$
18–30	$(15.3 \times wt) + 679$	$(14.7 \times wt) + 496$
30–60	$(11.6 \times wt) + 879$	$(8.7 \times wt) + 829$
>60	$(13.5 \times wt) + 487$	$(10.5 \times wt) + 596$

wt, body weight (kg).

Table 3.3 Examples of metabolic equivalent (MET) values for various physical activities

Activity	MET
Basketball	8.0
Chopping wood	6.0
Cleaning house	2.0–4.0
Cycling for pleasure	8.0
Gardening	5.0
Kayaking	5.0
Mowing lawn (power mower)	4.5
Painting house	4.0–5.0
Playing musical instrument	2.0–4.0
Running slowly (8–11 km/h)	8.0–10.0
Running quickly (14–16 km/h)	16.0–18.0
Soccer	7.0–10.0
Strength training	6.0
Stretching	4.0
Tennis	6.0–8.0
Skiing	7.0–14.0
Swimming laps	6.0–12.0
Walking	3.0–5.0
Water skiing	6.0

digest, process, and metabolize the contents of the meal. The thermic effect of feeding is higher for protein and carbohydrate than for fat. This is because, for fat, the process of energy storage is very efficient, whereas, for carbohydrate and protein, additional energy is required for metabolic conversion to the appropriate storage form (i.e., excess glucose converted to glycogen for storage, and excess amino acids from protein converted to fat for storage). In addition to the obligatory energetic cost of processing and storage of nutrients, a more variable facultative thermogenic component has been described. This component is mainly pertinent to carbohydrates, which through increased insulin secretion produce a diphasic activation of the sympathoadrenal system. The initial phase is an insulin-mediated increase in sympathetic activity, which produces a β-adrenoceptor-mediated increase in energy expenditure. The second and later phase occurs when a counter-regulatory increase in plasma epinephrine is elicited by the falling blood glucose. This increase in epinephrine has a similar slight stimulatory effect on energy expenditure. As a result of the mediation by β-adrenoceptors the thermic effect of carbohydrate-rich meals can be slightly reduced by pharmacological β-adrenoceptor antagonists.

Energy expenditure related to physical activity

Physical activity energy expenditure encompasses all types of activity, including sports and leisure, work-related activities, general activities of daily living, and fidgeting. The metabolic rate of physical activity is determined by the amount or duration of activity (i.e., time), the type of physical activity (e.g., walking, running, typing), and the intensity at which the particular activity is performed. The metabolic cost of physical activities is frequently expressed as metabolic equivalents (METs), which represent multiples of RMR. Thus, by definition, sitting quietly after a 12 hour fast is equivalent to 1 MET. Table 3.3 provides MET values for other typical physical activities. The cumulative total daily energy cost of physical activity is highly variable both within and between individuals. Therefore, physical activity provides the greatest source of plasticity or flexibility in the energy expenditure system, and is the component through which large changes in energy expenditure can be achieved.

Total energy expenditure: measurement by doubly labeled water

The integrated sum of all components of energy expenditure is termed total energy expenditure. Until recently, there was no good way to measure total energy expenditure in humans living under their habitual conditions. Total energy expenditure can be measured over 24 hours or longer in a metabolic chamber, but this environment is artificial and is not representative of the normal daily pattern of physical activity. The DLW technique can be used to obtain an integrated measure of all components of daily energy expenditure over extended periods, typically 7–14 days, while subjects are living in their usual environment. The technique was first introduced in the 1950s as an isotopic technique for measuring the carbon dioxide production rate in small animals. Unfortunately, it was not possible to apply the technique to humans because the dose required was cost prohibitive given the relatively poor sensitivity of the required instrumentation at that time. It was not for another 20 years that the inventors of this technique described the feasibility of applying the technique to measure free-living energy expenditure in humans, and 10 years later this concept became a reality.

The DLW method requires a person to ingest small amounts of "heavy" water that is isotopically labeled with deuterium and oxygen-18 (^2H_2O and $H_2^{18}O$). These forms of water are naturally occurring, stable (nonradioactive) isotopes of water that differ from the most abundant form of water. In deuterium-labeled water, the hydrogen is replaced with deuterium, which is an identical form of water except that deuterium has an extra neutron in its nucleus compared with hydrogen, and is thus a heavier form of water; similarly, ^{18}O-labeled water contains oxygen with an additional two extra neutrons. Thus, these stable isotopes act as molecular tags so that water can be tracked in the body. After a loading dose, deuterium-labeled water is washed out of the body as a function of body water turnover; ^{18}O is also lost as a function of water turnover, but is lost via carbon dioxide production as well. Therefore, using a number of assumptions, the rate of carbon dioxide production and energy expenditure can be assessed based on the different rates of loss of these isotopes from the body.

The major advantages of the DLW method are that the methodology is truly noninvasive and nonobtrusive (subjects are entirely unaware that energy expenditure is being measured), and measurement is performed under free-living conditions over extended periods (7–14 days). Moreover, when used in combination with indirect calorimetry for assessment of resting metabolic rate, physical activity-related energy expenditure can be assessed by the difference (i.e., total energy expenditure minus resting metabolic rate, minus the thermic effect of meals = physical activity energy expenditure). The additional power of assessing total energy expenditure with the DLW method is that this approach can provide a measure of total energy intake in subjects who are in energy balance. This is because, by definition, in a state of

energy balance, total energy intake must be equivalent to total energy expenditure. This aspect of the technique has been used as a tool to validate energy intakes using other methods such as food records and dietary recall. For example, it has been known for some time that obese subjects report a lower than expected value for energy intake. At one time it was thought that this was due to low energy requirements in the obese due to low energy expenditure and reduced physical activity. However, using DLW, it has now been established that obese subjects systematically underreport their actual energy intake by 30–40% and actually have a normal energy expenditure, relative to their larger body size.

The major disadvantages of the technique are the periodic nonavailability and expense of the ^{18}O isotope (around €500–600 for a 70 kg adult), the need for and reliance on expensive equipment for analysis of samples, and that the technique is not well suited to large-scale epidemiological studies. Furthermore, although the technique can be used to obtain estimates of physical activity energy expenditure, it does not provide any information on physical activity patterns (i.e., type, duration, and intensity of physical activity periods during the day).

The DLW technique has been validated in humans in several laboratories around the world by comparison with indirect calorimetry in adults and infants. These studies generally show the technique to be accurate to within 5–10%, relative to data derived by indirect calorimetry for subjects living in metabolic chambers. The theoretical precision of the DLW technique is 3–5%. However, the experimental variability is ±12% under free-living conditions, owing to fluctuations in physical activity levels, and ±8% under more controlled sedentary living conditions. The good accuracy and reasonable precision of the technique therefore allow the DLW method to be used as a "gold standard" measure of free-living energy expenditure in humans against which other methods can be compared.

3.5 Energy requirements

How much energy do we need to sustain life and maintain our body energy stores? Why do some people require more energy and others less? In other words, what are the energy requirements of different types of people? Based on our earlier definition of energy balance, the energy needs or energy requirements of the body to maintain energy balance must be equal to total daily energy expenditure. Total daily energy expenditure is the sum of the individual components of energy expenditure as discussed previously, and represents the total energy requirements of an individual that are required to maintain energy balance. Until recently, there was no accurate way to measure total energy expenditure or energy needs of humans. The DLW technique has provided a truly noninvasive means to measure accurately total daily energy expenditure, and thus energy needs, in free-living humans. Before DLW, energy requirements were usually assessed by measurement or prediction of RMR, the largest component of energy requirements. However, since the relationship between RMR and total energy expenditure is highly variable because of differences in physical activity, the estimation of energy needs from knowledge of RMR is not that accurate and requires a crude estimate of physical activity level. Nevertheless, reasonable estimates can be made to estimate daily energy budgets for individuals (Table 3.4).

Following the validation of DLW in humans, this technique has been applied to many different populations. Total energy expenditure is often compared across groups or individuals using the ratio of one's total energy expenditure to RMR, or physical activity level (PAL). Thus, for example, if the total energy expenditure was 12.6 MJ/day and the RMR was 6.3 MJ/day, the PAL factor would be 2.0. This value indicates that total energy expenditure is twice the RMR. The PAL factor has been assessed in a variety of types of individual. A low PAL indicates a sedentary lifestyle, whereas a high PAL represents a highly active lifestyle. The highest recorded sustained PAL in humans was recorded in cyclists participating in the Tour de France road race. These elite athletes could sustain a daily energy expenditure that was up to five times their RMR over extended periods. Smaller animals, such as migrating birds, have a much higher ceiling for achieving higher rates of total energy expenditure, which can reach up to 20 times their RMR.

Factors such as body weight, FFM, and RMR account for 40–60% of the variation in total energy expenditure. Total energy expenditure is similar between lean and obese individuals after taking into account differences in FFM. Thus, fatness has small, but important, additional effects on total energy expenditure, partly through RMR, as discussed previously, but also by increasing the energetic cost of any physical activity.

With regard to age, some studies suggest that only a limited change in total energy expenditure (relative to RMR) occurs from childhood to adulthood, but that a decline occurs in the elderly. Recent data also suggest a gender-related difference in total energy expenditure, in addition to that previously described for RMR. In a meta-analysis that examined data from a variety of published studies, absolute total energy expenditure was significantly higher in males than in females by 3.1 MJ/day (10.2 ± 2.1 MJ/day in females, 13.3 ± 3.1 MJ/day in males), and nonresting energy expenditure remained higher in men by 1.1 MJ/day.

Table 3.4 Typical daily energy budgets for a sedentary and a physically active individual of identical occupation, body weight, and resting metabolic rate of 6.0 MJ/day (4.2 kJ/min)

Activity	Activity index	Minutes per day		MJ per day	
		Sedentary	Active	Sedentary	Active
Sleep	1.0	480	480	2.0	2.0
Daily needs	1.06	120	120	5.3	5.3
Occupational	1.5	480	480	3.0	3.0
Passive recreation	2.0	360	300	3.0	2.5
Exercise	12.0	0	60	0	3.0
Total		1440	1440	8.6	11.1
				PAL = 1.4	PAL = 1.8

Thus, the sedentary individual would need to perform 60 min of vigorous activity each day at an intensity of 12.0 to increase the physical activity level (PAL) from a sedentary 1.4 to an active and healthy 1.8.

Individuals who have sedentary occupations and do not participate frequently in leisure pursuits that require physical activity probably have a PAL factor in the region of 1.4. Those who have occupations requiring light activity and participate in light physical activities in leisure time probably have a PAL around 1.6 (this is a typical value for sedentary people living in an urban environment). Individuals who have physically active occupations and lifestyles probably have a PAL greater than 1.75. It has been suggested that the optimal PAL that protects against the development of obesity is around 1.8 or higher. Increasing one's physical activity index from 1.6 to 1.8 requires 30 min of daily vigorous activity, or 60 min of light activity (Table 3.4).

3.6 Energy balance in various conditions

Infancy and childhood

Changes in energy intake during infancy have been well characterized. During the first 12 months of life, energy intake falls from almost 525 kJ/kg per day in the first month of life to a nadir of 399 kJ/kg per day by the eighth month, then rises to 441 kJ/kg per day by the 12th month. However, total energy expenditure in the first year of life is relatively constant at around 252–294 kJ/kg per day. In infants, the large difference between total energy expenditure and energy intake is explained by a positive energy balance to account for growth. In the first 3 months of life it is estimated that the energy accretion due to growth is 701.4 kJ/day, or approximately 32% of energy intake, falling to 151.2 kJ/day, or 4% of energy intake, by 1 year of age. Individual growth rates and early infancy feeding behavior are at least two known factors that would cause variation in these figures.

There is now substantial evidence to suggest that existing recommendations may overestimate true energy needs, based on measurement of total energy expenditure in infants. In the first year of life, traditional values of energy requirements overestimate those derived from measurement of total energy expenditure and adjusted for growth by 11%. Between 1 and 3 years of age the discrepancy is more striking, where the traditional values for requirements are 20% higher than those derived from total energy expenditure and adjusted for growth. For example, in 3 year old children total energy expenditure by DLW aver-ages 5.1 MJ/day, while the currently recommended intake for these children is 6.2 MJ/day. Thus, newer estimates of the energy requirements of infants are needed based on assessment of total energy expenditure data.

Several laboratories have reported measurements of total energy expenditure in young, healthy, free-living children around the world. Despite marked differences in geographical locations, the data are similar, although environmental factors such as season and sociocultural influences on physical activity can influence total energy expenditure and thus energy requirements. In the average 5 year old child weighing 20 kg, total energy expenditure is approximately 5.5–5.9 MJ/day, which is significantly lower than the existing recommended daily allowance for energy in children of this age, by approximately 1.7–2.1 MJ/day. Thus, as with infants, newer estimates of energy needs in children are needed based on assessment of total energy expenditure data.

Aging

In the elderly, two different problems related to energy balance can be recognized. In one segment of the elderly population there is a decline in food intake that is associated with dynamic changes in body composition where there is a tendency to lose FFM, which leads to loss in functionality. In others there is a tendency to gain fat mass, which increases the risk for obesity, cardiovascular disease, and noninsulin-dependent diabetes. These two opposing patterns suggest that the ability to self-regulate whole body energy balance may diminish with aging. Thus, prescription of individual energy requirements may serve as a useful tool to prevent the age-related deterioration of body composition. Other special considerations in the elderly relate to meeting energy needs in special populations, such as those with Alzheimer's and Parkinson's disease, which frequently can lead to malnourished states and a diminishing of body weight. It was thought that these neurological conditions may lead to body weight loss because of an associated hypermetabolic condition in which metabolic rate may increase above normal, thus increasing energy needs. However, more recent studies have clearly shown that the wasting or loss of body weight often associated with these conditions is explained by a reduction in food intake, probably owing to a loss in functionality.

Energy requirements in physically active groups

The DLW technique has been used to assess energy requirements in highly physically active groups of people. The most extreme case is a study that assessed the energy requirements of cyclists performing in the 3 week long Tour de France bicycle race. The level of total energy expenditure recorded (PAL factor of 5.3, or approximately 35.7 MJ/day) was the highest recorded sustained level in humans. In another study involving young male soldiers training for jungle warfare, energy requirements were 19.9 MJ/day (PAL factor of 2.6). The total energy expenditure of four mountaineers climbing Mount Everest was 13.6 MJ/day (PAL 2.0–2.7), which was similar to energy expenditure during on-site preparation prior to climbing (14.7 MJ/day). Total energy expenditure in free-living collegiate swimmers was almost 16.8 MJ/day in men and 10.9 MJ/day in women. In elite female runners previously performed studies of energy intake suggested unusually low energy requirements. However, in a study in nine highly trained young women, free-living energy expenditure was 11.9 ± 1.3 MJ/day, compared with the reported energy intake of 9.2 ± 1.9 MJ/day. This study suggests that elite female runners underreport true levels of energy intake and confirms the absence of energy-saving metabolic adaptations in this population.

Regular participation in exercise is traditionally thought to elevate energy requirements through the additional direct cost of the activity, as well as through an increase in RMR. However, in some situations energy requirements are not necessarily altered by participation in regular physical activity. For example, in a study of an elderly group of healthy volunteers, there was no significant change in total energy expenditure in the last 2 weeks of an 8 week vigorous endurance training program. The failure to detect an increase in total energy expenditure occurred despite a 10% increase in RMR (6703.2 ± 898.8 to 7404.6 ± 714 kJ/day), as well as an additional 630 kJ/day associated with the exercise program. These increases in energy expenditure were counteracted by a significant reduction in the energy expenditure of physical activity during nonexercising time (2.4 ± 1.6 versus 1.4 ± 1.9 MJ/day). The lack of increase in total energy expenditure in this study is probably explained by a compensatory energy-conserving adaptation to this vigorous training program leading to a reduction in spontaneous physical activity and/or a reduction in voluntary physical activities, similar to that observed in several animal studies. Thus, it should not automatically be assumed that energy requirements are elevated by participation in activity programs, and the ultimate change in energy requirements may be dictated by the intensity of the training program and the net sum of change in the individual components of energy expenditure. An important area of research is to identify the optimal program of exercise intervention in terms of exercise mode, type, duration, and intensity that can have optimal effects on all components of energy balance.

Energy requirements in pregnancy and lactation

Pregnancy and lactation are two other examples in which energy metabolism is altered in order to achieve positive energy balance. The specific changes in energy requirements during pregnancy are unclear and the various factors affecting this change are complex. Traditional government guidelines suggest that energy requirements are raised by 1.3 MJ/day during pregnancy. This figure is based on theoretical calculations based on the energy accumulation associated with pregnancy. However, these figures do not include potential adaptations in either metabolic efficiency or PAL during pregnancy. In a study that performed measures in 12 women every 6 weeks during pregnancy the average increase in total energy expenditure was 1.1 MJ/day. The average energy cost of pregnancy (change in total energy expenditure plus change in energy storage) was 1.6 MJ/day. However, there was considerable variation among the 12 subjects for the increase in average total energy expenditure (264.6 kJ/day to 3.8 MJ/day) and the average energy cost of pregnancy (147 kJ/day to 5.2 MJ/day).

Metabolic adaptations during lactation have been examined in well-nourished women using the DLW technique. The energy cost of lactation was calculated to be 3.7 MJ/day. Just over half of this energy cost was achieved by an increase in energy intake, while the remainder was met by a decrease in physical activity energy expenditure (3.2 MJ + 873.6 kJ/day at 8 weeks of lactation compared with 3.9 + 1.1 MJ/day in the same women prior to pregnancy).

Energy requirements in disease and trauma

The DLW technique has been used in various studies to assess the energy requirements of hospitalized patients. Information on energy requirements during hospitalization for disease or trauma is important because:

- energy expenditure can be altered by the disease or injury
- physical activity is often impaired or reduced
- both underfeeding and overfeeding of critically ill patients can lead to metabolic complications; therefore, correct assessment of energy requirements during recovery is an important part of therapy.

The metabolic response during recovery from a burn injury includes an increase in RMR, although this is not necessarily a function of the extent of the burn. The widely used formulae to predict energy needs in burn patients are not based on measurement of energy expenditure and estimate that most patients require 2–2.5 times their estimated RMR. However, using the DLW technique, total energy expenditure was 6.7 + 2.9 MJ/day in 8 year old children recovering from burn injury, which was equivalent to only 1.2 times the nonfasting RMR. The lower than expected values for total energy expenditure in children recovering from burns suggest that RMR is not as elevated in burn patients as previously speculated, and that RMR is not a function of burn size or time after the injury, probably owing to improvements in wound care which reduce heat loss. In addition, energy requirements in patients recovering from burn injury are reduced because of the sedentary nature of their hospitalization.

In a study of patients with anorexia nervosa, total energy expenditure was not significantly different than controls (matched for age, gender, and height). However, physical activity-related energy expenditure was 1.3 MJ/day higher in anorexia nervosa patients, which was compromised by a 1.3 MJ/day lower RMR. Thus, energy requirements in anorexia nervosa patients are normal, despite alterations in the individual components of total energy expenditure. In infants with cystic fibrosis, total energy expenditure was elevated by 25% relative to weight-matched controls, although the underlying mechanism for this effect is unknown.

Developmental disabilities appear to be associated with alterations in energy balance and nutritional status at opposite ends of the spectrum. For example, cerebral palsy is associated with reduced fat mass and FFM, whereas half of patients with myelodysplasia are obese. It is unclear whether the abnormal body composition associated with these conditions is the end-result of inherent alterations in energy expenditure and/or food intake, or whether alterations in body composition are an inherent part of the etiology of the specific disability. In addition, it is unclear how early in life total energy expenditure may be altered and whether reduced energy expenditure is involved with the associated obese state. Nevertheless, prescription of appropriate energy requirements may be a useful tool in the improvement of nutritional status in developmental disabilities.

Total energy expenditure has been shown to be lower in adolescents with both cerebral palsy and myelodysplasia, partly owing to reduced RMR but primarily to reduced physical activity. Based on measurements of total energy expenditure, energy requirements of adolescents with cerebral palsy and myelodysplasia are not as high as previously speculated. In nonambulatory patients with cerebral palsy, energy requirements are estimated to be 1.2 times RMR, and in the normal range of 1.6–2.1 times RMR in ambulatory patients with cerebral palsy.

3.7 Obesity

Basic metabolic principles

Obesity is the most common form of a disruption in energy balance and now constitutes one of the major and most prevalent disorders of nutrition. Because of the strong relationship between obesity and health risks, obesity is now generally considered a disease by health professionals.

Although the body continuously consumes a mixed diet of carbohydrate, protein, and fat, and sometimes alcohol, the preferred store of energy is fat. There is a clearly defined hierarchy of energy stores that outlines a preferential storage of excess calories as fat. For alcohol, there is no storage capacity in the body. Thus, alcohol that is consumed is immediately oxidized for energy. For protein, there is a very limited storage capacity and, under most situations, protein metabolism is very well regulated. For carbohydrate there is only a very limited storage capacity, in the form of glycogen, which can be found in the liver and in muscle. Glycogen provides a very small and short-term energy store, which can easily be depleted after an overnight fast or after a bout of exercise. Most carbohydrate that is consumed is immediately used for energy. Contrary to popular belief, humans cannot convert excess carbohydrate intake to fat. Instead, when excess carbohydrates are consumed, the body adapts by preferentially increasing its use of carbohydrate as a fuel, thus, in effect, burning off any excessive carbohydrate consumption. Large excesses of carbohydrate may induce *de novo* lipogenesis, but normally this process is quantitatively minor. However, no such adaptive mechanism for fat exists. In other words, if excess fat is consumed, there is no mechanism by which the body can increase its use of fat as a fuel. Instead, when excess fat calories are consumed, the only option is to accumulate the excess fat as an energy store in the body. This process occurs at a very low metabolic cost and is therefore an extremely efficient process. To store excess carbohydrate as glycogen is much more metabolically expensive and therefore a less efficient option. There is another important reason why the body would prefer to store fat rather than glycogen. Glycogen can only be stored in a hydrated form that requires 3 g of water for each gram of glycogen, whereas fat does not require any such process. In other words, for each gram of glycogen that is stored, the body has to store an additional 3 g of water. Thus, for each 4 g of storage tissue, the body stores only 16.8 kJ, equivalent to just 4.2 kJ/g, compared with the benefit of fat which can be stored as 37.8 kJ/g.

Thus, a typical adult with 15 kg of fat carries 567.0 MJ of stored energy. If the adult did not eat and was inactive, he or she might require 8.4 MJ/day for survival, and the energy stores would be sufficient for almost 70 days. This length is about the limit of human survival without food. Given that glycogen stores require 4 g to store 4.2 kJ (3 g of water plus 1 g of glycogen = 16.8 kJ), we can calculate that to carry this much energy in the form of glycogen requires 135 kg of weight. It is no wonder therefore that the body's metabolism favors fat as the preferred energy store.

Definition of obesity

Obesity has traditionally been defined as an excess accumulation of body energy, in the form of fat or adipose tissue. Thus, obesity is a disease of positive energy balance, which arises as a result of dysregula-tion in the energy balance system – a failure of the regulatory systems to make appropriate adjustments between intake and expenditure. It is now becoming clear that the increased health risks of obesity may be conferred by the distribution of body fat. In addition, the influence of altered body fat and/or body fat distribution on health risk may vary across individuals. Thus, obesity is best defined by indices of body fat accumulation, body fat pattern, and alterations in health risk profile.

The body mass index (BMI) is now the most accepted and most widely used crude index of obesity. This index classifies weight relative to height squared. The BMI is therefore calculated as weight in kilograms divided by height squared in meters, and expressed in the units of kg/m^2. Obesity in adults is defined as a BMI above 30.0 kg/m^2, while the normal range for BMI in adults is 18.5–24.9 kg/m^2. A BMI in the range of 25–30 kg/m^2 is considered overweight. In children, it is more difficult to classify obesity by BMI because height varies with age during growth; thus, age-adjusted BMI percentiles must be used.

One of the major disadvantages of using the BMI to classify obesity is that this index does not distinguish between excess muscle weight and excess fat weight. Thus, although BMI is strongly related to body fatness, at any given BMI in a population, there may be large differences in the range of body fatness. A classic example of misclassification that may arise from the use of the BMI is a heavy football player or body-builder with a large muscle mass who may have a BMI above 30 kg/m^2 but is not obese; rather, this man has a high body weight for his height resulting from increased FFM.

Since the health risks of obesity are related to body fat distribution, and in particular to excess abdominal fat, other anthropometric indices of body shape are useful in the definition of obesity. Traditionally, the waist-to-hip ratio has been used as a marker of upper versus lower body-fat distribution. More recent studies suggest that waist circumference alone provides the best index of central body-fat pattern and increased risk of obesity-related conditions. The recommended location for the measurement of waist circumference is at the midpoint between the lowest point of the rib cage and the iliac crest. The risk of obesity-related diseases is increased above a waist circumference of 94 cm in men and above 80 cm in women.

Etiology of obesity: excess intake or decreased physical activity

Stated simply, obesity is the end-result of positive energy balance, or an increased energy intake relative to expenditure. It is often stated, or assumed, that obesity is simply the result of overeating or lack of physical activity. However, the etiology of obesity is not as simple as this, and many complex and interrelated factors are likely to contribute to the development of obesity; it is extremely unlikely that any single factor causes obesity. Many cultural, behavioral, and biological factors drive energy intake and energy expenditure, and contribute to the homeostatic regulation of body energy stores, as discussed earlier in the chapter. In addition, many of these factors are influenced by individual susceptibility, which may be driven by genetic, cultural, and hormonal factors. Obesity may develop very gradually over time, such that the actual energy imbalance is negligible and undetectable.

Although there are genetic influences on the various components of body-weight regulation, and a major portion of individual differences in body weight can be explained by genetic differences, it seems unlikely that the increased global prevalence of obesity has been driven by a dramatic change in the gene pool. It is more likely and more reasonable that acute changes in behavior and environment have contributed to the rapid increase in obesity, and genetic factors may be important in the differing individual susceptibilities to these changes. The most striking behavioral changes that have occurred have been an increased reliance on high-fat and energy-dense fast foods, with larger portion sizes, coupled with an ever-increasing sedentary lifestyle. The more sedentary lifestyle is due to an increased reliance on technology and labor-saving devices, which has reduced the need for physical activity for everyday activities. Examples of energy-saving devices are:

- increased use of automated transport rather than walking or cycling
- central heating and the use of automated equipment in the household, e.g., washing machines
- reduction in physical activity in the workplace due to computers, automated equipment, and electronic mail, which all reduce the requirement for physical activity at work

- increased use of television and computers for entertainment and leisure activities
- use of elevators and escalators rather than using stairs
- increased fear of crime, which has reduced the likelihood of playing outdoors
- poor urban planning, which does not provide adequate cycle lanes or even pavements in some communities.

Thus, the increasing prevalence, numerous health risks, and astounding economic costs of obesity clearly justify widespread efforts towards prevention.

The relationship between obesity and lifestyle factors reflects the principle of energy balance. Weight maintenance is the result of equivalent levels of energy intake and energy expenditure. Thus, a discrepancy between energy expenditure and energy intake depends on either food intake or energy expenditure, and it is becoming clear that physical activity provides the main source of plasticity in energy expenditure. In addition, lifestyle factors such as dietary and activity patterns are clearly susceptible to behavioral modification and are likely targets for obesity prevention programs. A second, yet related, reason that control of the obesity epidemic will depend on preventive action is that both the causes and health consequences of obesity begin early in life and track into adulthood. For example, both dietary and activity patterns responsible for the increasing prevalence of obesity are evident in childhood.

Role of physical activity and energy expenditure in the development of obesity

Although it is a popular belief that reduced levels of energy expenditure and physical activity lead to the development of obesity, this hypothesis remains controversial and has been difficult to prove. There are certainly good examples of an inverse relationship between physical activity and obesity (e.g., athletes are lean and nonobese individuals), as well as good examples of the positive relationship between obesity and physical inactivity (obese individuals tend to be less physically active). However, not all studies provide supporting evidence. For example, several studies suggest that increased television viewing (as a marker for inactivity) increases the risk of obesity, whereas others do not. Similar to the results for physical activity, some studies suggest that a low level of energy expenditure predicts the development of obesity, and others do not support this hypothesis.

Physical activity is hypothesized to protect people from the development of obesity through several channels. First, physical activity, by definition, results in an increase in energy expenditure owing to the cost of the activity itself, and is also hypothesized to increase RMR. These increases in energy expenditure are likely to decrease the likelihood of positive energy balance. However, the entire picture of energy balance must be considered, particularly the possibility that increases in one or more components of energy expenditure can result in a compensatory reduction in other components (i.e., resting energy expenditure and activity energy expenditure). Secondly, physical activity has beneficial effects on substrate metabolism, with an increased reliance on fat relative to carbohydrate for fuel utilization, and it has been hypothesized that highly active individuals can maintain energy balance on a high-fat diet.

Cross-sectional studies in children and adults have shown that energy expenditure, including physical activity energy expenditure, is similar in lean and obese subjects, especially after controlling for differences in body composition. Children of obese and lean parents have also been compared as a model of preobesity. Some studies show that children of obese parents had a reduced energy expenditure, including physical activity energy expenditure, whereas another study did not. A major limitation of the majority of studies that have examined the role of energy expenditure in the etiology of obesity is their cross-sectional design. Because growth of individual components of body composition is likely to be a continuous process, longitudinal studies are necessary to evaluate the rate of body fat change during the growing process. Again, some longitudinal studies support the idea that reduced energy expenditure is a risk factor for the development of obesity, whereas others do not. Finally, intervention studies have been conducted to determine whether the addition of physical activity can reduce obesity. These studies tend to support the positive role of physical activity in reducing body fat.

Several possibilities could account for such discrepant findings. First, the ambiguous findings in the literature may be explained by the possibility that differences in energy expenditure and physical activity and their impact on the development of obesity are different at the various stages of maturation. This hypothesis is supported by previous longitudinal studies in children, showing that a reduced energy expenditure is shown to be a risk factor for weight gain in the first 3 months of life, but not during the steady period of prepubertal growth. Secondly, there could be individual differences in the effect of altered energy expenditure on the regulation of energy balance. Thus, the effect of energy expenditure on the etiology of obesity could vary among different subgroups of the population (e.g., boys versus girls, different ethnic groups) and could also have a differential effect within individuals at different stages of development. It is conceivable that susceptible individuals fail to compensate for periodic fluctuations in energy expenditure. Third, explanations related to the methodology can also be offered because of the complexity of the nature of physical activity and its measurement. The success of controlled exercise interventions in improving body composition indicates an extremely promising area for the prevention of obesity. However, further studies are required to elucidate the specific effects of different types of exercise on the key features of body weight regulation.

3.8 Perspectives on the future

Much is known about how the body balances energy intake and expenditure. There are, however, areas that need further research. The technology to determine total energy expenditure with doubly labeled water has been standardized. Most of the data from using this method have been obtained in populations living in industrialized countries. More studies on infants, children, adolescents, adults, pregnant and lactating women, and the elderly living in developing countries are indicated. Doubly labeled water is an expensive method. There is a need to develop more cost-effective methods that can be used in field studies and to determine the energy cost of specific activities of people throughout the life cycle in developing countries. Obesity has recently been defined as a disease by the World Health Organization. The growing problem of obesity worldwide, and in children and in people who were previously food insecure and malnourished, needs to be addressed with better information about the behavioral and cultural factors that influence energy balance. This demands a more holistic, integrated approach to the study of obesity in the future.

Acknowledgment

This chapter has been revised and updated by Arne Astrup and Angelo Tremblay based on the original chapter by Michael I Goran and Arne Astrup.

Reference

Blundell JE, Rogers PJ, Hill AJ. Evaluating the satiating power of foods: implications for acceptance and consumption. In: Solms J, Booth DA, Pangbourne RM, Raunhardt O, eds. *Food Acceptance and Nutrition*. Academic Press, London, 1987: 205–219.

Further reading

Bray G, Bouchard. D, eds. *Handbook of Obesity*, 3rd edn. Informa Healthcare, New York, 2008.
DeFronzo RA, Ferrannini E, Keen H, Zimmet P. *International Textbook of Diabetes Mellitus*, 3rd edn. John Wiley & Sons, Chichester, 2004.

4
Nutrition and Metabolism of Proteins and Amino Acids

Naomi K Fukagawa and Yong-Ming Yu

Key messages

- Protein is the most abundant nitrogen-containing compound in the diet and the body. Proteins are formed when L-α-amino acids polymerize via peptide bond formation.
- Amino acids have similar central structures with different side-chains determining the multiple metabolic and physiological roles of free amino acids.
- Indispensable (essential) amino acids cannot be synthesized by humans from materials ordinarily available to cells at a speed commensurate with the demands of human growth and maintenance.
- The requirements for indispensable amino acids can be defined as "the lowest level of intake that achieves nitrogen balance or that balances the irreversible oxidative loss of the amino acid, without requiring major changes in normal protein turnover and where there is energy balance with a modest level of physical activity." For infants, children, and pregnant and lactating women, requirements would include protein deposited and secretion of milk proteins.
- "Conditionally" indispensable amino acids are those for which there are measurable limitations to the rate at which they can be synthesized because their synthesis requires another amino acid and because only a number of tissues are able to synthesize them, and probably only in limited amounts. The metabolic demands for these amino acids may rise above the biosynthetic capacity of the organism.
- Protein and amino acid requirements are determined by the processes of protein synthesis, and maintenance of cell and organ protein content, as well as the turnover rates of protein and amino acid metabolism, including synthesis, breakdown, inter-conversions, transformations, oxidation, and synthesis of other nitrogen-containing compounds and urea. These processes are influenced by genetics, phase of life cycle, physical activity, dietary intake levels, how energy needs are met, route of delivery of nutrients, disease, hormones, and immune system products.
- Protein and amino acid requirements can be determined by nitrogen excretion and balance, factorial estimations, and/or tracer techniques.
- Existing recommendations on requirements differ by various authorities because of a lack of data when some were formulated, different interpretations of data, and different criteria for judging adequate intakes.
- The United Nations plans to publish new recommendations for protein and amino acids in the near future. Those made by the Institute of Medicine, US National Academies of Science, in 2002 are cited in this chapter.
- Apparent protein digestibility, measured in the past as the difference between nitrogen intake and fecal nitrogen output, underestimates "true" digestibility because fecal nitrogen is derived, in part, from endogenous nitrogen sources.
- Tracer techniques have shown that "true" digestibility of most dietary proteins is high. The quality of food protein can be assessed as the protein digestibility-corrected amino acid score.
- Animal protein foods generally have higher concentrations of indispensable amino acids than plant foods. Lysine is often the most limiting amino acid, followed by sulfur amino acids (methionine and cystine) and tryptophan and threonine.

4.1 Introduction

Protein is the most abundant nitrogen-containing compound in the diet and in the body. It is one of the five classes of complex biomolecules present in cells and tissues, the others being DNA, RNA, polysaccharides, and lipids. The polymerization of L-α-amino acids through synthesis of peptide bonds contributes to the formation and structural framework of proteins. These may contain two or more polypeptide chains forming multimeric proteins, with the individual chains being termed subunits. Proteins are the workhorses in cells and organs and their building blocks are the amino acids, which are joined together according to a sequence directed by the base sequence of the DNA (the genome), and so they serve as the currency of protein nutrition and metabolism. The Human Genome Project completed in 2000 revealed that the human genome consists of only 30 000 genes, whereas there may be hundreds of thousands of proteins that are responsible for giving a human its particular characteristics and uniqueness. A new field of nutrition research has now opened up and is referred to as "nutrigenomics," which is the study of how nutrition and genomics interact to influence health. Proteins and amino acids fulfill numerous functions, many of which are summarized in Table 4.1. Some

amino acids, such as glutamine (Tables 4.2 and 4.3), play multiple roles. It is not surprising, therefore, that inappropriate intakes of proteins and/or of specific amino acids can have important consequences for tissue and organ function, and the maintenance of health and the well-being of the individual.

This chapter begins with a short historical perspective and then moves in Sections 4.3 and 4.4 to discuss the structure, chemistry, and classification of amino acids. Section 4.5 is concerned with the biology of protein and amino acid requirements, with Sections 4.6 and 4.7 describing how the requirements are established and how they may be met, respectively. Finally, Section 4.8 examines how factors other than dietary protein can influence the requirements for proteins and amino acids.

4.2 A historical perspective

The early history of protein metabolism and nutrition is closely tied to the discovery of nitrogen and its distribution in nature. The reason for this is that proteins, on average, contain about 16% nitrogen by weight (to convert nitrogen to protein it is necessary to multiply by 6.25). Daniel Rutherford, in Edinburgh, can be regarded as the discoverer of nitrogen, which he called "phlogisticated air" in his Doctorate in

Table 4.1 Some functions of amino acid and proteins

Function	Example
Amino acids	
Substrates for protein synthesis	Those for which there is a codon
Regulators of protein turnover	Leucine; cysteine; arginine; glutamine
Regulators of enzyme activity (allosteric)	Glutamate and NAG synthase
Phenylalanine and PAH activation	
Precursor of signal transducer	Arginine and nitric oxide
Methylation reactions	Methionine
Neurotransmitter	Tryptophan (serotonin); glutamine
Ion fluxes	Taurine; glutamate
Precursor of "physiologic" molecules	Arg (creatinine); Glu-(NH_2) purines
	Histidine/β-alanine (carnosine)
	Cysteine/glycine/glutamate (glutathione)
Transport of nitrogen	Alanine; glu-(NH_2)
Regulator of gene transcription	Amino acid depletion and asparagine synthase gene activation
Regulator of mRNA translation	Leucine: alters activity of initiation factor 4E-BP and P70 (6SK) via mTOR signaling pathway
Proteins	
Enzymatic catalysis	Branched chain ketoacid dehydrogenase
Transport	B_{12} binding proteins; ceruloplasmin; apolipoproteins; albumin
Messengers/signals	Insulin; growth hormone; IGF-1
Movement	Kinesin; actin; myosin
Structure	Collagens; elastin; actin
Storage/sequestration	Ferritin; metallothionein
Immunity	Antibodies; cytokine, chemokines
Growth; differentiation; gene expression	Peptide growth factors; transcription factors

IGF-1, insulin-like growth factor-1; NAG, *N*-acetyl glutamate; PAH, phenylalanine hydroxylase; glu-(NH_2), glutamine.

Table 4.2 Multiple functions of an amino acid; glutamine as an example

Substrate of protein synthesis (codons: CAA, CAG)
Anabolic/trophic substance for muscle; intestine ("competence factor")
Controls acid–base balance (renal ammoniagenesis)
Substrate for hepatic ureagenesis
Substrate for hepatic/renal gluconeogenesis
Fuel for intestinal enterocytes
Fuel and nucleic acid precursor and important for generation of cytotoxic products in immunocompetent cells
Ammonia scavenger
Substrate for citrulline and arginine synthesis
Nitrogen donor (nucleotides, amino sugars, coenzymes)
Nitrogen transport (1/3 circulating N) (muscle; lung)
Precursor of GABA (via glutamate)
Shuttle for glutamate (CNS)
Preferential substrate for GSH production?
Osmotic signaling mechanism in regulation of protein synthesis?
Stimulates glycogen synthesis
L-Arginine NO metabolism
Taste factor (umami)

CNS, central nervous system; GABA, γ-aminobutyric acid; GSH, growth-stimulating hormone; NO, nitric oxide.

Table 4.3 Biochemical roles of amino acids not directly related to protein metabolism

Amino acid	Biochemical function
Integration of carbon and nitrogen metabolism	
Leucine, isoleucine, valine	Ubiquitous nitrogen donors and metabolic fuel
	Ubiquitous nitrogen donor, extracellular
Glutamate	Transporter of four-carbon units
Glutamine	See Table 4.2
Alanine	Ubiquitous nitrogen donor, extracellular
	Transporter of three-carbon units
Aspartate	Ubiquitous nitrogen donor
	Transfer form of nitrogen from cytoplasmic amino acids to urea
Single carbon metabolism	
Methionine	Donor and acceptor of methyl groups
	Important role in single-carbon metabolism
Glycine	Donor of methylene groups
Serine	Donor of hydroxymethylene groups
Neurotransmitter synthesis	
Histidine	Precursor for histamine synthesis
Phenylalanine and tyrosine	Precursors for tyramine, dopamine, epinephrine, and norepinephrine synthesis
Tryptophan	Precursor for serotonin synthesis
Glutamate	Precursor for γ-aminobutyric acid synthesis
Miscellaneous	
Arginine	Immediate precursor for urea
	Precursor for nitric oxide synthesis
Cysteine	Potential intracellular thiol buffer
	Precursor for glutathione and taurine synthesis
Glycine	Nitrogen donor for heme synthesis
Histidine/β-alanine	Precursors for carnosine synthesis

Medicine thesis in 1792. The first amino acid to be discovered was cystine, which was extracted from a urinary calculus by Wallaston in England in 1810. It was not until 1935 that threonine, the last of the so-called nutritionally indispensable (essential) amino acids for mammals, including man, was discovered by WC Rose at the University of Illinois. Finally, the term "protein" was invented by the Swedish chemist Jons Jakob Berzelius (1779–1848) and this was later accepted and promoted by the influential Dutch chemist Gerhardus Mulder in 1838.

The nutritional importance of nitrogenous components in the diet was first recognized in 1816 by Magendie. He described experiments in dogs that received only sugar and olive oil until they died within a few weeks. It was concluded that a nitrogen source was an essential component of the diet. Magendie's insightful views on nitrogen metabolism and nutrition were followed by studies carried out by the French scientific school, including Justus von Leibig, who investigated the chemical basis of protein metabolism and discovered that urea was an end-product of protein breakdown in the body. Later, Leibig founded a school of biochemical studies in Gissen and later in Munich, Germany, from which Carl Voit emerged as a distinguished scientist and laid the foundations of modern studies of body nitrogen balance. He, in turn, trained many famous scientific celebrities, including Max Rubner, from Germany, who studied the specific dynamic action of proteins and their effects on energy metabolism, and Wilbur Atwater and Graham Lusk, from the USA, who studied food composition, protein requirements, and energy metabolism. Through their work, and that of others, theories of protein metabolism were proposed and challenged, leading to the more or less contemporary view which was established through the seminal work of Rudolf Schoenheimer, conducted at Columbia University, New York, in the mid-1930s and early 1940s. He applied the new tracer tool of stable isotope-enriched compounds, especially amino acids, in the study of dynamic aspects of protein turnover and amino acid metabolism. Stable isotopes (such as ^{13}C, ^{18}O, and ^{15}N) are naturally present in our environment, including the foods we eat, and they are safe to use in human metabolic studies. Using this approach, Schoenheimer established the fundamental biological principle of a continued tissue and organ protein loss and renewal, which forms the basis for the dietary need for protein or supply of amino acids and a utilizable form of nitrogen.

4.3 Structure and chemistry of amino acids

With the exception of proline, the amino acids that make up peptides and proteins have the same central structure (Figure 4.1; the A in this figure and

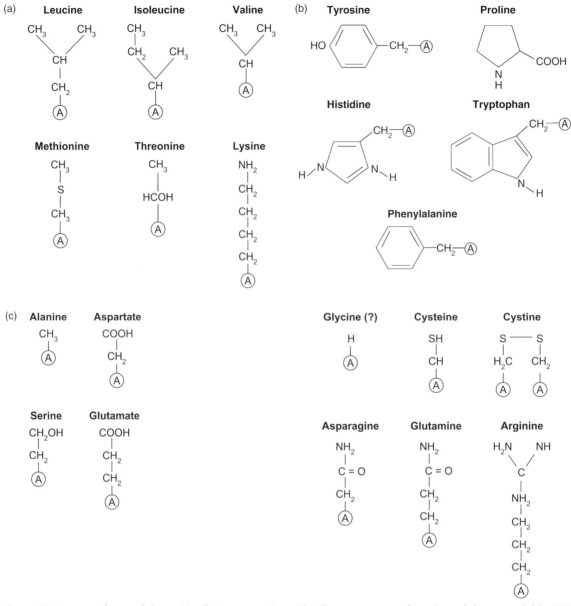

Figure 4.1 Structures of some of the nutritionally important amino acids. All are components of proteins and they are coded by DNA. (a) Nutritionally indispensable (essential) includes also tryptophan and histidine; (b) nutritionally conditionally indispensable; (c) nutritionally dispensable.

subsequent figures represent the $-\overset{\displaystyle H}{\underset{\displaystyle NH_2}{C}}-$ COOH moiety).

The carboxylic acid and amino nitrogen groups are the components of the peptide bond that links the amino acids within the linear peptide structure, while the side-chains distinguish the physical and chemical properties of each chemical class of amino acid. In addition, some features of the amino acid side-chains are critical to the metabolic and physiological roles of free, as opposed to protein-bound, amino acids (Table 4.3; Figures 4.1 and 4.2). These roles are reflections of

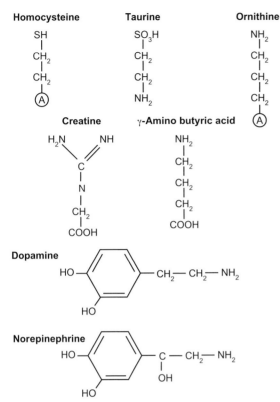

Figure 4.2 Physiologically important amino acid metabolites. Both the metabolic relationship between alanine and glutamic acid and their transamination partners, the keto acids pyruvate and α-ketoglutarate, and the similarity between the catabolic oxidation pathway of the branched-chain amino acids and the β-oxidation pathway of saturated fatty acids are shown.

either their specific chemical properties or specific metabolic interrelationships. Examples of the former are the facility of methionine to donate a methyl group in one-carbon metabolism, the propensity for the amide group of glutamine to serve as a nitrogen source for pyrimidine synthesis, or the sulfhydryl group of cysteine forming disulfide bonds for cross-linking. The former metabolic relationship allows alanine and glutamate (and glutamine) to provide a link between carbohydrate and protein metabolism; the latter enables the branched amino acids to function when required, as a "universal" fuel throughout the body.

Some of these amino acid and nitrogen compounds are derivatives of other amino acids:

• creatine is formed from glycine, arginine, and methionine and serves in intracellular energy transduction

• dopamine is formed from tyrosine and fulfills a neurotransmitter function

• ornithine can be formed from glutamate and serves as both an intermediate in the urea cycle and a precursor of the polyamines spermine and spermidine, which are used in DNA packaging.

Finally, other amino acids (Figure 4.3) appear in proteins via a post-translational modification of a specific amino acid residue in the polypeptide chain that is being formed during protein synthesis.

In addition to serving the function as precursors for protein synthesis, amino acids also serve as signaling molecules modulating the process of protein synthesis. The translation of mRNA into protein in skeletal muscle is initiated from (1) the binding of met-tRNA to the 40S ribosomal subunit to form the 43S preinitiation complex; (2) the subsequent binding of this complex to mRNA and its localization to the AUG start codon; and (3) the release of the initiation factors from the 40S ribosomal complex to allow the formation of the 80S ribosomal complex via the joining of the 60S ribosomal subunit. Then the 80S ribosomal complex proceeds to the elongation stage of translation. The formation of the 43S preinitiation complex is mediated by a heterotrimeric complex of eIF–4F proteins. The signaling pathway regulating mRNA translation involves the protein kinase termed the mammalian target of rapamycin (mTOR). mTOR regulates the formation of the eIF–4F complex via a series of phosphorylation–dephosphorylation processes of the downstream targets. The mTOR signaling pathway is traditionally considered to be solely involved in mediating the action of hormones. Recent studies revealed that the branched-chain amino acids, especially leucine, serve a unique role in regulating mRNA translation via the same mTOR-signaling pathway. Increased availability of leucine activates the mTOR and its downstream targets. However, inhibition of the mTOR pathway by rapamycine partially inhibits the stimulatory effect of leucine on protein synthesis, indicating the involvement of an mTOR-independent signaling pathway by leucine in the regulation of protein synthesis. The detailed mechanisms involved in these regulations, especially those of the mTOR-independent pathways, remain an active field of research.

Furthermore, individual amino acids play multiple regulatory roles in health and diseased conditions.

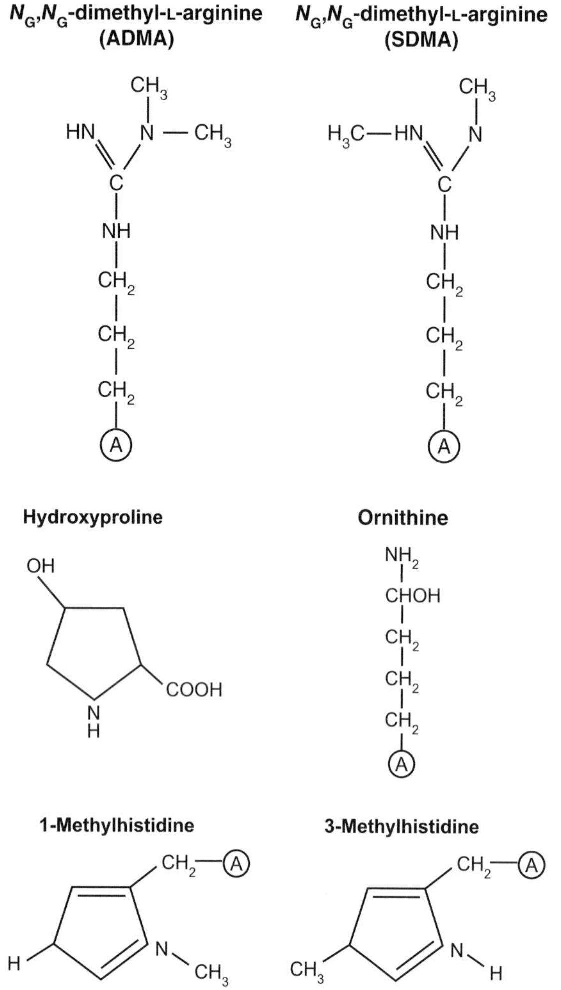

N_G,N_G-dimethyl-L-arginine (ADMA)

N_G,N_G-dimethyl-L-arginine (SDMA)

Hydroxyproline

Ornithine

1-Methylhistidine

3-Methylhistidine

Figure 4.3 Some amino acids that arise via a post-translational modification of a polypeptide-bound amino acid. These amino acids are not coded by DNA but are important determinants of the structural and functional characteristics of proteins. Shown are (1) the formation of hydroxyproline, from proline, involved in the maturation of the different types of collagens in cells; (2) the methylation of a specific histidine in the muscle protein actin (it could be that this modification gives this protein its ability to function effectively in the contractile activities of the skeletal muscles that help us to move about); and (3) the methylation of arginine to form asymmetric and symmetric dimethylarginine, which serve as an endogenous nitric oxide synthase inhibitor and play important roles in modulating nitric oxide production and organ blood flow in health and diseased conditions.

For example, glycine is an important anti-inflammatory, immunomodulatory, and cytoprotective agent through the glycine receptor on the cell surface. The role of cysteine in regulating glutathione synthesis and its role in protection against oxidative damage has been well established. The physiology of the arginine–nitric oxide pathway has also been an active area of investigation. In general, these nonprotein functions of amino acids serve important functions in the maintenance of (1) immune and other protective functions; (2) digestive function; and (3) cognitive and neuromuscular function. It is also worth noting that these functions are primarily exerted by nutritionally dispensable amino acids. Hence, the *de novo* synthesis pathways and/or the amount of exogenous supply of these amino acids or their precursors are important in modulating the physiological and pathophysiological conditions.

4.4 Classification of amino acids

"Indispensability" as a basis of classification

For most of the past 65 years amino acids have been divided into two general, nutritional categories: indispensable (essential) and dispensable (nonessential). This categorization provided a convenient and generally useful way of viewing amino acid nutrition at the time. The original definition of an indispensable amino acid was:

> One which cannot be synthesized by the animal organism out of materials *ordinarily available* to the cells *at a speed* commensurate with the demands for *normal growth*.

There are three important phrases in this definition: *ordinarily available*, *at a speed* and for *normal growth*.

The phrase "ordinarily available" is an important qualifier within this definition because a number of nutritionally essential amino acids, for example the branched-chain amino acids, phenylalanine and methionine, can be synthesized by transamination of their analogous α-keto acids. However, these keto acids are not normally part of the diet and so are not "ordinarily available to the cells." They may be used in special situations such as in nitrogen-accumulating diseases, including renal failure, where they may assist in maintaining a better status of body nitrogen metabolism.

The phrase "at a speed" is equally important because there are circumstances in which the rate of synthesis of an amino acid may be constrained, such as by the availability of appropriate quantities of "nonessential" nitrogen. Further, the rate of synthesis becomes of particular importance when considering a group of amino acids, exemplified by arginine, cysteine, proline, and probably glycine. These amino acids are frequently described as being conditionally indispensable. That is, their indispensability is dependent upon the physiological or pathophysiological condition of the individual.

Finally, the phrase "normal growth" is critical in two respects. First, it serves to emphasize that the definitions were originally constructed in the context of growth. For example, for the growing rat arginine is an indispensable amino acid, but the adult rat does not require the presence of arginine in the diet and so it becomes a dispensable amino acid at that later stage of the life cycle. Of course, if the capacity to synthesize arginine is compromised by removing a significant part of the intestine which produces citrulline, a precursor of arginine, then the adult rat once again requires arginine as part of an adequate diet. Second, by confining the definition to growth, this fails to consider the importance of amino acids to pathways of disposal other than protein deposition. This aspect of amino acid utilization will be considered below.

Chemical and metabolic characteristics as bases of classification

It is also possible to classify amino acids according to their chemical and metabolic characteristics rather than on the basis of their need for growth. Examination of the amino acids that are generally considered to be nutritionally indispensable for humans and most other mammals indicates that each has a specific structural feature, the synthesis of which cannot be accomplished owing to the absence of the necessary mammalian enzyme(s) (Table 4.4). Indeed, in obliga-

tory carnivores, such as cats, the further loss of some critical enzyme(s) renders these animals particularly dependent on dietary sources of specific amino acids, such as arginine. The lack of arginine in a single meal when given to a cat can be fatal. However, even within this view, the important term is "*de novo* synthesis" because some amino acids can be synthesized from precursors that are structurally very similar. For example, methionine can be synthesized both by transamination of its keto acid analogue and by remethylation of homocysteine. According to this metabolic assessment of amino acids, threonine and lysine are the only amino acids that cannot be formed via transamination or via conversion from another carbon precursor. In this narrower metabolic view, they are truly indispensable amino acids. A contemporary nutritional classification of amino acids in human nutrition is given in Table 4.5.

Strictly speaking, a truly dispensable amino acid is one that can be synthesized *de novo* from a nonamino acid source of nitrogen (e.g., ammonium ion) and a carbon source (e.g., glucose). Accordingly, and from a knowledge of biochemical pathways, the only true metabolically indispensable amino acid is glutamic acid, and possibly also glycine. This is because they can be synthesized from glucose and ammonium ions, in the case of glutamate, and from carbon dioxide and ammonium ions, in the case of glycine. However, the *in vivo* conditions may differ in both qualitative and quantitative terms from studies in test-tubes or in isolated cells in culture; amino acid metabolism *in vivo* is inherently more complex than is immediately evident from a simple consideration of biochemical pathways alone.

Table 4.4 Structural features that render amino acids indispensable components of the diet of mammals

Amino acid	Structural feature
Leucine, isoleucine, valine	Branched aliphatic side-chain
Lysine	Primary amine
Threonine	Secondary alcohol
Methionine	Secondary thiol
Tryptophan	Indole ring
Phenylalanine	Aromatic ring
Histidine	Imidazole ring

Table 4.5 The dietary amino acids of nutritional significance in humans

Indispensable	Conditionally indispensable	Dispensable
Valine	Glycine	Glutamic acid (?)
Isoleucine	Arginine	Alanine
Leucine	Glutamine	Serine
Lysine	Proline	Aspartic acid
Methionine	Cystine	Asparagine
Phenylalanine	Tyrosine	
Threonine	(Taurine)[a]	
Tryptophan	(Ornithine)[a]	
Histidine	(Citrulline)[a]	

[a] Nonproteinogenic amino acids, which have nutritional value in special cases.

Sources of nonspecific nitrogen for humans

In earlier texts it would have been stated that, given a sufficient intake of the indispensable amino acids, all that is then additionally needed to support body protein and nitrogen metabolism would be a source of "nonspecific" nitrogen (NSN) and that this could be in the form of a simple nitrogen-containing mixture, such as urea and diammonium citrate. However, this is no longer a sufficient description of what is actually required to sustain an adequate state of protein nutriture in the human. This can be illustrated by considering the nitrogen cycle, on which all life ultimately depends (Figure 4.4). From this it can be seen that some organisms are capable of fixing atmospheric nitrogen into ammonia, and plants are able to use either the ammonia or soluble nitrates (which are reduced to ammonia) produced by nitrifying bacteria. However, vertebrates, including humans, must obtain dietary nitrogen in the form of amino acids or other organic compounds, possibly as urea and purine and pyrimidines. Glutamate and glutamine provide a critical entry of the ammonia from the nitrogen cycle into other amino acids. It is, therefore, important to examine briefly the way in which the human body may obtain this NSN so as to maintain the nitrogen economy of the individual.

Ammonia can be introduced into amino acids by ubiquitous glutamate ammonia ligase (glutamine synthetase) that catalyzes the following reaction:

$$\text{Glutamate} + \text{NH}_4^+ + \text{ATP} \rightarrow \text{Glutamine} + \text{ADP} + \text{P}_i + \text{H}^+ \tag{4.1}$$

and (2) via the glutamate dehydrogenase reaction:

$$\alpha\text{-Ketoglutarate} + \text{NH}_4^+ + \text{NADPH} \rightleftharpoons \text{L-Glutamate} + \text{NADP} + \text{H}_2\text{O} \tag{4.2}$$

However, because K_m for NH_4^+ in this reaction is high (>1 mM), this reaction is thought to make only a modest contribution to net ammonia assimilation in the mammal.

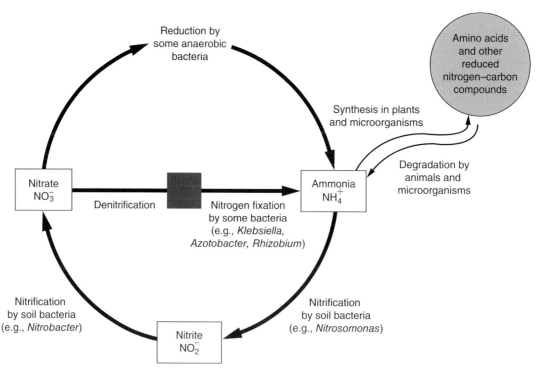

Figure 4.4 The nitrogen cycle. The most abundant form of nitrogen is present in air, which is four-fifths molecular nitrogen (N_2). The total amount of nitrogen that is fixed in the biosphere exceeds 10^{11} kg annually. Reproduced from Lehninger AL, Nelson DL, Cox MM. *Principles of Biochemistry*, 2nd edn. New York: Worth, 1993.

In bacteria and plant chloroplasts, glutamate is produced by the action of glutamate synthase, according to the reaction:

$$\alpha\text{-Ketoglutarate} + \text{glutamine} + \text{NADPH} + \text{H}^+$$
$$\rightarrow 2 \text{ Glutamate} + \text{NADP} \qquad (4.3)$$

The sum of the glutamate synthase (eqn 4.3) and glutamine synthetase (eqn 4.1) reactions is, therefore:

$$\alpha\text{-Ketoglutarate} + \text{NH}^+_4 + \text{NADPH} + \text{ATP}$$
$$\rightarrow \text{Glutamate} + \text{NADP} + \text{ADP} + \text{P}_i \qquad (4.4)$$

Hence, the two reactions combined (eqn 4.4) give a net synthesis of one molecule of glutamate. However, because glutamate synthetase is not present in animal tissues, a net incorporation of ammonia nitrogen via this nitrogen cycle arises primarily from glutamate rather than from glutamine. A net accumulation of glutamine would be achieved via the glutamine synthetase reaction that uses ammonia, which would be derived from various sources including glutamate or other amino acids or via hydrolysis of urea by the microflora on the intestinal lumen.

A net incorporation of ammonia into glycine might also be achieved via the glycine synthase (glycine cleavage) reaction, as follows:

$$\text{CO}_2 + \text{NH}^+_4\text{H}^+ + \text{NAD} + N_5,N_{10}\text{-}$$
$$\text{Methylenetetrahydrofolate}$$
$$\rightleftharpoons \text{Glycine} + \text{NAD}^+ + \text{Tetrahydrofolate} \qquad (4.5)$$

The glycine could then be incorporated into proteins and into such compounds as glutathione, creatine, and the porphyrins, as well as being converted to serine. The nitrogen of serine would then either be available for cysteine (and taurine) synthesis or be released as ammonia via the serine dehydratase reaction. However, the glycine cleavage reaction appears to be more important in glycine catabolism than for its synthesis. Therefore, the glycine–serine pathway of ammonia incorporation into the amino acid economy of the organism would appear to have only a limited effect on a net nitrogen input into the amino acid economy of the body. Serine can be formed from glucose via 3-phosphoglycerate, which comes from carbohydrate metabolism, and its nitrogen obtained from glutamic acid synthesis via transamination with 2-ketoglutarate.

This suggests, therefore, the possibility that glutamate is a key amino acid in making net amino nitrogen available to the mammalian organism; this glutamate would be derived ultimately from plant protein. In this sense, glutamate or its lower homologue, aspartic acid, which could supply the α-amino nitrogen for glutamate, or its derivative, glutamine, would be required as a source of α-amino nitrogen. While additional research is necessary to determine whether glutamate, or one of these metabolically related amino acids, would be the most efficient source of α-amino nitrogen, these considerations potentially offer a new perspective on the NSN component of the total protein requirement. In 1965, a United Nations expert group stated:

> The proportion of nonessential amino acid nitrogen, and hence the E/T [total essential or indispensable amino acids to total nitrogen] ratio of the diet, has an obvious influence on essential amino acid requirements … . To make the best use of the available food supplies there is an obvious need to determine the minimum E/T ratios for different physiological states … . Finally, the question arises whether there is an optimal pattern of nonessential amino acids.

This statement can just as well be repeated today, but clearly recent studies are beginning to provide deeper metabolic insights into the nature of the NSN needs of the human body.

"Conditional" indispensability

A contemporary nutritional classification of amino acids in human nutrition is given in Table 4.5 and some points should be made here about the "conditionally" indispensable amino acids, a term that is used to indicate that there are measurable limitations to the rate at which they can be synthesized. There are several important determinants. First, their synthesis requires the provision of another amino acid, either as the carbon donor (e.g., citrulline in the case of arginine synthesis or serine in the case of glycine synthesis) or as a donor of an accessory group (e.g., the sulfur group of methionine for cysteine synthesis). The ability of the organism to synthesize a conditionally essential amino acid is, therefore, set by the availability of its amino acid precursor. Second, some of these amino acids are synthesized in only a limited number of tissues. The best example of this is the crucial dependence of the synthesis of proline and arginine on intestinal metabolism. Third, most evidence suggests that, even in the presence of abundant quantities of the appropriate precursors, the quantities of conditionally essential amino acids that can be synthesized may be quite limited. Thus, there are circumstances, for example in immaturity and during stress, under which the metabolic demands for the amino acids rise to values that are beyond the biosynthetic capacity of the organism. This appears to be the case with regard to the proline and arginine nutrition of severely burned individuals, and cysteine and perhaps glycine in the nutrition of prematurely delivered infants.

4.5 Biology of protein and amino acid requirements

Body protein mass

A major and fundamental quantitative function of the dietary α-amino acid nitrogen and of the indispensable amino acids is to furnish substrate required for the support of organ protein synthesis and the maintenance of cell and organ protein content. Therefore, in the first instance the body protein mass is a factor that will influence the total daily requirement for protein. Adult individuals of differing size but who are otherwise similar in age, body composition, gender, and physiological state would be expected to require proportionately differing amounts of nitrogen and indispensable amino acids. Changes in the distribution and amount of body protein that occur during growth and development and later on during aging may be considered, therefore, as an initial approach for understanding the metabolic basis of the dietary protein and amino acid needs. (For more detailed considerations of body composition please refer to Chapter 2.)

Direct measures of total body protein cannot yet be made in living subjects, although there are various indirect measures from which it is possible to obtain a picture of the body nitrogen (protein) content at various stages of life. From these approaches it is clear that body nitrogen increases rapidly from birth during childhood and early maturity, reaching a maximum by about the third decade. Thereafter, body nitrogen decreases gradually during the later years, with the decline occurring more rapidly in men than in women. A major contributor to this age-related erosion of body nitrogen is the skeletal musculature. Strength training during later life can attenuate or partially reverse this decline in the amount of protein in skeletal muscles and improve overall function.

The protein requirement of adults is usually considered to be the continuing dietary intake that is just sufficient to achieve a "maintenance" of body nitrogen, often measured only over relatively short experimental periods. For infants and growing children and pregnant women an additional requirement is needed for protein deposition in tissues. However, this concept is oversimplified since the chemical composition of the body is in a dynamic state and changes occur in the nitrogen content of individual tissues and organs in response to factors such as diet, hormonal balance, activity patterns, and disease. Thus, proteins are being continually synthesized and degraded in an overall process referred to as turnover. The rate of turnover and the balance of synthesis and degradation of proteins, in addition to the mass of protein, are also important determinants of the requirements for nitrogen and amino acids, and these aspects will be discussed in the following section.

Turnover of proteins and amino acid metabolism

Protein synthesis, degradation, and turnover

The principal metabolic systems responsible for the maintenance of body protein and amino acid homeostasis are shown in Figure 4.5. They are:

- protein synthesis
- protein breakdown or degradation
- amino acid interconversions, transformation, and eventually oxidation, with elimination of carbon dioxide and urea production
- amino acid synthesis, in the case of the nutritionally dispensable or conditionally indispensable amino acids.

Dietary and nutritional factors determine, in part, the dynamic status of these systems; such factors include the dietary intake levels relative to the host's protein and amino acid requirements, the form and route of delivery of nutrients, i.e., parenteral (venous) and enteral (oral) nutritional support, and timing of intake during the day, especially in relation to the intake of the major energy-yielding substrates, which are the carbohydrates and fats in foods. Other factors, including hormones and immune system products, also regulate these systems. This will be a topic for discussion in the following volume. Changes in the

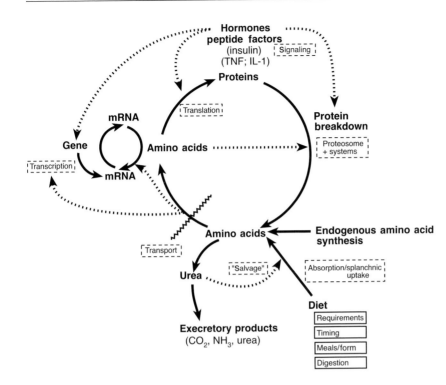

Figure 4.5 The major systems in amino acid uptake, utilization, and catabolism, with an indication of the processes involved and some factors that can affect them. TNF, tumor necrosis factor, IL, interleukin.

rates and efficiencies of one or more of these systems lead to an adjustment in whole body nitrogen (protein) balance and retention, with the net direction and the extent of the balance depending upon the sum of the interactions occurring among the prevailing factor(s).

In effect, there are two endogenous nitrogen cycles that determine the status of balance in body protein:

- the balance between intake and excretion
- the balance between protein synthesis and breakdown (Figure 4.6).

In the adult these two cycles operate so that they are effectively in balance (nitrogen intake = nitrogen excretion and protein synthesis = protein breakdown), but the intensity of the two cycles differs, the flow of nitrogen (and amino acids) being about three times greater for the protein synthesis/breakdown component than for nitrogen intake/excretion cycle.

Protein synthesis rates are high in the premature newborn, possibly about 11–14 g protein synthesized per kilogram of body weight per day, and these rates decline with growth and development so that in term babies and young adults these rates are about 7 g and

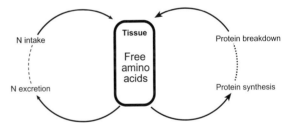

Figure 4.6 The two endogenous nitrogen cycles that determine the status of body protein (nitrogen) balance. (Adapted from Waterlow JC. The mysteries of nitrogen balance. *Nutr Res Rev* 1999; **12**: 25–54, with permission of Cambridge University Press.)

4–5 g protein/kg per day, respectively. Three points relevant to nutritional requirements may be drawn from these data. First, the higher rate of protein synthesis in the very young, compared with that in the adult, is related not only to the fact that a net deposition of protein occurs during growth, which may account for about 30% of the total amount of protein synthesized in the 6 month old infant, but also to a high rate of protein turnover (synthesis and breakdown) associated with tissue remodeling and repair, as well as to removal of abnormal proteins. In the adult the protein turnover is associated with cell and organ protein maintenance since there is no net tissue growth under most circumstances. Second, as will be seen later, at all ages in healthy subjects the rates of whole body protein synthesis and breakdown are considerably greater than usual intakes (the latter are about 1–1.5 g protein/kg per day in adults) or those levels of dietary protein thought to be just necessary to meet the body's needs for nitrogen and amino acids (about 0.8 g protein/kg per day). It follows, therefore, that there is an extensive reutilization within the body of the amino acids liberated during the course of protein breakdown. If this were not the case it might be predicted that we would be obligate carnivores and this, undoubtedly, would have changed the course of human evolution. Third, although not evident from this discussion alone, there is a general as well as functional relationship between the basal energy metabolism or resting metabolic rate and the rate of whole body protein turnover. Protein synthesis and protein degradation are energy-requiring processes, as will be described elsewhere in these volumes, and from various studies, including interspecies components, it can be estimated that about 15–20 kJ (4–5 kcal) of basal energy expenditure is expended in association with the formation of each gram of new protein synthesis and turnover. In other words, protein and amino acid metabolism may be responsible for about 20% of total basal energy metabolism. Because basal metabolic rate accounts for a significant proportion of total daily energy expenditure, it should be clear from this discussion that there are significant, quantitative interrelationships between energy and protein metabolism and their nutritional requirements. For these reasons it would not be difficult to appreciate that both the level of dietary protein and the level of dietary energy can influence the balance between rates of protein synthesis and protein breakdown and so affect body nitrogen balance. Their effects are interdependent and their interactions can be complex. This can be illustrated by the changes in body nitrogen balance that occur for different protein and energy intakes (Figure 4.7); as seen here, the level of energy intake, whether above or below requirements, determines the degree of change in the nitrogen balance that occurs in response to a change in nitrogen intake. Conversely, the level of nitrogen intake determines the quantitative effect of energy intake on nitrogen balance. Therefore, optimum body protein nutrition is achieved when protein and

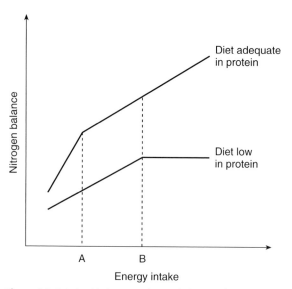

Figure 4.7 Relationship between nitrogen balance and energy intake with diets of different protein levels. Between energy intake A (low) and B (higher) the two lines are parallel. (Reproduced from Munro HN, Allison JB, eds. *Mammalian Protein Metabolism*, vol. I. New York: Academic Press, 1964: 381 with permission.)

energy intakes (from sources such as carbohydrates and lipids) are sufficient to meet or balance the needs for amino acids, nitrogen, and the daily energy expenditure or, in the case of growth, the additional energy deposited in new tissues.

Amino acids as precursors of physiologically important nitrogen compounds

As already pointed out, amino acids are also used for the synthesis of important nitrogen-containing compounds that, in turn, play critical roles in cell, organ, and system function. In carrying out these particular roles the amino acid-derived metabolites also turn over and they need to be replaced ultimately by the nitrogen and indispensable amino acids supplied by protein intake. Estimates on the quantitative utilization of these precursor and nonproteinogenic roles of amino acids in human subjects are limited but it is possible to give some examples.

- Arginine is the precursor of nitric oxide (NO); the total amount of NO synthesized (and degraded) per day represents less than 1% of whole body arginine flux and less than 1% of the daily arginine intake.

- In contrast, the rate of synthesis and degradation of creatinine is relatively high and accounts for 10% of the whole body flux of arginine and for 70% of the daily intake of arginine.
- Similarly, the synthesis and turnover of glutathione (a major intracellular thiol and important antioxidant, formed from glutamate, glycine, and cysteine) accounts for a high rate of cysteine utilization such that it greatly exceeds the equivalent of the usual daily intake of cysteine. Since continued glutathione synthesis involves a reutilization of endogenous cysteine, a low intake of dietary methionine and cyst(e)ine would be expected to have an unfavorable influence on glutathione status and synthesis. This has been shown experimentally to be the case, especially in trauma patients and those suffering from acquired immunodeficiency syndrome (AIDS). Because glutathione is the most important intracellular antioxidant that protects cells against damage by reactive oxygen species, this would mean that particular attention should be paid to such amino acids in nutritional therapy in these groups of patients.

Urea cycle enzymes and urea production

Finally, with reference to the major processes shown in Figure 4.5, the urea cycle enzymes, which are distributed both within the mitochondrion and in the cytosol (Figure 4.8), are of importance. The production of urea may be viewed largely, but not entirely, as a pathway involved in the removal of amino nitrogen and contributing to an adjustment of nitrogen loss to nitrogen intake under various conditions. The five enzymes of urea biosynthesis associate as a tightly connected metabolic pathway, called a metabalon, for conversion of potentially toxic ammonia as well as removal of excess amino acids via their oxidation with transfer of the nitrogen to arginine and ultimately urea. This is especially important when the supply of protein or amino acids is high owing to

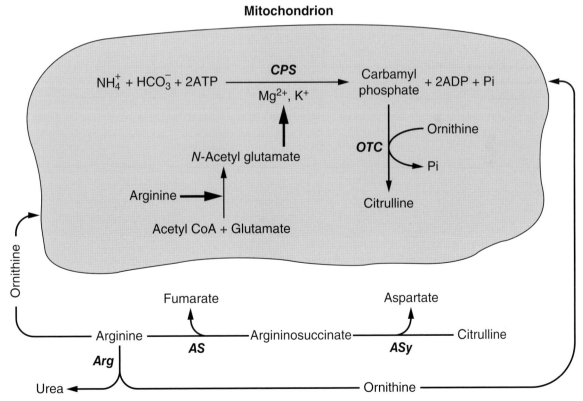

Figure 4.8 The urea cycle enzymes and their distribution in the liver. CPS, carbamoyl phosphate synthetase; OTC, ornithine transcarbamylase; Asy, argininosuccinic synthetase; AS, argininosuccinate; Arg, arginase.

variations in the exogenous intake or when there is a high rate of whole body protein breakdown in catabolic states, as occurs in severe trauma and following overwhelming infection.

Altered intakes of indispensable amino acids and of total nitrogen result in changes in rates of amino acid oxidation and the output of urea nitrogen in urine. There is a roughly parallel change in urea production and excretion throughout a relatively wide range of change in the level of dietary nitrogen intake above and below physiological requirement levels. Part of this urea enters the intestinal lumen, where there is some salvaging of urea nitrogen, via intestinal hydrolysis of urea to form ammonia. This ammonium nitrogen can be made available to the host for the net synthesis of dispensable or conditionally indispensable amino acids. However, the quantitative extent to which this pathway of nitrogen flow serves to maintain whole body N homeostasis and retention under normal conditions is a matter of uncertainty. The ammonia from urea could also enter the nitrogen moiety of the indispensable amino acids, but this would be essentially by an exchange mechanism and so would not contribute to a net gain of these amino acids in the body.

The reutilization of urea nitrogen starts from the hydrolysis of the intact urea molecule. By constantly infusing the $[^{15}N_2]$-urea tracer, the appearance of the singly labeled $[^{15}N]$-urea should represent the extent of urea hydrolysis. A 24 hour constant infusion of $[^{15}N_2]$-urea revealed a minimal amount of $[^{15}N]$-urea appearance in the plasma, and a linear relationship over a wide range of protein intake versus total urea production and urea hydrolysis. Furthermore, the possible metabolic pathways involved in the assimila-tion of ammonia generated from urea nitrogen include (1) citrulline synthesis, (2) L-glutamate dehydrogenase pathway in the mitochondria, and (3) glycine synthase. The net formation of amino nitrogen from these pathways is quantitatively minimal compared with the metabolic fluxes of these amino acids through their major pathways, such as protein turnover, dietary intake, and de novo synthesis (of the nutritionally dispensable amino acids only).

Summary of the metabolic basis for protein and amino acid requirements

It should be evident from this account of the underlying aspects of the needs for α-amino nitrogen and indispensable amino acids, that the "metabolic" requirement can usefully be divided: first, into those needs directly associated with protein deposition, a critical issue in infants, early childhood nutrition, and during recovery from prior depletion due to disease or malnutrition; and, second, into those needs associated with the maintenance of body protein balance, which accounts for almost all of the amino acid requirement in the healthy adult, except for that due to the turnover and loss of the various physiologically important nitrogen-containing products, some of which were mentioned above. Quantifying the minimum needs for nitrogen and for indispensable amino acids to support growth should be relatively easy, in principle, because these needs are simply the product of the rate of protein nitrogen deposition and the amino acid composition of the proteins that are deposited. Here, it may be pointed out that the gross amino acid composition of whole body proteins shows essentially no difference among a variety of mammals, including humans (Table 4.6). Thus, at the

Table 4.6 Essential amino acid composition of mixed body protein of immature mammals

	Amino acid composition (mg/g protein)							
	Lysine	Phenylalanine	Methionine	Histidine	Valine	Isoleucine	Leucine	Threonine
Rat	77	43	20	30	52	39	85	43
Human	72	41	20	26	47	35	75	41
Pig	75	42	20	28	52	38	72	37
Sheep	75	42	17	23	53	33	79	47
Calf	69	39	18	27	42	30	74	43

From Reeds PJ. Dispensable and indispensable amino acids for humans. J Nutr 2000; **130**: 1835S–1840S. Reprinted with permission of The American Society for Nutrition.

Table 4.7 The involvement of amino acids in physiological systems and metabolic function

System	Function	Product	Precursor
Intestine	Energy generation	ATP	Glu, Asp, Glutamine
	Proliferation	Nucleic acids	Glutamine, Gly, Asp
	Protection	Glutathione	Cys, Glu, Gly
		Nitric oxide	Arg
		Mucins	Thr, Cys, Ser, Pro
Skeletal muscle	Energy generation	Creatine	Gly, Arg, Met
	Peroxidative protection	Taurine (?)	Cys
Nervous system	Transmitter synthesis	Adrenergic	Phe
		Serotinergic	Try
		Glutaminergic	Glu
		Glycinergic	Gly
		Nitric oxide	Arg
	Peroxidative protection	Taurine (?)	Cys
Immune system	Lymphocyte proliferation	(?)	Glutamine, Arg, Asp
	Peroxidative protection	Glutathione	Cys, Glu, Gly
Cardiovascular	Blood pressure regulation	Nitric oxide	Arg
	Peroxidative protection (?)	Red cell glutathione	Cys, Glu, Gly

major biochemical level the qualitative pattern of the needs of individual amino acids to support protein deposition would be expected to be generally similar.

In humans, in contrast to rapidly growing mammals such as the rat and pig, the obligatory amino acid needs for the purposes of net protein deposition are for most stages in life a relatively minor portion of the total amino acid requirement. Hence, most of the requirement for nitrogen and amino acids is associated with the maintenance of body protein stores (or body nitrogen equilibrium). A major portion of the maintenance nitrogen and amino acids needs is directly associated with protein metabolism and reflects two related factors.

- Amino acids released from tissue protein degradation are not recycled with 100% efficiency.
- Amino acid catabolism is a close function of the free amino acid concentration in tissues, and so the presence of the finite concentrations of free amino acids necessary to promote protein synthesis inevitably leads to some degree of amino acid catabolism and irreversible loss.

The other metabolic component of the requirement for nitrogen and amino acids, as mentioned above, is due to the turnover of functionally important products of amino acid metabolism, which are also necessary to maintain health. Although this may not necessarily be a major quantitative component of the daily requirement, it is qualitatively and functionally of considerable importance; health depends on the maintenance of this component of the protein need.

Finally, four physiological systems appear to be critical for health: the intestine, to maintain absorptive and protective function; the immune and repair system and other aspects of defense; the skeletal musculature system; and the central nervous system. Within each system it is possible to identify critical metabolic roles for some specific amino acids (Table 4.7). Also of note is that, with certain exceptions (the involvement of phenylalanine and tryptophan in the maintenance of the adrenergic and serotinergic neurotransmitter systems, and methionine as a methyl group donor for the synthesis of creatine, as well as the branched-chain amino acids as nitrogen precursors for cerebral glutamate synthesis), the necessary precursors shown here are the dispensable and conditionally indispensable amino acids.

4.6 Estimation of protein and amino acid requirements

Having considered the biology of protein and protein requirements, this section now considers how these factors may be used to estimate the requirement for protein and for amino acids. The first section discusses nitrogen balance and the definition of protein requirements, before discussing how these vary with age and for various physiological groups. Subsequent sections cover the estimation of the requirements for the indispensable amino acids.

Nitrogen balance and definition of requirement

The starting point for estimating total protein needs has been, in most studies, the measurement of the amount of dietary nitrogen needed for zero nitrogen balance, or equilibrium, in adults. In the growing infant and child and in women during pregnancy and lactation, or when repletion is necessary following trauma and infection, for example, there will be an additional requirement associated with the net deposition of protein in new tissue and that due to secretion of milk. Thus, a United Nations (UN) Expert Consultation in 1985 defined the dietary need for protein as follows.

> The protein requirement of an individual is defined as the lowest level of dietary protein intake that will balance the losses from the body in persons maintaining energy balance at modest levels of physical activity. In children and pregnant or lactating women, the protein requirement is taken to also include the needs associated with the deposition of tissues or the secretion of milk at rates consistent with good health.

Most estimates of human protein requirements have been obtained directly, or indirectly, from measurements of nitrogen excretion and balance (Nitrogen balance = Nitrogen intake – Nitrogen excretion via urine, feces, skin, and other minor routes of nitrogen loss). It must be recognized that the nitrogen balance technique has serious technical and interpretative limitations and so it cannot serve as an entirely secure or sufficient basis for establishing the protein and amino acid needs for human subjects. Thus, there are:

- a number of inherent sources of error in nitrogen balance measurements that should be considered
- a number of experimental requirements that must be met if reliable nitrogen balance data are to be obtained.

These include

- the need to match closely energy intake with energy need, for the various reasons discussed earlier

- an appropriate stabilization period to the experimental diet and periods long enough to establish reliably the full response to a dietary change
- timing and completeness of urine collections
- absence of mild infections and of other sources of stress.

Reference to detailed reviews of the concepts behind and techniques involved in the nitrogen balance approach is given in the reading list at the end of this chapter.

When direct nitrogen balance determinations of the protein requirement data are lacking, as is the case for a number of age groups, an interpolation of requirements between two age groups is usually made simply on the basis of body weight considerations. A factorial approach may also be applied; here, the so-called obligatory urine and fecal nitrogen losses are determined (after about 4–6 days of adaptation to a protein-free diet in adults), summated together with other obligatory losses, including those via sweat and the integument. For children, estimates of nitrogen deposition or retention are also included. In the case of very young infants the recommendations for meeting protein requirements are usually based on estimated protein intakes by fully breast-fed infants.

Protein requirements for various age and physiological groups

The protein requirements for young adult men and women have been based on both short- and long-term nitrogen balance studies. This also applies to healthy elderly people, whose protein requirements have been judged not to be different from those of younger adults. In order to make practical recommendations to cover the requirements for most individuals, it is necessary to adjust the average or mean requirement for a group by a factor that accounts for the variation in protein requirements among apparently similar individuals in that group. This factor is usually taken to be the coefficient of variation (CV) around the mean requirement and traditionally a value of $2 \times CV$ (SD/mean) is added to the mean physiological requirement, so that the needs of all but 2.5% of individuals within the population would be covered. This adjusted requirement value is taken to be the safe practical protein intake for the healthy adult (Table 4.8). Most individuals would require less

Table 4.8 The United Nations (1985 FAO/WHO/UNU) and Institute of Medicine (2002/2005) recommendations for a safe practical protein intake for selected age groups and physiological states. Reproduced with permission from WHO

Group	Age (years)	Safe protein level (g/kg/day)	
		UNU	IOM
Infants	0.3–0.5	1.47	1.5
	0.75–1.0	1.15	1.1
Children	3–4	1.09	0.95
	9–10	0.99	0.95
Adolescent	13–14 (girls)	0.94	0.85
	13–14 (boys)	0.97	0.85
Young adults	19+	0.75	0.80
Elderly		0.75	0.80
Women: pregnant	2nd trimester	+6 g daily	~1.1
	3rd trimester	+11 g daily	~1.1
lactating	0.6 months	~+16 g daily	~1.1
	6–12 months	12 g daily	~1.1

Values are for proteins such as those of quality equal to a hen's egg, cow's milk, meat, or fish.

than this intake to maintain an adequate protein nutritional status.

It is worth emphasizing two points. First, the current UN recommendations shown in Table 4.8 apply to healthy individuals of all ages. However, it is highly likely that the needs of sick or less healthy patients would differ from and usually exceed those of healthy subjects. In this case, the values given in this table can be regarded only as a basis from which to begin an evaluation of how disease and stress, including surgery, affect the needs for dietary protein. Unfortunately, the quantitative needs for protein (total nitrogen) in sick, hospitalized patients can be only very crudely approximated at this time.

Second, the values shown in Table 4.8 apply to high-quality food proteins, such as eggs, milk, meat, and fish. The differing nutritional value of food proteins will be considered below.

Definition and determination of indispensable amino acid requirements

Definition

It is possible to modify slightly the earlier definition for the requirements for protein (nitrogen) for a specific, indispensable amino acid, which can be stated, therefore, as:

. . . . the lowest level of intake of an indispensable amino acid that achieves nitrogen balance or that balances the irreversible oxidative loss of the amino acid, without requiring major changes in normal protein turnover and where there is energy balance with a modest level of physical activity. For infants, children and pregnant and lactating women, the requirements for the amino acid will include the additional amount of the amino acid needed for net protein deposition by the infant, child or fetus and conceptus and for the synthesis and secretion of milk proteins.

The foregoing is an operational definition of requirement, as in the case of protein. Ideally, a functional definition and determination of these requirements inherently would be preferable. However, the choice and nature of the functional index or (indices) (such as maximum resistance to disease or enhanced physical performance) and its quantitative definition remain a challenge for future nutrition and health-related research.

Determination

In general, the approaches and methods that have been most often used to determine specific indispensable amino acid requirements are similar to those used for estimation of total protein needs, i.e., nitrogen excretion and balance and factorial estimation. Thus, amino acid requirements have been assessed by nitrogen balance in adults, and by determining the amounts needed for normal growth and nitrogen balance in infants, preschool children, and school-aged children. For infants, they have also been approached by assessment of the intakes provided by breast milk or those supplied from intakes of good-quality proteins. In addition, factorial predictions of the amino acid requirements of infants and adults have been made. One such factorial approach for use in adults includes the following assumptions.

- The total obligatory nitrogen losses (those losses occurring after about 4–6 days of adjustment to a protein-free diet) are taken to be approximately 54 mg/kg nitrogen per day in an adult, or equivalent to 0.36 g protein/kg/day.
- The average amino acid composition of body proteins can be used to estimate the contribution made

by each amino acid to this obligatory nitrogen output (equivalent, therefore, to the obligatory amino acid losses).

- At requirement intake levels, an absorbed amino acid is used to balance its obligatory oxidative loss with an assumed efficiency of about 70%.

This predictive or factorial approach is analogous to the factorial method for estimating the total nitrogen (protein) requirement of individuals at various ages (where various routes of nitrogen excretion and nitrogen gains are summated and an efficiency factor is used to estimate the intake needed to balance this summation).

Tracer techniques

With advances in the routine measurement of stable isotope enrichment in biological matrices and the expanded use of tracers enriched with these isotopes in human metabolic research, a series of tracer studies was begun at the Massachusetts Institute of Technology, USA, in the early 1980s to determine amino acid requirements in adults. Since that time several research groups have used different paradigms in tracer-based studies of human amino acid requirements. These can be distinguished according to the choice of tracer and protocol design applied:

- studies involving the use of a labeled tracer of the dietary amino acid being tested and with its rate of oxidation (O) at various test intake levels [the direct amino acid oxidation (DAAO) technique, e.g., [^{13}C]-lysine as a tracer to determine the lysine requirement]; this technique has been used to assess the requirements in adults for leucine, valine, lysine, threonine, and phenylalanine
- studies involving use of an "indicator" tracer to assess the status of indicator amino acid oxidation (IAAO) or indicator amino acid balance (IAAB) with varying levels of a test amino acid; examples of the IAAO and IAAB approaches are where the rate of [^{13}C]-phenylalanine oxidation (Figure 4.9) is measured or a [^{13}C]-leucine balance determined at varying levels of lysine intake to estimate the lysine requirement
- kinetic studies designed to assess the retention of protein during the postprandial phase of amino acid metabolism, using [^{13}C]-leucine as a tracer: the postprandial protein utilization (PPU) approach; this last and promising approach has not yet found

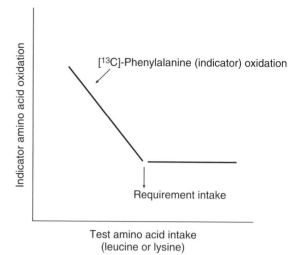

Figure 4.9 Outline of the concept of the indicator amino acid oxidation technique for estimation of indispensable amino acid requirements. Here the indicator is [^{13}C]-phenylalanine and the dietary requirement is being estimated for either leucine or lysine.

an extensive use in studies of human amino acid requirements.

None of these methods is without its limitations, but at present the IAAO and IAAB approaches, involving tracer studies lasting for a continuous 24 hour day, would appear to be the "reference method" for estimating amino acid requirements in adults.

Indispensable amino acid requirement values

There is still debate and uncertainty about the precise requirements for amino acids in humans of all ages. Three major sets of proposed amino acid requirement values for healthy subjects should be noted in this text. First, there are the requirements proposed by the UN in 1985 for the various age groups, which are presented in Table 4.9. Second, another expert group in 1994 (International Dietary Energy Consultancy Group; IDECG) also assessed the amino acid needs of infants by using a factorial method and these turned out to be much lower than those shown in Table 4.9 for infants. It should be noted, however, that the 1994 IDECG values approximate the average requirements, whereas the requirement intakes derived from estimates of breast milk intake (shown in Table 4.9) would be expected to be well above the requirement for virtually all infants and certainly well

Table 4.9 1985 FAO/WHO/UNU[a] estimates of amino acid requirements at different ages (mg/kg/day). Reproduced with permission from WHO

Amino acid	Infants (3–4 months)	Preschool children (2 years)	School boys (10–12 years)	Adults
Histidine	28	?	?	[8–12]
Isoleucine	70	31	28	10
Leucine	161	73	44	14
Lysine	103	64	44	12
Methionine and cystine	58	28	22	13
Phenylalanine and tyrosine	125	69	22	14
Threonine	87	37	28	7
Tryptophan	17	12.5	3.3	3.5
Valine	93	38	25	10
Total	714	352	216	84
Total per g protein[b]	434	320	222	111

[a] FAO/WHO/UNU. Technical Report Series No. 724. Geneva: World Health Organization, 1985. Data taken from Table 4, p. 65, and Table 38, p. 121, and based on all amino acids minus histidine.
[b] Total mg per g crude protein.

above the mean or average requirement. It is not surprising, therefore, that the UN and IDECG requirements disagreed. This also shows why recommendations by different national and international expert groups differ; they interpret the same data differently, use different data, and also may choose to set different criteria for judging the adequacy of intake.

Further, as is characteristic of various estimates of human nutrient requirements in general, it must be appreciated that the values given in Table 4.9 are based on limited data; the values for the preschool children are derived from a single set of investigations carried out at the Institute for Central America and Panama, while those for the school-aged children come from studies conducted by a single group of investigators in Japan. Those for adults are based primarily on the nitrogen balance studies in men carried out in the 1950s and 1960s. There are multiple reasons for questioning the precise reliability and nutritional significance of the adult values, and they include the facts that adult amino acid requirement values (Table 4.9) are greatly influenced by:

- the inappropriate experimental design used earlier for estimation of requirements
- the inadequacy of the nitrogen balance technique and the criterion of nitrogen balance that has been used to judge the nutritional adequacy of the levels of amino acid intake tested.

Therefore, some contemporary and newly proposed amino acid requirement estimates for adults are shown in Table 4.10. The more recent values are generally very different from the recommendations made in 1985. It is important to remain alert in nutrition, as these texts will emphasize. At the time of writing the original text, a new UN expert group was meeting to consider all of the new data that had been accumulated in the past 20 years. It was expected that new recommendations would be made in 2002 or 2003, but, since they have not been published, the recommendations by the Institute of Medicine of the US Academies of Science have been added as a separate column in Table 4.10. The important point, however, is that all is not set in stone. Nutritional knowledge continues to advance, and with it the recommendations must change or at least be responsive to this new information.

4.7 Meeting protein and amino acid needs

Knowledge of the requirements for the specific indispensable amino acids and for total protein provides the basis for evaluating the relative capacity (or quality) of individual protein foods or mixtures of food protein sources to meet human amino acid requirements.

The two major determinants of the nutritional quality of food proteins are:

- the content of indispensable amino acids in the protein

Table 4.10 The earlier and three contemporary suggested patterns of amino acid requirements in healthy adults

Amino Acid	United Nations[a] 1985	University of Surrey[b] 1999	MIT[c] 2000	IOM[d] 2002
Isoleucine	10[e] (13)[f]	18 (30)	23 (35)	(25)
Leucine	14 (19)	26 (44)	23 (65)	(55)
Lysine	12 (16)	19 (31)	30 (50)	(51)
Methionine and cystine	13 (17)	16 (27)	13 (25)	(25)
Phenylalanine and tyrosine	14 (19)	20 (33)	39 (65)	(47)
Threonine	7 (9)	16 (26)	15 (25)	(27)
Tryptophan	3.5 (5)	4 (6)	6 (10)	(7)
Valine	10 (13)	14 (23)	20 (35)	(32)

[a]FAO/WHO/UNU. Technical Report Series No. 724. Geneva: World Health Organization, 1985.
[b]Millward DJ. The nutritional value of plant-based diets in relation to human amino acid and protein requirements. *Proc Nutr Soc* 1999; **58**: 249–260.
[c]Young VR, Borgonha S. Nitrogen and amino acid requirements: the Massachusetts Institute of Technology Amino Acid Requirement Pattern. *J Nutr* 2000; **130**: 1841S–1849S, reproduced with permission of the American Society of Nutrition.
[d]US National Academies of Science Institute of Medicine.
[e]Values expressed as mg/kg/d.
[f]Values expressed as mg amino acid/protein required for effectively meeting total protein and amino acid needs.

- the extent to which the indispensable amino acids are available to the host metabolism.

Digestibility and intestinal amino acid metabolism

Traditionally, the assessment of the availability of dietary proteins and amino acids under practical conditions has been based on "apparent digestibility," i.e., the difference between nitrogen intake and fecal nitrogen output. However, for two reasons, this method is unsatisfactory for the precise estimation of the digestibility of individual amino acids. First, fecal nitrogen consists largely of bacterial protein, and because the composition of bacterial protein differs markedly from that of common dietary proteins, it gives very little information on the digestibility of different food-derived amino acids. Second, the bacterial nitrogen is not only derived from undigested protein. This is because proteins secreted into the intestinal lumen, as well as the urea nitrogen that has diffused from the blood, are important contributors to colonic nitrogen flow. Studies in both animals and humans using ^{15}N-labeled amino acids suggest that at least 50% of the fecal nitrogen is derived from the body rather than directly from undigested dietary protein.

Recently, ^{15}N-labeled dietary proteins have been given to adults and by measuring the flow of ^{15}N from the terminal ileum it is possible to calculate the "true" digestibility of the dietary source. There have also been a number of studies in pigs in which ^{15}N-labeled

amino acids have been infused intravenously for prolonged periods. This labels the host proteins so that the ^{15}N labeling of ileal proteins allows the calculation of the endogenous contribution of the luminal protein pool. By and large, the results of all these studies lead to the same conclusion; namely, that the true digestibility of most dietary proteins is very high and that at least 50% of the fecal nitrogen is derived from host metabolism rather than from the diet.

Most of the evidence favors the conclusion that there is an almost complete digestion of most dietary proteins in the small bowel. It is also quite clear that a considerable amount of amino acid metabolism occurs in the tissue of the splanchnic bed, in general, and in the intestinal mucosa, in particular, before the amino acids, liberated from food proteins during the digestive process, reach organs such as the liver, kidneys, and skeletal muscles. Calculations based on recent isotopic studies suggest that intestinal amino acid utilization (both from the diet and via the blood supply to the intestine; the mesenteric arterial circulation) can account for as much as 50% of the body's utilization of amino acids. It is also important to note that the degree to which individual amino acids are utilized by the gut varies markedly (Table 4.11). Among the indispensable amino acids, threonine utilization is particularly high and virtually all of the dietary glutamate and aspartate are utilized within the mucosa. In addition, the magnitude of splanchnic amino acid metabolism varies with age, being apparently greater in infants and also perhaps in the elderly.

This can affect the efficiency with which the amino acids derived from the protein ingested are used to support overall body nitrogen and amino acid homeostasis and balance.

Protein nutritional quality

Not all proteins have the same capacity to meet the physiological requirements for total nitrogen and the indispensable amino acids. The concentration and availability of the individual indispensable amino acids are major factors responsible for the differences in the nutritive values of food proteins. Thus, the content and balance of indispensable amino acids differ among plant and animal protein foods. For the present purpose a summary is given in Table 4.12, listing the four indispensable amino acids that are most likely to be limiting, or in shortest supply and especially in food proteins of plant origin. As can be seen, lysine is present in a much lower concentration in all the major plant food groups than in animal protein foods and is most frequently the most limiting amino acid.

The nutritional significance of these differences can be assessed in a number of ways. One useful approach is an amino acid scoring procedure that compares the content of amino acids in a protein with a reference human amino acid requirement pattern.

In 1991 a UN Expert Consultation reviewed the appropriate methods for measuring quality of food proteins for the nutrition of human populations. This consultation concluded that the most appropriate method available was the protein digestibility-corrected amino acid score (PDCAAS) method, and it was recommended for international use. This amino acid scoring procedure, including a correction for digestibility, uses the amino acid requirement pattern for a 2–5 year old child (as shown in Table 4.9). This is the reference amino acid requirement pattern for this purpose, expressing the amino acid requirement in relation to the total protein requirement.

The PDCAAS is estimated from the following equation:

$$PDCAAS = \frac{\text{Concentration of most limiting, digestibility-corrected amino acid in a test protein}}{\text{Concentration of that amino acid in the 1991 FAO/WHO amino acid scoring reference pattern (preschool child: see Table 4.9)}}$$

In addition to establishing the amino acid reference pattern for use in the PDCAAS method, the UN Consultation considered the procedures for measuring and estimating amino acids and digestibility. This approach offers considerable benefits over that of animal bioassays, which traditionally have been used

Table 4.11 The uptake of dietary amino acids by the visceral tissues

Amino acid	Percentage of intake	
	Utilization by the liver and gut (human)	Utilization by the gut (piglet)
Leucine	26	37
Lysine	32	45
Phenylalanine	39	53
Threonine	No data	65
Glutamine	53	50
Glutamate	88	95

Table 4.12 The amino acid content of different food protein sources

Food source	mg/g protein (mean ± SD)			
	Lysine	Sulfur amino acids	Threonine	Tryptophan
Legumes	64 ± 10	25 ± 3	38 ± 3	12 ± 4
Cereals	31 ± 10	37 ± 4	32 ± 4	12 ± 2
Nuts, seeds	45 ± 14	46 ± 17	36 ± 3	17 ± 3
Fruits	45 ± 12	27 ± 6	29 ± 7	11 ± 2
Animals foods	85 ± 9	38	44	12

From Young VR, Scrimshaw NS, Pellett PL. Significance of dietary protein source in human nutrition: Animal and/or plant proteins? In: Waterlow JC, Armstrong DG, Fowder L, Riley, eds. *Feeding a World Population of More Than Eight Billion People.* Oxford University Press in association with the Rank Prize Funds, Oxford, 1998: 206.

to assess the quality of food protein in human diets. An important benefit is that the PDCAAS approach uses human amino acid requirements as the basis of evaluation, which ensures that appropriate levels of indispensable amino acids will be provided in the diet. In addition, use of the proposed amino acid scoring procedure facilitates an evaluation of blending of foods to optimize nitrogen utilization and meet

Table 4.13 Protein digestibility-corrected amino acid score (PDCAAS) of wheat, rice, maize, sorghum, and millet

Protein source	PDCAAS
Wheat	40 (L)
Rice	56 (L)
Maize	43 (L)
Sorghum	33 (L)
Millet	53 (L)
Beef	>100 (S)

From Young VR, Scrimshaw NS, Pellett PL. Significance of dietary protein source in human nutrition: Animal and/or plant proteins? In: Waterlow JC, Armstrong DG, Fowder L, Riley, eds. *Feeding a World Population of More Than Eight Billion People.* Oxford University Press in association with the Rank Prize Funds, Oxford, 1998: 207.
L, lysine first limiting amino acid; S, sulfur amino acids (methionine and cystine).

protein and amino acid needs. A listing of some calculated PDCAAS values for selected food protein sources is given in Table 4.13 and a worked example for a mixture of food proteins is presented in Table 4.14.

The development of an internationally derived procedure for evaluating protein quality using the amino acid scoring concept is a step that had long been required. This PDCAAS procedure can be modified as new knowledge about specific amino acid requirements emerges, as the determination of availability of dietary amino acids is improved, and as the factors affecting digestibility and availability are better understood. For the present, the PDCAAS procedure would appear to be very useful for evaluating the nutritional quality of human food protein sources.

Major sources of food proteins in the diet

The relative proportions in the diet of food proteins of animal and plant origin differ according to geographical region and other socioeconomic and cultural factors. Broadly, animal protein foods account for 60–70% of the total protein intake in the developed regions (Table 4.15). In contrast, plant proteins make up about 60–80% of the total protein intake in developing regions, with cereals being the dominant source in this case. Given the differences in amino acid content of

Table 4.14 Worked example of a protein digestibility-corrected amino acid score (PDCAAS) for a mixture of wheat, chickpea, and milk powder

	Analytical data (mg/g protein)							Quantities in mixture (mg)				
	Weight (g)	Protein (g/100 g)	Lys	SAA	Thr	Trp	Digestibility factor	Protein (g)	Lys	TSAA	Thr	Trp
								A × B = P				
	A	B	C	D	E	F	G	100	P × C	P × D	P × E	P × F
Wheat	350	13	25	35	30	11	0.85	45.5	1138	1593	1365	501
Chickpea	150	22	70	25	42	13	0.80	33.0	2310	825	1386	429
Milk powder	50	34	80	30	37	12	0.95	17.0	1360	510	629	204
Totals								95.5	4808	2928	3380	1134
Amino acids mg/g protein (total for each amino acid/total protein)									50	31	35	12
Reference scoring pattern used			58	25	34	11						
Amino acids scoring for mixture amino acid/g protein divided by reference pattern									0.86	1.24	1.03	1.09
Weighted average protein digestibility sum of [protein × factor (P × G)] divided by protein total								0.85				
Score adjusted for digestibility (PDCAAS) (0.85 × 0.86)									0.73 (or 73%) with lysine limiting			

From Food and Agriculture Organization of the United Nations. *Protein Quality Evaluation.* FAO Food and Nutrition Paper 51. FAO, Rome, 1991: table 10.
Lys, lysine; SAA, sulfur amino acids; Thr, threonine; Trp, tryptophan; TSAA, total sulfur amino acids.

Table 4.15 Protein supplies per caput per day for selected regions

Region	Plant protein		Animal protein		Cereal protein		Total protein (g)
	Total (g)	%	Total (g)	%	Total (g)	%	
World	26	36	46	64	33	46	72
Developing regions							
Africa	11	20	46	80	31	54	58
Asia	16	25	49	75	36	56	65
Latin America	32	45	39	55	25	36	70
Developed regions							
North America	72	64	41	36	25	22	113
Western Europe	62	60	41	40	25	24	103
Oceania	71	69	32	31	19	19	102

From Young VR, Scrimshaw NS, Pellett PL. Significance of dietary protein source in human nutrition: Animal and/or plant proteins? In: Waterlow JC, Armstrong DG, Fowder L, Riley, eds. *Feeding a World Population of More Than Eight Billion People.* Oxford University Press in association with the Rank Prize Funds, Oxford, 1998: 212.

Table 4.16 Calculated mean values per caput for the availability of specific indispensable amino acids in developed and developing regions

Region	Amino acid per day (mg)				mg/g protein			
	Lys	SAA	Try	Thr	Lys	SAA	Try	Thr
Developing[a]	2947	2160	693	2204	49	36	11	37
Developed and transitional[b]	6149	3619	1177	3799	64	38	12	40

From Young VR, Scrimshaw NS, Pellett PL. Significance of dietary protein source in human nutrition: Animal and/or plant proteins? In: Waterlow JC, Armstrong DG, Fowder L, Riley, eds. *Feeding a World Population of More Than Eight Billion People.* Oxford University Press in association with the Rank Prize Funds, Oxford, 1998: 212.
[a]Data for 61 countries.
[b]Data for 29 countries.
SAA, sulfur amino acids; TSAA, total sulfur amino acids.

food proteins mentioned above it is not surprising that there are distinct differences in the intakes of the indispensable amino acids by different population groups worldwide. An example of such differences is given in Table 4.16. As already noted, the four amino acids of greatest importance and those most likely to be most limiting in intake, relative to requirements, are lysine, the sulfur amino acids (methionine and cystine), tryptophan, and threonine.

4.8 Factors other than diet affecting protein and amino acid requirements

Not everyone of the same age, body build, and gender has the same nutrient requirements. These differences may be due, in part, to variations in genetic background. Various environmental, physiological, psychological, and pathological influences affect the variability in physiological requirements for nutrients among individuals (Table 4.17). For example, as already discussed, the growing infant or child requires higher nutrient intakes per unit of body weight than does the adult. Besides energy, for which the daily requirement declines with age because of reduced physical activity, it appears that the nutrient needs of healthy aged subjects do not differ significantly from those of young adults. Nevertheless, a characteristic of aging is an increased incidence of disease and morbidity, which is likely to be far more important than age per se in determining practical differences between the nutrient requirements of younger adults and elderly people.

Table 4.17 Agent, host, and environment factors that affect protein and amino acid requirements and the nutritional status of the individual

Agent (dietary) factors
  Chemical form of nutrition (protein and amino acid source)
  Energy intake
  Food processing and preparation (may increase or decrease dietary needs)
  Effect of other dietary constituents
Host factors
  Age
  Sex
  Genetic makeup
  Pathologic states
  Drugs
  Infection
  Physical trauma
  Chronic disease, cancer
Environmental factors
  Physical (unsuitable housing, inadequate heating)
  Biologic (poor sanitary conditions)
  Socioeconomic (poverty, dietary habits and food choices, physical activity)

Thus, superimposed infection, altered gastrointestinal function, and metabolic changes that often accompany chronic disease states would all be expected to reduce the efficiency of dietary nitrogen and amino acid utilization. The metabolic response to acute infection in healthy young men has been characterized in experiments involving different types of intracellular infection, and involves an increased loss of body nitrogen, together with increased losses of several other nutrients including potassium, magnesium, phosphorus, and vitamin C. This increased loss clearly implies increased needs for nitrogen, amino acids, and other nutrients.

In addition to the catabolic response of body nitrogen metabolism to infection and trauma, there is a corresponding anabolic component that is of major importance during recovery from these stressful conditions. Anabolic responses occur not only during recovery but also in the early phase of illness, when anabolism is associated with increased production of immunocompetent cells such as phagocytes and other leukocytes, and the induction of several tissue enzymes and immunoglobulins.

During recovery from infection two characteristics of the anabolic period that follows are that the increased nitrogen retention seen during this period is greater than that measured during the preincubation phase, and its duration is much longer than the catabolic period. This may be due, in part, to the effect of protein depletion antedating an acute episode, which may be the case in poor communities. However, in spite of the potential for disease states to increase protein and amino acid needs there are too few studies that help to assess precisely their quantitative influence on nutrient utilization and dietary requirements.

4.9 Perspectives on the future

The purpose of this chapter was to provide a general overview of human protein and amino acid metabolism and a basis for an improved appreciation of the metabolic determinants of the requirements for protein (nitrogen) and for specific amino acids. With the recent beginning of the postgenome era, functional genomics, proteomics, and metabolomics will take on an increasingly important basic and applied research focus in biology. Thus, it will be even more critical for students to understand the physiology of human protein metabolism at its various levels of biological complexity (cell, organ, and whole body) and its nutritional corollaries.

There are certain areas of research in protein nutrition where more knowledge will equip nutritionists to make the best use of available food supplies. An example is the influence of the ratio of total essential or indispensable amino acids to total nitrogen and amino acid requirements for different physiological states. Another is the need for a functional definition of protein requirements (e.g., indices) for maximum resistance to disease and enhanced physical performance. These are some of the challenges facing nutritionists in the future. It is hoped that this chapter will serve as an appropriate catalyst for further learning in this area of human nutrition.

Acknowledgment

This chapter has been revised and updated by Naomi K Fukagawa and Yong-Ming Yu based on the original chapter by Vernon R Young and Peter J Reeds. It is dedicated to their memory. For more information on this topic visit www.nutritiontexts.com

References

FAO/WHO/UNU. Energy and protein requirements. Report of a Joint FAO/WHO/UNU Expert Consultation.Technical Report Series No. 724. World Health Organization, Geneva, 1985, 1–206.

Institute of Medicine, US National Academies of Science. *Dietary Reference Intakes for Energy, Carbohydrate, Fiber, Fat, Fatty Acids, Cholesterol, Protein, and Amino Acids*. Institute of Medicine, US National Academies of Science, Washington, DC, 2002.

Millward DJ. The nutritional value of plant-based diets in relation to human amino acid and protein requirements. *Proc Nutr Soc* 1999; **58**: 249–260.

Munro HN, Allison JB, eds. *Mammalian Protein Metabolism*, vols I and II. Academic Press, New York, 1964.

Reeds PJ. Dispensable and indispensable amino acids for humans. *J Nutr* 2000; **130**: 1835S–1840S.

Waterlow JC. The mysteries of nitrogen balance. *Nutr Res Rev* 1999; **12**: 25–54.

Young VR, Borgonha S. Nitrogen and amino acid requirements: the Massachusetts Institute of Technology Amino Acid Requirement Pattern. *J Nutr* 2000; **130**: 1841S–1849S.

Young VR, Scrimshaw NS, Pellett PL. Significance of dietary protein source in human nutrition: Animal and/or plant proteins? In: Waterlow JC, Armstrong DG, Fowder L, Riley, eds. *Feeding a World Population of More Than Eight Billion People*. Oxford University Press in association with the Rank Prize Funds, Oxford, 1998, 205–222.

Further reading

Cohen PP. Regulation of the ornithine-urea cycle enzymes. In: Waterlow JC, Stephen JML, eds. *Nitrogen Metabolism in Man*. Applied Science, London, 1981: 215.

Food and Agriculture Organization of the United Nations. *Protein Quality Evaluation*. Food and Nutrition Paper 51. FAO: Rome, 1991.

Garrow JS, Halliday D, eds. *Substrate and Energy Metabolism in Man*. John Libbey, London, 1985.

Lehninger AL, Nelson DL, Cox MM. *Principles of Biochemistry*, 2nd edn. Worth, New York, 1993.

Munro HN, ed. *Mammalian Protein Metabolism*, vol. III. Academic Press, New York, 1969.

Munro HN, ed. *Mammalian Protein Metabolism*, vol. IV. Academic Press, New York, 1970.

Waterlow JC, Garlick PJ, Millward DJ. *Protein Turnover in Mammalian Tissues and in the Whole Body*. North-Holland, Amsterdam, 1978.

Wolfe RR. *Radioactive and Stable Isotope Tracers in Biomedicine: Principles and Practice of Kinetic Analysis*. Wiley-Liss, New York, 1992.

Young VR, Yu Y-M, Fukagawa NK. Energy and Protein Turnover. In: Kinney JM, Tucker HN, eds. *Energy and Protein Turnover in Energy Metabolism: Tissue Determinants and Cellular Corollaries*. Raven Press, New York, 1992: 439–466.

5
Digestion and Metabolism of Carbohydrates

John Mathers and Thomas MS Wolever

Key messages

- Carbohydrates are the single most abundant and economic sources of food energy in the human diet, constituting 40–80% of total energy intake in different populations.
- Carbohydrates are classified according to their degree of polymerization into sugars, oligosaccharides, and polysaccharides – the last consisting of starches with different degrees of resistance to digestion – and dietary fibers or nonstarch polysaccharides.
- Glycemic carbohydrates are digested (hydrolyzed by enzymes) to sugars (monosaccharides) in the small bowel and absorbed and metabolized.
- Nonglycemic carbohydrates are fermented in varying degrees to short-chain fatty acids (SCFAs), carbon dioxide, hydrogen, and methane in the large bowel. Absorbed SCFAs are metabolized in colonic epithelial, hepatic, and muscle cells.
- For optimum function of the nervous system and other cells, blood glucose concentrations are tightly controlled by a group of hormones (insulin in the absorptive phase; glucagon, epinephrine, and cortisol in the postabsorptive phase), utilizing several possible metabolic pathways for glucose anabolism and catabolism.
- Intakes of optimum amounts of different types of carbohydrates are associated with good health through effects on energy balance, digestive functions, blood glucose control, and other risk factors for several chronic diseases.

5.1 Introduction: carbohydrates in foods

Carbohydrates are one of the four major classes of biomolecules and play several important roles in all life forms, including:

- sources of metabolic fuels and energy stores
- structural components of cell walls in plants and of the exoskeleton of arthropods
- parts of RNA and DNA in which ribose and deoxyribose, respectively, are linked by N-glycosidic bonds to purine and pyrimidine bases
- integral features of many proteins and lipids (glycoproteins and glycolipids), especially in cell membranes where they are essential for cell–cell recognition and molecular targeting.

Carbohydrates are very diverse molecules that can be classified by their molecular size (degree of polymerization or DP) into sugars (DP 1–2), oligosaccharides (DP 3–9), and polysaccharides (DP > 9). The physicochemical properties of carbohydrates and their fates within the body are also influenced by their monosaccharide composition and the type of linkage between sugar residues. Examples of food carbohydrates and an overview of their digestive fates are given in Table 5.1.

From birth, carbohydrate provides a large part of the energy in human diets, with approximately 40% of the energy in mature breast milk being supplied as lactose. After weaning, carbohydrates are the largest source (40–80%) of the energy in many human diets, with most of this derived from plant material except when milk or milk products containing lactose are consumed. The carbohydrate contents of some vegetable dishes are summarized in Table 5.2.

5.2 Digestive fate of dietary carbohydrates

As with other food components, the digestive fate of particular carbohydrates depends on their inherent chemical nature and on the supramolecular structures within foods of which they are a part. To be absorbed from the gut, carbohydrates must be broken

Table 5.1 Classes of food carbohydrates and their likely fates in the human gut

Class	DP	Example	Site of digestion	Absorbed molecules
Monosaccharides	1	Glucose	Small bowel	Glucose
	1	Fructose	Small bowel[a]	Fructose
	2	Sucrose	Small bowel	Glucose + fructose
	2	Lactose[b]	Small bowel	Glucose + galactose
Oligosaccharides	3	Raffinose	Large bowel	SCFA
	3–9	Inulin	Large bowel	SCFA
Polysaccharides	>9	Starches	Predominantly small bowel[c]	Glucose
	>9	Nonstarch polysaccharides	Large bowel	SCFA

[a] Except where very large doses are consumed in a single meal.
[b] Except in lactose-intolerant subjects, in whom lactose flows to the large bowel.
[c] Some starch escapes small bowel digestion (resistant starch). In all these cases, the carbohydrate entering the large bowel becomes a substrate for bacterial fermentation to short-chain fatty acids (SCFAs).
DP, degree of polymerization.

down to their constituent monosaccharide units, and a battery of hydrolytic enzymes capable of splitting the bonds between sugar residues is secreted within the mouth, from the pancreas, and on the apical membrane of enterocytes. While these carbohydrases ensure that about 95% of the carbohydrate in most human diets is digested and absorbed within the small intestine, there is considerable variation in bioavailability between different carbohydrate classes and between different foods. Carbohydrates that are digested to sugars and absorbed as such in the small bowel are called "glycemic" carbohydrates.

Hydrolysis in the mouth and small bowel

The major carbohydrase secreted by the salivary glands and by the acinar cells of the pancreas is the endoglycosidase α-amylase, which hydrolyzes (digests) internal α-1,4-linkages in amylose and amylopectin molecules to yield maltose, maltotriose, and dextrins. These oligosaccharides, together with the food disaccharides sucrose and lactose, are hydrolyzed by specific oligosaccharidases expressed on the apical membrane of the epithelial cells that populate the small intestinal villi. Sucrase–isomaltase is a glycoprotein anchored via its amino-terminal domain in the apical membrane that hydrolyzes all of the sucrose and most of the maltose and isomaltose. The resulting monomeric sugars are then available for transport into the enterocytes.

Absorption and malabsorption in the small bowel

Glucose and galactose are transported across the apical membrane by the sodium–glucose transport protein-1 (SGLT1), a process that is powered by Na$^+$/K$^+$-ATPase on the basolateral membrane (Figure 5.1). In contrast, fructose is absorbed by facilitated transport via the membrane-spanning GLUT5 protein. A member of the same family of transporter proteins, GLUT2, is the facilitated transporter on the basolateral membrane which shuttles all three monosaccharides from the enterocyte towards the blood vessels linking with the portal vein for delivery to the liver.

The capacity of the human intestine for transport of glucose, galactose, and fructose is enormous – estimated to be about 10 kg per day – so that this does not limit absorption in healthy individuals. Carbohydrate malabsorption is usually caused by an inherited or acquired defect in the brush border oligosaccharidases. More than 75% of human adults are lactose intolerant because of a loss (possibly genetically determined) of lactase activity after weaning (primary lactose intolerance). In such individuals, ingestion of more than very small amounts of lactose leads to the passage of the sugar to the large bowel, where it is fermented to produce short-chain fatty acids (SCFAs) and gases as end-products. The appearance of hydrogen in the breath after ingestion of lactose is the basis for diagnosis of malabsorption of this carbohydrate. Diseases of the intestinal tract, such as protein-energy malnutrition, intestinal infections, and celiac disease, which reduce expression of lactase on the enterocyte apical membrane, can result in secondary lactase insufficiency. Sucrase–isomaltase activity, which rises rapidly from the pylorus towards the jejunum and then declines, is inducible by sucrose feeding. About 10% of Greenland Eskimos and 0.2% of North Americans have sucrase–isomaltase deficiency. A missense

Table 5.2 Carbohydrate composition (g/100 g) of some vegetable dishes

Dish	Water	Carbohydrate	Starch	Total sugars	Glucose	Fructose	Galactose	Sucrose	Maltose	Lactose	Oligosaccharides	NSPs	Cellulose
Bhaji, okra	77.7	7.6	0.4	5.5	1.9	1.7	0	1.9	0	Tr	1.7	3.2	1.0
Cannelloni, spinach	73.4	12.6	10.4	2.2	0.1	0.1	0	0.1	0.1	1.7	Tr	1.2	0.8
Chili, beans and lentils	72.6	13.1	7.9	4.3	1.3	1.4	0	1.6	0	0	0.8	3.6	1.1
Curry, chickpea	52.7	21.3	18.7	1.2	Tr	0.1	0	1.0	0	0	1.4	4.5	1.1
Flan, cheese and mushroom	49.1	18.7	16.4	2.3	0.2	0.2	0	0.1	Tr	1.8	Tr	0.9	0.1
Pizza, cheese and tomato	51.0	25.2	23.0	2.2	0.6	0.6	0	0.9	0.1	Tr	0	1.4	0.2
Shepherd's pie, vegetable	71.7	15.8	14.0	1.4	0.5	0.4	0	0.6	0	0	0.4	2.4	0.8

Data from Holland et al. (1992). Reproduced with permission from HMSO.
NSPs, nonstarch polysaccharides (Englyst method; Englyst et al. 1999); Tr, trace.

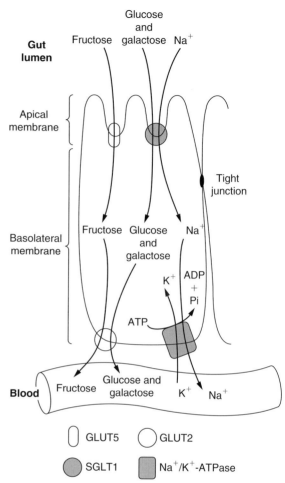

Figure 5.1 Sugar transporters on enterocytes, showing the transport of glucose and galactose across the apical membrane.

mutation in SGLT1 is responsible for the very rare glucose–galactose malabsorption syndrome, but such individuals absorb fructose well. In up to 60% of adults, the capacity for facilitated diffusion of fructose appears to be limited, resulting in symptoms of "intestinal distress" when challenged by consumption of 50 g fructose.

5.3 Glycemic carbohydrates

The rate of uptake of glucose (and other sugars) from the gut is determined by the rate of hydrolysis of oligosaccharides and polysaccharides that are susceptible to pancreatic and brush border enzymes. In addition to the primary structure of the polymers, many factors intrinsic to the ingested foods and to the consumer influence these rates, including:

- food factors
  - particle size
  - macrostructure and microstructure of food, especially whether cell walls are intact
  - amylose–amylopectin ratio of starches
  - lipid content of food
  - presence (or otherwise) of enzyme inhibitors
- consumer factors
  - degree of comminution in the mouth
  - rate of gastric emptying
  - small bowel transit time.

All three main sugars absorbed from the gut (glucose, galactose, and fructose) are transported via the portal vein to the liver (glucose concentrations in the portal vein after a meal can rise to almost 10 mM), but only glucose appears in significant concentrations in the peripheral circulation. Most of the galactose and fructose is removed during first pass through the liver via specific receptors on hepatocytes, so that the blood concentration of these sugars rarely exceeds 1 mM. Within the hepatocytes, galactose is converted to galactose-1-phosphate by the enzyme galactokinase and then to glucose-1-phosphate in three further steps. Fructose is also phosphorylated in hepatocytes (by fructokinase) to fructose-1-phosphate, which is subsequently split by aldolase B to yield one molecule of each of the glycolytic intermediates dihydroxyacetone phosphate and glyceraldehyde. Although the liver removes some glucose, using the bidirectional transporter GLUT2, most is transported in the peripheral circulation for utilization by muscle, adipose, and other tissues.

Metabolic utilization of carbohydrate

Peripheral tissues utilize glucose and the above-mentioned intermediates from fructose and galactose via glycolysis and the citric acid or Krebs cycle pathways. Glycolysis, a sequence of reactions in which glucose is converted to pyruvate, with concomitant production of ATP, is the prelude to the citric acid cycle and electron transport chain, which together release the energy contained in glucose. Under aerobic conditions pyruvate enters mitochondria, where it is completely oxidized to carbon dioxide and water. If the supply of oxygen is limited, as in actively contracting muscle, pyruvate is converted to lactate. Therefore,

complete oxidation of glucose to carbon dioxide and water occurs under aerobic conditions through the reactions of the glycolytic pathway (in the cell's cytoplasm), the Krebs cycle, and oxidative phosphorylation (in the mitochondrion). The overall reaction can be summarized stoichiometrically as:

$$C_6H_{12}O_6 + 6O_2 \rightarrow 6CO_2 + 6H_2O$$

Approximately 40% of the free energy (ΔG) released by this transformation is captured by the production of ATP (38 moles of ATP per mole of glucose oxidized), which is used for a wide variety of purposes, including powering muscle contraction, transporting substances across membranes against a concentration gradient, and synthesis of cell macromolecules. The remainder of the free energy is released as heat.

When the demand for oxygen exceeds supply, as in muscle during intense exercise, anaerobic glycolysis produces lactic acid as a major end-product. The relative lack of oxygen means that oxidative phosphorylation cannot keep up with the supply of reduced dinucleotides and, for glycolysis to proceed, NADH must be recycled back to NAD$^+$. This is achieved by the reaction:

$$\text{Pyruvate} + \text{NADH} + \text{H}^+ \rightarrow \text{Lactate} + \text{NAD}^+$$

which is catalyzed by the enzyme lactate dehydrogenase. Anaerobic glycolysis provides some or all of the ATP needs for some cells and tissues; for example, erythrocytes, white blood cells, lymphocytes, the kidney medulla, and eye tissues. The lactate released from tissues undergoing anaerobic glycolysis is taken up by other tissues that have a high number of mitochondria per cell, such as heart muscle, in which the lactate is converted back to pyruvate and then enters the Krebs cycle via acetyl coenzyme A.

In hepatic and muscle cells some glucose is converted to glycogen in the glycogenesis pathway. Glycogen is a readily mobilized storage form of glucose residues linked with α-1,4-glycosidic bonds into a large, branched polymer. Glycogen is a reservoir of glucose for strenuous muscle activity and its synthesis and degradation are important for the regulation of blood glucose concentrations.

Regulation of blood glucose concentration

The exocrine pancreas (and other tissues) is primed to expect a rise in blood glucose concentration by peptide hormones such as gastric inhibitory peptide

(GIP) that are secreted from enteroendocrine cells within the mucosa of the small bowel. As the glucose concentration in blood rises above 5 mM after a meal, these peptide hormones amplify the response of the β-cells of the endocrine pancreas, resulting in the discharge of the hormone insulin from secretory granules which fuse with the cell membrane. Insulin has several effects on metabolism, including facilitating the transport, by GLUT4, of glucose into adipocytes and muscle cells.

In healthy people, blood glucose concentration (glycemia) is homeostatically controlled within a fairly narrow range. It seldom falls below about 5 mM, even after a prolonged fast, and returns to this value within a couple of hours of a meal. In the absence of uptake from the gut (the postabsorptive state), about 8 g glucose per hour is provided for those tissues with an obligatory demand for glucose – namely, the brain, red blood cells, mammary gland, and testis – by breakdown of stores of glycogen in the liver and muscle and by gluconeogenesis. The brain of an adult has a glucose requirement of about 120 g/day. The amount readily available in glycogen approximates 190 g. In long periods of fasting and starvation glucose must be formed from noncarbohydrate sources by a process known as gluconeogenesis. Gluconeogenesis occurs in the liver (responsible for about 90% of gluconeogenesis) and kidney and is the synthesis of glucose from a range of substrates including pyruvate, lactate, glycerol, and amino acids. Amino acids are derived by catabolism of the body's proteins. All amino acids, with the exceptions of lysine and leucine, are glucogenic. Triacylglycerols (from adipose tissue) are catabolized to release glycerol. These gluconeogenic processes are triggered by a fall in blood glucose concentration below about 5 mM and are signaled to the tissues by the secretion of glucagon and the glucocorticoid hormones.

Diabetes and its consequences

Diabetes may be diagnosed as an exaggerated response in blood glucose concentration following ingestion of a fixed amount of glucose (glucose tolerance test). The most common forms of diabetes are type 1 diabetes (T1DM) and type 2 diabetes (T2DM). T1DM results from the autoimmune destruction of the β-cells of the endocrine pancreas (possibly following viral exposure), the consequence of which is insulin insufficiency. Control of blood glucose concentra-

tions in T1DM requires the exogenous supply of insulin by injection. Implanted insulin minipumps or pancreatic β-cells may offer alternative forms of treatment in the future. Symptoms of type 1 diabetes include the presence of glucose in urine, passage of large volumes of urine, body weight loss, and, in extreme cases, ketosis (excess production of acetone, acetoacetate, and β-hydroxybutyrate). Although there is good evidence of genetic predisposition to T2DM, expression of the disease is due mainly to lifestyle (excess energy intakes and low physical activity), resulting in obesity, especially when the extra fat is accumulated on the trunk. The early stages of T2DM are characterized by insulin insensitivity/resistance, i.e., failure of the tissues to produce a normal response to insulin release that can be seen as relatively wide swings in blood glucose concentrations following a carbohydrate-containing meal. Raised blood glucose concentration sustained for several years is believed to be fundamental to the spectrum of complications, including macrovascular (atherosclerosis) and microvascular diseases and problems with the kidneys (nephropathy), nerves (neuropathy), and eyes (retinopathy and cataract) experienced by diabetics.

Dietary management of blood glucose concentration

Glycemic index

As an aid to the dietary management of blood glucose concentrations in diabetics, Jenkins and colleagues (1981) introduced the concept of the glycemic index (GI), which provides a means of comparing quantitatively the blood glucose responses (determined directly by *in vivo* experiments) following ingestion of equivalent amounts of digestible carbohydrate from different foods. When a range of carbohydrate-containing foods was ranked according to their GI values, there was a strong linear relationship with the rapidly available glucose (RAG) from similar foods determined *in vitro* as the sum of free glucose, glucose from sucrose, and glucose released from starches over a 20 minute period of hydrolysis with a battery of enzymes under strictly controlled conditions (Englyst method; Englyst *et al.* 1999). This offers the possibility of assaying foods *in vitro* for their RAG content, which will be quicker and cheaper than the current approach based on GI measurements *in vivo*.

Studies with glucose and starches enriched with the stable isotope carbon-13 have demonstrated that glucose absorption from the gut following a meal continues for several hours after blood concentrations have returned to fasting levels. In this later postprandial period, insulin secretion is sufficient to ensure that the rate of glucose absorption is matched by the rate of glucose removal from the circulation. ^{13}C-Labeled substrates are being used increasingly to investigate the kinetics of digestion, absorption, and metabolic disposal of glucose and other sugars from a range of foods. When continued over several years, high rates of glucose absorption and the subsequent challenge to the capacity of the pancreatic β-cells to secrete insulin may be the primary determinants of insulin resistance and eventual pancreatic failure that contribute strongly to the etiology of diabetes and cardiovascular disease. Such kinetic studies are likely to be helpful in identifying foods with slower rates of intestinal hydrolysis – information that can be used in public health advice or in counseling of individuals.

Fructose

When glucose and fructose are available simultaneously after a meal containing sucrose, how does the body select which fuel to use first for oxidative purposes? This question has been resolved by experiments in which volunteers consumed, on two separate occasions, high-sucrose test meals which were identical except that one or other of the constituent monomeric sugars was ^{13}C-labeled in each meal. The volunteers blew into tubes at intervals after the meals to provide breath samples for measurement of enrichment of expired carbon dioxide with ^{13}C. The results showed that, after the high sucrose meal, fructose was oxidized much more rapidly and extensively than was glucose (Figure 5.2).

This rapid oxidation of fructose may be explained by the fact that, because it is phosphorylated in hepatocytes, it bypasses 6-phosphofructokinase, one of the key regulatory enzymes in glycolysis.

5.4 Nonglycemic carbohydrates

Carbohydrates that are not absorbed in the small intestine enter the large bowel, where they are partially or completely broken down by bacteria in the colon by a process called fermentation. McCance and Lawrence in 1929 were the first to classify carbohydrates as "available" and "unavailable." They realized that not all carbohydrates provide "carbohydrates for

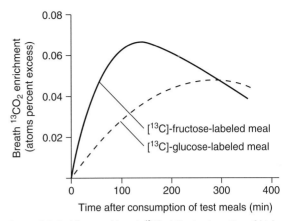

Figure 5.2 Enrichment of breath ^{13}CO$_2$ following ingestion of high-sucrose test meals labeled with [^{13}C]-fructose and [^{13}C]-glucose. (Redrawn from Daly *et al.*, 2000, with permission of the American Society for Nutrition.)

metabolism" to the body. They called these carbohydrates "unavailable." This was a very useful concept because it drew attention to the fact that some carbohydrate is not digested and absorbed in the small intestine, but rather reaches the large bowel where it is fermented. However, it is now realized that it is misleading to talk of carbohydrate as unavailable because some indigestible carbohydrate can provide the body with energy through fermentation in the colon. Thus, "unavailable carbohydrates" are not really unavailable. For this reason, it has been suggested by the Food and Agriculture Organization (FAO 1998) of the United Nations and World Health Organization that the term "nonglycemic carbohydrates" is more appropriate.

Nature of carbohydrates that enter the colon

Carbohydrates that enter the colon can be classified either physiologically or chemically. Neither of these classifications is entirely satisfactory because it is difficult to measure the physiologically indigestible carbohydrate and this varies in different people. Further, the chemical structure of carbohydrates does not always predict their physiological behavior.

Physiological classification of carbohydrates entering the colon

Carbohydrates enter the colon because (1) monosaccharide transporters do not exist in the intestinal mucosa or do not function at a high enough rate; (2)

the enzymes needed to digest the carbohydrates are not present in the small intestine; (3) the enzymes are present but cannot gain access to the carbohydrates; or (4) the enzymes do not digest the carbohydrates rapidly enough for them to be completely absorbed. In addition, a small amount of carbohydrate entering the colon consists of carbohydrate residues occurring on mucopolysaccharides (mucus) secreted by the small and large intestinal mucosal cells.

Some carbohydrates are always nonglycemic because the human species lacks the enzymes necessary for their digestion. However, a significant proportion (perhaps up to half) of all carbohydrates that escape digestion in the small intestine have a chemical structure which is such that they could potentially be digested or absorbed in the small intestine, but they are variably absorbed for various reasons, examples of which are given below.

First, some monosaccharides and sugar alcohols are only partially absorbed because of low affinity for intestinal transporters. Xylose is taken up by the glucose transporter, but is only partly absorbed because of a low affinity. Fructose is poorly absorbed on its own, but readily absorbed in the presence of glucose. The surface area of the small intestine available for absorption is reduced by diseases that cause atrophy of the intestinal mucosa, such as tropical sprue or celiac disease, or surgical resection of a portion of the intestine (e.g., for Crohn's disease). An increased rate of intestinal transit (e.g., high osmotic load in the small intestinal lumen from undigested sugars) reduces the time available for absorption to occur.

Second, some individuals have a low or absent intestinal lactase activity; thus, lactose is partly or completely nonabsorbed in these individuals. The availability of pancreatic amylase may be reduced in cystic fibrosis or in individuals whose pancreatic mass has been destroyed by, for example, recurrent pancreatitis.

Third, although starch (amylopectin or amylose) is potentially digested in the small intestine, if it is trapped inside intact cell walls or other plant cell structures, intestinal enzymes may not be able to gain access to it, and therefore it remains undigested. The digestibility of the carbohydrates in banana depends on the degree of ripeness. The starch in green banana is very indigestible, but, as the banana ripens, the starch is converted to digestible sugars.

Finally, there are many reasons why carbohydrates may not be digested rapidly enough to be completely absorbed. Some forms of retrograded or resistant starch, or foods with a large particle size, are digested so slowly that the time spent in the small intestine is not long enough for their complete digestion. Digestion of these carbohydrates can be altered by factors that affect transit time. The presence of osmotically active and unabsorbed molecules (such as unabsorbed sugars) will draw water into the intestine and speed the rate of transit. Substances that increase bulk, such as wheat bran, will have similar effects. Transit rate is slowed in old age and in the presence of viscous fibers. Drugs may increase or decrease the rate of transit. Certain disorders can also affect transit time, such as gastroparesis, a complication of type I diabetes.

Chemical classification of carbohydrates entering the colon

The chemical classification of carbohydrates entering the colon is as follows:

- *Monosaccharides*: all except for glucose, fructose, and galactose are partly or completely unabsorbed. Fructose in the absence of a source of glucose (mono-, di-, or polysaccharide) is partly unabsorbed.
- *Sugar alcohols*: all are partly or completely unabsorbed.
- *Disaccharides*: all except for maltose, sucrose, and lactose are unabsorbed. Lactose is completely or partly unabsorbed in individuals with low intestinal lactase activity.
- *Oligosaccharides*: all are unabsorbed except for maltodextrins.
- *Polysaccharides*: all nonstarch polysaccharides are unabsorbed.
- *Resistant starch.*

Amount of carbohydrate entering the colon

It is difficult to measure the amount of carbohydrate entering the human colon. However, it has been estimated that at least 30 g of carbohydrate is required to support the growth of the bacterial population in the colon of an individual on a typical Western diet producing about 100 g stool per day. About half of that amount will come from nonstarch polysaccharide (NSP, also known as dietary fiber), 1–2 g from indigestible oligosaccharides, and probably about 1–2 g from intestinal mucopolysaccharides. These components add up to only 18–20 g. Where does the other 10–12 g come from? It is believed to come from starch, because experiments in humans show that about 5–15% of the starch in foods enters the colon. Typical Western diets contain about 120–150 g starch per day, and, if 8% of this enters the colon, this will provide the additional 10–12 g carbohydrate. The amount of carbohydrate entering the colon, however, can be increased several-fold, up to 100 g/day or more, by changes in diet such as increased intake of NSP, non-digestible or partially digestible carbohydrates (ingredients in functional foods), total starch, resistant starch, or slowly digested, low-GI foods.

Resistant starch

Resistant starch is starch that escapes digestion in the small intestine and enters the colon. However, there is controversy over the amounts of resistant starch in foods because there is no universally accepted method for measuring it (different methods yield different results). The amount of resistant starch measured chemically is generally less than that observed to enter the colon (or leave the small intestine) in experiments in human volunteers.

In the 1970s and early 1980s it first became apparent that appreciable amounts of starch are not digested in the small bowel, from experiments showing that breath hydrogen increased after eating normal starchy foods. The only source of hydrogen gas in the human body is as a product of the anaerobic fermentation of carbohydrates by colonic bacteria (see below). If a person consumed a load of an absorbable sugar such as glucose, breath hydrogen did not go up. In contrast, if lactulose (an unabsorbed disaccharide of fructose and galactose) was consumed, breath hydrogen increased rapidly, and the area under the breath hydrogen curve over an 8–12 hour period was directly proportional to the amount of lactulose consumed. If subjects ate common starchy foods such as white bread or potato, breath hydrogen levels increased to an extent that suggested that 5–10% of the starch was fermented in the colon. Subsequently, other ways of measuring carbohydrate entering the colon were developed. In one technique, subjects swallowed a tube that was passed through the stomach and along to the end of the small intestine so that the material leaving the small intestine and about to enter the

colon could be sampled. Another method was to study people who have had their colons removed surgically and in whom the end of the ileum was sutured to a stoma in the body wall. In this way, the material leaving their small intestine could be collected quantitatively in a bag attached to their abdomen. With these methods, the amount of carbohydrate leaving the small intestine can be measured directly. These methods confirmed that a substantial amount of starch enters the colon.

The main forms of resistant starch (RS) are physically enclosed starch, for example within intact cell structures (known at RS_1); raw starch granules (RS_2); and retrograded amylose (RS_3). These kinds of starch can be identified chemically using methods developed by Englyst and colleagues (Englyst *et al.* 1996).

Dietary fiber

Major interest in dietary fiber began in the early 1970s with the proposal by Burkitt and Trowell (1975) that many Western diseases were due to a lack of fiber in the diet. However, the definition of dietary fiber has been, and continues to be, a source of scientific controversy. Indeed, two consecutive reports from the FAO (1997 and 1998) recommended that the term "dietary fiber" be phased out. Nevertheless, the term appears to be here to stay because it is accepted by consumers, the food industry, and governments.

A definition and method of measuring fiber is important for scientific studies and for food-labeling purposes. The student must be aware that the definitions and methods of measuring fiber have changed over time, and differ in different parts of the world. Knowledge of what is meant by the term "fiber" and what is included in the measurement is essential for proper interpretation of the scientific literature (but often is not given in the methods section of papers and reports).

Originally, Burkitt and Trowell (1975) defined fiber as the components of plant cell walls that are indigestible in the human small intestine. Later, the definition was expanded to include storage polysaccharides within plant cells (e.g., the gums in some legumes). Many different methods were developed to measure dietary fiber, but they measured different things. All of the methods start with the drying and grinding of the food and extraction of the fat using an organic solvent. If the remaining material is treated with strong acid, the chemical bonds in starch and many (but not all) polysaccharides will be broken down to release their component sugars. If these are filtered away, the residue is "crude fiber." For many years this was the way in which fiber was measured for food tables. However, acid hydrolysis breaks down many carbohydrates that would not be digested in the small intestine. So, in more modern methods, the food residue is digested with amylase to hydrolyze the starch to soluble sugars and oligosaccharides. The latter are removed by filtration or by centrifugation to leave a residue containing mainly dietary fiber, proteins, and inorganic materials.

The two main methods used to determine dietary fiber are chemical and gravimetric. In the chemical method (used in the UK), the residue is subjected to acid hydrolysis and the resultant sugars are measured colorimetrically, by gas chromatography or by high-performance liquid chromatography. The sum of all these sugars constitutes the NSP. The chemical method includes only carbohydrates in the NSP. In the gravimetric method (used in the USA and elsewhere), the residue is dried and weighed, and the amounts of protein and mineral materials present are subtracted (after separate analyses). The gravimetric method includes the NSP, plus other noncarbohydrate components such as lignin and waxes. Recently, all countries in Europe have recognized the gravimetric method as an approved method for measuring fiber in foods.

The main areas of disagreement now with respect to fiber are whether indigestible oligosaccharides and sugars and nonplant compounds should be included and whether the definition of fiber should include a physiological component. In Japan, fructooligosaccharides (FOSs) are classified as dietary fiber for food-labeling purposes. However, FOSs and similar compounds, being soluble in water, are not included in the dietary fiber methods, because they are filtered out along with the sugars resulting from the starch hydrolysis. Specific methods exist for FOSs and related compounds, and they could be included as fiber. Certain animal-derived compounds, such as chitin and chitosan, derived from the shells of shrimp and crabs, are indigestible, would be included in the gravimetric fiber analysis, and could be classified as fiber. Chitin has some physiological properties, such as cholesterol lowering, which are associated with dietary fiber. There are many other indigestible carbohydrate and noncarbohydrate compounds, both natural and artificial, that could be classified as "fiber" (e.g., polydextrose, sucrose polyester, styrofoam). Should these be included in dietary fiber? In favor of this is the argument that some of these materials have physiological properties associated with fiber, such as stool bulking, or effects on satiety or blood glucose and cholesterol. Against this is the feeling that dietary fiber should include only plant materials that are normally present in the diet. These are not easy issues and they have not been resolved.

Intakes of dietary fiber, oligosaccharides, and other indigestible sugars

Vegetarians tend to have higher fiber intakes than omnivores. The typical intake of dietary fiber in North America and northern and central Europe is about 15 g/day. In Scandinavia and Italy, fiber consumption is 20–30 g/day, whereas in African countries such as Uganda, Kenya, Malawi, and Nigeria intakes may be as high as 50 g/day or more. Naturally occurring oligosaccharides are consumed in legumes, onions, fennel, chicory, and similar foods. Intakes in Western countries are probably up to 2–4 g/day. Fructo- and galactooligosaccharides are now being added to certain "functional foods" in a number of countries, and intakes from such sources may increase substantially (up to 10–20 g/day). Many kinds of indigestible or partially digested carbohydrates are entering the food supply in dietetic, diabetic, or functional foods, including sugar alcohols (polyols, e.g., sorbitol, mannitol, lactitol), polydextrose, resistant starch, hydrogenated starch, and other chemically modified starches and carbohydrates. Thus, the total amount of carbohydrate entering the colon could become very substantial for people using these foods. Individually, these ingredients are generally recognized as safe, and evidence from populations consuming 50 g and more NSP per day suggests that the colon has the capacity to adapt to large increases in the load of carbohydrate. However, safe upper limits of intake are unknown and the health implications of an increased supply of a wide range of carbohydrates to the colon are currently based on inference rather than scientific data.

Fermentation in the colon

The colon contains a complex ecosystem consisting of over 400 known species of bacteria that exist in a symbiotic relationship with the host. The bacteria obtain the substrates that they require for growth from the host, and return to the host the by-products of their metabolism. The major substrate that the bacteria receive from the host is carbohydrate, mostly in the form of polysaccharides. They obtain nitrogen from urea (which diffuses into the colon from the blood) and undigested amino acids and proteins. Fermentation is the process by which microorganisms break down monosaccharides and amino acids to derive energy for their own metabolism. Fermentation reactions do not involve respiratory chains that use molecular oxygen or nitrate as terminal electron acceptors. Most of the fermentation in the human colon is anaerobic, i.e., it proceeds in the absence of a source of oxygen. Different bacteria use different substrates via different types of chemical reaction. However, as a summary of the overall process, fermentation converts carbohydrates to energy, plus various end-products, which include the gases carbon dioxide, hydrogen, and methane, and the SCFAs acetic (C2), propionic (C3), and butyric (C4) acids. Acetate, propionate, and butyrate appear in colonic contents in approximate molar ratios of 60:20:20, respectively. Most of the SCFAs produced are absorbed and provide energy for the body (Figure 5.3).

The roles of SCFAs in metabolism are discussed later in this chapter. Formic acid (C1) and minor amounts of longer chain SCFAs and branched-chain SCFAs may also be produced. In addition, lactic and succinic acids and ethanol or methanol may be intermediate or end-products depending on the conditions of the fermentation. For example, rapid fermentation in an environment with a low pH results in the accumulation of lactic and succinic acids.

The first step in fermentation is the breakdown of polysaccharides, oligosaccharides, and disaccharides to their monosaccharide subunits. This is achieved either by the secretion of hydrolytic enzymes by bacteria into the colonic lumen or, more commonly, by expression of such enzymes on the bacterial surface so that the products of hydrolysis are taken up directly by the organism producing the enzyme. To degrade the NSP of dietary fiber, the bacteria may need to attach themselves to the surface of the remnants of the plant cell walls or other particulate material.

Once the monosaccharide is internalized, the majority of carbohydrate-fermenting species in the colon use the glycolytic pathway to metabolize carbohydrate to pyruvate. This pathway results in the reduction of NAD^+ to NADH. Fermentation reactions are controlled by the need to maintain redox balance between reduced and oxidized forms of pyridine nucleotides. The regeneration of NAD^+ may be achieved in a number of different ways (Figure 5.4).

Electron sink products such as ethanol, lactate, hydrogen, and succinate are produced by some bacteria to regenerate oxidized pyridine nucleotides. These fermentation intermediates are subsequently fermented to SCFAs by other gut bacteria, and are important factors in maintaining species diversity in the ecosystem.

Fate of short-chain fatty acids

Colonic fermentation can be viewed as a way in which the human host can recover part of the energy of malabsorbed carbohydrates. The amount of energy recovered from fermentation depends on the fermentability of the carbohydrate (which can range from 0% to 100%) and the nature of the products of fermentation. On a typical Western diet, about 40–50% of the energy in carbohydrate that enters the colon is available to the human host as SCFAs. The rest of the energy is unavailable to the host, being lost as heat or unfermented carbohydrate or used to produce gases or for bacterial growth (Figure 5.5).

SCFAs are almost completely absorbed and, while some butyrate is oxidized by colonocytes (the epithelial cells lining the colon), most arrives at the liver via the portal vein. Propionate and butyrate are removed in first pass through the liver, but increased concentrations of acetate can be observed in peripheral blood several hours after consumption of indigestible but fermentable carbohydrates. These absorbed

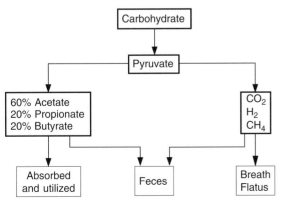

Figure 5.3 Overview of carbohydrate fermentation in the human colon.

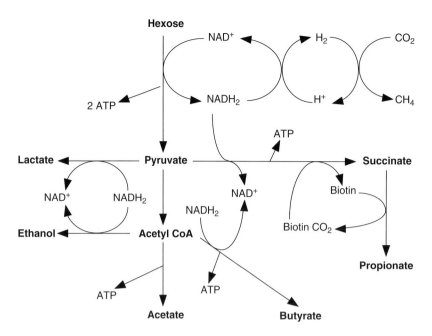

Figure 5.4 Summary of biochemical pathways used by the anaerobic bacteria in the colon. Acetyl CoA, acetyl coenzyme A.

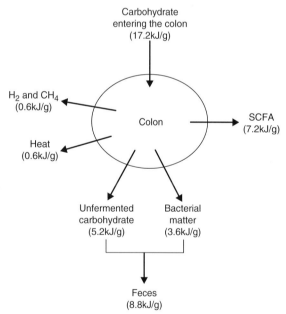

Figure 5.5 Quantitative fate of carbohydrate in the colon. SCFA, short-chain fatty acid.

SCFAs are readily oxidized and contribute modestly (up to 10%) to the body's energy supply.

There is considerable interest in the possible effects of individual SCFAs on the health of the colon and the whole body. The strongest evidence to date is for an anticancer effect of butyrate, which may be due to the ability of butyrate to induce differentiation and apoptosis (programmed cell death) of colon cancer cells. There is some support for the hypothesis that propionate may help to reduce the risk of cardiovascular disease by lowering blood cholesterol concentration and/or by an effect on hemostasis, but the evidence so far is not conclusive.

5.5 Carbohydrates and dental caries

The resident bacteria in the mouth ferment carbohydrates to yield acidic end-products (mainly lactic acid but also some formic, acetic, and propionic acids), which result in a drop in dental plaque pH. When the pH falls below 5.5, the dental enamel dissolves in the plaque fluid and repeated exposure to periods of very low pH can lead to caries. Not all carbohydrates are equally cariogenic. The sugars found commonly in human foods, e.g., sucrose, fructose, glucose, and maltose, are all readily fermented by bacteria in the mouth. Lactose, galactose, and starches are less cariogenic, while sugar alcohols such as xylitol (used as a sweetener in some confectionery and chewing gums) are noncariogenic. Eating sugars with meals reduces the risk of caries, as does the consumption of cheese, which provides phosphates to prevent demineralization and to encourage demineralization of the enamel. Fluoride ingestion in foods and drinking water or topical application via toothpastes and mouth rinses prevents dental caries. Too much fluoride in drinking water can cause fluorosis, which damages the skeleton and teeth. The optimum concentration of fluoride in temperate areas of the world is 1 mg/l, falling to 0.6 mg/l in tropical climates where fluid intake is likely to be greater.

5.6 Perspectives on the future

The carbohydrate structure and amounts in many foods and ingredients can be manipulated to achieve specific physicochemical properties of benefit for food structure and organoleptic effects and to produce a diverse range of physiological effects. It can be expected that many functional foods of the future will contain such specially selected or modified carbohydrates, but the metabolic and health consequences of these carbohydrates should be examined in more detail before health claims can be justified.

Future research on carbohydrate nutrition should also focus on the physiological and biochemical (metabolic) effects of the SCFAs produced from nonglycemic carbohydrates.

To provide a sound evidence base for recommendations for intakes of specific carbohydrates, the relationships between intakes of different types and quantities of carbohydrate with health and disease, for example during transition of traditional people and consequent lowering of intakes, should be a fruitful area for research.

References

Burkitt DP, Trowell HC. *Refined Carbohydrate Foods and Disease.* Academic Press, London, 1975.

Englyst KN, Englyst HN, Hudson GL *et al.* Rapidly available glucose in foods: an in vitro measurement that reflects the glycemic response. *Amer J Clin Nutr* 1999; **69**: 448–454.

Englyst HN, Kingman SM, Hudson GJ *et al.* Measurement of resistant starch in vitro and in vivo. *Br J Nutr* 1996; **75**: 749–755.

Food and Agriculture Organization of the United Nations. FAO food and nutrition paper 66. Carbohydrates in human nutrition. Report of an FAO/WHO Expert Consultation on Carbohydrates, 14–18 April, 1997, Rome, Italy. FAO, Rome, 1998.

Holland B, Unwin ID, Buss DH. *Vegetable Dishes.* Second supplement to McCance and Widdowson's *The Composition of Foods*, 5th edn. Cambridge: Royal Society of Chemistry, 1992.

Jenkins DJA, Wolever TMS, Taylor RH *et al.* Glycemic index of foods: a physiological basis for carbohydrate exchange. *Am J Clin Nutr* 1981;**34**:362–366.

Mccance RA, Lawrence RD. The carbohydrate content of foods. *MRC Special Report Series* 1929, No. 135.

Further reading

Asp N-G. Development of dietary fibre methodology. In: McCleary BV, Prosky L, eds. *Advanced Dietary Fibre Technology*. Blackwell Science, Oxford, 2001: 77–88.

Brody T. *Nutritional Biochemistry*, 2nd edn. Academic Press, San Diego, CA, 1999.

Daly ME, Vale C, Walker M *et al.* Acute fuel selection in response to high-sucrose and high-starch meals in healthy men. *Am J Clin Nutr* 2000; **71**: 1516–1524.

Johnson LR. *Gastrointestinal Physiology*, 5th edn. Mosby, St Louis, MO, 1997.

Rugg-Gunn AJ. *Nutrition and Dental Health.* Oxford University Press, Oxford, 1993.

Wolever TMS. *The Glycaemic Index: A Physiological Classification of Dietary Carbohydrate.* CABI, Wallingford, 2006.

6
Nutrition and Metabolism of Lipids

Bruce A Griffin and Stephen C Cunnane

Key messages

- Lipids are organic compounds composed of a carbon skeleton with hydrogen and oxygen substitutions. The most abundant lipids are sterols or esters of fatty acids with various alcohols such as glycerol and cholesterol.
- Fatty acids are the densest dietary source of energy, but lipids also have important structural roles in membranes. The processes controlling the synthesis, modification, and degradation of fatty acids contribute to the fatty acid profile of membrane and storage lipids.
- By enhancing the taste of cooked foods, some dietary lipids are potentially significant risk factors for obesity and other chronic, degenerative diseases that influence human morbidity and mortality.

- Dietary lipids (fats) are emulsified, lipolyzed (hydrolyzed), and solubilized in the upper small gut before they are absorbed in the ileum, entering enterocytes with the help of fatty acid-binding proteins.
- Lipids are precursors to hormones such as steroids and eicosanoids, and dietary lipids are carriers for fat-soluble vitamins.
- Lipids are transported in the blood circulation as lipoprotein particles: the chylomicrons, very low-density, low-density, and high-density lipoproteins.
- Some polyunsaturated fatty acids are vitamin like because they cannot be synthesized *de novo* (linoleate, α-linolenate).

6.1 Introduction: the history of lipids in human nutrition

The term "lipid" was introduced by Bloor in 1943, by which time the existence of cholesterol had been known for nearly 200 years and individual fats for 130 years. Cholesterol was named "cholesterine" (Greek for bile-solid) by Chevreul in 1816, although he did not discover it. Cholesterol's association with aortic plaques dates at least to Vogel's work in 1843. Chevreul isolated a mixture of 16- to 18-carbon saturated fatty acids in 1813 that was called margarine because he thought it was a single 17-carbon fatty acid, margarate. The mixed triacylglycerol (TAG) of palmitate (16:0) and stearate (18:0) was also called margarine, whereas the triglyceride of oleate, stearate, and palmitate became known as oleomargarine. Phospholipids were discovered by Thudicum, who isolated and named sphingosine in 1884 and also lecithin (phosphatidylcholine) and kephalin (phosphatidylethanolamine). The difference in polarity across phospholipids is a key attribute of these molecules and was termed "amphipathic" by Hartley in 1936 and renamed "amphiphilic" by Winsor in 1948.

The first understanding of how fat was absorbed emerged in 1879 when Munk studied fat emulsions and showed that lymph contained TAG after a fatty meal, and even after a meal not containing TAG. In 1905, Knoop deduced that fatty acid β-oxidation probably occurred by stepwise removal of two carbons from the fatty acid. The probable role of two carbon units as building blocks in the synthesis of fatty acids was recognized by Raper in 1907, but it took until the 1940s for Schoenheimer, Rittenberg, Bloch, and others to confirm this, using tracers such as deuterated water and carbon-13. The late 1940s was a seminal period in our understanding of how fatty acid oxidation occurs. Green and colleagues discovered that ketones were fatty acid oxidation products, and Lehninger demonstrated the role of mitochondria as the cellular site of fatty acid oxidation. Microsomal desaturases were shown to introduce an unsaturated bond into long-chain fatty acids by Bloomfield and Bloch in 1960.

In 1929, Mildred and George Burr discovered that the absence of fat in a diet otherwise believed to contain all essential nutrients impaired growth and caused hair loss and scaling of the skin of rats. This led to the isolation of the two primary "essential" polyunsaturated fatty acids, linoleate (18:2n-6) and α-linolenate (18:3n-3). The prostaglandins are a subclass of eicosanoids that were discovered in the early 1930s by Von Euler, who mistakenly believed that they originated from the prostate gland. The link between the eicosanoids and polyunsaturates, principally arachidonate, was established in the 1960s.

6.2 Terminology of dietary fats

Lipids

Like other organic compounds, all lipids are composed of a carbon skeleton with hydrogen and oxygen substitutions. Nitrogen, sulfur, and phosphorus are also present in some lipids. Water insolubility is a key but not absolute characteristic distinguishing most lipids from proteins and carbohydrates. There are some exceptions to this general rule, since short- to medium-chain fatty acids, soaps, and some complex lipids are soluble in water. Hence, solubility in a "lipid solvent" such as ether, chloroform, benzene, or acetone is a common but circular definition of lipids.

There are four categories of lipids, as classified by Bloor: simple, compound (complex), derived, and miscellaneous (Table 6.1). Simple lipids are esters of fatty acids with various alcohols such as glycerol or cholesterol. They include triacylglycerols (TAG = neutral fats and oils), waxes, cholesteryl esters, and vitamin A and D esters. Compound lipids are esters of fatty acids in combination with both alcohols and other groups. They include phospholipids, glycolipids, cerebrosides, sulfolipids, lipoproteins, and lipopolysaccharides. Derived lipids are hydrolysis products of simple or compound lipids, including fatty acids, monoacylglycerols and diacylglycerols, straight-chain and ring-containing alcohols, sterols, and steroids. Miscellaneous lipids include some wax lipids, carotenoids, squalene, and vitamins E and K.

Saturated and unsaturated fatty acids

The main components of dietary fat or lipids are fatty acids varying in length from one to more than 30 carbons. They are carboxylic acids with the structure

Table 6.1 Classification of lipids

Simple lipids (fatty acids esterified with alcohols)	Fats (fatty acids esterified with glycerol)
	Waxes (true waxes, sterol esters, vitamin A and D esters)
Complex lipids (fatty acids esterified with alcohols plus other groups)	Phospholipids (contain phosphoric acid and, usually, a nitrogenous base)
	Glycolipids (lipids containing a carbohydrate and nitrogen but no phosphate and no glycerol)
	Sulfolipids (lipids containing a sulfur group)
	Lipoproteins (lipids attached to plasma or other proteins)
	Lipopolysaccharides (lipids attached to polysaccharides)
Derived lipids (obtained by hydrolysis of simple or complex lipids)	Fatty acids (saturated, monounsaturated, or polyunsaturated)
	Monoacylglycerols and diacylglycerols
	Alcohols (include sterols, steroids, vitamin D, vitamin A)
Miscellaneous lipids	Straight-chain hydrocarbons
	Carotenoids
	Squalene
	Vitamins E and K

RCOOH, where R is hydrogen in formic acid, CH_3 in acetic acid, or else a chain of one to over 30 CH_2 groups terminated by a CH_3 group. The various names for individual fatty acids (common, official) and their abbreviations are complicated, and the use of one or other form is somewhat arbitrary. The basic rule for the abbreviations is that there are three parts: number of carbons, number of double bonds, and position of the first double bond. Thus, the common dietary saturated fatty acid palmitate is 16:0 because it has 16 carbons and no double bonds. The common dietary polyunsaturated fatty acid linoleate is 18:2n-6 because it has 18 carbons, two double bonds, and the first double bond is at the sixth carbon from the methyl-terminal (n-6). Beyond six carbons in length, most fatty acids have an even number of carbons (Table 6.2). Older fatty acid terminology referring to saturated or unsaturated carbons in lipids that still occasionally appears includes: aliphatic (a saturated carbon), olefinic (an unsaturated carbon), allylic (a saturated carbon adjacent to an unsaturated carbon), and doubly allylic carbon (a saturated carbon situated between two unsaturated carbons).

Table 6.2 Nomenclature of common fatty acids

Saturated	Monounsaturated	Polyunsaturated
Formic (1:0)	Lauroleic (12:1n-3)	Linoleic (18:2n-6)
Acetic (2:0)	Myristoleic (14:1n-5)	γ-Linolenic (18:3n-6)
Propionic (3:0)	Palmitoleic (16:1n-7)	Dihomo-γ-linolenic (20:3n-6)
Butyric (4:0)	Oleic (18:1n-9)	Arachidonic (20:4n-6)
Valeric (5:0)	Elaidic (trans-18:1n-9)	Adrenic (22:4n-6)
Caproic (6:0)	Vaccenic (18:1n-7)	n-6 Docosapentaenoic (22:5n1-6)
Caprylic (8:0)	Petroselinic (18:1n-12)	α-Linolenic (18:3n-3)
Capric (10:0)	Gadoleic (20:1n-11)	Stearidonic (18:4n-3)
Lauric (12:0)	Gondoic (20:1n-9)	Eicosapentaenoic (20:5n-3)
Myristic (14:0)	Euricic (22:1n-9)	n-3 Docosapentaenoic (22:5n-3)
Palmitic (16:0)	Nervonic (24:1n-9)	Docosahexaenoic (22:6n-3)
Margeric (17:0)		
Stearic (18:0)		
Arachidic (20:0)		
Behenic (22:0)		
Lignoceric (24:0)		

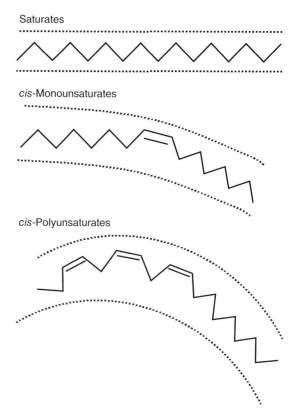

Saturates

cis-Monounsaturates

cis-Polyunsaturates

Figure 6.1 Stick models illustrating the basic structural differences between saturated, *cis*-monounsaturated, and *cis*-polyunsaturated fatty acids. As shown in two dimensions, the increasing curvature caused by inserting one or more double bonds increases the area occupied by the fatty acid. The physical area occupied by unsaturated fatty acids is further accentuated in three dimensions because esterified fatty acids rotate around the anchored terminal.

Lengthening of the chain and the introduction of additional double bonds beyond the first one occur from the carboxyl-terminal. The presence of one or more double bonds in a fatty acid defines it as "unsaturated," compared with a saturated fatty acid which contains no double bonds. A saturated fatty acid generally occupies less space than an equivalent chain length unsaturated fatty acid (Figure 6.1). Double bonds allow for isomerization or different orientation (*cis* or *trans*) of the adjoining carbons across the double bond (Figure 6.2). In longer chain fatty acids, double bonds can also be at different positions in the molecule. Hence, unsaturation introduces a large amount of structural variety in fatty acids and the resulting lipids. Further details about the features of the different families of fatty acids are given in Sections 6.6 and 6.8.

Short- and medium-chain fatty acids

Short-chain fatty acids (less than eight carbons) are water soluble. Except in milk lipids, they are not commonly esterified into body lipids. Short-chain fatty acids are found primarily in dietary prod-

ucts containing ruminant milk fat. Hence, although they are produced in relatively large quantities from the fermentation of undigested carbohydrate in the colon, as such, they do not become part of the body lipid pools. Medium-chain fatty acids (8–14 carbons) arise as intermediates in the synthesis of long-chain fatty acids or by the consumption of coconut oil or medium-chain TAG derived from it. Like short-chain fatty acids, medium-chain fatty acids are present in milk but they are also rarely esterified into body lipids, except when consumed in large amounts in clinical situations requiring alternative energy sources. Medium-chain fatty acids (8–14 carbons) are rare in the diet except for coconut and milk fat.

cis-Monounsaturates

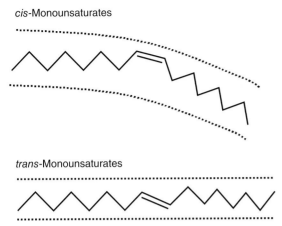

trans-Monounsaturates

Figure 6.2 Stick models comparing a *cis*- with a *trans*-unsaturated fatty acid. A *cis*-unsaturated double bond creates a U-shaped space and confers curvature to the molecule because, relative to the longitudinal axis of the fatty acid, the two hydrogens at the double bond are on the same side of the molecule. A *trans*-unsaturated double bond does not confer curvature to the molecule because the hydrogens are on opposite sides of the double bond. A *trans*-double bond therefore tends to give the fatty acid physicochemical properties more like that of a saturated fatty acid.

Long-chain saturated and monounsaturated fatty acids

Long-chain fatty acids (>14 carbons) are the main constituents of dietary fat. The most common saturated fatty acids in the body are palmitate and stearate. They originate from three sources: directly from the diet, by complete synthesis from acetyl-coenzyme A (CoA), or by lengthening (chain elongation) of a pre-existing shorter-chain fatty acid. Hence, dietary or newly synthesized palmitate can be elongated within the body to form stearate and on to arachidate (20:0), behenate (22:0), and lignocerate (24:0). In practice, little stearate present in the human body appears to be derived by chain elongation of pre-existing palmitate. In humans, saturates longer than 24 carbons do exist but usually arise only during genetic defects in fatty acid oxidation, as will be discussed later.

Palmitate and stearate are important membrane constituents, being found in most tissue phospholipids at 20–40% of the total fatty acid profile. Brain membranes contain 20- to 24-carbon saturates that, like palmitate and stearate, are synthesized within the brain and have little or no access to the brain from the circulation. The normal membrane content of long-chain saturates can probably be sustained without a dietary source of these fatty acids. Compared with all other classes of dietary fatty acid, especially monounsaturated or polyunsaturated fatty acids, excess intake or synthesis of long-chain saturates is associated with an increased risk of cardiovascular disease.

The most common long-chain *cis*-monounsaturated fatty acids in diet and in the body are oleate (18:1n-9) and palmitoleate (16:1n-7), with the former predominating by far in both the body's storage and membrane lipids. As with stearate, most oleate in the human body appears to be of dietary origin. Hence, although humans have the capacity to desaturate stearate to oleate, dietary oleate is probably the dominant source of oleate in the body. Only plants can further desaturate oleate to linoleate and again to α-linolenate. As with saturates of >18 carbons in length, 20-, 22-, and 24-carbon monounsaturates derived from oleate are present in specialized membranes such as myelin.

Polyunsaturated fatty acids (PUFAs)

Linoleate and α-linolenate are the primary dietary *cis*-polyunsaturated fatty acids in most diets. Neither can be synthesized *de novo* (from acetate) in animals so are 'essential' fatty acids. They can be made by chain elongation from the two respective 16-carbon precursors, hexadecadienoate (16:2n-6) and hexadecatrienoate (16:3n-3), which are found in common edible green plants at up to 13% of total fatty acids. Hence, significant consumption of green vegetables will provide 16-carbon polyunsaturates that contribute to the total available linoleate and α-linolenate.

Linoleate is the predominant polyunsaturated fatty acid in the body, commonly accounting for 12–15% of adipose tissue fatty acids. In the body's lean tissues there are at least three polyunsaturates present in amounts >5% of the fatty acid profile (linoleate, arachidonate, docosahexaenoate). In addition, at least two other biologically active polyunsaturates are present in body lipids [dihomo-γ-linolenate (20:3n-6) and eicosapentaenoate (20:5n-3)], although usually in amounts between 1% and 3% of total fatty acids. Marine fish are the richest source of 20- to 22-carbon polyunsaturates. α-Linolenate and its precursor, hexadecatrienoate (16:3n-3), are the only n-3 polyunsaturates in common terrestrial plants.

Hydrogenated and conjugated fatty acid isomers

The introduction of unsaturation with one double bond creates the possibility of both positional and geometric isomers in fatty acids. Among long-chain unsaturated fatty acids, positional isomers exist because the double bond can be introduced into several different locations, i.e., 18:1n-7, 18:1n-9, 18:1n-11, etc. Geometric isomers exist because the two remaining hydrogens at each double bond can be opposite each other (*trans*) or on the same side of the molecule (*cis*; Figure 6.2). Thus, there is *cis*-18:1n-9 (oleate) and *trans*-18:1n-9 (elaidate), and so on for all unsaturated fatty acids, with the combinations mounting exponentially as the number of double bonds increases.

Trans isomers of monounsaturated or polyunsaturated fatty acids arise primarily from partial hydrogenation during food processing of oils, but some also occur naturally in ruminants. The number of *trans* isomers increases with the number of double bonds, so there is only one *trans* isomer of oleate but there are three *trans* isomers of linoleate and seven of α-linolenate. Virtually all naturally occurring polyunsaturated fatty acids have double bonds that are methylene interrupted, i.e., have a CH_2 group between the two double bonds. However, methylene interruption between double bonds can be lost, again, through food processing, and the bonds moved one carbon closer together, becoming conjugated. Thus, the double bonds in linoleate are at the 9–10 and 11–12 carbons, but in conjugated linoleate they are at the 9–10 carbons and the 11–12 carbons. Some degree of further desaturation and chain elongation can occur in conjugated fatty acids, but much less than with methylene-interrupted polyunsaturates. Thus, conjugated linoleate is the main conjugated fatty acid that has attracted considerable attention with respect to its potential role in nutritional health.

Fats and oils

Fats are esters of fatty acids with glycerol (Table 6.1). They usually occur as triesters or triacylglycerols (TAGs), although monoacylglycerols and diacylglycerols occur during fat digestion and are used in food processing. Most common dietary fats contain a mixture of 16- to 18-carbon saturated and unsaturated fatty acids. By convention, fats that are liquid at room temperature are called oils, a feature arising from their lower proportion of saturated (straight-chain) and higher proportion of unsaturated (bent-chain) fatty acids. Unsaturated fatty acids usually have a lower melting point; this facilitates liquefaction of the fats of which they are a component. TAGs of animal origin are commonly fats, whereas those of fish or plant origin are usually oils. Animal fats and fish oils frequently contain cholesterol, whereas plant oils do not contain cholesterol but usually contain other "phyto" sterols.

TAGs are primarily used as fuels, so dietary fats (mostly TAGs) are commonly associated with energy metabolism rather than with structural lipids found in membranes. However, membrane lipids as well as TAGs are extracted with lipid solvents used to determine the fat content of foods, tissues, or plant material. Hence, because organs such as brain are rich in membrane phospholipids, when the total lipids are extracted to determine the organ's chemical composition, these organs are said to have a certain fat content. On a chemical basis this is true, but this description often misconstrues the nature of the lipid because the brain in particular contains virtually no TAG.

Phospholipids

Phospholipids contain two nonpolar, hydrophobic acyl tail groups and a single functional head group that is polar and hydrophilic. Hence, they are relatively balanced amphiphilic lipids and, in this capacity, are crucial components of biological membranes. The head groups contain phosphorus and amino acids (choline, serine, ethanolamine), sugars (inositol), or an alcohol (glycerol). Phosphatidylcholine (lecithin) is the most abundant phospholipid in animal tissues but phosphatidylglycerols (glycosides) predominate in plant lipids. Phospholipids containing a fatty acid amide are sphingolipids. Various phospholipases can hydrolyze the acyl groups or head group during digestion or metabolism.

One of the outstanding characteristics that make phospholipids suitable as major constituents of biological membranes is that, in water, they naturally aggregate into spherical or rod-like liposomes or vesicles, with the hydrophilic portion facing outwards and the hydrophobic portion facing inwards (Figure 6.3). Changing the constituent acyl groups from saturated to polyunsaturated changes the fluidity of these aggregates because of the greater amount of space

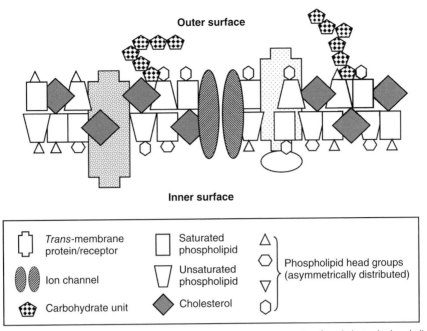

Figure 6.3 Simplified schematic view of a membrane bilayer. The main components are proteins, free cholesterol, phospholipids, and carbohydrates. There are many different proteins with a myriad of shapes, membrane distribution, and functions, of which three are illustrated. Membrane phospholipids principally help to create the bilayer. They have four types of "head groups" (choline, ethanolamine, serine, and inositol) that are located at or near the membrane's two surfaces. The two fatty acids in phospholipids are mixtures of 16- to 22-carbon saturates, monounsaturates, and polyunsaturates in all combinations, with those rich in unsaturated fatty acids occupying more space; hence, their trapezoid shape compared with the narrower, rectangular shape of the more saturated phospholipids. Free cholesterol represents 30–40% of the lipid in most membranes. The many different carbohydrates are on the membrane's surfaces and are bound to lipids and/or proteins in the membrane.

occupied by more unsaturated fatty acids. At interfaces between non-miscible polar and non-polar solvents, phospholipids also form a film or monolayer.

Sterols

The main sterol of importance in human nutrition is cholesterol. It has multiple roles including being:

- a vital component of biological membranes
- a precursor to bile salts used in fat digestion
- a precursor to steroid hormones.

Sterols are secondary alcohols belonging to the poly-isoprenoids or terpinoids (terpenes), which have a common precursor, isopentenyl diphosphate. Other members of the terpinoids include squalene, carotenoids, and dolichols. Bacteria appear to be the only life forms not containing cholesterol. Sterols have a common cyclopentano(a)perhydrophenanthrene skeleton with different substitutions giving rise to the multiple sterols and steroids.

6.3 Lipids as components of the diet

Food or dietary sources of lipids are listed in Table 6.3. Cholesterol is found only in animal lipids, while a variety of other phytosterols occur in plants. Soyabeans, leafy plants, and lean animal meat are rich in dietary phospholipids. Animal fat and plant oils from seeds or nuts are rich in TAG.

The leafy and fruit components of plants contain phospholipids and sterols, whereas seeds contain triglycerides. With rare exceptions such as flaxseed (linseed), edible green leaves are proportionally much richer in α-linolenate than are seeds. Seed oils are usually rich in either linoleate or oleate. Common plant sterols include β-sitosterol, β-sitostanol, and campesterol. Foods enriched with esters of plant sterols are used widely to lower blood cholesterol via the inhibition of cholesterol absorption in the gut.

Phospholipids and cholesterol constitute the majority of lipids in tissues (gut, kidney, brain,

Table 6.3 Common food sources of lipids

Cholesterol	Eggs, shellfish, organ meats
Phytosterols	Soya products, olive oil
Short-chain fatty acids (1–6 carbons)	Milk fat
Medium-chain fatty acids (8–14 carbons)	Milk fat, coconut fat
Long-chain fatty acids (16–20 carbons)	Saturates: animal fat, shortening, butter, palm oil, peanuts
	Monounsaturates: olive, canola oils
	Linoleate: sunflower, safflower, corn oils, soyabean
	α-Linolenate: flaxseed oil, canola, soyabean oil, walnuts
	γ-Linolenate: evening primrose oil, borage oil, blackcurrant seed oil
	Stearidonate: blackcurrant seed oil
	Arachidonate: lean meat and organ lipids
	Eicosapentaenoate: marine cold-water fish, shellfish, some seaweeds
	Docosahexaenoate: marine cold-water fish, shellfish
	Trans fatty acids: partially hydrogenated fats and oils

skeletal muscle, etc.) of lean, undomesticated animals. By contrast, in domesticated animals, TAGs or non-membrane lipids present in subcutaneous and intramuscular adipose tissue deposits are the dominant form of lipid on a weight basis. This is because domestication usually involves rearing animals with minimal exercise and on higher energy intakes, leading to more subcutaneous and visceral TAG obtained through both fat synthesis and deposition of dietary fat. Animal meat lipids are the main dietary source of arachidonate (20:4n-6), although it can also be obtained from tropical marine fish.

Lipoproteins are the main form of lipid in the blood (see Section 6.5). Like lipoproteins, milk lipids also occur as globules consisting of a combination of a mainly TAG core surrounded by a membrane containing proteins, cholesterol, and phospholipids.

Phospholipids and cholesterol constitute the main lipids of undomesticated edible fish, which usually have low amounts of TAG or stored body fat. As in domesticated animals, it is likely that subcutaneous and intramuscular fat deposits of TAG will increase in commercially farmed fish. Cold-water marine fish are the main dietary source of the long-chain n-3 (omega-3) polyunsaturates eicosapentaenoate (20:5n-3), and docosahexaenoate (22:6n-3), but the former

is also found in several types of edible seaweed. Tropical fish generally have higher arachidonate than do cold-water fish.

Partial hydrogenation is a common feature of unsaturated fatty acids in processed foods. Complete hydrogenation makes fats very hard and is more expensive than partial hydrogenation. Depending on the applications and the source of the original oil or fat, partial hydrogenation is an economical way to control the properties of fats or oils used in food production. Dietary diacylglycerols and monoacyl-glycerols are used by the food industry for emulsification of water- and oil-based components in foods such as ice cream and mayonnaise.

6.4 Digestion, absorption, and transport of dietary fat

The average daily intake of fat in a Western diet ranges between 50 and 100 g and provides between 35% and 40% of total energy. It consists mainly of TAG, which forms the principal component of visible oils and fats, and minor quantities of phospholipids and cholesterol esters (CEs). The physical properties of dietary fat, such as their hardness at room temperature (melting point) and subsequent metabolic properties once in the body, are determined by the number of double bonds in their constituent fatty acids (degree of saturation or unsaturation) and length of the fatty acid carbon chain (see Tables 6.2 and 6.3). As mentioned in Section 6.2, fats that are solid at room temperature tend to consist of long-chain saturated fats (>14 carbons, no double bonds), whereas oils consist of long-chain unsaturated fats with several double bonds. It has become conventional to refer to dietary fats as "lipids" once they have been absorbed into the body via the small intestine, although it is not incorrect to refer to dietary fat as "dietary lipid."

Reception, emulsification, lipolysis, solubilization, and absorption

The digestion of dietary fat takes place in three phases, known as the gastric, duodenal, and ilial phases. These involve crude emulsification in the stomach, lipolytic breakdown by lipases and solubilization with bile salts in the duodenum and, finally, absorption into the epithelial cells or enterocytes lining the walls of the small intestine or ileum. Digestion may actually be initiated in the mouth under the influence of a lingual lipase secreted by the palate, although its contribution to lipolysis in adults is questionable and thought to be more important in young suckling infants, in which its release is stimulated by suckling and the presence of milk. It is possible that this lingual lipase is carried into the stomach, where it acts as a human gastric lipase (HGL) that has been shown to degrade up to 10% of ingested fat. Although these early products of fat digestion, fatty acids and monoacylglycerols, represent a relatively minor component of fat digested, their entry into the duodenum is believed to supply a major stimulus for the production of the hormone cholecystokinin (CCK), which inhibits gut motility.

The stomach serves mainly as an organ of mechanical digestion and, by churning its contents, produces a coarse creamy emulsion known as chyme. The circular pyloric sphincter muscle that separates the stomach from the duodenum and, with other factors, controls the rate of gastric emptying opens twice a minute to release approximately 3 ml of chyme. Since emulsified fat in chyme is less dense than the aqueous material, the two fractions separate with the fat collecting above the aqueous layer. As a result, the entry of emulsified fat into the duodenum is delayed, allowing sufficient time for the minor breakdown products to act on CCK.

The duodenal phase involves the breakdown of the emulsified fat by a process known as lipolysis and the solubilization of the products of lipolysis. The entry of chyme containing minor lipolytic products into the duodenum stimulates the:

- release of CCK, which inhibits gut motility
- secretion of bile acids from the gall bladder
- release of pancreatic juice containing a battery of lipases.

Lipolysis is an enzyme-catalyzed hydrolysis that releases fatty acids from lipids (TAGs, phospholipids, and CEs). It involves the hydrolytic cleavage of bonds between a fatty acid and the glycerol backbone of TAGs and phospholipids, and cholesterol in CEs, and occurs not only in the digestive tract but also in circulating and intracellular lipids (Figure 6.4). The hydrolysis of emulsified dietary fat entering the duodenum is catalyzed by a battery of pancreatic enzymes including a pancreatic lipase that acts chiefly on TAG and phospholipase A_2 and a cholesterol ester hydrolase acting on phospholipids and CEs. The hydrolysis of TAG by pancreatic lipase occurs in a sequential

fashion with the initial removal of a fatty acid from position 1 and then position 3 from the glycerol backbone, generating a 2,3-diacylglycerol, followed by a 2-monoacylglycerol (2-MAG).

Solubilization of emulsified fat

With the notable exceptions mentioned previously (Section 6.2), fats are insoluble in water and must be rendered soluble before they can be absorbed in the gut and transported within cells and in the circulation. In each of these situations, this is achieved by the hydrophobic fat or lipid associating with molecules that are capable of interfacing with both hydrophobic and hydrophilic environments. Molecules with these characteristics are called amphipathic molecules, examples of which are phospholipids, bile salts, and specialized proteins known as apoproteins (Figure 6.5). In the small intestine emulsified fats are solubilized by associating with bile salts produced in the liver and stored and released from the gallbladder, and phospholipids to form complex aggregates known as mixed micelles. Lipids within cells and in the circulation are solubilized by combining with specific proteins known as fatty acid-binding proteins (FABPs) and apolipoproteins (ApoA, B, C, E), respectively. Further details of the structure and function of these specialized proteins are given in Section 6.5.

The action of pancreatic lipase on TAG yields free fatty acids and 2-MAG. Fatty acids of short- and medium-chain length ($\leq$14 carbons) are absorbed directly into the portal circulation with free glycerol and transported bound to albumin to the liver, where they are rapidly oxidized. In contrast, long-chain fatty acids (LCFAs; >14 carbons) associate with bile salts in bile juice from the gallbladder and are absorbed into the enterocyte for further processing and packaging into transport lipoproteins. The primary bile salts, cholic and chenodeoxycholic acids, are produced from cholesterol in the liver under the action of the rate-limiting enzyme 7-α-hydroxylase. These bile salts act effectively as detergents, solubilizing lipids by the formation of mixed micelles. These are spherical associations of amphipathic molecules (with hydrophobic and hydrophilic regions) with a hydrophilic surface of bile salts and phospholipids that encapsulates a hydrophobic core of more insoluble LCFAs and 2-MAG (see Figure 6.4). The micelle core will also contain some lipid-soluble vitamins including tocopherols and carotenoids. The formation of mixed

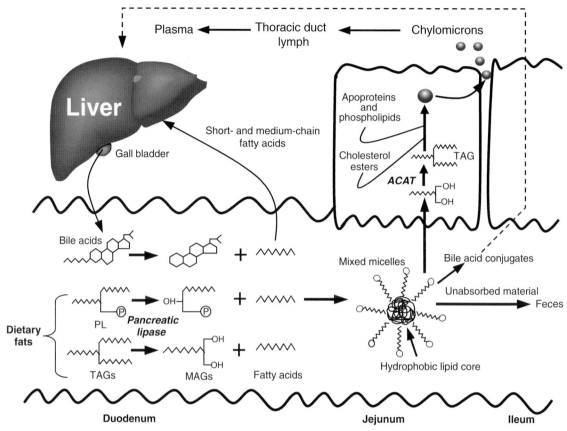

Figure 6.4 Reception, emulsification, lipolysis, solubilization, and absorption of fats. ACAT, acyl-CoA-cholesterol acyltransferase; MAG, mono-acylglycerol; TAG, triacylglycerol; PL phospholipid; P, phosphate.

micelles increases the solubility of fat by 100- to 1000-fold. They create an acidic microenvironment for the lipid core which, through protonation, facilitates the dissociation of LCFAs and 2-MAG from the micelle and diffusion into the enterocyte.

Absorption of solubilized fat

The ilial or absorptive phase involves the transit of dietary fats from mixed micelles into the enterocyte. Although originally believed to be a purely passive process, dependent on factors such as the rate of gastric emptying, extent of mixing, and gut motility, the translocation of LCFAs and 2-MAG from the micelle into the enterocyte is now known to be assisted by the presence of FABPs within the cell membrane and the cell. These maintain a diffusion gradient down which LCFAs and MAGs can flow into the cell. FABPs have numerous roles within cells and specific-

ity for different types of LCFAs. Thus, the absorption of LCFAs and 2-MAG derived from dietary TAGs occurs by facilitated diffusion via FABP, which increases membrane permeation and promotes cellular uptake of LCFAs and monoglycerides. An additional factor that drives the diffusion gradient is the rapid re-esterification of LCFAs into 2-MAG and 2-MAG into TAGs within the enterocyte by the enzyme acyl-CoA-cholesterol acyltransferase (ACAT). The absorption of dietary TAGs in the small intestine is extremely efficient, with up to 90% being absorbed. Dietary cholesterol also associates within mixed micelles and is absorbed in a similar manner by specific sterol-carrying proteins resident in the enterocyte membrane. Thus, cholesterol is also absorbed by a protein-facilitated mechanism but, in contrast to dietary TAGs, only about 40% of dietary cholesterol will be absorbed directly.

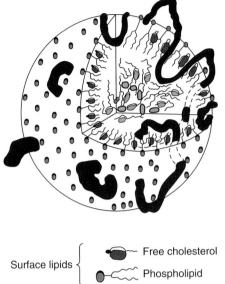

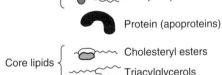

Figure 6.5 General lipoprotein structure. (Reproduced from Durrington PN. *Hyperlipidaemia Diagnosis and Management*, 2nd edn. Elsevier Science, Oxford, copyright 1995 with permission of Elsevier.)

Enterohepatic circulation

The absorption of fat in the small intestine is dependent on the availability of bile acids from biliary secretions which also contain free cholesterol. Both bile acids (>95%) and biliary cholesterol are salvaged by an energy-dependent process in the terminal ileum. This active process of reabsorption via the enterohepatic circulation is tightly controlled by a feedback mechanism that is sensitive to hepatic levels of cholesterol. Thus, the reabsorption of cholesterol downregulates the activity of 7-α-hydroxylase in the liver, shutting down the further production of bile acids. Substances in the lumen of the gut that are capable of binding or competing with bound bile acids, such as naturally occurring plant sterols or soluble nonstarch polysaccharides (NSPs), prevent their reabsorption which, in effect, interrupts the enterohepatic circulation. This depletes the supply of cholesterol and accelerates the production of bile acids, depleting the liver of cholesterol (Figure 6.6). To replenish this loss, liver cells respond by increasing their uptake of cholesterol from circulating lipoproteins in the blood, with the result of a decrease in blood cholesterol. Interruption of the enterohepatic circulation helps to explain the cholesterol-lowering action of some of the earliest known cholesterol-lowering drugs, but also such dietary constituents as the phytosterols (sitosterol and stanol esters) and soluble fiber or NSPs. For further details of the control mechanism see Section 6.5.

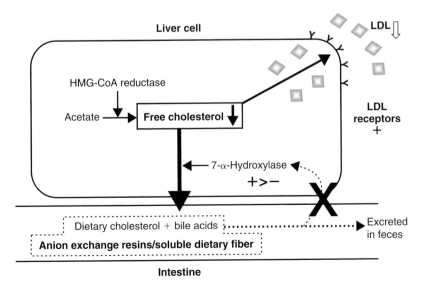

Figure 6.6 Interruption of the enterohepatic circulation. LDL, low-density lipoprotein; HMG-CoA, 3-hydroxy-3-methyl-glutaryl-coenzyme A.

Re-esterification of triacylglycerols in the enterocyte

Once LCFAs have entered the cell they are activated by acyl-CoA and are re-esterified with glycerol back into TAG and phospholipids by two distinct biochemical pathways, the 2-MAG and glycerol-3-phosphate (G-3-P) pathways. The difference between these two pathways lies in:

- their substrates of activation
- the former using 2-MAG and the latter α-glycero-3-phosphate
- their location within different cellular organelles: the 2-MAGs reside in the smooth endoplasmic reticulum and the G-3-P in the rough endoplasmic reticulum
- the periods during which they are most active.

The 2-MAG pathway is quantitatively of greater importance in the enterocyte of the intestine and thus predominates in the postprandial period, whereas the G-3-P pathway is more active in the postabsorptive phase in tissues such as liver, muscle, and adipose tissue. Following the absorption of a fatty meal and uptake of 2-MAG into the enterocyte, up to 90% of these molecules are rapidly acylated back to 1,2-diacylglycerol and finally TAGs by the sequential actions of three enzymes: CoA ligase, monoglycerol acyltransferase, and diacylglycerol acyltransferase. In a similar fashion, lysophosphatidylcholine, produced by the action of pancreatic phospholipase 'A' on dietary phospholipids, is absorbed by the enterocyte and re-esterified back to phosphatidylcholine in the enterocyte by direct acetylation (Figure 6.7). The bulk of free cholesterol absorbed from the intestinal lumen is also re-esterified in the enterocyte by the enzyme ACAT.

Lipoprotein assembly and secretion

Plasma lipoproteins are a family of spherical, macromolecular complexes of lipid and protein, the principal function of which is to transport endogenous lipids (synthesized in the liver) and exogenous lipids (synthesized in the gut from dietary fats) from these sites of production and absorption to peripheral sites of utilization (e.g., oxidation in muscle, incorporation in membranes, or as precursors of biologically active metabolites) and storage (e.g., adipose tissue).

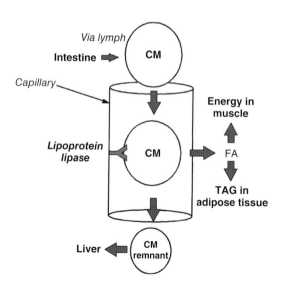
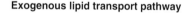
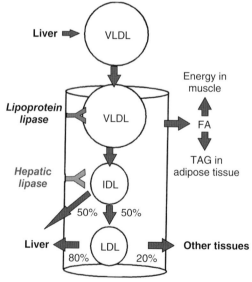

Figure 6.7 Re-esterification of triacylglycerides in enterocytes. CM, chylomicron; FA, fatty acid; IDL, intermediate-density lipoprotein; LDL, low-density lipoprotein; TAG, triacylcerol; VLDL, very low-density lipoprotein. (Reproduced from Mangiapane EH, Salter AM, eds. *Diet, Lipoproteins and Coronary Heart Disease. A Biochemical Perspective.* Nottingham University Press, Nottingham, 1999, with permission of Nottingham University Press.)

In the small intestine, the newly re-esterified TAGs and CEs associate with specific amphipathic proteins and phospholipids in the enterocyte to form the largest and most TAG-rich lipoproteins, known as chylomicrons. The enterocyte is capable of synthesizing three different apoproteins (apo): apoA-I, apoA-IVs and apoB (B-48). The last apoprotein is expressed in two isoforms, the arbitrarily named apoB-100, which is synthesized in the liver, and a shorter relative of B-100, which is produced by the enterocyte and is approximately 48% of the size of B-100 and thus appropriately named apoB-48. While both apoproteins are products of the same gene, the mRNA undergoes post-transcriptional editing in the enterocyte to produce a truncated polypeptide. ApoB-48 is produced in the rough endoplasmic reticulum and transferred to the smooth endoplasmic reticulum, where it combines with a lipid droplet, or nascent chylomicron, and then migrates to the Golgi apparatus. Here, the apoproteins (A-I, A-IV, and B-48) are glycosylated before the chylomicrons eventually leave the enterocyte by exocytosis through the basement membrane, across the intracellular space between the enterocyte and the lacteal, and are finally discharged into the lymphatic vessels.

Postprandial lipemia

The turbidity or milkiness of serum or plasma following the ingestion of fat marks the arrival of dietary fat now contained in chylomicrons in the blood. The milky appearance of plasma or serum after the ingestion of fat arises from the chylomicrons, which are of a sufficient size physically to scatter light and create the milky appearance of serum or plasma after a meal. The size and composition of the chylomicrons produced after a fatty meal are determined by the fat content of the meal. Hence, the nature of fatty acids in chylomicron TAG reflects the nature of fatty acid in the meal. Each chylomicron particle carries a single molecule of apoB-48 which, unlike its other smaller counterparts A-I and A-IV, remains with the chylomicron throughout its life in the circulation. There is little evidence to suggest that the production of apoB-48, and thus the number of particles, increases in response to an increased flux of dietary fat. Instead, the enterocyte incorporates more TAG into each chylomicron and expands the size of each chylomicron to facilitate the transport of larger amounts of absorbed dietary fat. There is evidence to suggest that

chylomicrons containing lipids enriched with poly-unsaturated fatty acids (PUFAs) are larger than chylomicrons enriched with saturated fat, since the former occupy more space when packaged into a lipoprotein. This has implications for the subsequent metabolism and fate of these lipoproteins in the circulation, since TAGs associated with larger chylomicrons are known to be hydrolyzed more rapidly. It is thought that apoB-48 is produced continuously in the enterocyte-forming pools of apoB-48 in readiness for the sudden reception of dietary fat and production of chylomicrons. Nevertheless, small chylomicrons can be detected throughout the postabsorptive phase.

The onset, duration, and magnitude of postprandial lipemia can be monitored in the laboratory after a standard fat-containing meal by making serial measurements of serum TAG or more specifically TAG associated with TAG-rich lipoproteins over a postprandial period of up to 8 or 9 hours (remnants of chylomicrons can be detected 12 hours after a meal). Alternatively, the levels of apoB-48 or retinyl esters in serum act as useful markers or tracer molecules for following the metabolism of chylomicrons in the postprandial period. In normal subjects postprandial lipemia peaks between 3 and 4 hours and subsides to baseline concentration after 5–6 hours. In some cases, postprandial TAG (mainly in chylomicrons) can appear in the blood within 30 min and peak as early as 1 hour after the ingestion of fat. So rapid is this rise in TAG that it is believed to represent preformed lipid in the enterocyte from the previous meal that is shunted into the circulation by the incoming fat load. Note that, in addition to the time taken to emulsify, hydrolyze, and absorb dietary fat, re-esterification of TAG in the enterocyte and lipoprotein assembly alone takes about 15 min, although shunting means that the first TAG can appear within 30 min, with the first peak after 1 hour. This shunting phenomenon is particularly noticeable during the day and gives rise to two or even more peaks, whereas postprandial peaks following an overnight fast are usually monophasic.

Chylomicrons are not the only TAG-rich lipoproteins in the postprandial phase. Chylomicrons clearly contribute significantly to the extent of postprandial lipemia, and the rate at which the TAGs in these lipoproteins are hydrolyzed is known to be a critical determinant of the extent and time-course of postprandial lipemia. The TAGs in circulating chylomicrons are

Table 6.4 Plasma lipoproteins: classes, composition, and distribution

	Chylomicrons	VLDLs	LDLs	HDLs
Mass (10^6 Da)	0.4–3.0	10–100	2–3.5	0.2–0.3
Density (g/ml)	>0.95	<1.006	1.02–1.063	1.063–1.210
Particle diameter (nm)	>90	30–90	22–28	5–12
Apoproteins	B-48, A-I, C-I, C-II, C-III, E	B-100, E	B-100	A-I, A-II
Lipids % mass (molecules/particle)				
Cholesterol	8 (60 000)	22 (10 000)	48 (2000)	20 (100)
Triacylglycerols	83 (500 000)	50 (24 000)	10 (300)	8 (20)
Ratio of particles				
Postabsorptive	1	40	1000	10 000
Postprandial	1	25	250	250 000

VLDL, very low-density lipoprotein; LDL, low-density lipoprotein; HDL, high-density lipoprotein.

lipolyzed by a rate-limiting lipase known as lipoprotein lipase (LPL). LPL is tethered to the endothelial lining of blood vessels in peripheral tissues, most notably muscle and adipose tissue, by proteoglycan fibers, and as such is known as an endothelial lipase. Several molecules of LPL can interact and lipolyze the TAG from a single chylomicron particle to generate a chylomicron remnant which is removed by specific cell membrane receptors in the liver. The situation is complicated by the fact that TAG-rich lipoproteins from the liver, known as very low-density lipoprotein (VLDL), also contribute to this postprandial lipemia to variable extents in health and disease states. These VLDLs containing endogenously produced TAG are similar in lipid composition to chylomicrons but considerably smaller (Table 6.4). While chylomicrons carry up to 80% of measurable plasma TAG during the postprandial period, VLDL particles can carry up to 80% of the measurable protein (mainly as apo-B), and significantly outnumber chylomicrons at all times. VLDL-TAG are also metabolized by LPL, which creates competition for the clearance of endogenously and exogenously derived TAG carried by VLDLs and chylomicrons respectively.

Postprandial lipemia: relevance to atherosclerosis

It was suggested by Zilversmit in 1979 that atherosclerosis was a postprandial phenomenon. This concept was based on the finding that patients either with or at high risk of developing coronary heart disease (CHD) showed an impaired capacity to remove TAG-rich lipoproteins from the circulation after a meal. This resulted in enhanced postprandial lipemia, which also became known as the TAG intolerance hypothesis. At

about the same time, evidence emerged that TAG-rich lipoproteins, and especially remnants of chylomicrons, were directly atherogenic, meaning that they can damage the endothelial lining of arteries and promote the deposition of cholesterol in coronary arteries. For this reason, there is considerable research interest in the metabolic determinants of postprandial lipemia. This includes the mechanisms that underlie the production and removal of TAG-rich lipoproteins, not only in the intestine but also in the liver, since the production and removal of VLDL can clearly influence postprandial events. The quality and, to a lesser extent, quantity of dietary fat are extremely important in this respect and have a major role to play in modulating lipid-mediated atherosclerosis.

6.5 Circulating lipids: lipoprotein structures and metabolism

Circulating blood lipids are insoluble in water and must be solubilized for transportation in the extracellular fluid by combining with bipolar molecules with charged and uncharged regions (apoproteins and phospholipids). This property, known as amphipathicity, enables these molecules to associate with aqueous (hydrophilic) and nonaqueous (hydrophobic) environments and thus renders them perfect for enveloping insoluble lipids, chiefly TAG and CE, in macromolecular lipid–protein complexes called lipoproteins. It is worth remembering that, in the absence of lipoproteins, TAG would exist in aqueous blood as immiscible oil droplets, while free fatty acids liberated from TAG and phospholipids in the absence of the blood protein albumin would act as detergents and dissolve cell membranes.

Lipoprotein structure: a shopping bag and groceries

The general structure of a lipoprotein consists of a central core of hydrophobic, neutral lipid (TAG and CE) surrounded by a hydrophilic coat of phospholipids, free cholesterol, and apoproteins. A useful analogy for this arrangement of molecules is that of a "shopping bag and groceries," with the lipid core representing the groceries and the outer coat the fabric of the bag. The apoproteins weave in and out of the lipid core and outer surface layer and form the thread of the fabric which holds the bag together (see Figure 6.5). This clever arrangement of molecules renders the hydrophobic lipids soluble for the purpose of transport in blood. In addition to conferring structural integrity on the lipoprotein particle, apoproteins have a vital role in controlling the metabolism of lipoproteins by acting as ligands for cell membrane receptors and cofactors for key enzymes.

Plasma lipoproteins can be subdivided into distinct classes on the basis of their physical properties and/or composition, both of which reflect the physiological role in the transport of lipids from sites of synthesis (endogenous lipids) and absorption (exogenous lipids, absorbed in the gut) to sites of storage (adipose tissue) and utilization (skeletal muscle). The principal classes of lipoproteins are traditionally defined by density, which is determined by the ratio of lipid to protein in the lipoprotein particle. Since lipids tend to occupy a greater molecular volume than proteins, they are lighter and less dense. Thus, particles with high lipid content are larger and less dense (carry more lipid groceries) than lipoproteins enriched with protein. This property relates directly to the transport function and metabolic interrelationships between lipoprotein classes in blood. It can also be used to separate lipoproteins of different densities because lipoproteins of different density have different flotation characteristics in the ultracentrifuge (note that plasma lipoproteins will float when subjected to centrifugal force, whereas pure proteins sink). Other classification schemes for plasma lipoproteins have exploited differences in their net electrical charge (electrophoretic mobility), particle size (exclusion chromatography, gradient gel electrophoresis), and immunological characteristics conferred upon the lipoprotein by the types of apoproteins in each lipoprotein subclass (see Table 6.4). Some of these techniques permit the further resolution of VLDL, low-density lipoproteins (LDLs), and high-density lipoproteins (HDLs) into discrete subclasses, the distribution of which relates to cardiovascular risk and is determined by genetic and lifestyle factors.

Lipoprotein transport pathways

Lipoprotein transport can be described in terms of the production, transport, and removal of cholesterol or TAG from the circulation. In reality, these two processes are inseparable because both TAG and cholesterol are transported together in lipoproteins. Lipoproteins are in a constant state of change, with lipids and apoproteins constantly shuttling between different lipoproteins that interrelate through integrated metabolic pathways. A useful analogy here is to think of lipoproteins as railway trains, transporting passengers that represent lipids and apoproteins within a complex rail network. The trains and passengers are in a constant state of flux within and between stations. Lipoprotein metabolism is controlled by the activity of functional proteins (enzymes, cell surface receptors, receptor ligands) that determine the rate at which lipoproteins enter and leave the system, and by the physicochemical properties of the lipoprotein themselves. This corresponds to all of the rate-limiting features of a train journey, the number of trains, and type of passengers.

All lipoproteins, with the notable exception of HDLs, begin life as TAG-rich particles The principal transport function of these lipoproteins in the first instance is to deliver fatty acids liberated from the TAG to tissues. The enterocytes in the gut are the producers of lipoproteins which deliver dietary fats into the blood as chylomicrons (exogenous lipid), whereas the liver is the central terminus for the production of VLDLs and removal of their cholesterol-rich end-products, LDLs. VLDLs, although smaller than chylomicrons, resemble the latter in many ways and are often referred to as the liver's chylomicrons. While the rate at which the gut produces chylomicrons depends largely on the amount of absorbed dietary fat, the rate of production of VLDL is determined by the supply of fatty acids in the liver that can be re-esterified back to TAG for incorporation into VLDL. These fatty acids are derived chiefly from the systemic circulation in the form of nonesterified fatty acids (NEFAs), and to a lesser extent from the uptake of circulating lipoprotein remnants. It is noteworthy that, although the liver has the capacity to synthesize fatty acids, the amount synthesized by *de novo* lipogenesis is relatively small in humans on a mixed Western diet. However, the contribution of fatty acids from this source may increase in conditions associated with an overproduction of VLDLs, and has been shown to occur on low-fat, high-carbohydrate diets, and in metabolic disease.

Metabolic determinants of lipoprotein metabolism

The metabolism of serum lipoproteins and fate of their transport lipids is controlled by:

- the physical and chemical characteristics of the lipoprotein, such as its size and lipid and apoprotein content
- the activity of the endothelial LPL and hepatic lipase (HL), so called because they are attached to the surface of endothelial cells lining blood vessels in peripheral tissues, such as adipose tissue and skeletal muscle, and the liver, respectively
- lipid transfer proteins; cholesteryl ester and phospholipid transfer proteins, (CETP and PLTP respectively).
- apoproteins that act as activators of enzymes and ligands for specific lipoprotein receptors on the surfaces of cells (apoB-100 and apoE as ligands for the LDLs and remnant receptors in the liver, respectively)
- the activity of specific lipoprotein receptors on cell surfaces.

Lipoprotein transport is traditionally described in terms of the forward and reverse transport of cholesterol. Forward transport encompasses the exogenous and endogenous pathways, which describes the arrival of cholesterol in the blood from either the gut or the liver and carriage back to the liver for processing; the liver has the unique capacity to secrete cholesterol either as free cholesterol or as bile acids. Conversely, reverse transport describes the HDL pathway and the efflux of cholesterol out of peripheral tissues back to the liver. This directionality can be misleading because each pathway can direct cholesterol back to the liver. Both the exogenous and endogenous pathways share a common saturable lipolytic pathway that consists of a delipidation cascade in which the TAG-rich lipoproteins (chylomicrons and VLDLs), after receiving apoC (C-II) from HDL, an essential cofactor for the

activation of LPL, are progressively depleted of their TAG in a stepwise fashion by LPL to become cholesterol-rich remnants that are removed by specific, high-affinity receptors found chiefly in the liver. Several molecules of LPL may bind to a single chylomicron or VLDL particle, although LPL shows greater affinity for chylomicrons in preference to VLDL. This situation leads to competition between these TAG-rich lipoproteins and provides a mechanism to explain how VLDL can influence the clearance of TAG in the postprandial period.

Lipolyzed chylomicrons form chylomicron remnants which, during passage through the liver, bind to specific receptors on the surface of hepatocytes that recognize apoE, an apoprotein that is also acquired at an early stage from HDLs. Remnant receptors are maintained at a very high level of activity and are not downregulated through a feedback mechanism (see low-density lipoprotein receptor pathway). This is fortunate, since chylomicron remnants have been shown to be capable of depositing their cholesterol in artery walls, thus promoting coronary atherosclerosis. The secretion of VLDL from the liver is again followed by the sequential lipolysis of TAG by LPL and generation of VLDL remnants or, in this case, the further lipolysis of these remnants into LDL. The remnants and LDLs bind to another receptor in the liver that recognizes both apoE exclusively in VLDL remnants and apoB-100 in LDLs, namely the LDL receptor. Approximately 60% of LDL is removed by the LDL receptor. The remainder is internalized into cells via scavenger receptors. This latter route has been associated with the development of atherosclerotic disease.

Whether a VLDL particle is removed as a remnant or transcends to LDL largely depends on its pedigree, i.e., its size and lipid composition. Experiments with radioactively labeled VLDL have shown that larger, TAG-rich VLDL particles are less likely to be converted into LDL and are removed as partially delipidated VLDL remnants, whereas smaller VLDLs are precursors of LDL.

The low-density lipoprotein receptor pathway

The incontrovertible link between plasma cholesterol and CHD is directly responsible for the rapid growth, and occasional quantum leaps, in our understanding of cholesterol homeostasis in relation to diet and

Serum LDL

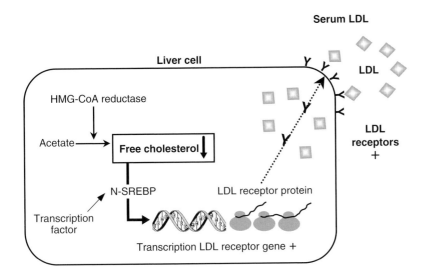

Figure 6.8 Low-density lipoprotein (LDL) receptor pathway. HMG-CoA, 3-hydroxy-3-methyl-glutaryl-coenzyme A; SREBP, sterol regulatory element binding protein.

disease, the most prolific of which was the discovery of the LDL receptor pathway by the Nobel Prize winners Goldstein and Brown (1977) (Figure 6.8). All cells, most notably those in the liver, have a highly developed and sensitive mechanism for regulating intracellular and intravascular levels of cholesterol. Cells in the liver synthesize approximately 500 mg of cholesterol a day and, although they can import the same quantity from the blood in the form of LDL, in the complete absence of LDL, cells could theoretically manufacture sufficient cholesterol to meet their metabolic needs. However, when stressed, cells will always import cholesterol in preference to synthesizing it themselves as the former process takes less energy. Cells acquire cholesterol from the blood by the uptake and degradation of LDL particles. As the requirement for free cholesterol increases within the cell, it increases its production and thus activity of LDL receptors, so that more LDL is extracted from the blood, lowering blood cholesterol. Conversely, if the cell becomes overloaded with cholesterol, it senses that it requires less cholesterol and produces fewer LDL receptors, causing blood cholesterol to increase. Since the production of LDL receptors is regulated by the intracellular level of free cholesterol, anything that increases free cholesterol within the cell will inadvertently lower blood LDL cholesterol. Intracellular free cholesterol represses the activity of a sterol regulatory element binding protein (SREBP), a positive nuclear transcription factor that promotes the transcription of the LDL receptor gene when free cholesterol levels fall.

The metabolic effects of intracellular free cholesterol are:

- it decreases the production of LDL receptors via SREBP
- it inhibits the synthesis of cholesterol by the enzyme 3-hydroxy-3-methylglutaryl (HMG)-CoA reductase
- it increases the re-esterification of cholesterol for storage as cholesterol esters.

Goldstein and Brown were aided in the discovery of the LDL receptor by studying a condition known as familial hypercholesterolemia, a genetic abnormality in the LDL receptor gene that produces defects in the LDL receptor pathway and considerably elevated blood cholesterol concentrations in early life (15–20 mmol/l) and premature cardiovascular disease. They also initiated pioneering studies on the influence of dietary fats on the activity of the LDL pathway, which led to a widely accepted explanation for the cholesterol-raising properties of saturated fatty acids.

Reverse cholesterol transport (high-density lipoprotein pathway)

The removal of cholesterol from tissues back to the liver via HDLs represents the only route of elimination for cholesterol from the body. This physiological role of HDLs explains, in part, the cardioprotective effects of these lipoproteins, as indicated by a strong inverse relationship between serum HDL cholesterol

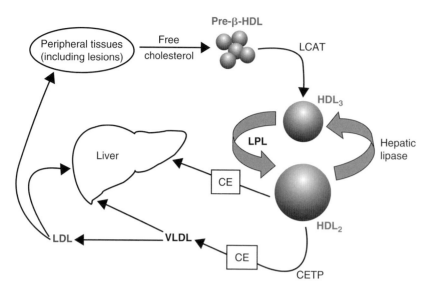

Figure 6.9 Reverse cholesterol transport. CE, cholesterol ester; CETP, cholesterol ester transfer protein; HDL, high-density lipoprotein; LCAT, lecithin–cholesterol acyltransferase; LDL, low-density lipoprotein; LPL, lipoprotein lipase; VLDL, very low-density lipoprotein.

and CHD risk in prospective cohort studies. The activity of the HDL pathway is influenced by genetic and dietary factors that can interact to either increase or reduce the efficiency of cholesterol removal. This, in turn, may be reflected in changes in the concentration of serum HDLs and their functional properties.

HDLs are synthesized in the gut and liver, and increase their particle size in the circulation as a result of the acquisition of cholesterol from two principal sources: (1) surface material released from TAG-rich lipoproteins during lipolysis and (2) peripheral tissues. The particles, which are responsible for removing cholesterol from cells, are very small pre-HDLs and are disk-shaped particles composed of phospholipid and apoA-I (ApoA-I is capable of this function on its own). The efflux of free cholesterol from tissue sites, including deposits of cholesterol in the coronary arteries, is facilitated by the formation of a free cholesterol gradient from the cell across the cell membrane to pre-HDLs. The gradient is generated by the re-esterification of free cholesterol by the enzyme lecithin–cholesterol acyltransferase (LCAT) and via the migration of these newly formed cholesterol esters into the hydrophobic core of what becomes mature, spherical HDL. The newly acquired cholesterol is transported back to the liver either directly by HDL or indirectly by transfer to apoB-containing lipoproteins VLDL and LDL. Blood vessels in the liver contain a close relative of LPL, i.e., HL. This enzyme acts on smaller lipoproteins and especially the surface

phospholipid of HDL, where it effectively punches a hole in the surface coat to facilitate access to the lipid core and delivery of CE to the hepatocyte (Figure 6.9).

Interrelationships among serum triacylglycerols and low- and high-density lipoproteins

Lipids are constantly moving between lipoprotein particles. This movement is not totally random but influenced by the relative lipid composition of the lipoproteins and by specific lipid transfer proteins (LTPs) that act as lipid shuttles. In a normal, healthy individual, TAG-rich lipoproteins transfer TAG to LDL and HDL in equimolar exchange for CE. This is mediated through an LTP called cholesteryl transfer protein (CETP). In this way, CEs are transferred from HDL to VLDL for passage back to the liver. Conversely, when the concentration of serum TAG and thus TAG-rich lipoproteins is increased, for example by either the overproduction of TAG in the liver or the impaired removal of TAG by LPL, the result is a net transfer of TAG into LDL and HDL. As LDL and HDL are overloaded with TAG they become favored substrates for the action of HL and are remodeled into smaller and denser particles. While small, dense HDL is catabolized rapidly in the liver, lowering serum HDL and impairing reverse cholesterol transport, small, dense LDLs are removed less effectively by LDL receptors and accumulate in serum. Small, dense LDL, by virtue of its size, has a much greater potential to infiltrate the artery wall and deposit its cholesterol. Even a moderately raised concentration of serum TAG (>1.5 mmol/l) may be inversely associated with reduced HDL cholesterol (<1 mmol/l) and a predominance of small, dense LDL. This collection of findings is known as the atherogenic lipoprotein phenotype (ALP) and is a very common but modifiable source of increased CHD risk in free-living populations.

Endocrine control of lipoprotein metabolism

All hormones exert an influence on lipoprotein metabolism. However, with respect to diet and the control of postprandial lipid metabolism, insulin has by far the greatest impact. Although classically associated with carbohydrate metabolism and the uptake of glucose into cells, the actions of insulin are critical to the control of postprandial lipid metabolism. Insulin is secreted in response to the reception of food in the gut and it:

- stimulates LPL in adipose tissue
- suppresses the intracellular lipolysis of stored TAG in adipose tissue by inhibiting hormone-sensitive lipase
- suppresses the release of VLDL from the liver.

Insulin coordinates the lipolysis of dietary TAG and uptake of NEFA into adipose tissue. It achieves this by minimizing the release of NEFA from TAG stores in adipose tissue and TAGs produced in the liver by suppressing the secretion of VLDL. The sensitivity of the target tissues – liver, adipose tissue, and, perhaps to a lesser extent, skeletal muscle – to insulin is critical to the maintenance of these effects. Failure of insulin action, insulin resistance, in conditions such as obesity and diabetes results in dyslipidemia characterized by an impaired capacity to lipolyze TAG-rich lipoproteins (TAG intolerance or enhanced postprandial lipemia). This effect is compounded by the failure of insulin to suppress the mobilization of NEFA from adipose tissue TAG, which increases the flux of NEFA to the liver and stimulates the overproduction of VLDL ('portal hypothesis'). The suppression of VLDL secretion is also abolished so that VLDL is released into the postprandial circulation and is free to compete with chylomicrons, augmenting postprandial lipemia still further. This series of events gives rise to a dyslipidemia or ALP, which is found frequently in insulin-resistant conditions. Insulin also stimulates the synthesis of cholesterol by activating HMG-CoA reductase and the activity of LDL receptors, although the overall effect on cholesterol homeostasis is small in relation to the control of the LDL pathway described above.

Sex hormones

The effect of sex hormones on serum lipoproteins is best illustrated by the pronounced differences in lipid and lipoprotein profiles between adult men and premenopausal women. Men present with higher total serum and LDL cholesterol, higher serum TAG, and lower HDL cholesterol concentrations than premenopausal women. This difference in lipid profiles confers protection against CHD on premenopausal women so that their CHD risk lags some 10 years behind that of men of the same age. This applies until estrogen failure at the menopause, when CHD risk in women overtakes that of men. Estrogen was the first compound shown to stimulate LDL receptor activity in cell culture, an effect that not only accounts for lower LDL levels in women but also the sharp increase in LDL cholesterol after the menopause, to levels above those of men. Estrogens also stimulate the production of TAG and VLDL, but any adverse effects must be outweighed by the efficiency of TAG removal mechanisms that maintain lower serum TAG levels in women than in men until the menopause. In addition to these effects, estrogen selectively inhibits the activity of HL, which contributes to the HDLs in women. In direct contrast, the androgenic male hormone testosterone suppresses LDL receptor activity, raising LDL cholesterol. It is also a powerful stimulant of HL activity, and is responsible for lowering HDL cholesterol in men, most notably in male body builders on anabolic steroids, in whom serum HDL can be almost absent.

The triacylglycerol hypothesis

Dietary effects on serum cholesterol or LDLs alone provide an inadequate basis on which to explain the relationship between diet and CHD within populations. The ability of humans to protect themselves against an overaccumulation of cholesterol in their vascular system through nutritional changes depends to a much greater extent on increasing the efficiency of the HDL pathway and utilization of TAG-rich lipoproteins. The latter represent the precursors of potentially harmful cholesterol-rich remnants and LDLs that contribute to coronary atherosclerosis. The effects of diet, and in particular dietary fats, in modulating the clearance of TAG-rich lipoproteins in the postprandial period is of paramount importance in preventing the accumulation of atherogenic remnants and development of proatherogenic abnormalities in LDL and HDL. The actions of insulin coordinate the metabolism of TAG-rich lipoproteins but can become defective through energy imbalance, weight gain, and ultimately obesity. As a consequence, the most common abnormalities in lipoproteins to increase risk in populations arise from a primary defect in the metabolism of TAG, induced through insulin resistance and not cholesterol per se. Equally important is the fact that these metabolic defects originate, in part, through nutrient–gene interactions and are thus highly amenable to dietary modification.

6.6 Body lipid pools

Lipids in the human body exist in two major pools: structural lipids in membranes and storage lipids in body fat. The lipid composition and metabolic fate of these two pools are quite distinct, although many of the fatty acids occupying both pools are the same. The main components of both membrane and storage lipids are the long-chain (16–24 carbons) saturated, monounsaturated, and polyunsaturated fatty acids. Although several of the major long-chain fatty acids in the body are common to both membrane and storage lipids, namely palmitate, stearate, oleate, and linoleate, three important distinctions exist between membrane and storage lipids.

1 Membrane lipids are not usually hydrolyzed to release free fatty acids for energy metabolism.
2 Membrane lipids contain a much higher proportion of long-chain PUFAs.
3 Membrane lipids are more diverse and rarely include TAGs, which are the main component of storage lipids.

Structural lipid pool

Biological membranes surrounding cells and subcellular organelles exist primarily as lipid bilayers (Figure 6.3). The lipids in both the inner and outer surfaces of membranes are composed mainly of phospholipids and free cholesterol, which interface with a myriad of proteins functioning as receptors, transporters, enzymes, ion channels, etc. Some lipids, i.e., PUFAs, confer the feature of "fluidity" to membranes, whereas others, i.e., cholesterol and saturated fatty acids, have the opposite rigidifying effect. Membranes have extraordinarily diverse fatty acid profiles and phospholipid composition depending on their tissue and subcellular location. They are also the body's reservoir of both fat-soluble vitamins and eicosanoid precursors such as arachidonate.

Most of the body's cholesterol is present in the unesterified form in membranes, where it represents 35–45% of total lipids. Skin, plasma, and adrenal cortex contain 55–75% of cholesterol in the esterified form. Bile also contains free cholesterol and bile salts derived from cholesterol.

Storage lipid pool

Triacylglycerols are the main energy storage form of lipids and they are the principal component of body fat. TAG-containing fatty acids destined for oxidation are also present in measurable but much lower amounts in all tissues that can oxidize long-chain fatty acids, i.e., muscle and heart. TAG is synthesized by the intestine and liver, where it is subsequently incorporated into lipoproteins (see Section 6.4) for the transport of lipids to and from other tissues.

The main fatty acids in the TAG of adult human body fat are palmitate (20–30%), stearate (10–20%), oleate (45–55%), and linoleate (10–15%). The fatty acid profile of adult body fat always reflects the profile of dietary fat. Only rarely would this result in other fatty acids being more prevalent in body fat than the four listed here. At birth, the fatty acid profile of body fat is unusual in having very low linoleate (<3%) and α-linolenate (<1%) but a higher proportion of long-chain polyunsaturates than later in life. Body fat occupies several discrete sites that expand and contract as needed. Body fat is about 82% by weight TAG, making it by far the main body pool of palmitate, stearate, oleate, and linoleate.

The main sites of body fat are subcutaneous and intravisceral, and they have different rates of response to stimuli for accumulation or release of fatty acids. Within a given site, growing evidence suggests that PUFAs are more easily released from adipose tissue TAG than are saturated fatty acids, especially during fasting or longer term energy deficit.

Plasma and milk lipids

In a way, plasma and milk lipids are an exception to the general rule distinguishing membrane and storage lipids. Plasma and milk lipids are present mostly as lipoproteins, comprising mostly phospholipids and cholesterol in the surrounding membrane and TAG in the core (see Section 6.5). Plasma lipids contain the only significant pool of free fatty acids or NEFAs in the body. Free fatty acids are not components of lipoproteins but are transported bound to albumin. They are liberated mostly from adipose tissue when plasma glucose and insulin are low. Plasma also contains proportionally more fatty acids esterified to cholesterol (cholesteryl esters) than are found in tissues.

Whole body content and organ profile of fatty acids

An estimate of the whole body content of lipids in a healthy adult human is given in Table 6.5. Additional body fat is deposited during pregnancy, but the fatty acid composition remains similar to that of nonpregnant adults and reflects dietary fat intake. The total lipid content of plasma rises in the third trimester, with a proportionally greater increase in saturated fatty acids than PUFAs. This downward trend in the percentage of PUFA towards term has led to some concern about the possible adverse consequences for the fetus of deficiency of PUFA. However, the actual amount of PUFA in blood lipids rises but less so than for saturated fatty acids; resulting in a proportional decrease in PUFA.

Soon after birth, body lipid composition starts to change. Brain cholesterol rises moderately from under 40% to nearly 50% of brain lipids. Docosahexaenoate

Table 6.5 Body fat content of major fatty acids in humans

Fatty acid	Content (g)
Palmitic acid	3320
Stearic acid	550
Oleic acid	6640
Linoleic acid	1560
Arachidonic acid	80
α-Linolenic acid	130
Eicosapentaenoic acid	<10
Docosahexaenoic acid	<10
Total	12 300

Data are based on a 70 kg adult human with 20% (14 kg) body fat. Fat tissue contains about 88% actual fatty acids by weight, yielding about 12.3 kg fatty acids in this example.

also rises rapidly in brain lipids, followed a little later by an increasing content of long-chain saturates and monounsaturates as myelin develops. Adipose tissue contains very little linoleate or α-linolenate at birth but their content increases rapidly with milk feeding. Plasma cholesterol is relatively low at birth and in infancy, but increases by more than twofold by adulthood.

In general, regardless of the profile of dietary fatty acids, saturated and monounsaturated fatty acids predominate in adipose tissue, whereas there is a closer balance between saturates, monounsaturates, and polyunsaturates in structural lipids. Long-chain PUFAs such as docosahexaenoate are present in high concentrations in specialized membranes, including those of the retina photoreceptor, in synapses of the brain, and in sperm.

6.7 Long-chain fatty acid metabolism

Synthesis

Synthesis of fatty acids occurs in the cytosol. It begins with acetyl-CoA being converted to malonyl-CoA by acetyl-CoA carboxylase, an enzyme dependent on biotin. Malonyl-CoA and a second acetyl-CoA then condense via β-ketothiolase. This is subsequently reduced, dehydrated, and then hydrogenated to yield a four-carbon product that recycles through the same series of steps until the most common long-chain fatty acid product, palmitate, is produced (Figure 6.10). Acetyl-CoA is primarily an intramitochondrial product. Thus, the transfer of acetyl-CoA to the cytosol for fatty acid synthesis appears to require its conversion to citrate to exit the mitochondria before being reconverted to acetyl-CoA in the cytosol.

There are three main features of long-chain fatty acid synthesis in mammals:

1 inhibition by starvation
2 stimulation by feeding carbohydrate after fasting
3 general inhibition by dietary fat.

Carbohydrate is an important source of carbon for generating acetyl-CoA and citrate used in fatty acid synthesis. Enzymes of carbohydrate metabolism also help to generate the NADPH needed in fatty acid synthesis. Acetyl-CoA carboxylase is a key control point in the pathway and is both activated and induced to polymerize by citrate. Acetyl-CoA carboxylase is

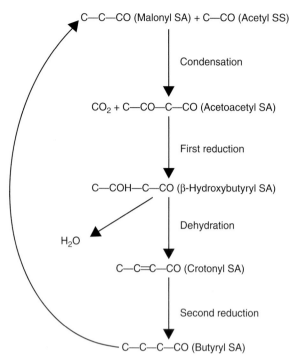

Figure 6.10 Principal steps in fatty acid synthesis. The individual steps occur with the substrate being anchored to the acyl carrier protein. SA, *S*-acyl carrier protein; SS, *S*-synthase.

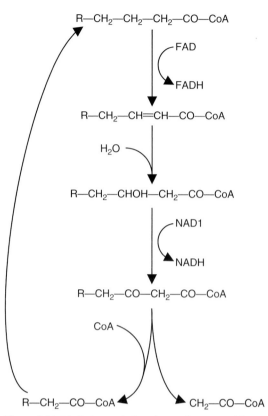

Figure 6.11 Principal steps in β-oxidation of a saturated fatty acid. The steps shown follow fatty acid "activation" (binding to coenzyme A) and carnitine-dependent transport to the inner surface of the mitochondria. Unsaturated fatty acids require additional steps to remove the double bonds before continuing with the pathway shown. FAD, flavin adenine dinucleotide; FADH reduced flavin adenine dinucleotide; R, 12 carbons.

inhibited by long-chain fatty acids, especially PUFAs such as linoleate. This is probably one important negative feedback mechanism by which both starvation and dietary fat decrease fatty acid synthesis. High amounts of free long-chain fatty acids would also compete for CoA, leading to their β-oxidation. Elongation of palmitate to stearate, etc., can occur in mitochondria using acetyl-CoA, but is more commonly associated with the endoplasmic reticulum where malonyl-CoA is the substrate.

Humans consuming >25% dietary fat synthesize relatively low amounts of fat (<2 g/day). Compared with other animals, humans also appear to have a relatively low capacity to convert stearate to oleate and linoleate or α-linolenate to the respective longer chain polyunsaturates. Hence, the fatty acid profiles of most human tissues generally reflect the intake of dietary fatty acids; when long-chain n-3 PUFAs are present in the diet, this is evident in both free-living humans as well as in experimental animals. Nevertheless, fatty acid synthesis is stimulated by fasting/refeeding or weight cycling, so these perturbations in

normal food intake can markedly alter tissue fatty acid profiles.

Oxidation

β-Oxidation is the process by which fatty acids are utilized for energy. Saturated fatty acids destined for β-oxidation are transported as CoA esters to the outer leaflet of mitochondria by FABP. They are then translocated inside the mitochondria by carnitine acyl-transferases. The β-oxidation process involves repeated dehydrogenation at sequential two-carbon steps and reduction of the associated flavoproteins (Figure 6.11). Five ATP molecules are produced during production of each acetyl-CoA. A further 12 ATP molecules are produced after the acetyl-CoA condenses with oxaloacetate to form citrate and goes through the tricarboxylic acid cycle.

The efficiency of fatty acid oxidation depends on the availability of oxaloacetate and, hence, concurrent carbohydrate oxidation. β-Oxidation of saturated fatty acids appears to be simpler than oxidation of unsaturated fatty acids because, before the acetyl-CoA cleavage, it involves the formation of a *trans* double bond two carbons from the CoA. In contrast, β-oxidation of unsaturated fatty acids yields a double bond in a different position that then requires further isomerization or hydrogenation. From a biochemical perspective, this extra step appears to make the oxidation of unsaturated fatty acids less efficient than that of saturated fatty acids. However, abundant *in vivo* and *in vitro* research in both humans and animals clearly shows that long-chain *cis*-unsaturated fatty acids with one to three double bonds (oleate, linoleate, α-linolenate) are more readily β-oxidized than saturated fatty acids of equivalent chain length, such as palmitate and stearate. The oxidation of PUFA and monounsaturates in preference to saturates has potential implications for chronic diseases such as coronary artery disease because their slower oxidation implies slower clearance from the blood, thereby providing more opportunity for esterification to cholesterol and subsequent deposition in the vessel wall.

In peroxisomes, fatty acid β-oxidation is a truncated process by which long-chain PUFAs are chain shortened. This peroxisomal detour has been identified as an obligatory step in the endogenous synthesis of docosahexaenoate from eicosapentaenoate.

Odd-carbon long-chain fatty acids are relatively uncommon but, when β-oxidized, yield propionyl-CoA, the further β-oxidation of which requires biotin and vitamin B_{12} as coenzymes.

Ketogenesis and ketosis

Large amounts of free fatty acids inhibit glycolysis and the enzymes of the tricarboxylic acid cycle, thereby impairing production of oxaloacetate. When insufficient oxaloacetate is available to support the continued oxidation of acetyl-CoA, two acetyl-CoA molecules condense to form a ketone, acetoacetate. Acetoacetate can be spontaneously decarboxylated to form acetone, a volatile ketone, or converted to a third ketone, β-hydroxybutyrate. When glucose is limiting, ketones are an alternative source of energy for certain organs, particularly the brain. They are also efficient substrates for lipid synthesis during early postnatal development. Conditions favoring ketogenesis include starvation, diabetes, and a very high-fat, low-carbohydrate "ketogenic" diet.

Carbon recycling

Carbon recycling is the process by which acetyl-CoA derived from β-oxidation of one fatty acid is incorporated into another lipid instead of completing the β-oxidation process to carbon dioxide. In principle, all fatty acids undergo this process to some extent but it is most clearly evident for two PUFAs, linoleate and α-linolenate. Carbon recycling captures the overwhelming majority of α-linolenate carbon, i.e., about 10 times more than is incorporated into docosahexaenoate, which remains in the body of suckling rats 48 hours after dosing with uniformly ^{13}C-labeled α-linolenate. Carbon recycling of linoleate in the rat captures similar amounts of the linoleate skeleton to those of arachidonate, the main desaturation and chain-elongation product of linoleate. Hence, carbon recycling appears to be a ubiquitous feature of the metabolism of PUFA, although its biological significance is still unclear.

Peroxidation

Peroxidation (auto-oxidation) is the nonenzyme-catalyzed reaction of molecular oxygen with organic compounds to form peroxides and related breakdown products. PUFAs are particularly vulnerable to peroxidation at the double bonds. Initiating agents such as pre-existing peroxides, transition metals, or ultraviolet or ionizing radiation produce singlet oxygen. Singlet oxygen can then abstract hydrogen at the double bonds of polyunsaturates to produce free (peroxy) radicals, which abstract further hydrogens from the same or different fatty acids and propagate the peroxidation process. Eventually, this leads to termination by the formation of stable degradation products or hydroperoxides (Figure 6.12). *Trans* isomers are frequently formed during the process. Hydroperoxides can form further hydroperoxy radicals or can be reduced by antioxidants, which contain thiol groups, i.e., glutathione and cysteine. Peroxidation of dietary fats gives rise to aldehydes, i.e., 2-undecenal, 2-decenal, nonanal, or octanal, which have a particular odor commonly known as rancidity.

Since peroxidation is a feature of polyunsaturates, it is a potential hazard facing most membranes and dietary lipids. Antioxidants such as vitamin E are usually present in sufficient amounts to prevent or

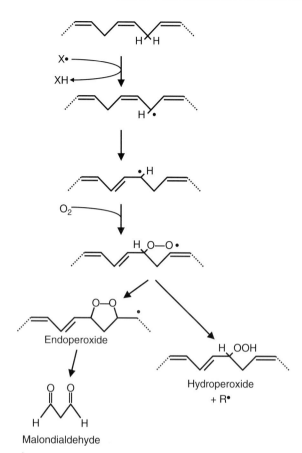

Endoperoxide

Hydroperoxide
+ R•

Malondialdehyde

Figure 6.12 Principal steps in peroxidation of a polyunsaturated fatty acid.

block peroxidation in living tissues. Humans and animals readily detect peroxidized fats in foods by their disagreeable odor and avoid them. However, modeling the effects of peroxides produced *in vivo* and *in vitro* is particularly challenging because lipid peroxidation undoubtedly is an important part of several necessary biological processes such as activation of the immune response.

Desaturation, chain elongation, and chain shortening

One important characteristic of long-chain fatty acid metabolism in both plants and animals is the capacity to convert one to another via the processes of desaturation, chain elongation, and chain shortening.

Plants and animals use desaturases to insert a double bond into long-chain fatty acids. There are several desaturases, depending on the position in the acyl chain into which the double bond is inserted. Although myristate (14:0) and palmitate can be converted to their monounsaturated derivatives, myristoleate (14:1n-5) and palmitoleate (16:1n-7) respectively, commonly it is only the fatty acids of 18 or more carbons that undergo desaturation. The Δ^9 desaturases in all organisms, except for anaerobic bacteria, use oxygen and NADPH to introduce a *cis* double bond at carbons 9 and 10 of stearate. This is accomplished by an enzyme complex consisting of a series of two cytochromes and the terminal desaturase itself. The acyl-CoA form of fatty acids is the usual substrate for the desaturases, but fatty acids esterified to phospholipids can also be desaturated *in situ*.

All mammals that have been studied can convert stearate to oleate via Δ^9 desaturase. However, in the absence of dietary oleate, young rats may have insufficient capacity to sustain normal tissue oleate levels. Normal values depend on the reference, which can vary widely depending on the source and amount of oleate in the diet. Nevertheless, it is important to distinguish between the existence of a given desaturase and the capacity of that pathway to make sufficient of the necessary product fatty acid. Hence, as with the long-chain polyunsaturates and, indeed, with other nutrients such as amino acids (see Chapter 4), it is important to keep in mind that the existence of a pathway to make a particular fatty acid or amino acid does not guarantee sufficient capacity of that pathway to make that product. This is the origin of the concept of "conditional essentiality" or "indispensability." Both plants and animals are capable of desaturating at the 9–10 carbon (Δ^9 desaturase) of stearate, resulting in oleate. However, only plants are capable of desaturating oleate to linoleate and then to α-linolenate. Once linoleate and α-linolenate are consumed by animals, their conversion to the longer chain PUFAs of their respective families proceeds primarily by an alternating series of desaturation (Δ^6 and Δ^5 desaturases) and chain-elongation steps (Figure 6.13). Sequential desaturations or chain elongations are also a possibility, resulting in a large variety, though low abundance, of other PUFAs.

During dietary deficiency of linoleate or α-linolenate, oleate can also be desaturated and chain elongated to the PUFA eicosatrienoate (20:3n-9). Hence, most but not all PUFAs are derived from linoleate or α-linolenate.

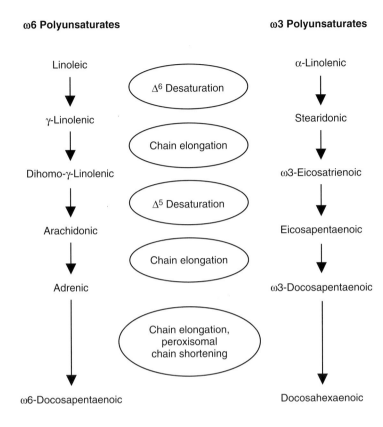

ω6 Polyunsaturates

Linoleic

Δ^6 Desaturation

γ-Linolenic

Chain elongation

Dihomo-γ-Linolenic

Δ^5 Desaturation

Arachidonic

Chain elongation

Adrenic

Chain elongation,
peroxisomal
chain shortening

ω6-Docosapentaenoic

ω3 Polyunsaturates

α-Linolenic

Stearidonic

ω3-Eicosatrienoic

Eicosapentaenoic

ω3-Docosapentaenoic

Docosahexaenoic

Figure 6.13 Conversion of linoleic (18:2n-6) and α-linolenic (18:3n-3) acids to their respective longer chain, more unsaturated polyunsaturates. In membranes, linoleic and arachidonic acids are the principal n-6 polyunsaturates, while docosahexaenoic acid is the principal n-3 polyunsaturate. Hence, these two families of fatty acids have different affinities for the desaturation and chain-elongation enzymes. This pathway is principally based in the endoplasmic reticulum but appears to depend on peroxisomes for the final chain shortening, which involves 24 carbon intermediates that are not illustrated.

Chain elongation of saturated and unsaturated fatty acids occurs primarily in the endoplasmic reticulum, although it has also been demonstrated to occur in mitochondria. Unlike the desaturation steps immediately before and after, the elongation steps do not appear to be rate limiting in the metabolism of linoleate or α-linolenate.

Despite the capacity to insert at least three double bonds in both n-3 and n-6 polyunsaturates, there is no proof that a Δ^4 desaturase exists to insert the final double bond in docosapentaenoate (22:5n-6) or docosahexaenoate (Figure 6.13). Rather, it appears that the precursors to these two fatty acids undergo a second elongation, repeated Δ^6 desaturation followed by chain shortening in peroxisomes. This unexpectedly convoluted series of steps is corroborated by the docosahexaenoate deficiency observed in disorders of peroxisomal biogenesis such as Zellweger's syndrome.

Hydrogenation

Opposite to the desaturation process is hydrogenation or removal of unsaturated bonds in lipids. Rumen bacteria are the only organisms known to have this capability. As in chemical hydrogenation practiced by the food industry, biohydrogenation in the rumen can be incomplete, resulting in the formation of small amounts of *trans* isomers, particularly of oleate, linoleate, and α-linolenate, which are found in milk fat.

Eicosanoids

Eicosanoids are 20-carbon, oxygen-substituted cyclized metabolites of dihomo-γ-linolenate, arachidonate, or eicosapentaenoate. They are produced via a cascade of steps starting with the cyclooxygenase or lipoxygenase enzymes present in microsomes. The main cyclooxygenase products comprise the classical prostaglandins, prostacyclin and the thromboxanes. The main lipoxygenase products are the leukotrienes (slow-reacting substances of anaphylaxis) and the noncyclized hydroperoxy derivatives of arachidonate that give rise to the hepoxylins and lipoxins (Figure 6.14).

Eicosanoids are considered to be fast-acting local hormones, the presence of which in the plasma and urine is largely a spillover from localized production,

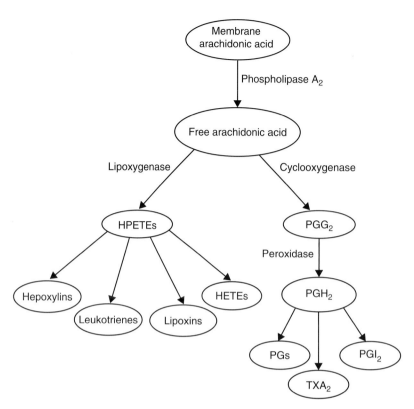

Figure 6.14 The arachidonic acid cascade is a fundamental component of cell signaling during injury. Phospholipase A_2 is immediately activated and the free arachidonic acid thus released is accessible to a controlled peroxidation process involving several cyclooxygenases (constitutive or inducible) and lipoxygenases. Over 50 metabolically active products are potentially produced, depending on the tissue involved, the type of cell that has been stimulated, and the type of injury. Only the main classes of these metabolites are shown. Before excretion, they are further metabolized to stable products that are not shown. Several of the cyclooxygenase products are competitive with each other, such as the platelet-aggregating and blood vessel wall-constricting effects of thromboxane A_2 (TXA$_2$) produced in platelets, versus the opposite effects of prostacyclin (PGI$_2$) derived from the blood vessel wall. HETE, hydroxyeicosatetraenoic acid; HPETE, hydroperoxyeicosatetraenoic acid; PG, prostaglandin; TX, thromboxane.

usually in response to an injury or a stimulus that releases the free precursor, most commonly arachidonate. The site of highest eicosanoid concentration appears to be the seminal fluid, although some species have no detectable eicosanoids in semen. Eicosanoids are second messengers modulating, among other pathways, protein phosphorylation. The lung is a major site of eicosanoid inactivation.

Four important characteristics of eicosanoid action should be noted. First, individual eicosanoids often have biphasic actions as one moves from very low through to higher, often pharmacological, concentrations. Thus, effects can vary dramatically depending not only on the experimental system but also on the eicosanoid concentration used. Second, several of the more abundant eicosanoids arising from the same precursor fatty acid have opposite actions to each other. For instance, prostacyclin and thromboxane A_2 are both derived from arachidonate but the former originates primarily from the endothelium and inhibits platelet aggregation, while the latter originates primarily from platelets and is a potent platelet-aggregating agent. Third, competing eicosanoids

derived from dihomo-γ-linolenate (1 series) and from eicosapentaenoate (3 series) often have effects that oppose those derived from arachidonate (2 series) (Figures 6.14 and 6.15). Thus, unlike prostaglandin E_2, prostaglandin E_1 has anti-inflammatory actions, reduces vascular tone, and inhibits platelet aggregation. Fourth, varying the ratio of the precursor fatty acids in the diet is an effective way to modify eicosanoid production. Thus, eicosapentaenoate and dihomo-γ-linolenate inhibit the synthesis of 2 series eicosanoids derived from arachidonate. This occurs by inhibiting arachidonate release from membranes by phospholipase A_2 and its cascade through the cyclooxygenases and lipoxygenases. The overproduction of 2 series eicosanoids is associated with higher blood pressure, increased platelet aggregation, and inflammatory processes, and can be effectively inhibited by dietary approaches using oils rich in eicosapentaenoate and γ-linolenate (18:3n-6), the precursor to dihomo-γ-linolenate.

Stable analogues of some classical prostaglandins have specialized medical applications, including the termination of pregnancy and the closing of a patent

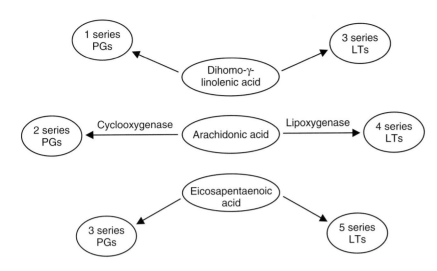

Figure 6.15 Arachidonic acid is not the only 20-carbon polyunsaturated fatty acid that can be metabolized via the cyclooxygenases and lipoxygenases; both dihomo-γ-linolenic acid (20:3n-6) and eicosapentaenoic acid (20:5n-3) are well-established precursors as well, and produce prostaglandins (PGs) and leukotrienes (LTs) that are frequently competitive with those produced from arachidonate, thereby neutralizing the effects of the arachidonate cascade (see Figure 6.14). This provides a critical balance in the overall reaction to cell injury.

ductus arteriosus shortly after birth. Many anti-inflammatory and anti-pyretic drugs are inhibitors of eicosanoid synthesis. One potentially dangerous side-effect of inhibiting eicosanoid synthesis is gastric erosion and bleeding. Receptor antagonists of leukotrienes are effective in reducing the symptoms of asthma.

6.8 Nutritional regulation of long-chain fatty acid profiles and metabolism

Phospholipids of all cellular and subcellular membranes contain a diverse range of long-chain fatty acids, the profile of which is subject to both dietary influence and endogenous control. A few organs, notably the brain, maintain extraordinarily strict control of their membrane composition. However, the fatty acid profile of most organs is usually responsive to the influence of changes in dietary fatty acid composition and other nutritional variables, yet maintains the vital "gatekeeper" functions of all membranes. Hence, when changes in dietary fat alter membrane fatty acid profiles, appropriate membrane fluidity can be maintained by the addition or removal of other lipids such as cholesterol. Insufficient energy intake and the presence of disease have important consequences for fatty acid synthesis, desaturation, and chain elongation and, consequently, tissue fatty acid profiles.

Saturates and monounsaturates

Inadequate energy intake increases macronutrient oxidation, including fatty acids. Short-term fasting

followed by refeeding a carbohydrate-rich meal is the classic way to stimulate fatty acid synthesis. Insulin is implicated in this process. When repeated, fasting/refeeding or weight cycling induces a gradual increase in the proportion of saturated and monounsaturated compared with PUFAs in tissues, especially body fat. This shift occurs because of the increase in fatty acid synthesis, easier oxidation of polyunsaturates, and the inhibition of desaturation and chain elongation by fasting. The implications of such an alteration in tissue fatty acid profiles have not yet been extensively studied, but probably involve changes in insulin sensitivity and other hormone effects. Protein deficiency also inhibits desaturation and chain elongation of PUFAs.

Copper supplementation increases Δ^9 desaturase activity in animals, resulting in higher oleate levels. This effect was first observed when copper was used to reduce gastrointestinal infection in pigs, but also led to softer back fat. Opposite to the effects of copper supplementation, copper deficiency inhibits synthesis of both oleate and docosahexaenoate.

Polyunsaturated fatty acids

There are four key features of the nutritional regulation of the profiles and metabolism of PUFAs. These attributes govern the effects of deficiency or excess of one or more of these families of fatty acids almost as much as their level in the diet. These key features are:

1 specificity within families
2 competition between families

3 substrate and end-product inhibition
4 cofactor nutrients.

Specificity

An n-6 PUFA cannot be converted to an n-3 or n-9 PUFA. Thus, deficiency of one family of polyunsaturates cannot be corrected by excess of those in a different family and, indeed, is exacerbated by excess intake of the other families.

Competition

The three families of PUFAs appear to use a common series of desaturases and chain elongases. The preference of these enzymes is for the more unsaturated fatty acids so, everything else being equal, more α-linolenate will be desaturated than linoleate or oleate. However, in practice, more linoleate is consumed than α-linolenate and, as a result, more arachidonate is produced endogenously than eicosapentaenoate. Furthermore, this competition for desaturation and chain elongation between linoleate and α-linolenate can lead to exacerbation of symptoms of deficiency of one or other fatty acid family. Thus, as has been demonstrated both clinically and experimentally, excess linoleate intake using sunflower oil is a common way to accelerate deficiency of n-3 PUFA.

Inhibition

Excess linoleate or α-linolenate intake appears to inhibit production of the respective long-chain products in the same fatty acid family, i.e., high α-linolenate intake inhibits synthesis of docosahexaenoate. Likewise, the main end-products of desaturation and chain elongation tend to inhibit further metabolism through this pathway, so arachidonate inhibits its own synthesis. Similarly, dietary deficiency of linoleate increases activity of the Δ^6 and Δ^5 desaturases, presumably to restore depleted levels of long-chain n-6 polyunsaturates such as arachidonate.

Cofactors

The cofactor requirements of the desaturation chain-elongation enzymes are not yet well understood, but a few relationships are known. The desaturases are metalloenzymes containing iron, and iron deficiency therefore inhibits desaturase activity. Magnesium is needed for microsomal desaturase activity *in vitro*. Zinc deficiency inhibits Δ^6 and Δ^5 desaturation, apparently by interrupting the flow of electrons from NADH. This effect is severe enough that inherited forms of zinc deficiency such as acrodermatitis enteropathica cause a precipitous decline in plasma arachidonate, greater than usually observed with dietary deficiency of n-6 polyunsaturates.

6.9 Nutritional and metabolic effects of dietary fatty acids

Two types of issue exist in relation to the nutritional and health implications of individual dietary lipids.

1 Whether synthesized endogenously or only obtained from the diet, what are the specific membrane, precursor, or metabolic effects of dietary lipids beyond that of providing energy?
2 Whether synthesized endogenously or obtained from the diet, does an excess amount of a dietary lipid have beneficial or deleterious implications for health?

Short- and medium-chain fatty acids

Short-chain fatty acids (1–6 carbons) are mostly derived from carbohydrate fermentation in the large bowel and appear to be mainly used for energy, although they are also substrates in several pathways. Butyrate may have an important role as an energy substrate for enterocytes. Medium-chain fatty acids (8–14 carbons) naturally appear in mammalian milk and are almost exclusively used as energy substrates. They may also be chain elongated to palmitate.

Saturated fatty acids

Palmitate and stearate constitute a major proportion of the acyl groups of membrane phospholipids and all mammals have the capacity to synthesize them. Hence, empirically, they presumably have an important function in energy metabolism, cell structure, normal development, and growth. The 20- to 24-carbon saturates are also important constituents of myelin. However, in any of these functions, it is unlikely that a dietary source of saturates is necessary. In fact, the brain is unable to acquire saturated fatty acids from the circulation and relies on its own endogenous synthesis for these fatty acids. Furthermore, chronic excess intake and/or synthesis of palmitate and stearate is associated with an increased risk of diabetes and coronary artery disease.

Monounsaturated fatty acids

Little is known about the nutritional or health implications of palmitoleate (16:1n-7), but there is a burgeoning interest in the main dietary monounsaturated fatty acid, oleate, and the health implications of olive oil. In the context of the same total fat intake, the main benefit of higher oleate intake seems to be that this reduces intake of palmitate and stearate and that this helps to lower serum cholesterol.

Partially hydrogenated fatty acids

Partially hydrogenated fatty acids contain a large proportion of *trans* fatty acids that are not naturally occurring but arise directly from food processing. Hence, unlike saturates and *cis*-unsaturated fatty acids, they are not a necessary component of the diet except in the small amounts found in cow's milk. Their physical characteristics make them economically suitable for inclusion in a wide variety of baked, fried, and oil-based foods, from which they can easily contribute up to 10% of dietary fat depending on food selection. Epidemiological evidence and some experimental studies show that common dietary *trans* fatty acids raise LDL cholesterol and lower HDLs in healthy adults, so the main nutritional concern is that they may contribute to an increased risk of cardiovascular disease (see Section 6.11).

Trans fatty acids have also been experimentally shown to compete with and impair the metabolism of other dietary long-chain fatty acids, but the relevance of these observations in humans is unclear. *Trans* fatty acids can be present in baby foods at relatively high concentrations but, so far, there is no evidence of deleterious effects on growth or development. Some information on the metabolism of *trans* fatty acids in humans has been gained from tracer studies, but fundamental information, such as the rate at which they are oxidized, is still unknown.

Polyunsaturated fatty acids

Unlike saturates and monounsaturates, a dietary source of n-6 and n-3 polyunsaturates is a necessity for normal growth and development. As with other essential nutrients, this has given rise to assessment of the dietary requirements for polyunsaturates and the implications of inadequate dietary intake of them.

It has been accepted for over 50 years that n-6 polyunsaturates, particularly linoleate, are required in the diet of all mammals, including humans. Official dietary guidelines generally recommend a dietary source of linoleate at 1–2% of energy intake. It has taken much longer to demonstrate that n-3 PUFAs are required by humans. Although this now seems widely accepted among nutrition researchers, some countries, including the USA, still do not yet officially recognize that, as a minimum, α-linolenate is a required nutrient. As with other nutrients, the requirement for polyunsaturates varies according to the stage of the life cycle, with pregnancy, lactation, and infancy being the most vulnerable. Symptoms of linoleate deficiency are virtually impossible to induce in healthy adult humans, so the concept of "conditional indispensability or dispensability" of PUFAs has recently emerged to replace the older but ambiguous term "essential fatty acid." Linoleate appears to be conditionally dispensable in healthy nonpregnant adults, but is not in pregnancy, lactation, or infancy.

Because of the competition between the two families of PUFAs, deficiency of n-3 PUFA is commonly induced by an excess of dietary linoleate. Hence, discussion of the requirements for linoleate and α-linolenate has focused on their ratio in the diet. The ratio of n-6 to n-3 polyunsaturates in human milk (5:1 to 10:1) has been widely viewed as a suitable reference for this ratio in the general diet. In most affluent countries, this ratio remains much higher, at about 20:1, and has been implicated in subclinical deficiency of n-3 polyunsaturates. There is recent evidence to suggest that it is the absolute amounts of long-chain n-3 and n-6 fatty acids that are important in predicting health outcomes, and not the dietary ratio of these PUFAs.

Essential fatty acid deficiency

The first experimental model of deficiency of polyunsaturates was total fat deficiency. The elimination of dietary fat had to be extreme because the traces of fat found in starch and dietary proteins were sufficient to prevent reproducible symptoms of fat deficiency. The deficiency symptoms are now well known and involve dry, scaly skin, growth retardation, and reproductive failure. Most of these gross symptoms are relieved by linoleate and arachidonate. Although α-linolenate cannot be synthesized *de novo*, it has little effect on these gross symptoms. However, careful studies using a diet that is extremely deficient in n-3 polyunsaturates and contains an excess of n-6 polyunsaturates led to deficiency of n-3 polyunsaturates, characterized by delayed and impaired neuronal development and impaired vision. These symptoms have been traced in many species to the inadequate accumulation of docosahexaenoate in the brain and eye. Hence, the main function of n-3 polyunsaturates appears to hinge on synthesis of docosahexaenoate. In contrast, the function of n-6 polyunsaturates involves independent roles of at least linoleate and arachidonate.

Human cases of deficiency of PUFAs, usually involve a clinical disorder, often involving weight loss, trauma such as surgery, or a disease requiring parenteral nutrition. However, reports of these cases are uncommon and describe dissimilar characteristics, leading one to question whether the same deficiency exists. Recent investigations into the amount of PUFA in the whole body and the rate at which they can be oxidized suggest that traumatic or disease-related processes leading to weight loss affect metabolism of polyunsaturates more severely than simple dietary deficiency in a weight-stable, healthy individual. For example, deficiency of linoleate has been long suspected but difficult to demonstrate in cystic fibrosis. Despite poor fat digestion, intake levels of linoleate may not be inadequate but its β-oxidation could well be abnormally high owing to the chronic infectious challenge.

Clinical importance of polyunsaturates

Infant brain and visual development is dependent on adequate accumulation of docosahexaenoate. The 1990s saw intense clinical and experimental assessment of the role of docosahexaenoate in early brain development and a widespread concern that many infant formulae do not yet contain docosahexaenoate. Several clinical studies and extensive use of formulae containing docosahexaenoate and arachidonate have shown that they are safe. Many but not all such studies show an improvement in visual and cognitive scores compared with matched formulae containing no docosahexaenoate or arachidonate. The infant brain and body as a whole clearly acquire less docosahexaenoate when only α-linolenate is given. As a whole, these data suggest that docosahexaenoate is a conditionally indispensable fatty acid.

Aside from questionable deficiency of polyunsaturates in cystic fibrosis (see above), one of the most graphic examples of their deficiency being caused by

an inherited disease is Zellweger's syndrome. This condition causes severe mental retardation and early death. It is a disorder of peroxisomal biogenesis and one outcome is markedly impaired synthesis of docosahexaenoate. Dietary supplementation with docosahexaenoate appears to partially restore neurological development.

Epidemiological evidence shows that chronic degenerative diseases of affluence are directly associated with the deficiency of n-3 PUFAs. Indeed, countries with relatively high rates of these diseases usually have an adequate to perhaps unnecessarily higher intake of linoleate. High intakes of linoleate have been implicated in death from coronary artery disease and several types of cancer because these diseases are associated with low intakes of n-3 polyunsaturates. Mental illnesses such as schizophrenia may also be associated with low intake of n-3 polyunsaturates and respond to supplements of n-3 polyunsaturates. A more balanced ratio of intake of n-6 and n-3 polyunsaturates might achieve a reduction in the rate of these degenerative diseases but has not yet been widely investigated.

Diets in Paleolithic times contained no processed food and probably balanced amounts of n-3 to n-6 polyunsaturates and a lower level of saturates. Such diets would be predicted to lead to a lower incidence of degenerative disease. Since the brain has a very high energy requirement, it has also been speculated that human brain evolution beyond that of other primates was dependent on a reliable and rich source of dietary energy and a direct source of long-chain polyunsaturates, particularly docosahexaenoate.

6.10 Cholesterol synthesis and regulation

Cholesterol and the brain

Mammalian brain function is dependent on specialized membranes designed for signal transmission. Greater cognitive sophistication in humans appears to depend on a much greater number of connections and, consequently, greater potential for signal processing. Like the membrane lipids of most other mammalian organs, brain lipids contain a relatively high proportion of cholesterol, which increases from about 40% of the lipid content in neonates to nearly 50% in adults.

Unlike other organs, the mammalian brain is probably unique in being unable to acquire appreciable amounts of cholesterol from the circulation, i.e., from the diet or from synthesis outside the brain. This has been extensively studied in the young rat and supporting, although inconclusive, evidence is also available for the pig. The brain has sufficient capacity to synthesize cholesterol from acetyl-CoA derived primarily from either glucose or ketones. Hence, it achieves the required level of cholesterol apparently entirely by endogenous synthesis. In neonates, ketones appear to play a greater role as substrates for brain cholesterol than in adults, in whom their main function seems to be as an alternative fuel to glucose. Among the common dietary long-chain fatty acids that would give rise to ketones during fat oxidation, PUFAs, particularly linoleate and α-linolenate, appear to be the best substrates for ketogenesis, since carbon from these fatty acids readily appears in brain cholesterol in suckling rats.

6.11 Effect of diet on serum lipids and lipoproteins

Diet and serum cholesterol

Diet exerts a profound influence on blood lipids and lipoproteins and, as such, should always be a major component of strategies for the primary prevention of diseases in which lipids play an etiological role, such as CHD. Nevertheless, despite convincing epidemiological evidence and the existence of credible biochemical mechanisms to support a relationship between dietary fat and serum cholesterol, the outcome of prospective intervention trials designed to test this relationship within populations has been disappointing.

Over 30 years ago Keys and Hegsted made the landmark observation that variation in the concentration of serum cholesterol across seven different countries was positively related to the amount of energy derived from saturated fat. Conversely, they found that intake of dietary PUFA was inversely related to serum cholesterol. From this finding they were able to formulate equations that enabled them to predict the quantitative effect of saturated and polyunsaturated fat on serum cholesterol (Figure 6.16). In simpler terms, the ratio of PUFAs to saturated fatty acids (SFAs), the P : S ratio, was used with effect to predict changes in serum cholesterol. Although still effective today, the equations and P:S ratio are being superseded by advanced knowledge of the biological effects of individual fatty acids. It is now well established that saturated fats with between 12 and 16 carbon atoms, namely lauric, myristic, and palmitic acids, are particularly hypercholesterolemic, whereas stearic acid, an extremely abundant SFA in most diets, is relatively neutral in its effects on serum cholesterol. [Note that stearic acid is desaturated to monounsaturated fatty acids (MUFAs) by Δ^9 desaturase]. The cholesterol-raising effect of SFAs arises chiefly from an increase in LDL cholesterol and is about twice as potent as the hypocholesterolemic effect of dietary PUFAs. Paradoxically, SFAs actually increase serum HDL cholesterol. The polyunsaturates are divisible into two main series on the basis of the position of the first double bond from the methyl end of the fatty acid chain, the parent fatty acids being linoleic (C18:2n-6) and α-linolenic (C18:3n-3) acids. The cholesterol-lowering effects of dietary PUFA is largely attributable to the effects of linoleic acid in lowering LDL. Historically,

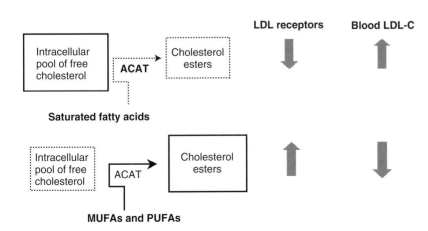

Figure 6.16 Influence of dietary fatty acids on serum cholesterol through differential effects on free cholesterol and low-density lipoprotein (LDL) receptor activity. ACAT, acyl-CoA-cholesterol acyltransferase; LDL-C, LDL cholesterol; MUFA, monounsaturated fatty acid; PUFA, polyunsaturated fatty acid.

monounsaturated fat was considered to be neutral with respect to its effects on lipids and lipoproteins and was omitted from the predictive formulae of Keys and Hegsted. However, further studies, prompted by interest in the role of MUFAs in the Mediterranean diet, have shown that MUFA-enriched diets may decrease LDL cholesterol, although possibly to a lesser extent than linoleic acid, and increase HDL cholesterol. An additional benefit of MUFAs is thought to be conferred by the presence of a single double bond in MUFAs, which when incorporated into the membrane phospholipids of LDL, protect this lipoprotein from oxidative modification, an essential prerequisite step in the deposition of cholesterol in the artery wall. In this regard, there has been concern that increasing dietary PUFA will impose additional oxidative stress on LDL. While this idea forms part of the rationale for limiting the amount of dietary PUFA to less than 10% of energy intake, there is as yet no convincing evidence of adverse effects from increasing the level of PUFA in tissues and circulating lipoproteins.

Trans *fatty acids*

While saturated fats consist of straight chains of carbon atoms which pack together tightly in the phospholipids of cell membranes and lipoproteins, in contrast, carbon double bonds in the *cis* configuration in MUFAs and PUFAs introduce a bend or kink into the carbon chain. This alters the physical properties of the phospholipids containing these fatty acids, by, for example, increasing their packing volume, a physical property that contributes to an increase in membrane fluidity. The partial hydrogenation of MUFAs and PUFAs, most notably during the industrial processing of foods for the purpose of solidifying unsaturated oils, results in a loss of this kink as the fatty acid assumes a straighter, *trans* configuration that resembles that found in SFAs. This likeness in chemical structure is thought to account for the SFA-like effects of *trans* fatty acids such as elaidic acid (*trans* isomer of oleic acid) on serum lipids (see Figures 6.1 and 6.2). The results of prospective cohort studies such as the Nurses' Health Study showed that high levels of *trans* fats in excess of 7% energy increased serum LDLs and reduced HDLs (Willet *et al.* 1993). However, despite the continued use of partially hydrogenated fats in food products, the average intake of *trans* fatty acids in most Western diets does not exceed 2% of total energy intake, and at this level

of intake these fats are unlikely to exert adverse effects on serum lipoproteins.

Plant sterols and soluble nonstarch polysaccharides

These compounds may be grouped together as they share a similar mode of action on LDL cholesterol, which is to reduce the availability of dietary and biliary cholesterol for absorption in the gut. This action interrupts the enterohepatic circulation and upregulates the production and activity of LDL receptors (see Section 6.5). Plant sterols and their esters such as those incorporated into margarines (stanols and stanol esters), despite being nearly identical in structure to cholesterol, are poorly absorbed and interfere with the reabsorption of cholesterol originating from bile (~1 g/day) and dietary sources (300 mg/day) by either coprecipitation or competition. Margarines or spreads (30–40 g/day) containing plant sterols or their derivatives have been shown to reduce LDL cholesterol by up to 14% in controlled trials. Soluble NSPs such as those found in gums and gelling agents from fruit (gum arabic and pectins) act in a similar way and have been shown to be equally efficacious in reducing LDL cholesterol.

Dietary cholesterol

There is a popular misconception that dietary cholesterol correlates directly with serum cholesterol, when in fact dietary cholesterol, within a range of normal dietary consumption (100–400 mg/day), has only a very small impact on blood cholesterol levels. Eggs represent the principal source of dietary cholesterol in most diets (1 egg yolk = 150–250 mg cholesterol); in their absence, most Western diets would contain considerably less than 100 mg cholesterol/day. The classic but extreme egg-feeding studies showed that feeding of up to six eggs per day (900 mg cholesterol) increased LDL cholesterol acutely. However, the body effectively counters this effect with sensitive, compensatory mechanisms to deal with an increasing load of dietary cholesterol, one of which is to reduce the amount of cholesterol absorbed in the gut. This compensation effectively abolishes any dose–response relationship between dietary cholesterol, over a practically realistic range of intakes, and serum cholesterol. Two factors that may influence the variability in response to dietary cholesterol are dietary saturated fatty acids, which have been shown to augment the cholesterol-raising effects of dietary cholesterol, and a phenomenon of increased susceptibility to dietary cholesterol in some individuals for some, as yet, unknown reason.

To place these dietary influences on blood cholesterol in perspective with other cholesterol-lowering strategies, a metaanalysis of dietary intervention trials undertaken by the World Health Organization (WHO) revealed that dietary modification could achieve reductions in serum cholesterol of between only 4% and 5%. This finding is in sharp contrast to the potent effects of cholesterol-lowering drugs, which can reduce serum cholesterol by 30–40% and have been shown, unequivocally, to reduce the incidence of death from CHD. It also highlights the need to address other risk factors which are more responsive to dietary change.

Fat quantity versus quality: importance of the ratio of n-6:n-3 polyunsaturated fatty acids

The underlying principle for a reduction in total fat intake is to reduce energy intake from the consumption of the most energy-dense macronutrient in order to prevent weight gain and ultimately obesity. The current recommendation for the UK is to reduce energy derived from fat to 35% or less. Since weight gain is associated with raised plasma TAGs and abnormalities in circulating lipoproteins, reducing total fat intake should, in theory, reduce blood lipids. However, in practice there is little evidence to support such an effect within populations. Metaanalyses have revealed that little benefit is to be gained, at least in terms of changes in blood lipids, by reducing total fat without altering the composition of dietary fatty acids. Metaanalyses have also helped to resolve the issue of what represents the most appropriate replacement nutrient for SFAs. Since PUFAs, and specifically linoleic acid, were shown to counter the actions of SFAs and were abundant in natural sources such as sunflower and corn oils, they were an obvious first choice. The alternative was to substitute fat with dietary carbohydrate. There have been problems associated with both of these approaches. First, increasing dietary linoleic acid excludes the lesser abundant, but more metabolically active, n-3 PUFA, and especially the longer chain (C20–C22) members of this series derived from marine oils [C20:5 (eicosapentaenoic acid) and C22:6 (docosahexaenoic acid)]. Overemphasis on linoleic

acid in the food industry, together with a widespread resistance to the consumption of fish, has increased the ratio of n-6 to n-3 PUFAs in northern Europe and the USA since the 1970s. This situation has major implications for the development of abnormalities in circulating lipoproteins, since deficiency in eicosapentaenoic acid and docosahexaenoic acid could help to promote an increase in plasma TAG. This could occur through an overproduction of endogenous TAG (VLDL) in the liver and intolerance to dietary (exogenous) fat, and lead to the development of dyslipidemia known as an ALP (see Section 6.5). The frequency of this dyslipidemia is believed to be very rare in Mediterranean countries that have a high intake of dietary n-3 PUFA and an n-6:n-3 ratio closer to 1. High-carbohydrate diets have been shown to increase plasma TAG. Carbohydrate-induced hypertriacylglycerolemia is not, as was originally thought, a short-term adaptive response in the liver, as it changes its pattern of oxidation from fat to carbohydrate, but a real phenomenon associated with the overconsumption of the non-milk extrinsic sugars, sucrose and fructose, most notably in individuals with insulin-resistant dyslipidemia. There is evidence to suggest that this effect can be avoided by limiting the intake of sucrose and increasing the intake of slowly absorbed carbohydrate with a low impact on blood glucose.

The results of several metaanalyses of dietary intervention trials support dietary MUFAs as the most favored substitute for dietary saturated fatty acids, and even linoleic acid in areas of high intake.

Effects of n-3 polyunsaturated fatty acids from plants and fish

The current dietary recommendation for the intake of long-chain n-3 PUFAs (eicosapentaenoic acid/docosahexaenoic acid) in the UK is 450 mg/day (SACN, 2004). This was to increase intake by consuming two portions of fish per week, one of which should be oily (e.g., mackerel, sardines). This recommendation was based on evidence from a host of epidemiological and intervention studies, which showed that regular fish consumption could reduce the risk of sudden cardiac death. Since this an acute end-point of CHD, the benefits of fish oil have been ascribed to the prevention of fatal cardiac arrhythmia, and, to a lesser extent, coronary thrombosis, but not to any favorable effects on blood lipids. However, there is also convincing evidence to show that fish oil supplementation (1 g/

day for 3 years) reduces the incidence of death from CHD in healthy, free-living subjects. This longer term benefit may be linked to the effects of eicosapentaenoic acid/docosahexaenoic acid on a host of other cardiovascular risk factors, including plasma TAGs and lipoproteins.

Long-chain n-3 PUFAs exert multiple effects on lipid metabolism, the most notable of which is the capacity to decrease postabsorptive plasma TAG levels by 20–30%. Fish oil-enriched diets have also been shown to attenuate the magnitude and duration of postprandial lipemia following the ingestion of a fat-containing meal. These effects are frequently accompanied by beneficial changes in circulating LDLs and HDLs, and the correction of an ALP.

Widespread knowledge of the favorable effects of eicosapentaenoic acid and docosahexaenoic acid has raised awareness of the need to increase intakes of these fatty acids, and to reduce the amount of n-6

PUFA at the same time. However, in practice, this will be difficult to achieve, not least because of a mass resistance to the increased consumption of oily fish and diminishing fish stocks. An obvious alternative would be to increase the intake of the shorter chain precursor of eicosapentaenoic acid/docosahexaenoic acid, α-linolenic acid (C18:3n-3). The latter is derived from plant seeds such as flax and rapeseed, and is desaturated and elongated to its longer chain relatives in the body. Unfortunately, the rate of conversion to eicosapentaenoic acid and especially docosahexaenoic acid is slow, and the efficiency of conversion is reduced by high levels of linoleic acid, which competes more effectively than α-linolenic acid for desaturation. There is, as yet, no evidence to suggest that the rate of conversion of dietary α-linolenic acid to eicosapentaenoic acid and especially docosahexaenoic acid is sufficient to achieve fish oil-like effects on blood lipids (Table 6.6).

Table 6.6 Effects on plasma lipids of substituting dietary saturated fats with polyunsaturated fatty acids, monounsaturated fatty acids, and carbohydrates

[a] n-6 PUFA in excess of 10% energy.
[b] Increase in response to redistribution of LDL subclasses.
PUFA: polyunsatruated fatty acids; MUFA: monounsaturated fatty acids.
SFA: saturated fatty acids; LC: long chain; EPA: eicosapentaenoic acid; DHA: docosahexaenoic acid; short chain;
LDL-C: low-density lipoprotein cholesterol; HDL-C: high-density lipoprotein cholesterol; TAG: triacylglycerols; TC: total cholesterol.

How do dietary fatty acids influence serum cholesterol and triacylglycerols?

In common with other physiological systems, lipoprotein metabolism is coordinated by interplay between the activity of specific genes and hormones that determines the production and activity of functional proteins (enzymes, receptors, lipid transfer, and apoproteins). Effects on these functional proteins ultimately regulate the quantity and quality of circulating lipids and lipoproteins. While there have been significant advances in knowledge of the modulatory effects of dietary fatty acids on hormones and gene expression, evidence for the effects of dietary fats on functional proteins is by far the most advanced.

Saturated fatty acids and low-density lipoprotein cholesterol

The most well-elucidated mechanism to explain how different dietary fats produce variable effects on LDL-cholesterol is through the LDL receptor pathway, the control of which has already been described (see Section 6.5). The ability of the cell to regulate its pool of free cholesterol depends to a large extent on the nature of the fatty acids available for esterification by the enzyme ACAT, an intracellular relative of LCAT. ACAT favors unsaturated fatty acids (MUFAs and PUFAs) as substrates for esterification, which utilizes free cholesterol within the cell. The resulting reduction in intracellular free cholesterol stimulates the transcription of the LDL receptor gene and production of new LDL receptors through the SREBP mechanism, and fall in circulating LDL as already described. Conversely, SFAs are poor substrates for ACAT, and their presence in the cell exerts the opposite effect on free cholesterol levels, thus increasing circulating LDL cholesterol and total serum cholesterol (Figure 6.8). Fatty acids may also exert direct effects on the activity of LDL receptors by altering the composition of membrane phospholipids and thus membrane fluidity. Alternatively, there is evidence to suggest that dietary PUFA could upregulate LDL receptors indirectly, by increasing the cholesterol content (lithogenicity) of bile and in this way accelerate the excretion of cholesterol.

Long-chain n-3 polyunsaturated fatty acids and serum triacylglycerols

Long chain n-3 PUFAs have potent effects in the liver, where they suppress the production of endogenous TAG by inhibiting the enzymes phosphatidic acid phosphatase and diacylglycerol acyltransferase. They may also selectively increase the degradation of apoB-100, further reducing the production of TAG-rich VLDLs. (Note that apoB-100 is produced constitutively, so that the production of VLDL is driven by the supply of substrates for the synthesis of TAG). In addition, long-chain n-3 PUFAs accelerate the clearance of TAG-rich lipoproteins from the circulation in the postprandial phase by stimulating the activity of LPL. Together, these effects are thought to underlie the ability of these fatty acids to correct the lipoprotein abnormalities associated with an ALP. It is also possible that many of the effects of eicosapentaenoic acid/docosahexaenoic acid on blood lipids and other cardiovascular risk factors are mediated through an increase in the sensitivity of tissues to the action of insulin. However, there is, as yet, no convincing evidence to support such an effect in adipose tissue, liver, or skeletal muscle.

Nutrient–gene interactions

It has been estimated that diet could account for up to 50% of the variation in blood lipids and lipoprotein levels between individuals. This would mean that genetic differences must explain the remaining 50%. In real terms, interactions between diet and genes represent a sizeable proportion of each of these unrealistically discrete fractions.

Fixed genetic polymorphisms

Variation in the structure of specific genes between individuals (genetic heterogeneity) has been shown to give rise to differences in dietary responsiveness. A few common polymorphisms have been identified in genes associated with lipoprotein metabolism, the best example of which is apoE. ApoE facilitates the uptake of TAG-rich lipoproteins (chylomicron remnants and VLDL) via the remnant and LDL receptors and, thus, in part, determines the removal of TAG from the circulation. The gene for apoE is polymorphic, which means that it exists in multiple forms between individuals. This polymorphism generates several isoforms of the protein that express variable affinities for their receptors and thus variable potential to remove TAG-rich lipoproteins from the circulation. In this way, apoE genotype can modulate the response of an individual to any dietary fat that exerts an influence on TAG-rich lipoproteins, giving rise to

Table 6.7 Effect of apoprotein E phenotype on serum cholesterol

Phenotype (gene frequency)	Receptor binding affinity	Hepatic free cholesterol	LDL receptor activity	LDL-C
E4 (ϵ_4 15%)	+ + +	↑ (feedback)	↓	↑
E3 (ϵ_3 77%)	+ +	→	→	→
E2 (ϵ_2 8%)	+	↓ (feedback)	↑	↓

Carriage of ϵ_4 allele is associated with increased risk of coronary heart disease and greater changes in low-density lipoprotein cholesterol (LDL-C) in response to increased dietary fat and cholesterol in men.

the concept of genetic susceptibility to diet (Table 6.7).

Modulation of gene expression

Dietary fatty acids and/or their intracellular (eicosanoid) derivatives can also influence the expression of genes (rate of gene transcription) by interacting with specific nuclear receptors within the nucleus of cells. These nuclear receptors control the rate of gene transcription by binding to specific regions of DNA known as responsive elements. Genes associated with the production of functional proteins can be either stimulated or repressed according to the nature of the nuclear transcription factor and its binding substrate (PUFAs or derivative). Peroxisome proliferator-activated receptors (PPARs) represent examples of nuclear receptors that may utilize long-chain PUFAs as substrates. PPARs can be found in all tissues of the body, but notably in the liver, where they control the synthesis of lipid and apoproteins (PPAR-α), and in adipose tissue (PPAR-γ), where they control the differentiation of adipocytes and insulin-sensitive mobilization and synthesis of TAG. SREBPs represent another example of nuclear transcription proteins that control cholesterol and fatty acid metabolism within the cell.

6.12 Perspectives on the future

Future research on fatty acids and their role in health and disease will be largely dictated by progress in intervention studies using fatty acid supplements in chronic diseases of inflammation, brain degeneration, cancer, and heart disease. Some of these studies will be based on effects of dietary fats on gene expression that have yet to be discovered; others will be based on information that we already have. No doubt the search

for the "ideal" fat intake will continue, but this seems misguided because humans in good health in different cultures and geographical locations ultimately consume a wide range of total fat and fatty acid ratios; their overall health is based on much more than their fat intake. Nevertheless, pursuit of an ideal fat intake or composition will satisfy the thirst of many researchers, consumers, and government agencies but, in all likelihood, will not greatly alter the impact of fats on disease processes. These would include:

- the role of the quantity and quality of dietary fat on postprandial lipemia, specific lipoproteins, and the risk of CHD
- the metabolic roles of the short-chain fatty acids (1–6 carbons)
- the effect of *trans* fatty acids in baby foods, and the level of intake of *trans* fatty acids that will increase the risk of CHD in adults
- the appropriate amounts of n-6 to n-3 polyunsaturates to prevent, reverse, and/or treat chronic degenerative diseases
- the requirements of docosahexaenoate and other long-chain PUFA in infant and enteral feeding
- the conditional indispensability of particular fatty acids throughout the life cycle (especially during pregnancy and lactation, and in the aged)
- the effects of particular dietary fatty acids and combinations of fatty acids on hormone and gene expression.

More knowledge in all of these areas will lead to a better understanding of the mechanisms through which dietary lipids influence blood lipids and lipoproteins and therefore the risk of chronic diseases. It will also lead to improved recommendations regarding the quantity and quality of dietary fats that are commensurate with optimum human health.

Acknowledgment

This chapter has been revised and updated by Bruce Griffin based on the original chapter by Bruce Griffin and Stephen Cunnane.

References

Bloomfield DK & Bloch K. The formation of Δ^9-unsaturated fatty acids. *J Biol Chem* 1960; **235**: 337-345.

Burr MM & Burr GO. A new deficiency disease produced by the rigid exclusion of fat from the diet. *J Biol Chem* 1929; **82**: 345-367.

Goldstein JL & Brown MS. Atherosclerosis: the LDL receptor hypothesis. *Metabolism* 1977; **26**: 1257-1275.

Hegsted DM, McGrandy RB, Myers ML et al. Quantitative effects of dietary fat on serum cholesterol in man. *Am J Clin Nutr* 1965; **17**: 281-295.

Keys A, Anderson JT & Grande F. Prediction of serum cholesterol responses of man to changes in fats in the diet. *Lancet* 1977; **2**: 959-966.

Ponticorvo L, Rittenberg D & Bloch K. The utilisation of acetate for the synthesis of fatty acids, cholesterol and protoporphyrin. *J Biol Chem* 1949; **179**: 839-842.

Scientific Advisory Committee on Nutrition (SACN) 2004. Report published for the Food Standards Agency and the Department of Health by TSO. ISBN 0-11-243083-X.

Willet WC, Stamfer MJ, Manson JE et al. Intake of trans fatty acids and risk of coronary heart disease among women, *Lancet* 1993; **341**: 581–585.

Zilversmit DB. Atherogenesis is a postprandial phenomenon. *Circulation* 1979; **60**: 473-485.

Further reading

Cunnane SC. Alpha-linolenate acid in human nutrition. In: Cunnane SC, Thompson LU, eds. *Flaxseed in Human Nutrition.* AOCS Press, Champaign, IL, 1995: 99–127.

Dolecek TA. Epidemiological evidence of relationships between dietary polyunsaturated fatty acids and mortality in the Multiple Risk Factor Intervention Trial. *Proc Soc Exp Biol Med* 1992; **200**: 177–182.

Durrington PN. *Hyperlipidaemia Diagnosis and Management*, 2nd edn. Elsevier Science, Oxford, 1995.

Griffin BA The effects of n-3 PUFA on LDL subfractions. *Lipids* 2001; **36**: S91–S97.

Griffin BA How relevant is the ratio of dietary n-6 to n-3 polyunsaturated fatty acids to cardiovascular disease risk? Evidence from the OPTILIP Study. *Curr Opin Lipidol* 2008; **19**: 57–62.

Lands WEM. Impact of daily food choices on health promotion and disease prevention. In: Hamazaki H, Okuyama H, eds. *Fatty Acids and Lipids: New Findings.* Karger, Basel, 2001: 1–5.

Lee A, Griffin BA. Dietary cholesterol, eggs and coronary heart disease in perspective. *Br Nutr Found Bull* 2006; **31**: 21–27.

Mangiapane EH, Salter AM, eds. *Diet, Lipoproteins and Coronary Heart Disease. A Biochemical Perspective*. Nottingham University Press, Nottingham, 1999.

Simopoulos AP. Evolutionary aspects of diet and essential fatty acids. In: Hamazaki H, Okuyama H, eds. *Fatty Acids and Lipids: New Findings.* Karger, Basel, 2001: 18–27.

Willett WC. *Eat, Drink and Be Healthy: The Harvard Medical School Guide to Healthy Eating.* Simon and Schuster, New York, 2001.

7
Dietary Reference Standards

Kate M Younger

Key messages

- This chapter discusses the development of terminology and the change in conceptual approaches to setting nutrient recommendations from adequate to optimum nutrition.
- The interpretation and uses of dietary recommendations are discussed.
- The chapter describes how reference values can be used to assess the adequacy of the nutrient intakes of population groups.

- The methods used to determine requirements are discussed. These include deprivation studies, radioactive tracer studies, balance studies, factorial methods, measurement of nutrient levels in biological tissues, biochemical and biological markers, and animal experiments.

7.1 Introduction

The first attempt to set standards for nutrient intakes was by the Food and Nutrition Board of the National Research Council of the USA in 1941, which published recommended daily allowances (RDAs) in 1943 to "provide standards to serve as a goal for good nutrition." The first UK RDAs followed in 1950, published by the British Medical Association, and many other countries and international agencies now publish dietary standards that are intended to allow the adequacy of the nutrient intakes of groups or populations to be assessed by comparison with the standards.

As the amount known about human requirements and nutrient functions has increased, so too has the size of the documents describing the recommendations, from a mere six pages dealing with 10 nutrients in 1943 to the series of weighty books, each dealing with the dietary reference intakes (DRIs) of only a few of more than 30 nutrients, published by the Institute of Medicine of the USA. Furthermore, continuing research and the development of more informed interpretations of the expanding body of data available necessitate the regular revision and updating of the recommendations; thus, the "standards" of the past become obsolete as they are replaced by new figures based on new data or new interpretations of existing data.

7.2 Terminology and conceptual approaches to setting nutrient recommendations

From the time of their first issue in the 1940s and throughout the next 50 years, the concepts and terminology of RDAs remained unchanged. The basis on which these RDAs were built was the statistical distribution of individual requirements to prevent deficiency criteria for the target nutrient. The peak of the curve of the Gaussian distributions of such requirements is the "average requirement," with half the population having requirements above this value and the other half having lower requirements. The RDA was taken to be a point on that distribution that was equal to the mean or "average requirements" plus 2 standard deviations (SDs) (Figure 7.1). By setting the recommendation close to the upper end of the distribution of individual requirements, the needs of most of the population would be met. If the standard were set to meet the apparent needs of almost everyone, the resultant value would be so high as to be unat-

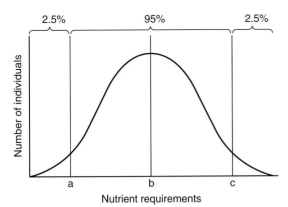

Figure 7.1 Frequency distribution of individual requirements for a nutrient. (a) The mean minus a notional 2 standard deviations (SDs); intakes below this will be inadequate for nearly all of the population. (b) The mean; the midpoint of the population's requirement. (c) The mean plus a notional 2 SDs; the intake that is adequate for nearly all of the population. Note that, in practice, because insufficient data exist to establish reliable means and SDs for many nutrient requirements, the reference intakes describing the points a and c on the curve are generally set, in the case of a, at the level that is judged to prevent the appearance of signs of deficiency (biochemical or clinical), and, in the case of c, at the level above which all individuals appear to be adequately supplied. Thus, it is unlikely that even 2.5% of the population would not achieve adequacy at intake level c.

tainable at population level. If the standard were set at the point of the average of all individual requirements, then half the population would have requirements in excess of the standard. In a normal distribution, some 2.5% of points lie at the upper and lower tails outside that range of the mean plus or minus 2 SDs. Thus, by setting the RDA to this point of the mean plus 2 SDs, we are setting the standard for 97.5% of the population. The consumption of most nutrients at levels somewhat greater than actually required is generally not harmful; hence, setting recommendations at the population average requirement plus a notional 2 SDs is logical if the aim is to describe an intake that is adequate for almost everyone. However, this is spectacularly inappropriate in the case of recommendations for energy intake, since even relatively small imbalances in energy intake over expenditure will lead, over time, to overweight and ultimately obesity, an increasing problem in most populations. Recommendations for energy intake are therefore given only as the estimated population average requirement.

Thus, for almost half a century, these were the terms used and the underlying conceptual approaches.

However, since the 1980s, changes have occurred in both of these areas.

Changes in terminology

Two basic changes occurred with regard to terminology. The first was that the term "recommended dietary allowance" was altered and the second was that new terms were introduced so that the adequacy of diets could be evaluated from several perspectives. The reason for changing the terminology was in effect to re-emphasize some of the basic concepts underlying the term RDA. "Recommended" has a prescriptive air about it and there were concerns that consumers might see this as something that had to be met daily and met precisely. The term "allowance" reinforces the perception of a prescriptive approach. Thus, the UK adopted the term dietary reference value (DRV), the EU introduced the term population reference intake (PRI), the USA and Canada introduced the term dietary reference intake (DRI), and Australia and New Zealand now use the term nutrient intake value (NIV). All are precisely equivalent to the original concept of the RDA, a term that many countries prefer to continue to use.

Two new terms were introduced: a minimum requirement and a safe upper level. The minimum requirement represents the average requirement minus 2 SDs (point a in Figure 7.1). A definition describing this point is given in Figure 7.1 along with the various terms used to define this point (Box 7.1). The concept of an upper safe limit of intake has gained importance in view of the increased opportunity for people to consume high levels of nutrients from fortified foods or supplements. The recently revised US DRI set "tolerable upper intake" levels (ULs) that are judged to be the highest level of nutrient intake that is likely to pose no risk of adverse health effects in almost all individuals in a group. The current European and UK recommendations also address this concern in the case of those nutrients for which toxic levels have been reported. The terms used by different recommending bodies to describe the various points on the distribution of individual requirements for a nutrient are given in Box 7.2, while precise definitions may be found in the relevant publications referred to.

The World Health Organization (WHO) has taken a rather different approach, defining population safe ranges of intake. "Normative requirement" is now

Box 7.1 Terms used to describe points a, b, and c on the frequency distribution

	a	b	c
European Communities Scientific Committee for Food **Population reference intakes** (1993)	Lowest threshold intake (**LTI**)	Average requirement (**AR**)	Population reference intake (**PRI**)
US Food and Nutrition Board, National Academy of Sciences, National Research Council **Recommended daily allowances** (1989)			Recommended daily allowance (**RDA**)
US Food and Nutrition Board, Institute of Medicine, National Academies of Health, Canada **Dietary reference intakes** (1997–2005)		Estimated average requirement (**EAR**)	Recommended daily allowance (**RDA**)
British Committee on Medical Aspects of Food Policy (COMA) **Dietary reference values** (1991)	Lower reference nutrient intake (**LRNI**)	Estimated average requirement (**EAR**)	Reference nutrient intake (**RNI**)
World Health Organization/Food and Agriculture Organization (WHO/FAO)			Recommended nutrient intake (**RNI**)
National Health and Medical Research Council (NHMRC), Australia and New Zealand **Nutrient reference values** (2006)		Estimated average requirement (**EAR**)	Recommended dietary intake (**RNI**)
United Nations University (UNU) **Nutrient intake values** (2007)		Average nutrient requirement (**ANR**)	Individual nutrient level (**INL$_x$**; in this case **INL$_{98}$**)

Box 7.2 Additional terms used

European population reference intake (1993)	Acceptable range of intakes
US recommended daily allowance (1989)	Safe intake and adequate intake
US dietary reference intake (1997–2005)	Adequate intake (**AI**) and tolerable upper intake level (**UL**), acceptable macronutrient distribution range (**AMDR**)
British dietary reference value (1991)	Safe and adequate intake
World Health Organization (1974–1996)	Recommended intake
World Health Organization (1996–)	Basal, normative, and maximum population requirement ranges, mean intake goals
National Health and Medical Research Council (2006)	Acceptable macronutrient distribution range (**AMDR**) and suggested dietary target (**SDT**)
United Nations University (2007)	Upper nutrient level (**UNL**)

used to describe the population mean normative requirement (which would allow the maintenance of, or a desirable, body store or reserve); "maximum" to refer to the upper limit of safe ranges of population mean intakes; and "basal" for the lower such limit, below which clinically detectable signs of inadequacy would be expected to appear. These WHO requirements are revised in groups of nutrients at different times (see Further reading), and in those that date from 1974 the term "recommended intake" or "recommended nutrient intake" is used to describe the average requirement plus an amount that takes into account interindividual variability and hence is considered to be sufficient for the maintenance of health in nearly all people.

More recently, the United Nations University (UNU) has published a suggested harmonized approach and methodologies for developing nutrient recommendations, together with proposed terminology (Box 7.1), that could be used worldwide to promote objectivity, transparency, and consistency among those setting and using nutrient recommendations. Their preferred term, nutrient intake value (NIV), refers to dietary intake recommendations based on research data; the term "nutrient" was chosen in order to distinguish these from dietary components such as cereals, and the term "value" is intended to emphasize the potential usefulness for both assessing dietary adequacy (and hence dietary planning) and policy-making. The individual nutrient level (INL_x) is flexible, in that x refers to the chosen percentile of the population for whom this intake is sufficient; for example 98% (mean or median requirement + 2 SDs), written as INL_{98}, but it could be set lower in the case of certain nutrients.

Changes in conceptual approach

When a committee sits to make a recommendation for a standard in relation to nutrient intakes, it begins with a distribution of requirements. In the past, although the choice of criteria for requirement might vary between committees, the orientation was always the same: requirements were set at a level that should prevent deficiency symptoms. More recently, the concern for health promotion through diet has led to the introduction of the concept of optimal nutrition, in which the optimal intake of a nutrient could be defined as that intake that maximizes physiological and mental function and minimizes the development of degenerative diseases. It should be borne in mind that, although this may appear simple enough to define in the case of single nutrients, things clearly become more complex when considering all nutrients together, in all possible physiological situations. Genetic variability may also, increasingly, be taken into account; for example, the requirement for folate of those carrying certain variants of the *MTHFR* gene (around 10% of the population tested thus far) might, arguably, need to be set higher than for the rest of the population.

It is now recognized that there are several levels for considering the concept of optimal nutrition, i.e., the level that:

- prevents deficiency symptoms, traditionally used to establish reference nutrient intakes
- optimizes body stores of a nutrient
- optimizes some biochemical or physiological function
- minimizes a risk factor for some chronic disease
- minimizes the incidence of a disease.

In the USA, the reference value for calcium is based on optimizing bone calcium levels, which is a move away from the traditional approach of focusing on preventing deficiency symptoms. An example of attempts to set the reference standard for optimizing a biochemical function is a level of folic acid that would minimize the plasma levels of homocysteine, a potential risk factor for cardiovascular disease. Another might be the level of zinc to optimize cell-mediated immunity. An example of a possible reference standard to optimize a risk factor for a disease is the level of sodium that would minimize hypertension or the level of n-3 polyunsaturated fatty acids (PUFAs) to lower plasma triacylglycerols (TAGs). The amount of folic acid to minimize the population burden of neural tube defect would be an example of a reference value to minimize the incidence of a disease. At present, there is much debate as to the best approach to choosing criteria for setting reference standards for minerals and vitamins, and this is an area that is likely to continue to court controversy. An important point to note in this respect is that, while minimizing frank deficiency symptoms of micronutrients is an acute issue in many developing countries, any evolution of our concepts of desirable or optimal nutrient requirements must lead to a revision of the estimate of the numbers of those with inadequate nutrition.

7.3 Interpretation and uses of dietary recommendations

When using dietary recommendations, several important points need to be considered.

The nutrient levels recommended are per person per day. However, in practice this will usually be achieved as an average over a period of time (days, weeks, or months) owing to daily fluctuations in the diet. As stated above, the setting of a range of dietary recommendations should encourage appropriate interpretation of dietary intake data, rather than the inappropriate assumption that the value identified to meet the needs of practically all healthy people is a minimum requirement for individuals. If an individual's nutrient intake can be averaged over a sufficient period then this improves the validity of the comparison with dietary recommendations. However, in the case of energy intakes, such a comparison is still inappropriate: dietary reference values for energy are intended only for use with groups, and it is more useful to compare an individual's energy intake with some measure or calculation of their expenditure in order to assess adequacy.

In the case of a group, the assumption can be made that the quality of the diet can be averaged across the group at a given time-point, and therefore that apparently healthy individuals within a group may compensate for a relative deficiency on one day by a relative excess on another. It should also be remembered that allowances may need to be made for body size, activity level, and perhaps other characteristics of the individual or group under consideration, since the recommended intakes are designed for "reference" populations.

Another assumption made when setting recommendations for a particular nutrient is that the intake of all other nutrients is adequate, which in an apparently healthy population eating a varied diet is probably reasonable.

Recommendations are not intended to address the needs of people who are not healthy: no allowance is made for altered nutrient requirements due to illness or injury. For example, patients confined to bed may require less energy owing to inactivity, and may require higher micronutrient intakes because of an illness causing malabsorption by the gut. Certain nutrients may also be used as therapeutic agents, for example n-3 fatty acids can have anti-inflammatory effects. These clinical aspects are considered elsewhere in these texts.

One complication arising in the formulation of dietary recommendations is caused by the fact that various groups of people within a population may have different nutrient requirements. Therefore, the population is divided into subgroups: children and adults by age bands, and by gender. For women, allowances are also made for pregnancy and lactation.

Infants are recommended to be fully breast-fed for the first few months of life. This poses a problem for the bodies setting the dietary recommendations, which have to set standards for those infants who are not breast-fed. The dietary recommendations for formula-fed infants are based on the energy and nutrients supplied in breast milk, but, because the bioavailability of some nutrients is lower in formula than in breast milk, the amounts stated appear higher than those that might be expected to be achieved by breast-feeding. This should not therefore be interpreted as an inadequacy on the part of human (breast) milk compared with formula milks, but rather the reverse.

The dietary recommendations for infants post-weaning and for children and adolescents are generally based on less robust scientific evidence than those for adults, for whom much more good information is available. In the absence of reliable data, values for children are usually derived by extrapolation from those of young adults. The calculation of nutrient requirements is generally based on energy expenditure because metabolic requirements for energy probably go hand in hand with those for nutrients in growing children. In the case of infants post-weaning on mixed diets, values are obtained by interpolation between values known for infants younger than 6 months and those calculated for toddlers aged 1–3 years. Thus, the dietary recommendations for children and adolescents need to be approached with some caution, being more suitable for planning and labeling purposes than as a description of actual needs.

Finally, assessment of the dietary adequacy of people at the other end of the population age range is made difficult by the lack of data on healthy elderly people. One of the normal characteristics of aging is that various body functions deteriorate to some extent, and disease and illness become more common as people age. Until more data are available, the assumption is made that, except for energy and a few nutrients, the requirements of the elderly (usually defined as those over 65 years old) are no different from those of younger adults.

Bearing the above points in mind, dietary recommendations can be useful at various levels.

- Governments and nongovernment organizations (NGOs) use dietary recommendations to identify the energy and nutrient requirements of populations and hence allow informed decisions on food policy. This could include the provision of food aid or supplements (or rationing) when the diet is inadequate, fortification of foods, providing appropriate nutrition education, introducing legislation concerning the food supply, influencing the import and export of food, subsidies on certain foods or for producers of food, and so on.
- The food industry requires this information in the development and marketing of products. The industry is aware of consumers' increasing interest in the nutritional quality of the food that they buy,

and has responded by providing foods to address particular perceived needs, and more informative food labels.

- Researchers and the health professions need to assess the nutritional adequacy of the diets of groups (or, cautiously, of individuals) by comparing dietary intake survey data with the dietary reference values (see below). Once the limitations of the dietary assessment data have been taken into account (see Chapter 10), this information can be used to attempt to improve people's nutrient intakes by bringing them more into line with the dietary recommendations. The formulation of dietary advice or guidelines depends on an appreciation of the existing situation: the solution can only be framed once the problem is characterized.

- Institutions and caterers use dietary recommendations to assess the requirements of groups and devise nutritionally adequate menus. This is a great deal more easily said than done, mainly because of the financial constraints involved and, often, the food preferences of the population being catered for.

- The public needs this information to help in the interpretation of nutrition information on food labels that may describe nutrient content in both absolute terms (g, mg, etc.) and as a percentage of the recommended dietary allowance (RDA) for that nutrient (usually per 100 g or per "serving"). It is thought that the latter is more meaningful to consumers, even though the concepts involved in setting the dietary recommendations are rather complex (making it difficult to judge which level of recommendation should be used as the standard) and they can be open to misinterpretation (see above). Since 1998, some UK manufacturers and retailers have provided information about guideline daily amounts (GDAs) for energy, some nutrients, salt, and fiber. These were developed by the Institute of Grocery Distribution (IGD, a UK research and training body for the food and grocery chain) and are derived from the DRVs [and the British Committee on Medical Aspects of Food Policy (COMA) and Scientific Advisory Council on Nutrition (SACN) recommendations for salt intake], but are much simplified. Unless consumers are provided with nutrition information in the most appropriate form on food labels, they cannot make informed choices as to what foods to buy and

eat to meet their own perceived needs. At the very least, consumers should be able to compare products to get their money's worth.

7.4 The use of reference values to assess the adequacy of the nutrient intakes of population groups

Ideally, this is accomplished by discovering the distribution of intakes of a nutrient in the population group (e.g., by carrying out a dietary survey), and comparing these intakes with the distribution of requirements for that nutrient within the same population. In practice, reliable data with which to plot the second of these distributions have rarely been collected, and therefore what must be used is an estimation of the average requirement together with an estimation of the variance in that requirement, i.e., the standard deviation (based on whatever scientific evidence is available), that is used to plot the population distribution of requirements as shown in Figure 7.1.

When considering how to assess the adequacy of nutrient intakes of populations it is important to compare the intakes with the most appropriate level of requirement as defined in dietary recommendations.

It is not useful to compare usual intakes with the RDA (PRI, RNI, i.e., the average requirement plus a notional 2 SDs) at the population level since this approach leads to overestimates of the prevalence of inadequacy. (It may, however, be justified to compare an individual's intake with the RDA.) Furthermore, this approach might be seen to encourage the consumption of higher intakes, which could be toxic in the case of certain nutrients.

Comparison of the population intake with the average requirement [AR; estimated average requirement (EAR)] is now considered to be the best estimation of dietary adequacy; if the average intake is less than the average requirement, then it is clear that there could be a problem in that population. Accordingly, using the average requirement as a cut-off point, the proportion of individuals in the group whose usual intakes are not meeting their requirements can be calculated, allowing the problem to be quantified. However, this approach cannot be used in the case of energy since energy intakes and requirements are highly correlated (the effects of an imbalance being quickly obvious to the individual).

The lowest defined intake level [lowest threshold intake (LTI), lower reference nutrient intake (LRNI), i.e., the average requirement minus a notional 2 SDs] is not regarded as being useful in the context of assessing the adequacy of population nutrient intakes. This is because it would identify only those individuals who were almost certainly not meeting their requirement, and by the same token would omit to include many in the population who would be at appreciable risk of nutrient inadequacy (in other words, those whose intake was below the average requirement).

Finally, the tolerable upper levels of intake defined for certain nutrients can also be used as cut-off points to identify those individuals at risk of consuming toxic levels of a nutrient.

7.5 Methods used to determine requirements and set dietary recommendations

In order to derive the most accurate and appropriate dietary recommendations, committees of experts are established that look at the scientific evidence and use their judgment to decide which nutrients to consider and then, for each nutrient, make decisions in respect of the:

- criterion by which to define adequacy
- estimation of the average amount required to meet that criterion of adequacy
- estimated standard deviation of requirement in the population under consideration (i.e., the shape of the frequency distribution over the range of requirements: broad, narrow, skewed, etc.).

The problem of different committees identifying different criteria of adequacy is illustrated by vitamin C (ascorbic acid). Experimental evidence (the Sheffield and Iowa studies) has shown that an intake of approximately 10 mg/day is required to prevent the deficiency disease scurvy in adult men. At intakes below 30 mg/day, serum levels are negligible, rising steeply with intakes of between 30 and 70 mg/day, after which they begin to plateau (and urinary excretion of the unmetabolized vitamin increases). The question facing the committees drafting dietary reference values is whether to choose a level of intake that allows some storage of the vitamin in the body pool (e.g., EU AR 30 mg/day for adults), or one that more nearly maximizes plasma and body pool levels (e.g.,

US EAR 60 and 75 mg/day for women and men, respectively). Similarly, variations in calcium recommendations exist because some committees choose to use zero calcium balance as the criterion of adequacy, while others use maximum skeletal calcium reserves.

In some cases, one recommending body will include a nutrient among its dietary recommendations while others will not; for example, vitamin E, the requirement for which depends directly on the dietary intake and tissue levels of PUFAs, which are highly skewed. The vitamin E requirement corresponding to the highest levels of PUFA intake would be much higher than that needed by those with much lower (but adequate) intakes. To set the high value as the recommendation might suggest to those with lower polyunsaturate intakes that they should increase their intake of vitamin E (unnecessarily). Thus, in Britain and Europe, only "safe and adequate" intakes have been set, based on actual intakes in healthy populations, which should be at least 3 mg/day for women and 4 mg/day for men. In contrast, the US RDA (DRI) has been raised to 15 mg/day as α-tocopherol, based on induced vitamin E deficiency studies in humans and measures of lipid peroxidation.

There are even some examples of dietary components that have not traditionally been regarded as essential nutrients having recommendations set for them, as in the case of choline. The US DRI defines an adequate intake for choline (of 450 and 550 mg/day for women and men, respectively), on the basis that endogenous synthesis of this compound is not always adequate to meet the demand for it (for the synthesis of acetylcholine, phospholipids, and betaine). Dietary intake data for choline and the scientific evidence for inadequacy are limited; thus, dose–response studies would need to be done before an average requirement could be derived. It is probable that further dietary components will be included in dietary recommendations as research data accumulate. Potential candidates include the flavonoids and some other antioxidant compounds.

7.6 Methods used to determine requirements

Deprivation studies

This is the most direct method and involves removing the nutrient from the diet, observing the symptoms of deficiency, and then adding back the nutrient until the symptoms are cured or prevented. Difficulties with this approach are as follows. First, that the experiment may need to continue for several years owing to the presence of body stores of the nutrient, and often requires a very limited and therefore boring dietary regimen. Second, unpredicted long-term adverse consequences may result. Third, such experiments are not ethical in vulnerable groups such as children (often the most relevant for study). In some cases, epidemiological data may be available; for example, the deficiency disease beriberi occurs in populations whose average thiamin intake falls below 0.2 mg/4.2 MJ (1000 kcal).

Radioactive tracer studies

This approach makes use of a known amount of the radioactively labeled nutrient, which is assumed to disperse evenly in the body pool, allowing the estimation of the total pool size by dilution of the isotope in samples of, for instance, plasma or urine (i.e., if the body pool is large, then the dilution will be greater than if the body pool is small). Specific activity, that is radioactivity per unit weight of the nutrient in the samples, can be used to calculate pool size as long as the total dose administered is known. The rate of loss can then be monitored by taking serial samples, allowing calculation of the depletion rate. In the case of vitamin C, the average body pool size of a healthy male was found to be 1500 mg, which, on a vitamin C-free diet, depleted at a rate of approximately 3% (of the body pool) per day. This fractional catabolic rate was independent of body pool size, and symptoms of scurvy appeared when the body pool fell below 300 mg. The estimated replacement intake needed to maintain the body pool above 300 mg was therefore 3% of 300 mg, i.e., 9 mg (similar to the 10 mg found to be needed to prevent scurvy in the earlier Sheffield experiment).

Balance studies

These rely on the assumption that, in healthy individuals of stable body weight, the body pool of some nutrients (e.g., nitrogen, calcium, and sodium) remains constant. Compensation mechanisms equalize the intake and output of the nutrient over a wide range of intakes, thereby maintaining the body pool. Thus, day-to-day variations of intake are compensated for by changes in either the rate of absorption

in the gut (generally in the case of those nutrients of which the uptake is regulated) or the rate of excretion in the urine (in the case of very soluble nutrients) or feces, or both. However, there comes a point beyond which balance cannot be maintained; therefore, it can be proposed that the minimum intake of a nutrient at which balance can be maintained is the subject's minimum required intake of that nutrient. However, this approach would need to be extended over time to investigate possible adaptive responses to reduced intakes, e.g., absorption could eventually be increased. In the case of calcium, the European consensus is that average daily losses are assumed to be 160 mg/day in adults, and absorption is assumed to be 30%; thus, around 530 mg would need to be consumed to balance the losses. Adding or subtracting 30% to allow for individual variation (the notional 2 SDs explained above) gives (rounded) dietary reference values of 400, 550 and 700 mg/day (LTI, AR, and PRI, respectively).

Factorial methods

These are predictions, rather than measurements, of the requirements of groups or individuals, taking into account a number of measured variables (factors, hence "factorial") and making assumptions where measurements cannot be made. For example, the increased requirements during growth, pregnancy, or lactation are calculated by this method; this approach is necessitated by the lack of experimental data in these physiological situations owing to ethical problems. The idea is that the rate of accumulation of nutrients can be calculated and hence the amount required in the diet to allow that accumulation can be predicted. In the case of pregnancy, the requirement is estimated to be the amount of the nutrient needed to achieve balance when not pregnant plus the amount accumulated daily during the pregnancy, all multiplied by a factor accounting for the efficiency of absorption and assimilation (e.g., 30% for calcium). For lactation, the calculation for energy is based on the amount in the milk secreted daily, which is increased by a factor accounting for the efficiency of conversion from dietary energy to milk energy (reckoned to be 95%), from which total is subtracted an allowance for the contribution from the extra fat stores laid down during pregnancy, which it is desirable to reduce in this way. The difficulty with this approach is that the theoretical predictions do not necessarily take account of physiological adaptations (e.g., increased efficiency of absorption in the gut) that may reduce the predicted requirement. This would apply particularly in the case of pregnancy, as shown by the ability of women to produce normal babies even in times of food shortage.

Measurement of nutrient levels in biological tissues

Some nutrient requirements can be defined according to the intakes needed to maintain a certain level of the nutrient in blood or tissue. For many water-soluble nutrients, such as vitamin C, blood levels reflect recent dietary intake, and the vitamin is not generally measurable in plasma at intakes less than about 40 mg/day. This level of intake has therefore been chosen as the basis for the reference in some countries such as the UK. This approach is not, however, suitable for those nutrients of which the plasma concentration is homeostatically regulated, such as calcium. In the case of the fat-soluble vitamin retinol, the dietary intake required to maintain a liver concentration of 20 μg/g has been used as the basis of the reference intake. To do this, the body pool size needed to be estimated; assumptions were made as to the proportion of body weight represented by the liver (3%) and the proportion of the body pool of retinol contained in the liver (90%). The fractional catabolic rate has been measured as 0.5% of the body pool per day, so this would be the amount needing to be replaced daily. The efficiency of conversion of dietary vitamin A to stored retinol was taken to be 50% (measured range 40–90%), giving an EAR of around 500 μg/day for a 74 kg man.

Biochemical markers

In many respects, biochemical markers represent the most satisfactory measure of nutrient adequacy since they are specific to the nutrient in question, are sensitive enough to identify subclinical deficiencies, and may be measured precisely and accurately. However, such markers are available for only a few nutrients, mostly vitamins, at present. One well-established example of a biochemical marker is the erythrocyte glutathione reductase activation test for riboflavin status. Erythrocytes are a useful cell to use for enzyme assays since they are easily obtainable and have a known life-span in the circulation (average 120 days), aiding the interpretation of results. Glutathione reductase depends on riboflavin and, when activity is measured in both the presence and absence of excess riboflavin, the ratio of the two activities (the erythrocyte glutathione reductase activation coefficient, EGRAC) reflects riboflavin status: if perfectly sufficient, the ratio would be 1.0, whereas deficiency gives values greater than 1.0.

Biological markers

These are measures of some biological function that is directly dependent on the nutrient of interest; again, not always easy to find, hence the recent suggestion that some functional indices be considered that are not necessarily directly dependent on the nutrient. Iron status is assessed according to a battery of biological markers, including plasma ferritin (which reflects body iron stores), serum transferrin saturation (the amount of plasma transferrin in relation to the amount of iron transported by it is reduced in deficiency), plasma-soluble transferrin receptor (an index of tissue iron status), and the more traditional tests such as blood hemoglobin (now considered to be a rather insensitive and unreliable measure of iron status since it indicates only frank anemia, and also changes as a normal response to altered physiological states such as pregnancy).

Vitamin K status is assessed by measuring prothrombin time (the length of time taken by plasma to clot), which is increased when vitamin K levels fall since the synthesis of prothrombin in the liver depends on vitamin K as a cofactor. This test is clinically useful in patients requiring anticoagulant therapy (e.g., using warfarin, which blocks the effect of vitamin K), in whom the drug dosage must be closely monitored.

Animal experiments

These are of limited use in defining human nutrient requirements because of species differences (e.g., rats can synthesize vitamin C, so it is not a "vitamin" for them), differences in metabolic body size (i.e., the proportions of metabolically active tissue, such as muscle, and less active tissue, such as adipose tissue, gut contents), and differences in growth rates (young animals generally grow far more rapidly than humans, e.g., cattle reach adult size in about 1 year). However, animals have provided much of the information on the identification of the essential nutrients, and their physiological and biochemical functions. Furthermore, animals can be used in experiments that would not be possible in humans, such as lifelong modifications in nutrient intake; it is merely the setting of human requirements for which they are inappropriate.

7.7 Perspectives on the future

As the amount known about human requirements and nutrient functions increases, so too will the complexity of dietary recommendations. It is probable that further dietary components will be included in dietary recommendations as research data accumulate. Potential candidates include the flavonoids and some other antioxidant compounds. Furthermore, continuing research and the development of more informed interpretations of the expanding body of data available necessitate the regular revision and updating of the recommendations.

The general conclusion that can be drawn here is that no single criterion of nutrient status can be used to define human requirements for all nutrients. This is not surprising when one considers the range of roles that the different essential nutrients play in humans.

Further reading

Department of Health. *Dietary Reference Values for Food Energy and Nutrients for the United Kingdom*. Report on Health and Social Subjects 41. Committee on Medical Aspects of Food Policy. HMSO, London, 1991.

Department of Health. *Nutrition and Bone Health: with Particular Reference to Calcium and Vitamin D*. Report on Health and Social Subjects 49. Committee on Medical Aspects of Food and Nutrition Policy. The Stationery Office, London, 1998.

Dietary reference intake texts available online at: http://lab.nap.edu/nap-cgi/discover.cgi?term=dietary%20reference%20intakes&restric=NAP.

EC Scientific Committee for Food Report. *Nutrient and Energy Intakes for the European Community*. 31st Series. Director General, Industry, Luxembourg, 1993.

Expert Group on Vitamins and Minerals. *Safe Upper Limits for Vitamins and Minerals*. Food Standards Agency, London, 2003.

Food and Agriculture Organization/World Health Organization. *Requirements for Vitamin A, Iron, Folate and Vitamin B$_{12}$*. Report of a Joint FAO/WHO Expert Consultation. Food and Nutrition Series. FAO, Rome, 1988.

Food and Agriculture Organization/United Nations University/World Health Organization. *Energy and Protein Requirements*. Report of a Joint FAO/WHO/UNU Expert Consultation. Technical Report Series 724. WHO, Geneva, 1985.

Food and Agriculture Organization/World Health Organization. *Human Vitamin and Mineral Requirements*. Report of a joint FAO/WHO expert consultation. Bangkok, Thailand. FAO, Rome, 2002.

Institute of Medicine (USA). *Dietary Reference Intakes for Calcium, Phosphorus, Magnesium, Vitamin D and Fluoride*. National Academy Press, Washington, DC, 1997.

Institute of Medicine (USA). *Dietary Reference Intakes for Thiamin, Riboflavin, Niacin, Vitamin B6, Folate, Vitamin B12, Pantothenic Acid, Biotin and Choline*. National Academy Press, Washington, DC, 1998.

Institute of Medicine (USA). *Dietary Reference Intakes for Water, Potassium, Sodium, Chloride and Sulfate*. National Academy Press, Washington, DC, 1998.

Institute of Medicine (USA). *Dietary Reference Intakes for Vitamin A, Vitamin K, Arsenic, Boron, Chromium, Copper, Iodine, Iron, Manganese, Molybdenum, Nickel, Silicon, Vanadium and Zinc*. National Academy Press, Washington, DC, 2000.

Institute of Medicine (USA). *Dietary Reference Intakes for Vitamin C, Vitamin E, Selenium and Carotenoids*. National Academy Press, Washington, DC, 2000.

Institute of Medicine (USA). *Dietary Reference Intakes for Energy, Carbohydrate, Fiber, Fat, Fatty Acids, Cholesterol, Protein and Amino Acids (Macronutrients)*. National Academy Press, Washington, DC, 2005.

Institute of Medicine (USA). *Dietary Reference Intakes: The Essential Guide to Nutrient Requirements*. National Academy Press, Washington, DC, 2006.

National Health and Medical Research Council. *Nutrient Reference Values for Australia and New Zealand Including Recommended Dietary Intakes*. Wickliffe Ltd, Wellington, 2006. Available online at http://www.nhmrc.gov.au/publications/synopses/_files/n35.pdf.

National Research Council, Food and Nutrition Board, Commission on Life Sciences. *Recommended Dietary Allowances*, 10th edn. National Academy Press, Washington, DC, 1989.

United Nations University. International harmonisation of approaches for developing nutrient-based dietary standards. In: King JC, Garza, C, eds. *Food and Nutrition Bulletin*, vol. 28, no. 1 (supplement). International Nutrition Foundation for The United Nations University, Tokyo, 2007. Available online at http://www.unu.edu/unupress/food/FNBv28n1_Suppl1_final.pdf.

World Health Organization. *Handbook on Human Nutritional Requirements*. Monograph Series No. 61. WHO, Geneva, 1974.

World Health Organization. *Diet, Nutrition and the Prevention of Chronic Diseases*. Technical Report Series 797. WHO, Geneva, 1990.

World Health Organization. *Trace Elements in Human Nutrition and Health*. WHO in collaboration with FAO, AEA, Geneva, 1996.

8
The Vitamins

David A Bender

Key messages

- The vitamins are a chemically disparate group of compounds with a variety of functions in the body.
- What they have in common is that they are organic compounds that are required for the maintenance of normal health and metabolic integrity.
- Vitamins are required in very small amounts, of the order of milligrams or micrograms per day, and thus can be distinguished from the essential fatty acids and the essential amino acids, which are required in larger amounts of grams per day.
- Where relevant, this chapter will deal with each of the vitamins under the following headings:
  - vitamers
  - absorption and metabolism
  - metabolic functions and other uses
  - deficiency
  - requirements
  - assessment of status
  - toxicity and drug interactions.

8.1 Introduction

In order to demonstrate that a compound is a vitamin, it is necessary to demonstrate both that deprivation of experimental subjects will lead to the development of a more or less specific clinical deficiency disease and abnormal metabolic signs, and that restoration of the missing compound will prevent or cure the deficiency disease and normalize metabolic abnormalities. It is not enough simply to demonstrate that a compound has a function in the body, since it may normally be synthesized in adequate amounts to meet requirements, or that a compound cures a disease, since this may simply reflect a pharmacological action and not indicate that the compound is a dietary essential.

The vitamins, and their principal functions and deficiency signs, are shown in Table 8.1; the curious nomenclature is a consequence of the way in which they were discovered at the beginning of the twentieth century. Early studies showed that there was something in milk that was essential, in very small amounts, for the growth of animals fed on a diet consisting of purified fat, carbohydrate, protein, and mineral salts.

Two factors were found to be essential: one was found in the cream and the other in the watery part of milk. Logically, they were called factor A (fat-soluble, in the cream) and factor B (water-soluble, in the watery part of the milk). Factor B was identified chemically as an amine, and in 1913 the name "vitamin" was coined for these "vital amines."

Further studies showed that "vitamin B" was a mixture of a number of compounds, with different actions in the body, and so they were given numbers as well: vitamin B_1, vitamin B_2, and so on. There are gaps in the numerical order of the B vitamins. When what might have been called vitamin B_3 was discovered, it was found to be a chemical compound that was already known, nicotinic acid. It was therefore not given a number. Other gaps are because compounds that were assumed to be vitamins and were given numbers, such as B_4 and B_5, were later shown either not to be vitamins, or to be vitamins that had already been described by other workers and given other names.

Vitamins C, D and E were named in the order of their discovery. The name "vitamin F" was used at one time for what we now call the essential fatty acids; "vitamin G" was later found to be what was already

Table 8.1 The vitamins, their principal functions and deficiency diseases

Vitamin		Functions	Deficiency disease
A	Retinol β-Carotene	Visual pigments in the retina; cell differentiation; β-carotene is an antioxidant	Night blindness, xerophthalmia; keratinization of skin
D	Calciferol	Maintenance of calcium balance; enhances intestinal absorption of Ca^{2+} and mobilizes bone mineral	Rickets (poor mineralization of bone); osteomalacia (demineralization of bone)
E	Tocopherols Tocotrienols	Antioxidant, especially in cell membranes	Extremely rare: serious neurological dysfunction
K	Phylloquinone Menaquinones	Coenzyme in formation of γ-carboxyglutamate in enzymes of blood clotting and bone matrix	Impaired blood clotting, hemorrhagic disease
B_1	Thiamin	Coenzyme in pyruvate and 2-keto-glutarate dehydrogenases, and transketolase; poorly defined function in nerve conduction	Peripheral nerve damage (beriberi) or central nervous system lesions (Wernicke–Korsakoff syndrome)
B_2	Riboflavin	Coenzyme in oxidation and reduction reactions; prosthetic group of flavoproteins	Lesions of corner of mouth, lips, and tongue; seborrheic dermatitis
Niacin	Nicotinic acid Nicotinamide	Coenzyme in oxidation and reduction reactions, functional part of NAD and NADP	Pellagra: photosensitive dermatitis, depressive psychosis
B_6	Pyridoxine Pyridoxal Pyridoxamine	Coenzyme in transamination and decarboxylation of amino acids and glycogen phosphorylase; role in steroid hormone action	Disorders of amino acid metabolism, convulsions
Folic acid		Coenzyme in transfer of one-carbon fragments	Megaloblastic anemia
B_{12}	Cobalamin	Coenzyme in transfer of one-carbon fragments and metabolism of folic acid	Pernicious anemia (megaloblastic anemia with degeneration of the spinal cord)
	Pantothenic acid	Functional part of coenzyme A and acyl carrier protein	Peripheral nerve damage (burning foot syndrome)
H	Biotin	Coenzyme in carboxylation reactions in gluconeogenesis and fatty acid synthesis	Impaired fat and carbohydrate metabolism, dermatitis
C	Ascorbic acid	Coenzyme in hydroxylation of proline and lysine in collagen synthesis; antioxidant; enhances absorption of iron	Scurvy: impaired wound healing, loss of dental cement, subcutaneous hemorrhage

known as vitamin B_2. Biotin is still sometimes called vitamin H. Vitamin K was discovered by Henrik Dam, in Denmark, as a result of studies of disorders of blood coagulation, and he named it for its function: *koagulation* in Danish.

As the chemistry of the vitamins was elucidated, so they were given names as well, as shown in Table 8.1. When only one chemical compound has the biological activity of the vitamin, this is quite easy. Thus, vitamin B_1 is thiamin, vitamin B_2 is riboflavin, etc. With several of the vitamins, a number of chemically related compounds found in foods can be interconverted in the body, and all show the same biological activity. Such chemically related compounds are called vitamers, and a general name (a generic descriptor) is used to include all compounds that display the same biological activity.

Some compounds have important metabolic functions, but are not considered to be vitamins, since, as far as is known, they can be synthesized in the body in adequate amounts to meet requirements. These include carnitine, choline, inositol, taurine, and ubiquinone.

Two compounds that are generally considered to be vitamins can be synthesized in the body, normally in adequate amounts to meet requirements: vitamin D, which is synthesized from 7-dehydrocholesterol in the skin on exposure to sunlight, and niacin, which is synthesized from the essential amino acid tryptophan. However, both were discovered as a result of studies of deficiency diseases that were, during the early twentieth century, significant public health problems: rickets (due to vitamin D deficiency and inadequate sunlight exposure) and pellagra (due to deficiency of both tryptophan and preformed niacin).

8.2 Vitamin A

Vitamin A was the first vitamin to be discovered, initially as an essential dietary factor for growth. It has a role in vision, as the prosthetic group of the light-sensitive proteins in the retina, and a major role in the regulation of gene expression and tissue differentiation. Deficiency is a major public health problem in large areas of the world, and prevention of vitamin A deficiency is one of the three micronutrient priorities of the World Health Organization (WHO) (the other two are iron and iodine).

Vitamers and international units

Two groups of compounds, shown in Figure 8.1, have vitamin A activity: retinol, retinaldehyde, and retinoic

acid (preformed vitamin A); and a variety of carotenes and related compounds (collectively known as carotenoids) that can be cleaved oxidatively to yield retinaldehyde, and hence retinol and retinoic acid. Those carotenoids that can be cleaved to yield retinaldehyde are known as provitamin A carotenoids.

Preformed vitamin A (mainly as retinyl esters) is found only in foods of animal origin. The richest source by far is liver, which may contain sufficient vitamin A to pose a potential problem for pregnant women, since retinol is teratogenic in excess. Carotenes are found in green, yellow, and red fruits and

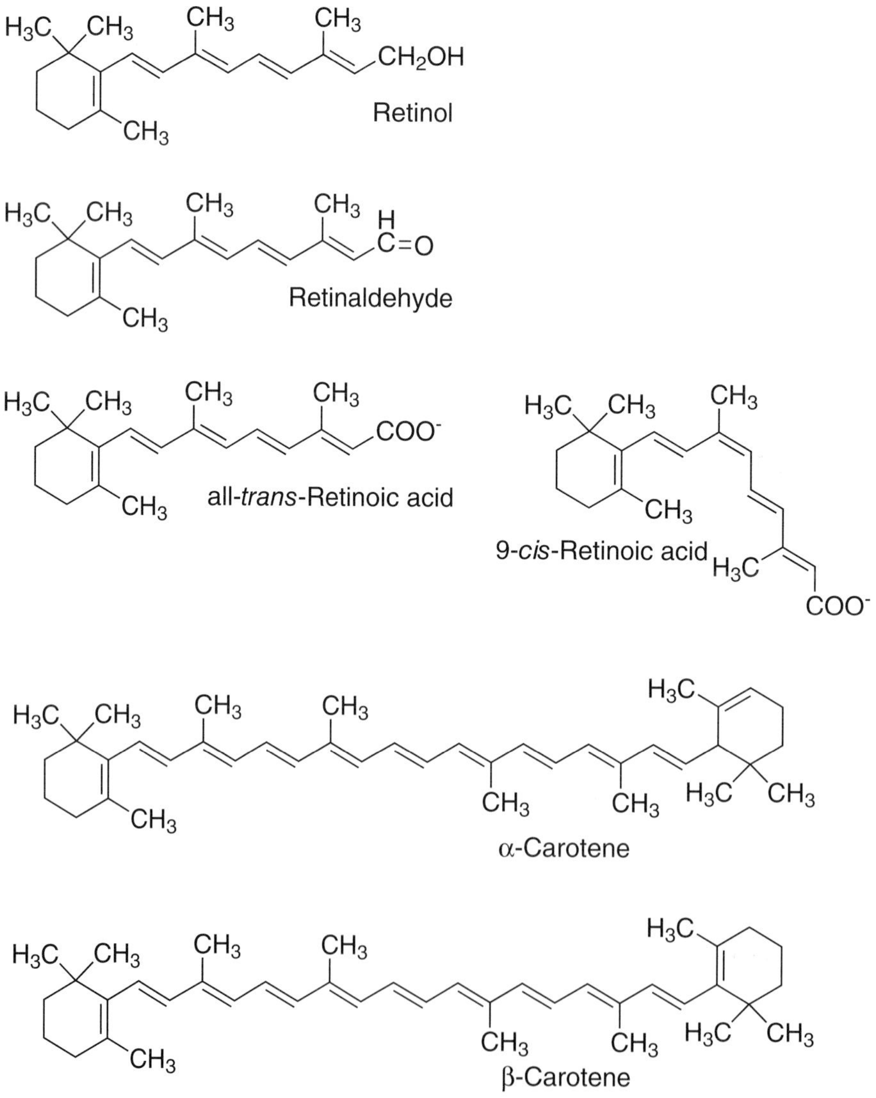

Figure 8.1 The major vitamin A vitamers and vitamin A active carotenoids.

vegetables, as well as in liver, margarine, and milk and milk products. In addition to their role as precursors of vitamin A, carotenoids have potentially useful antioxidant action, and there is epidemiological evidence that diets that are rich in carotenoids (both those that are vitamin A active and those that are not) are associated with a lower incidence of cancer and cardiovascular disease. However, intervention studies with β-carotene have been disappointing, and it is not possible to determine desirable intakes of carotene other than as a precursor of vitamin A.

Retinoic acid is a metabolite of retinol; it has important biological activities in its own right and will support growth in vitamin A-deficient animals. The oxidation of retinaldehyde to retinoic acid is irreversible. Retinoic acid cannot be converted *in vivo* to retinol, and does not support either vision or fertility in deficient animals.

Some 50 or more dietary carotenoids are potential sources of vitamin A: α-, β-, and γ-carotenes and cryptoxanthin are quantitatively the most important. Although it would appear from its structure that one molecule of β-carotene will yield two of retinol, this is not so in practice. Nutritionally, 6–12 μg of β-carotene is equivalent to 1 μg of preformed retinol. For other carotenes with vitamin A activity, 12–24 μg is equivalent to 1 μg of preformed retinol.

Conventionally, the total amount of vitamin A in foods is expressed as μg retinol equivalents, calculated from the sum of μg of preformed vitamin A + 1/6 × μg β-carotene + 1/12 × μg other provitamin A carotenoids. Recent studies on the absorption of carotenes and their bioefficacy as vitamin A precursors have led to the definition of retinol activity equivalents. 1 μg retinol activity equivalent = 1 μg preformed retinol, 12 μg β-carotene or 24 μg other provitamin A carotenoids.

Before pure vitamin A was available for chemical analysis, the vitamin A content of foods was determined by biological assays and the results were expressed in standardized international units (IU): 1 IU = 0.3 μg of retinol, or 1 μg of retinol = 3.33 IU. Although obsolete, IU are sometimes still used in food labeling.

Metabolism and storage of vitamin A and pro-vitamin A carotenoids

Retinol is absorbed from the small intestine dissolved in lipid. About 70–90% of dietary retinol is normally absorbed, and even at high levels of intake this falls only slightly. However, in people with a very low fat intake (less than about 10% of energy from fat), absorption of both retinol and carotene is impaired, and low-fat diets are associated with vitamin A deficiency.

Dietary retinyl esters are hydrolyzed by lipases in the intestinal lumen and mucosal brush border membrane, then re-esterified to form retinyl palmitate before release into the circulation in chylomicrons.

Tissues can take up retinyl esters from chylomicrons, but most retinol is in the chylomicron remnants that are taken up by the liver. Here retinyl esters are hydrolyzed, and the vitamin may either be secreted from the liver bound to retinol binding protein, or be transferred to stellate cells in the liver, where it is stored as retinyl esters in intracellular lipid droplets. Some 50–80% of the total body content of retinol is in the stellate cells of the liver, but a significant amount may also be stored in adipose tissue.

The main pathway for catabolism of retinol is oxidation to retinoic acid (which, as discussed below, has important biological activities in its own right, distinct from the activities of retinol). The main excretory product of both retinol and retinoic acid is retinoyl glucuronide, which is secreted in the bile.

As the intake of retinol increases, and the liver concentration rises above 70 μmol/kg, a different pathway becomes increasingly important for the catabolism of retinol in the liver. This is a microsomal cytochrome P_{450}-dependent oxidation, leading to a number of polar metabolites that are excreted in the urine and bile. At high intakes this pathway becomes saturated, and excess retinol is toxic since there is no further capacity for its catabolism and excretion.

Carotene dioxygenase

Like retinol, carotenoids are absorbed dissolved in lipid micelles. The biological availability and absorption of dietary carotene varies between 5% and 60%, depending on the nature of the food, whether it is cooked or raw, and the amount of fat in the meal.

As shown in Figure 8.2, β-carotene and other provitamin A carotenoids are cleaved in the intestinal mucosa by carotene dioxygenase, yielding retinaldehyde, which is reduced to retinol, then esterified and secreted in chylomicrons together with retinyl esters formed from dietary retinol.

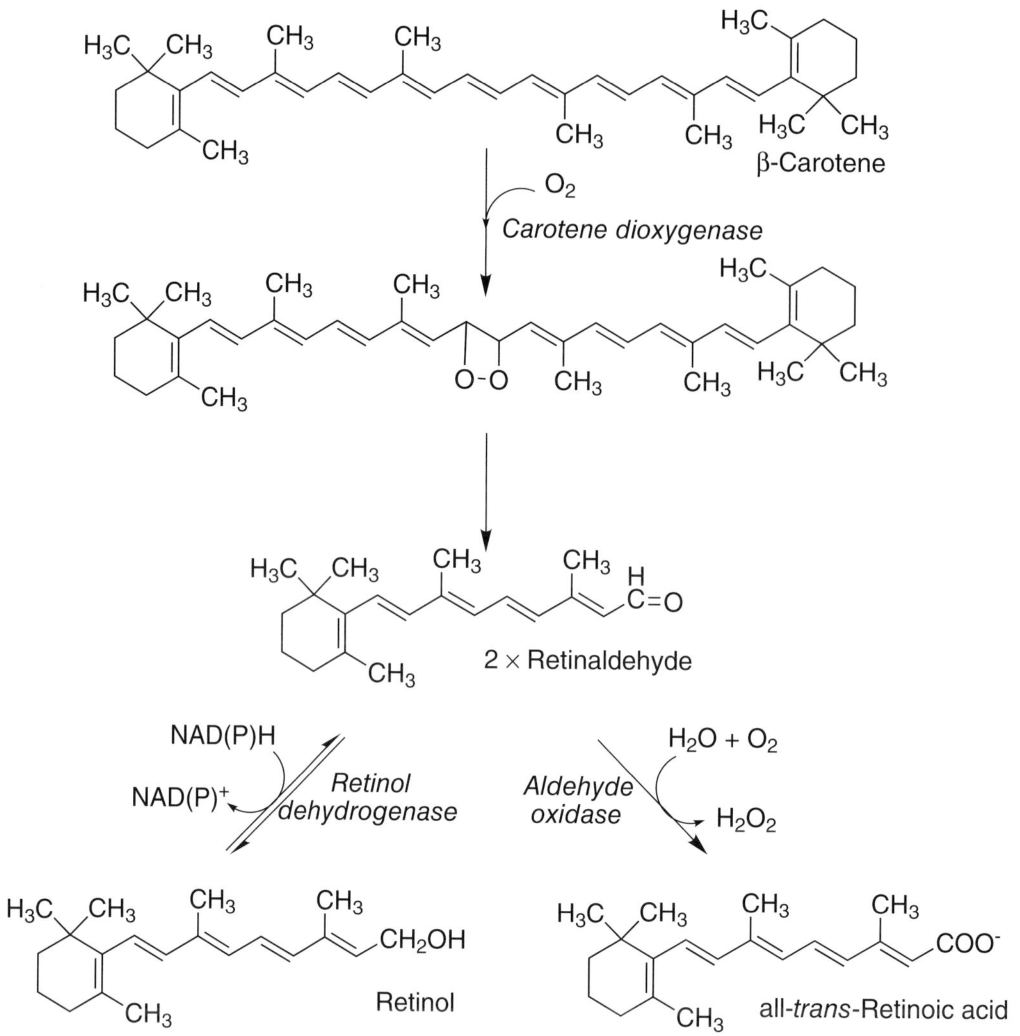

Figure 8.2 The oxidative cleavage of carotene to yield retinol and retinoic acid. Carotene dioxygenase (EC 1.13.11.21), retinol dehydrogenase (EC 1.1.1.105), retinaldehyde oxidase (EC 1.2.3.11).

Only a proportion of carotene undergoes oxidation in the intestinal mucosa, and a significant amount of carotene enters the circulation in chylomicrons. Carotene in the chylomicron remnants is cleared by the liver; some is cleaved by hepatic carotene dioxygenase, again giving rise to retinaldehyde and retinyl esters; the remainder is secreted in very low-density lipoproteins (VLDLs), and may be taken up and cleaved by carotene dioxygenase in other tissues.

Central oxidative cleavage of β-carotene, as shown in Figure 8.2, should yield two molecules of retinaldehyde, which can be reduced to retinol. However, as noted above, the biological activity of β-carotene, on

a molar basis, is considerably lower than that of retinol, not twofold higher as might be expected. In addition to poor absorption of carotene, three factors may account for this.

- The intestinal activity of carotene dioxygenase is relatively low, so that a relatively large proportion of ingested β-carotene may be absorbed unchanged.
- Other carotenoids in the diet may inhibit carotene dioxygenase and reduce the formation of retinol.
- The principal site of carotene dioxygenase attack is the central bond of β-carotene, but asymmetric cleavage also occurs, leading to the formation of 8′-,

10′- and 12′-apo-carotenals, which are oxidized to yield retinoic acid, but are not precursors of retinol or retinaldehyde.

Plasma retinol binding protein

Retinol is released from the liver bound to an α-globulin, retinol binding protein (RBP); this serves to maintain the vitamin in aqueous solution, protects it against oxidation and delivers the vitamin to target tissues. RBP is secreted from the liver as a 1:1 complex with the thyroxine-binding prealbumin, transthyretin. This is important to prevent urinary loss of retinol bound to the relatively small RBP, which would otherwise be filtered by the kidney, with a considerable loss of vitamin A from the body.

Cell surface receptors on target tissues take up retinol from the RBP–transthyretin complex, transferring it on to an intracellular RBP. The receptors also remove the carboxy-terminal arginine residue from RBP, so inactivating it by reducing its affinity for both transthyretin and retinol. As a result, apo-RBP is filtered at the glomerulus; most is reabsorbed in the proximal renal tubules and hydrolyzed. The apoprotein is not recycled.

During the development of vitamin A deficiency in experimental animals, the plasma concentration of RBP falls, whereas the liver content of apo-RBP rises. The administration of retinol results in release of holo-RBP from the liver. This provides the basis of the relative dose–response (RDR) test for liver reserves of vitamin A (see below).

Metabolic functions of vitamin A and carotenes

The first function of vitamin A to be defined was in vision. More recently, retinoic acid has been shown to have a major function in regulation of gene expression and tissue differentiation.

Vitamin A in vision

In the retina, retinaldehyde functions as the prosthetic group of the light-sensitive opsin proteins, forming rhodopsin (in rods) and iodopsin (in cones). Any one cone cell contains only one type of opsin, and hence is sensitive to only one color of light. Color blindness results from loss or mutation of one or other of the cone opsins.

In the pigment epithelium of the retina, all-*trans*-retinol is isomerized to 11-*cis*-retinol and then oxidized to 11-*cis*-retinaldehyde. This reacts with a lysine residue in opsin, forming the holoprotein rhodopsin. As shown in Figure 8.3, the absorption of light by rhodopsin causes isomerization of the retinaldehyde bound to opsin from 11-*cis* to all-*trans*, and a conformational change in opsin. This results in the release of retinaldehyde from the protein and the initiation of a nerve impulse. The overall process is known as bleaching, since it results in the loss of the color of rhodopsin. The all-*trans*-retinaldehyde released from rhodopsin is reduced to all-*trans*-retinol, and joins the pool of retinol in the pigment epithelium for isomerization to 11-*cis*-retinol and regeneration of rhodopsin. The key to initiation of the visual cycle is the availability of 11-*cis*-retinaldehyde, and hence vitamin A. In deficiency both the time taken to adapt to darkness and the ability to see in poor light are impaired.

The excited form of rhodopsin (metarhodopsin II) initiates a G-protein cascade leading to hyperpolarization of the outer section membrane of the rod or cone, caused by the closure of sodium channels through the membrane, and the initiation of a nerve impulse.

Retinoic acid and the regulation of gene expression

The main function of vitamin A is in the control of cell differentiation and turnover. All-*trans*-retinoic acid and 9-*cis*-retinoic acid are active in the regulation of growth, development, and tissue differentiation; they have different actions in different tissues. Like the steroid hormones and vitamin D, retinoic acid interacts with nuclear receptors that bind to response elements (control regions) of DNA, and regulate the transcription of specific genes.

There are two families of nuclear retinoid receptors: the retinoic acid receptors (RARs) bind all-*trans*-retinoic acid or 9-*cis*-retinoic acid, and the retinoid X receptors (RXRs) bind 9-*cis*-retinoic acid, and some of the other physiologically active retinoids as well. RXR can form active dimers with RARs, RXRs (homodimers), and the receptors for calcitriol (vitamin D), thyroid hormone, long-chain polyunsaturated fatty acid (PUFA) derivatives [the peroxisome proliferators-activated receptor (PPAR)], and one for which the physiological ligand has not yet been identified (the COUP receptor).

The result of this is that a very large number of genes are sensitive to control by retinoic acid in

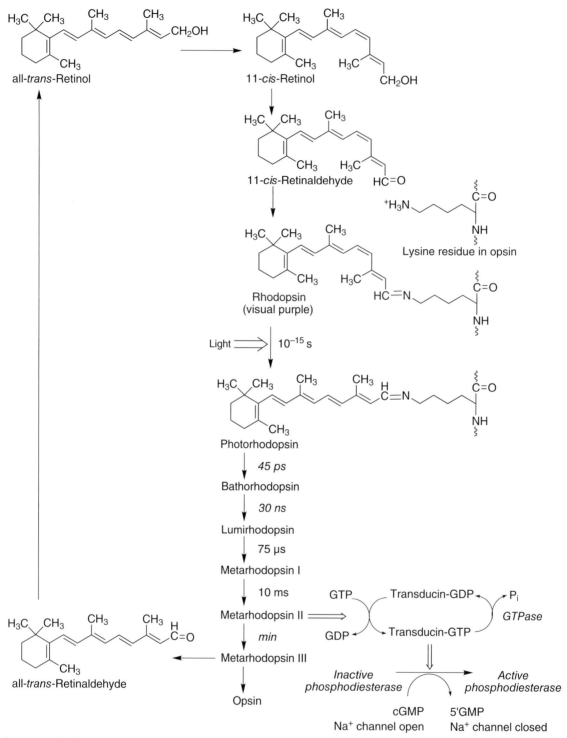

Figure 8.3 Role of vitamin A and the cyclic GMP cascade in the visual cycle. Retinol isomerase (EC 5.2.1.3), phosphodiesterase (EC 3.1.4.35).

different tissues, and at different stages in development, and retinoic acid is essential for the normal responses to vitamin D, thyroid hormone and long-chain PUFA derivatives.

Unoccupied RXRs can form dimers with calcitriol and other receptors; these bind to hormone response elements on DNA, but do not lead to activation of transcription. This means that vitamin A deficiency will impair responses to vitamin D and thyroid hormone more markedly than might be expected simply from lack of 9-*cis*-retinoic acid to form active heterodimers.

Vitamin A in excess may also impair responsiveness to vitamin D and other hormones, since high concentrations of 9-*cis*-retinoic acid will lead to the formation of RXR–RXR homodimers, leaving too few RXRs to form heterodimers with vitamin D and other receptors. There is epidemiological evidence that habitually high intakes of vitamin A are associated with poor bone health in later life as a result of impaired responsiveness to vitamin D.

The antioxidant function of carotenes

At least *in vitro*, and under conditions of low oxygen availability, carotenes can act as radical-trapping antioxidants. There is epidemiological evidence that high intakes of carotene are associated with a low incidence of cardiovascular disease and some forms of cancer, although the results of intervention trials with β-carotene have been disappointing, with an increased incidence of lung cancer among those taking carotene supplements.

The problem is that although carotene is an antioxidant at a low partial pressure of oxygen, as occurs in most tissues, at a high partial pressure of oxygen, as occurs in the lungs, it is an autocatalytic pro-oxidant, acting as a source of oxygen radicals. The UK Food Standards Agency specifically advises smokers not to take carotene supplements.

Vitamin A deficiency: night blindness and xerophthalmia

Worldwide, vitamin A deficiency is a major public health problem and the most important preventable cause of blindness; the WHO estimates that some 256 million children under 5 years old show subclinical deficiency and 2.7 million have xerophthalmia.

The earliest signs of clinical deficiency are associated with vision. Initially, there is a loss of sensitivity to green light; this is followed by impairment of the ability to adapt to dim light, then an inability to see at all in dim light: night blindness. More prolonged or severe deficiency leads to the condition called xerophthalmia: keratinization of the cornea, followed by ulceration – irreversible damage to the eye that causes blindness. At the same time there are changes in the skin, with excessive formation of keratinized tissue.

Vitamin A also plays an important role in the differentiation of immune system cells, and mild deficiency, not severe enough to cause any disturbance of vision, leads to increased susceptibility to a variety of infectious diseases. At the same time, the synthesis of RBP is reduced in response to infection (it is a negative acute-phase protein), so that there is a reduction in the circulating concentration of the vitamin, and hence further impairment of immune responses.

Signs of vitamin A deficiency also occur in protein–energy malnutrition, regardless of whether or not the intake of vitamin A is adequate. This is due to impairment of the synthesis of plasma RBP; functional vitamin A deficiency can occur secondary to protein–energy malnutrition; even if liver reserves of the vitamin are adequate, it cannot be mobilized.

Vitamin A requirements and reference intakes

There have been relatively few studies of vitamin A requirements in which subjects have been depleted of the vitamin for long enough to permit the development of clear deficiency signs. Current estimates of requirements are based on the intakes required to maintain a concentration in the liver of 70 µmol retinol/kg, as determined by measurement of the rate of metabolism of isotopically labeled vitamin A. This is adequate to maintain normal plasma concentrations of the vitamin, and people with this level of liver reserves can be maintained on a vitamin A-free diet for many months before they develop any detectable signs of deficiency.

The average requirement to maintain a concentration of 70 µmol/kg of liver is 6.7 µg retinol equivalents/kg body weight, and this is the basis for calculation of reference intakes.

Assessment of vitamin A status

The only direct assessment of vitamin A status is by liver biopsy and measurement of retinyl ester reserves.

This is an invasive procedure that cannot be considered for routine investigations and population surveys. Status can also be assessed by clinical and functional tests, the plasma concentrations of retinol and RBP, and the response to a test dose of vitamin A, the RDR test.

In field surveys, clinical signs of vitamin A deficiency, including Bitot's spots, corneal xerosis, corneal ulceration, and keratomalacia, can be used to identify those suffering from vitamin A deficiency. The earliest signs of corneal damage are detected by conjunctival impression cytology (CIC); however, abnormalities only develop when liver reserves are seriously depleted.

The ability to adapt to dim light is impaired early in deficiency, and dark adaptation time is sometimes used to assess vitamin A status. However, the test is not suitable for use on children (the group most at risk of deficiency) and the apparatus is not suited to use in the field.

The fasting plasma concentration of retinol remains constant over a wide range of intakes and only falls significantly when liver reserves are nearly depleted. Therefore, although less sensitive to subtle changes within the normal range than some methods of assessing nutritional status, measurement of plasma retinol provides a convenient and sensitive means of detecting people whose intake of vitamin A is inadequate to maintain normal liver reserves.

The RDR test is a test of the ability of a dose of retinol to raise the plasma concentration several hours after chylomicrons have been cleared from the circulation. It depends on the fact that apo-RBP accumulates in the liver in vitamin A deficiency. The RDR is the ratio of the plasma concentration of retinol 5 h after the dose to that immediately before it was given. An RDR greater than 20% indicates depletion of liver retinol to less than 70 µmol/kg.

Toxicity of vitamin A

There is only a limited capacity to metabolize vitamin A. Excessively high intakes lead to accumulation in the liver and other tissues, beyond the capacity of normal binding proteins, so that free, unbound, vitamin A is present. This leads to liver and bone damage, hair loss, vomiting, and headaches. Single doses of 60 mg of retinol are given to children in developing countries as a prophylactic against vitamin A deficiency: an amount adequate to meet the child's

needs for 4–6 months. About 1% of children so treated show transient signs of toxicity, but this is considered an acceptable risk in view of the high prevalence and devastating effects of deficiency.

The chronic toxicity of vitamin A is a more general cause for concern; prolonged and regular intake of more than about 7.5–9 mg/day by adults (and significantly less for children) causes signs and symptoms of toxicity affecting:

- the central nervous system: headache, nausea, ataxia and anorexia, all associated with increased cerebrospinal fluid pressure
- the liver: hepatomegaly with histological changes in the liver, increased collagen formation and hyperlipidemia
- bones: joint pains, thickening of the long bones, hypercalcemia and calcification of soft tissues
- the skin: excessive dryness, scaling and chapping of the skin, desquamation and alopecia.

The recommended upper limits of habitual intake of retinol, compared with reference intakes, are shown in Table 8.2. As discussed above, habitual high intakes of vitamin A, albeit below these prudent upper levels of intake, may be associated with impaired responsiveness to vitamin D, poor mineralization of bone and the early development of osteoporosis.

Teratogenicity of vitamin A

The synthetic retinoids (vitamin A analogues) used in dermatology are highly teratogenic. After women have been treated with them, it is recommended that contraceptive precautions be continued for 12 months, because of their retention in the body. By

Table 8.2 Prudent upper levels of habitual vitamin A intake

Age group	Upper limit of intake (µg/day)	Reference intakes[a] (µg/day)
Infants	900	350–375
1–3 years	1800	400
4–6 years	3000	400–500
6–12 years	4500	500–700
13–20 years	6000	600–700
Adult men	9000	600–1000
Adult women	7500	600–800
Pregnant women	3000–3300	700

[a] Reference intakes show range for various national and international authorities.

extrapolation, it has been assumed that retinol is also teratogenic, although there is little evidence. In case–control studies, intakes between 2400 µg/day and 3300 µg/day during pregnancy have been associated with birth defects. Other studies have not demonstrated any teratogenic effect at this level of intake, and it has been suggested that the threshold plasma concentration associated with teratogenic effects is unlikely to be reached with intakes below 7500 µg/day. Nevertheless, pregnant women are advised not to consume more than 3000 µg/day (American Pediatric Association recommendation) or 3300 µg (UK Department of Health recommendation).

Interactions of vitamin A with drugs and other nutrients

Historically, there was considerable confusion between vitamins A and D, and for many years it was not clear which acted in which system. By the 1950s it was believed that the problem had been solved, with clearly defined functions of vitamin A in vision, and vitamin D in calcium homeostasis and bone development. However, both have overlapping effects on a number of systems, including bone metabolism and immune system function. It is now known that this is the result of formation of retinoid–vitamin D receptor heterodimers, so that in some systems both are required in appropriate amounts for normal regulation of gene expression.

Chlorinated hydrocarbons, as contained in agricultural pesticides, deplete liver retinol. Metabolites of polychlorinated biphenyls bind to the thyroxine binding site of transthyretin, and in doing so impair the binding of RBP. As a result there is free RBP-bound retinol in plasma, which is filtered at the glomerulus and hence lost in the urine. Habitual use of barbiturates may also lead to deficiency as a result of induction of cytochrome P_{450}, which catalyzes the catabolism of retinol.

8.3 Vitamin D

Vitamin D is not strictly a vitamin, since it can be synthesized in the skin, and indeed under most conditions endogenous synthesis is the major source of the vitamin: it is only when sunlight exposure is inadequate that a dietary source is required. Its main function is in the regulation of calcium absorption and homeostasis; most of its actions are mediated by nuclear receptors that regulate gene expression. Deficiency, leading to rickets in children and osteomalacia in adults, continues to be a problem in northern latitudes, where sunlight exposure is poor.

There are relatively few sources of vitamin D, mainly oily fish, with eggs, liver, and butter providing modest amounts; fortified milk, containing ergocalciferol, is available in some countries. As a result, strict vegetarians are especially at risk of deficiency, especially in northern latitudes with little sunlight exposure.

Although meat provides apparently negligible quantities of vitamin D, it may be an important source, since what is present is largely the final active metabolite, calcitriol, which is many times more potent on a molar basis than is cholecalciferol.

Vitamers and international units

The normal dietary form of vitamin D is cholecalciferol (also known as calciol). This is also the compound that is formed in the skin by ultraviolet (UV) irradiation of 7-dehydrocholesterol. Some foods are enriched or fortified with (synthetic) ergocalciferol, which undergoes the same metabolism as cholecalciferol and has the same biological activity. Early studies assigned the name vitamin D_1 to an impure mixture of products derived from the irradiation of ergosterol; when ergocalciferol was identified it was called vitamin D_2, and when the physiological compound was identified as cholecalciferol it was called vitamin D_3.

Like vitamin A, vitamin D was originally measured in international units of biological activity before the pure compound was isolated: 1 IU = 25 ng of cholecalciferol; 1 µg of cholecalciferol = 40 IU.

Absorption and metabolism

Vitamin D is absorbed in lipid micelles and incorporated into chylomicrons; therefore, people on a low-fat diet will absorb little of such dietary vitamin D as is available. Indeed, it is noteworthy that at the time that rickets was a major public health problem in Scotland, herrings (a rich source) were a significant part of the diet: it can only be assumed that the diet was so low in fat that the absorption of the vitamin was impaired.

Synthesis of vitamin D in the skin
As shown in Figure 8.4, the steroid 7-dehydrocholesterol (an intermediate in the synthesis of cholesterol

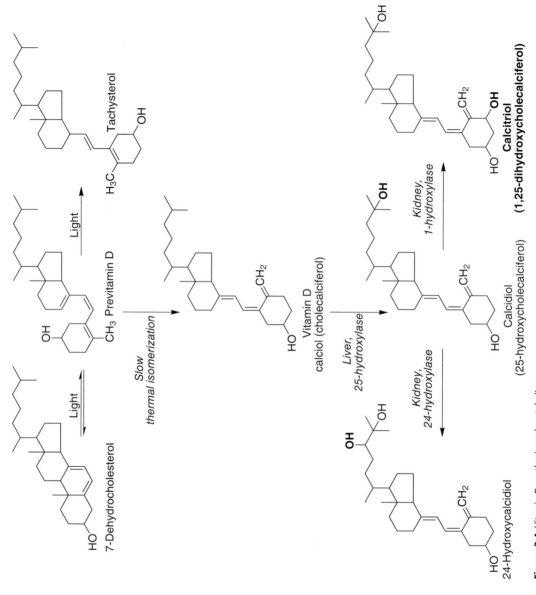

Figure 8.4 Vitamin D synthesis and metabolism.

Table 8.3 Nomenclature of vitamin D metabolites

Trivial name	Recommended name	Abbreviation
Vitamin D$_3$		
Cholecalciferol	Calciol	–
25-Hydroxycholecalciferol	Calcidiol	25(OH)D$_3$
1α-Hydroxycholecalciferol	1(S)-Hydroxycalciol	1α(OH)D$_3$
24,25-Dihydroxycholecalciferol	24(R)-Hydroxycalcidiol	24,25(OH)$_2$D$_3$
1,25-Dihydroxycholecalciferol	Calcitriol	1,25(OH)$_2$D$_3$
1,24,25-Trihydroxycholecalciferol	Calcitetrol	1,24,25(OH)$_3$D$_3$
Vitamin D$_2$		
Ergocalciferol	Ercalciol	–
25-Hydroxyergocalciferol	Ercalcidiol	25(OH)D$_2$
24,25-Dihydroxyergocalciferol	24(R)-Hydroxyercalcidiol	24,25(OH)$_2$D$_2$
1,25-Dihydroxyergocalciferol	Ercalcitriol	1,25(OH)$_2$D$_2$
1,24,25-Trihydroxyergocalciferol	Ercalcitetrol	1,24,25(OH)$_3$D$_2$

The abbreviations shown in column 3 are not recommended, but are frequently used in the literature.

that accumulates in the skin but not other tissues) undergoes a non-enzymic reaction on exposure to UV light, yielding previtamin D, which undergoes a further reaction over a period of hours to form cholecalciferol, which is absorbed into the bloodstream.

In temperate climates there is a marked seasonal variation in the plasma concentration of vitamin D; it is highest at the end of summer and lowest at the end of winter. Although there may be bright sunlight in winter, beyond about 40° N or S there is very little UV radiation of the appropriate wavelength for cholecalciferol synthesis when the sun is low in the sky. By contrast, in summer, when the sun is more or less overhead, there is a considerable amount of UV light even on a moderately cloudy day, and enough can penetrate thin clothes to result in significant formation of vitamin D.

In northerly climates, and especially in polluted industrial cities with little sunlight, people may well not be exposed to enough UV light to meet their vitamin D needs, and they will be reliant on the few dietary sources of the vitamin.

Metabolism to calcitriol

Cholecalciferol, either synthesized in the skin or from foods, undergoes two hydroxylations to yield the active metabolite, 1,25-dihydroxyvitamin D or calcitriol, as shown in Figure 8.4. Ergocalciferol from fortified foods undergoes similar hydroxylation to yield ercalcitriol. The nomenclature of the vitamin D metabolites is shown in Table 8.3.

The first stage in vitamin D metabolism occurs in the liver, where it is hydroxylated to form the 25-hydroxy derivative calcidiol. This is released into the circulation bound to a vitamin D binding globulin. There is no tissue storage of vitamin D; plasma calcidiol is the main storage form of the vitamin, and it is plasma calcidiol that shows the most significant seasonal variation in temperate climates.

The second stage of vitamin D metabolism occurs in the kidney, where calcidiol undergoes either 1-hydroxylation to yield the active metabolite 1,25-dihydroxyvitamin D (calcitriol) or 24-hydroxylation to yield an apparently inactive metabolite, 24,25-dihydroxyvitamin D (24-hydroxycalcidiol). Calcidiol 1-hydroxylase is also found in other tissues that are capable of forming calcitriol as an autocrine or paracrine agent.

Regulation of vitamin D metabolism

The main function of vitamin D is in the control of calcium homeostasis and, in turn, vitamin D metabolism in the kidney is regulated, at the level of 1- or 24-hydroxylation, by factors that respond to plasma concentrations of calcium and phosphate. In tissues other than the kidney that hydroxylate calcidiol to calcitriol, the enzyme is not regulated in response to plasma calcium.

- Calcitriol acts to reduce its own synthesis and increase formation of 24-hydroxycalcidiol, by regulating the expression of the genes for the two hydroxylases.
- Parathyroid hormone is secreted in response to a fall in plasma calcium. In the kidney it acts to increase the activity of calcidiol 1-hydroxylase and decrease that of 24-hydroxylase. In turn, both calcitriol and high concentrations of calcium repress the synthesis of parathyroid hormone; calcium also inhibits the secretion of the hormone from the parathyroid gland.
- Calcium exerts its main effect on the synthesis and secretion of parathyroid hormone. However, calcium ions also have a direct effect on the kidney, reducing the activity of calcidiol 1-hydroxylase.
- Phosphate also affects calcidiol metabolism; throughout the day there is an inverse fluctuation of plasma phosphate and calcitriol, and feeding people on a low-phosphate diet results in increased circulating concentrations of calcitriol.

Metabolic functions of vitamin D

The principal function of vitamin D is to maintain the plasma concentration of calcium; calcitriol achieves this in three ways:

- increased intestinal absorption of calcium
- reduced excretion of calcium by stimulating resorption in the distal renal tubules (due to increased calbindin D synthesis)
- mobilization of bone mineral.

There is a growing body of evidence that low vitamin D status (but not such a degree of deficiency as to disturb calcium homeostasis) is associated with impaired glucose tolerance, insulin resistance and non-insulin dependent diabetes mellitus, as well as obesity and the low grade chronic inflammation associated with (especially abdominal) obesity. There is also evidence poor vitamin D status is a factor in the etiology of some cancers. Calcitriol has a variety of permissive or modulatory effects; it is a necessary, but not sufficient, factor in:

- synthesis and secretion of insulin, parathyroid, and thyroid hormones;
- inhibition of production of interleukin by activated T-lymphocytes and of immunoglobulin by activated B-lymphocytes;

- differentiation of monocyte precursor cells;
- modulation of cell differentiation, proliferation and apoptosis.

In most of its actions, the role of calcitriol seems to be in the induction or maintenance of synthesis of calcium binding proteins, and the physiological effects are secondary to changes in intracellular calcium concentrations.

Calcitriol acts like a steroid hormone, binding to a nuclear receptor protein, commonly as a heterodimer with the RXR (vitamin A) receptor, then binding to hormone response elements on DNA and modifying the expression of one or more genes.

The best-studied actions of vitamin D are in the intestinal mucosa, where the intracellular calcium binding protein induced by vitamin D is essential for the absorption of calcium from the diet. Vitamin D also acts to increase the transport of calcium across the mucosal membrane by recruiting calcium transport proteins to the cell surface.

Calcitriol also raises plasma calcium by stimulating the mobilization of calcium from bone. It achieves this by activating osteoclast cells. However, it acts later to stimulate the laying down of new bone to replace the loss, by stimulating the differentiation and recruitment of osteoblasts.

Vitamin D deficiency: rickets and osteomalacia

Historically, rickets is a disease of toddlers, especially in northern industrial cities. Their bones are undermineralized as a result of poor absorption of calcium in the absence of adequate amounts of calcitriol. When the child begins to walk, the long bones of the legs are deformed, leading to bow-legs or knock knees. More seriously, rickets can also lead to collapse of the ribcage and deformities of the bones of the pelvis. Similar problems may also occur in adolescents who are deficient in vitamin D during the adolescent growth spurt, when there is again a high demand for calcium for new bone formation.

Osteomalacia is the adult equivalent of rickets. It results from the demineralization of bone, rather than the failure to mineralize it in the first place, as is the case with rickets. Women who have little exposure to sunlight are especially at risk from osteomalacia after several pregnancies, because of the strain that pregnancy places on their marginal reserve of calcium.

Osteomalacia also occurs in the older people. Here again the problem may be inadequate exposure to sunlight, but there is also evidence that the capacity to form 7-dehydrocholesterol in the skin decreases with advancing age, so that older people are more reliant on the few dietary sources of vitamin D.

Although vitamin D is essential for prevention and treatment of osteomalacia in older people, there is less evidence that it is beneficial in treating the other common degenerative bone disease of advancing age, osteoporosis, which is due to a loss of bone matrix, rather than enhanced release of calcium from bone with no effect on the organic matrix, as is seen in osteomalacia. The result is negative calcium balance and loss of bone mineral, but secondary to the loss of organic matrix, owing to progressive loss of estrogens and androgens, rather than failure of the vitamin D system.

Vitamin D requirements and reference intakes

It is difficult to determine requirements for dietary vitamin D, since the major source is synthesis in the skin. Before the development of methods for measurement of calcidiol the diagnosis of subclinical rickets was by detection of elevated alkaline phosphatase in plasma; nowadays, the main criterion of adequacy is the plasma concentration of calcidiol.

In older people with little sunlight exposure, a dietary intake of 10 μg of vitamin D/day results in a plasma calcidiol concentration of 20 nmol/l, the lower end of the reference range for younger adults at the end of winter. Therefore, the reference intake for older people is 10 μg/day, whereas average intakes of vitamin D from unfortified foods are less than 4 μg/day.

There is little evidence to establish what are appropriate plasma concentrations of calcidiol; certainly the lower end of the reference range for young adults at the end of winter in a temperate climate is a minimalist goal, and is not much higher than the level at which biochemical signs of deficiency occur. However, unfortified foods will not meet even this goal.

There is increasing evidence that high vitamin D status is associated with a lower incidence of various cancers, diabetes, and the metabolic syndrome, suggesting that desirable intakes are higher than current reference intakes. Widespread fortification of foods would improve vitamin D status, but might also put a significant proportion of the population at risk of hypervitaminosis and hypercalcemia. Increased sunlight exposure will improve vitamin D status without the risks of toxicity, but excessive sunlight exposure is a cause of skin cancer. The main problem in trying to balance improved vitamin D status through increased sunlight exposure, and increased risk of skin cancer, is that there is very little information on the amount of sunlight exposure required for the synthesis of a given amount of vitamin D.

Vitamin D toxicity

During the 1950s, rickets was more or less totally eradicated in Britain and other temperate countries. This was due to enrichment of a large number of infant foods with vitamin D. However, a small number of infants suffered from vitamin D poisoning, the most serious effect of which is an elevated plasma concentration of calcium. This can lead to contraction of blood vessels, and hence dangerously high blood pressure, and calcinosis, that is the calcification of soft tissues, including the kidney, heart, lungs, and blood vessel walls.

Some infants are sensitive to intakes of vitamin D as low as 50 μg/day. To avoid the serious problem of vitamin D poisoning in these susceptible infants, the extent to which infant foods are fortified with vitamin D has been reduced considerably. Unfortunately, this means that a small proportion, who have relatively high requirements, are now at risk of developing rickets. The problem is to identify those who have higher requirements and provide them with supplements.

The toxic threshold in adults is not known, but those patients suffering from vitamin D intoxication who have been investigated were taking supplements providing more than 250 μg/day.

Although excess dietary vitamin D is toxic, excessive exposure to sunlight does not lead to vitamin D poisoning. There is a limited capacity to form the precursor, 7-dehydrocholesterol, in the skin, and a limited capacity to take up cholecalciferol from the skin. Furthermore, prolonged exposure of previtamin D to UV light results in further reactions to yield lumisterol and other biologically inactive compounds.

Interactions with drugs and other nutrients

As discussed above, vitamin D receptors form heterodimers with RXR, so that vitamin D-dependent functions require adequate, but not excessive, vitamin A status. A number of drugs, including barbiturates and other anticonvulsants, induce cytochrome P_{450}, resulting in increased catabolism of calcidiol (and retinol), and cause drug-induced osteomalacia. The antituberculosis drug isoniazid inhibits cholecalciferol 25-hydroxylase in the liver, and prolonged administration can lead to the development of osteomalacia.

Strontium is a potent inhibitor of the kidney 1-hydroxylase, and strontium intoxication can lead to the development of vitamin D-resistant rickets or osteomalacia. Although there is normally little exposure to potentially toxic intakes of strontium, its salts are sometimes used to treat chronic lead intoxication.

8.4 Vitamin E

Although vitamin E was identified as a dietary essential for animals in the 1920s, it was not until 1983 that it was clearly demonstrated to be a dietary essential for human beings. Unlike other vitamins, no unequivocal physiological function for vitamin E has been defined; it acts as a lipid-soluble antioxidant in cell membranes, but many of its functions can be replaced by synthetic antioxidants. There is epidemiological evidence that high intakes of vitamin E are associated with lower incidence of cardiovascular disease, although in many intervention trials vitamin E supplements have been associated with increased all-cause mortality.

Vegetable oils are rich sources of vitamin E, but significant amounts are also found in nuts and seeds, most green leafy vegetables, and a variety of fish.

Vitamers and units of activity

Vitamin E is the generic descriptor for two families of compounds, the tocopherols and the tocotrienols (Figure 8.5). The different vitamers have different biological potency. The most active is α-tocopherol, and it is usual to express vitamin E intake in terms of mg α-tocopherol equivalents. This is the sum of mg α-tocopherol + 0.5 × mg β-tocopherol + 0.1 × mg γ-tocopherol + 0.3 × mg α-tocotrienol. The other vitamers have negligible vitamin activity.

The obsolete international unit of vitamin E activity is still sometimes used: 1 IU = 0.67 mg α-tocopherol equivalent; 1 mg α-tocopherol = 1.49 IU.

Synthetic α-tocopherol does not have the same biological potency as the naturally occurring compound. This is because the side-chain of tocopherol has three centers of asymmetry and when it is synthesized chemically the result is a mixture of the various isomers. In the naturally occurring compound all three centers of asymmetry have the R-configuration, and naturally occurring α-tocopherol is called all-R, or RRR-α-tocopherol.

Absorption and metabolism

Tocopherols and tocotrienols are absorbed unchanged from the small intestine, in micelles with other dietary lipids, and incorporated into chylomicrons. The major route of excretion is in the bile, largely as glucuronides and other conjugates.

There are two mechanisms for tissue uptake of vitamin E. Lipoprotein lipase releases the vitamin by hydrolyzing the triacylglycerols in chylomicrons and VLDLs, while separately there is uptake of low-density lipoprotein (LDL)-bound vitamin E by means of LDL receptors. Retention within tissues depends on intracellular binding proteins, and it is likely that the differences in biological activity of the vitamers are due to differences in the affinity of these proteins for the different vitamers.

Metabolic functions of vitamin E

The main function of vitamin E is as a radical-trapping antioxidant in cell membranes and plasma lipoproteins. It is especially important in limiting radical damage resulting from oxidation of PUFAs, by reacting with the lipid peroxide radicals before they can establish a chain reaction. The tocopheroxyl radical formed from vitamin E is relatively unreactive and persists long enough to undergo reaction to yield non-radical products. Commonly, the vitamin E radical in a membrane or lipoprotein is reduced back to tocopherol by reaction with vitamin C in plasma. The resultant monodehydroascorbate radical then undergoes enzymic or non-enzymic reaction to yield ascorbate and dehydroascorbate, neither of which is a radical.

The stability of the tocopheroxyl radical means that it can penetrate further into cells, or deeper into plasma lipoproteins, and potentially propagate a chain reaction. Therefore, although it is regarded as an antioxidant, vitamin E may, like other antioxidants, also have pro-oxidant actions at high

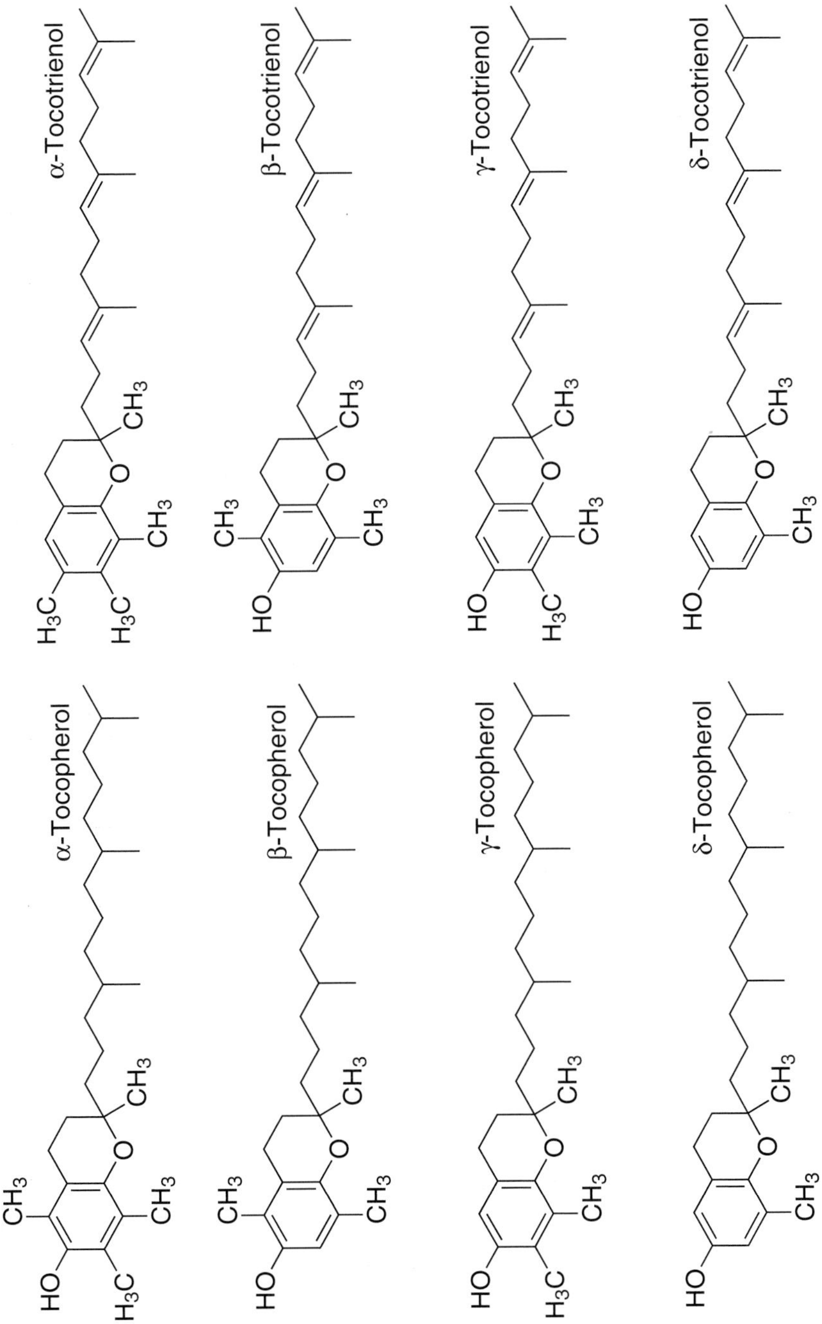

Figure 8.5 The vitamin E vitamers, tocopherols and tocotrienols.

concentrations. This may explain why, although epidemiological studies have shown a clear association between high blood concentrations of vitamin E and lower incidence of atherosclerosis, the results of intervention trials have generally been disappointing. In many trials there has been increased all-cause mortality among those taking vitamin E and other antioxidant supplements.

The tocotrienols have lower vitamin activity than tocopherols, and indeed it is conventional to consider only γ-tocotrienol as a significant part of vitamin E intake. However, because of their unsaturated side-chain, the tocotrienols also have a hypocholesterolemic action not shared by the tocopherols. They act to reduce the activity of 3-hydroxy-3-methylglutaryl-coenzyme A (HMG CoA) reductase, the rate-limiting enzyme in the pathway for synthesis of cholesterol, by repressing synthesis of the enzyme.

Vitamin E deficiency

In experimental animals vitamin E deficiency results in a number of different conditions.

- Deficient female animals suffer the death and reabsorption of the fetuses. This provided the basis of the original biological assay of vitamin E.
- In male animals deficiency results in testicular atrophy and degeneration of the germinal epithelium of the seminiferous tubules.
- Both skeletal and cardiac muscle are affected in deficient animals. This necrotizing myopathy is sometimes called nutritional muscular dystrophy – an unfortunate term, since there is no evidence that human muscular dystrophy is related to vitamin E deficiency.
- The integrity of blood vessel walls is affected, with leakage of blood plasma into subcutaneous tissues and accumulation under the skin of a green fluid: exudative diathesis.
- The nervous system is affected, with the development of central nervous system necrosis and axonal dystrophy. This is exacerbated by feeding diets rich in PUFAs.

Dietary deficiency of vitamin E in human beings is unknown, although patients with severe fat malabsorption, cystic fibrosis, some forms of chronic liver disease or (very rare) congenital lack of plasma β-lipoprotein suffer deficiency because they are unable to absorb the vitamin or transport it around the body.

They suffer from severe damage to nerve and muscle membranes.

Premature infants are at risk of vitamin E deficiency, since they are often born with inadequate reserves of the vitamin. The red blood cell membranes of deficient infants are abnormally fragile, as a result of unchecked oxidative radical attack. This may lead to hemolytic anemia if they are not given supplements of the vitamin.

Experimental animals that are depleted of vitamin E become sterile. However, there is no evidence that vitamin E nutritional status is in any way associated with human fertility, and there is certainly no evidence that vitamin E supplements increase sexual potency, prowess, or vigor.

Vitamin E requirements

It is difficult to establish vitamin E requirements, partly because deficiency is more or less unknown, but also because the requirement depends on the intake of PUFAs. It is generally accepted, albeit with little experimental evidence, that an acceptable intake of vitamin E is 0.4 mg α-tocopherol equivalent/g dietary PUFA.

Indices of vitamin E status

The plasma concentration of α-tocopherol is used to assess vitamin E status; since most vitamin E is transported in plasma lipoproteins, it is the concentration per gram total plasma lipid, or better per mole cholesterol, that is useful, rather than the simple concentration.

Erythrocytes are incapable of *de novo* lipid synthesis, so peroxidative damage resulting from oxygen stress has a serious effect, shortening red cell life and possibly precipitating hemolytic anemia in vitamin E deficiency. This has been exploited as a method of assessing status by measuring the hemolysis of red cells induced by dilute hydrogen peroxide relative to that observed on incubation in water. This gives a means of assessing the functional adequacy of vitamin E intake, albeit one that will be affected by other, unrelated, factors. Plasma concentrations of α-tocopherol below 2.2 mmol/mol cholesterol or 1.1 μmol/g total plasma lipid are associated with increased susceptibility of erythrocytes to induced hemolysis *in vitro*.

An alternative method of assessing functional antioxidant status, again one that is affected by both vitamin E and other antioxidants, is by measuring the exhalation of pentane arising from the catabolism of the products of peroxidation of n-6 PUFAs or ethane arising from n-3 PUFAs.

Higher levels of intake

There is good epidemiological evidence that intakes of vitamin E are associated with a lower risk of atherosclerosis and ischemic heart disease. High concentrations of vitamin E will inhibit the oxidation of PUFAs in plasma lipoproteins, and it is this oxidation that is responsible for the development of atherosclerosis. The plasma concentrations of α-tocopherol that appear to be beneficial would require an intake of 17–40 mg/day, which is above what could be achieved by eating normal diets. Individual intervention trials of vitamin E supplements have generally been disappointing, and metaanalysis shows a significant increase in all-cause mortality among people taking vitamin E (and other antioxidant) supplements. This presumably reflects the fact that the stable tocopheroxyl radical can penetrate deeper into tissues and plasma lipoproteins, and increase radical damage. However, it is also possible that the plasma concentration of α-tocopherol is a surrogate marker for some other protective factor in the diet.

Interactions with other nutrients

Vitamin C in plasma and extracellular fluid is important in reducing the tocopheroxyl radical in cell membranes and plasma lipoproteins back to tocopherol. There is also evidence that a variety of lipid-soluble antioxidants may be important in the antioxidant action of vitamin E in membranes and lipoproteins, including ubiquinone and synthetic antioxidants used in food processing, such as butylated hydroxytoluene and butylated hydroxyanisole. Synthetic antioxidants will prevent or cure a number of the signs of vitamin E deficiency in experimental animals.

There is a considerable overlap between the functions of vitamin E and selenium. Vitamin E reduces lipid peroxide radicals to unreactive fatty acids; the selenium-dependent enzyme glutathione peroxidase reduces hydrogen peroxide to water, thus lowering the intracellular concentration of potentially lipid-damaging peroxide. A membrane-specific isoenzyme of glutathione peroxidase will also reduce the tocopheroxyl radical back to tocopherol. Thus, vitamin E acts to remove the products of lipid peroxidation, whereas selenium acts both to remove the cause of lipid peroxidation and to recycle vitamin E.

8.5 Vitamin K

Vitamin K was discovered as a result of investigations into the cause of a bleeding disorder (hemorrhagic disease) of cattle fed on silage made from sweet clover and of chickens fed on a fat-free diet. The missing factor in the diet of the chickens was identified as vitamin K, whereas the problem in the cattle was that the feed contained dicumarol, an antagonist of the vitamin.

Since the effect of an excessive intake of dicumarol was severely impaired blood clotting, it was isolated and tested in low doses as an anticoagulant, for use in patients at risk of thrombosis. Although it was effective, it had unwanted side-effects, and synthetic vitamin K antagonists were developed for clinical use as anticoagulants. The most commonly used of these is warfarin, which is also used, in larger amounts, to kill rodents.

Vitamers

Three compounds have the biological activity of vitamin K (Figure 8.6):

- phylloquinone, the normal dietary source, found in green leafy vegetables;
- menaquinones, a family of related compounds synthesized by intestinal bacteria, with differing lengths of the side-chain;
- menadiol and menadiol diacetate, synthetic compounds that can be metabolized to phylloquinone.

Dietary sources, bacterial synthesis and metabolism

Phylloquinone has a role in photosynthesis, and therefore it is found in all green leafy vegetables; the richest sources are spring (collard) greens, spinach, and Brussels sprouts. In addition, soybean, rapeseed, cottonseed, and olive oils are relatively rich in vitamin K, although other oils are not.

About 80% of dietary phylloquinone is normally absorbed into the lymphatic system in chylomicrons, and is then taken up by the liver from chylomicron remnants and released into the circulation in VLDLs.

Intestinal bacteria synthesize a variety of menaquinones, which are absorbed to a limited extent from

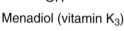

Phylloquinone (vitamin K$_1$)

Menaquinone (vitamin K$_2$)

Menadiol (vitamin K$_3$)

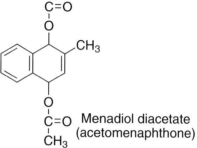

Menadiol diacetate (acetomenaphthone)

Figure 8.6 The vitamin K vitamers, phylloquinone (vitamin K$_1$), menaquinone (vitamin K$_2$), and menadiol (a synthetic compound, vitamin K$_3$).

the large intestine, again into the lymphatic system, cleared by the liver, and released in VLDLs. It is often suggested that about half of the requirement for vitamin K is met by intestinal bacterial synthesis, but there is little evidence for this, other than the fact that about half of the vitamin K in liver is phylloquinone and the remainder a variety of menaquinones. It is not clear to what extent the menaquinones are biologically active. It is possible to induce signs of vitamin K deficiency simply by feeding a phylloquinone-deficient diet, without inhibiting intestinal bacterial action.

The synthetic compound menadiol is absorbed largely into the hepatic portal system, and undergoes alkylation in the liver to yield menaquinone-4, which is released together with phylloquinone and other menaquinones in VLDLs.

Metabolic functions of vitamin K

Although it has been known since the 1920s that vitamin K was required for blood clotting, it was not until the 1970s that its precise function was estab-

lished. It is the cofactor for the carboxylation of glutamate residues in the postsynthetic modification of proteins to form the unusual amino acid γ-carboxyglutamate, abbreviated to Gla (Figure 8.7).

In the presence of warfarin, vitamin K epoxide cannot be reduced back to the active hydroquinone, but accumulates and is excreted as a variety of conjugates. However, if enough vitamin K is provided in the diet, the quinone can be reduced to the active hydroquinone by the warfarin-insensitive enzyme, and carboxylation can continue, with stoichiometric utilization of vitamin K and excretion of the epoxide. High doses of vitamin K are used to treat patients who have received an overdose of warfarin, and at least part of the resistance of some populations of rats to the action of warfarin is due to a high consumption of vitamin K from maram grass, although there are also genetically resistant populations of rodents.

Prothrombin and several other proteins of the blood clotting system (factors VII, IX and X, and proteins C and S) each contain between four and six γ-carboxyglutamate residues per mole. γ-Carboxy-

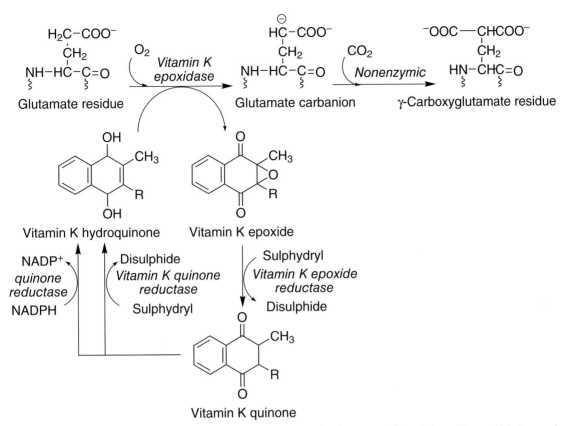

Figure 8.7 Role of vitamin K in the carboxylation of glutamate. Vitamin K epoxidase (EC 1.14.99.20), warfarin-sensitive epoxide/quinone reductase (EC 1.1.4.1), warfarin-insensitive quinone reductase (EC 1.1.4.2).

glutamate chelates calcium ions, and so permits the binding of the blood clotting proteins to lipid membranes. In vitamin K deficiency, or in the presence of an antagonist such as warfarin, an abnormal precursor of prothrombin (preprothrombin) containing little or no γ-carboxyglutamate is released into the circulation. Preprothrombin cannot chelate calcium or bind to phospholipid membranes, and so is unable to initiate blood clotting. Preprothrombin is sometimes known as PIVKA: the protein induced by vitamin K absence.

Other vitamin K-dependent proteins

It has long been known that treatment of pregnant women with warfarin or other anticoagulants can lead to bone abnormalities in the child: the fetal warfarin syndrome. Two proteins in bone matrix contain γ-carboxyglutamate: osteocalcin and a less well char-

acterized protein simply known as bone matrix Gla protein. Osteocalcin is interesting in that as well as γ-carboxyglutamate, it also contains hydroxyproline, so its synthesis is dependent on both vitamins K and C; in addition, its synthesis is induced by vitamin D, and the release into the circulation of osteocalcin provides a sensitive index of vitamin D action. It constitutes some 1–2% of total bone protein, and modifies the crystallization of bone mineral. The matrix Gla protein is found in a variety of tissues, and acts to prevent mineralization of soft connective tissue.

The fetal warfarin syndrome involves neurological as well as bone abnormalities. The vitamin K-dependent carboxylase is expressed in different brain regions at different times during embryological development, and the product of the growth arrest-specific gene 6 (*Gas6*) is a Gla-containing growth factor that is important in the regulation of growth and development, and the regulation of apoptosis and cell survival.

Vitamin K deficiency and requirements

Apart from deliberate experimental manipulation, vitamin K deficiency is unknown, and determination of requirements is complicated by a lack of information on the importance of menaquinones synthesized by intestinal bacteria.

The classical way of determining vitamin K status, and monitoring the efficacy of anticoagulant therapy, is by measuring the time required for the formation of a fibrin clot in citrated blood plasma after the addition of calcium ions and thromboplastin: the prothrombin time. A more sensitive index is provided by direct measurement of preprothrombin in plasma, most commonly by immunoassay using antisera against preprothrombin that do not react with prothrombin.

Based on determination of clotting time, and direct measurement of prothrombin and preprothrombin, an intake of 1 μg/kg body weight per day is considered adequate; this forms the basis of reference intakes of between 65 and 80 μg/day for adults.

A small number of newborn infants have very low reserves of vitamin K and are at risk of potentially fatal hemorrhagic disease. It is therefore generally recommended that all neonates should be given a single prophylactic dose of vitamin K.

Toxicity and drug interactions

There is no evidence that phylloquinone has any significant toxicity. However, high intakes can overcome the effects of warfarin and other anticoagulants. This means that patients who are being treated with warfarin could overcome the beneficial effects of their medication if they took supplements of vitamin K. The danger is that if their dose of warfarin is increased to counteract the effects of the vitamin supplements and they then stop taking the supplements, they would be receiving considerably too much warfarin and would be at risk of hemorrhage.

It is unlikely that a normal diet could provide a sufficient excess of vitamin K to lead to problems, but habitual consumption of especially rich sources could result in intakes close to those that antagonize therapeutic warfarin. A diet containing relatively large amounts of foods prepared with vitamin K-rich oils may pose a risk.

8.6 Vitamin B₁ (thiamin)

Historically, thiamin deficiency affecting the peripheral nervous system (beriberi) was a major public health problem in south-east Asia following the introduction of the steam-powered mill that made highly polished (and therefore thiamin-depleted) rice widely available. There are still sporadic outbreaks of deficiency among people whose diet is rich in carbohydrate and poor in thiamin. More commonly, thiamin deficiency affecting the heart and central nervous system is a problem in people with an excessive consumption of alcohol, to the extent that there was a serious suggestion in Australia at one time that thiamin should be added to beer.

The structures of thiamin and the coenzyme thiamin diphosphate are shown in Figure 8.8.

Thiamin is widely distributed in foods, with pork being an especially rich source; potatoes, whole-grain cereals, meat, and fish are the major sources in most diets. Like other water-soluble vitamins, thiamin is readily lost by leaching into cooking water; furthermore, it is unstable to light, and although bread and flour contain significant amounts of thiamin, much of this can be lost when baked goods are exposed to sunlight in a shop window.

Thiamin is also destroyed by sulfites, and in potato products that have been blanched by immersion in sulfite solution there is little or no thiamin remaining. Polyphenols, including tannic acid in tea and betel nuts, also destroy thiamin, and have been associated with thiamin deficiency.

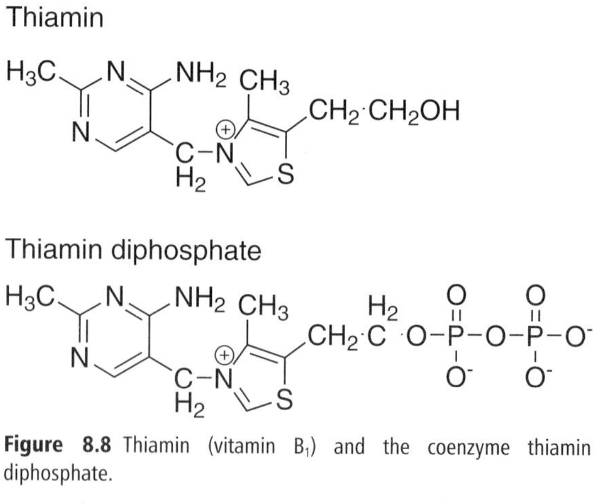

Figure 8.8 Thiamin (vitamin B₁) and the coenzyme thiamin diphosphate.

Thiaminases that catalyze base exchange or hydrolysis of thiamin are found in microorganisms (including some that colonize the gut), a variety of plants, and raw fish. The presence of thiaminase in fermented fish is believed to be a significant factor in the etiology of thiamin deficiency in parts of southeast Asia.

Absorption and metabolism of thiamin

Thiamin is absorbed in the duodenum and proximal jejunum, and then transferred to the portal circulation by an active transport process that is inhibited by alcohol. This may explain why alcoholics are especially susceptible to thiamin deficiency.

Tissues take up both free thiamin and thiamin monophosphate, then phosphorylate them further to yield thiamin diphosphate (the active coenzyme) and, in the nervous system, thiamin triphosphate.

Some free thiamin is excreted in the urine, increasing with diuresis, and a significant amount may also be lost in sweat. Most urinary excretion is as thiochrome, the result of non-enzymic cyclization, as well as a variety of products of side-chain oxidation and ring cleavage.

There is little storage of thiamin in the body, and biochemical signs of deficiency can be observed within a few days of initiating a thiamin-free diet.

Metabolic functions of thiamin

Thiamin has a central role in energy-yielding metabolism, and especially the metabolism of carbohydrates. Thiamin diphosphate (also known as thiamin pyrophosphate, see Figure 8.8) is the coenzyme for three oxidative decarboxylation reactions: pyruvate dehydrogenase in carbohydrate metabolism, α-ketoglutarate dehydrogenase in the citric acid cycle, and the branched-chain keto-acid dehydrogenase involved in the metabolism of leucine, isoleucine, and valine. These three enzymes are multienzyme complexes that catalyze oxidative decarboxylation of the substrate linked to reduction of enzyme-bound lipoamide, and eventually reduction of NAD^+ to NADH.

Thiamin diphosphate is also the coenzyme for transketolase, in the pentose phosphate pathway of carbohydrate metabolism. This is the major pathway of carbohydrate metabolism in some tissues, and an important alternative to glycolysis in all tissues, being the source of half of the NADPH required for fatty acid synthesis.

Thiamin triphosphate has a role in nerve conduction, as the phosphate donor for phosphorylation of a nerve membrane sodium transport protein.

Thiamin deficiency

Thiamin deficiency can result in three distinct syndromes:

- a chronic peripheral neuritis, beriberi, which may or may not be associated with heart failure and edema
- acute pernicious (fulminating) beriberi (shoshin beriberi), in which heart failure and metabolic abnormalities predominate, with little evidence of peripheral neuritis
- Wernicke's encephalopathy with Korsakoff's psychosis, a thiamin-responsive condition associated especially with alcohol and narcotic abuse.

In general, a relatively acute deficiency is involved in the central nervous system lesions of the Wernicke–Korsakoff syndrome, and a high energy intake, as in alcoholics, is also a predisposing factor. Dry beriberi is associated with a more prolonged, and presumably less severe, deficiency, and a generally low food intake, whereas higher carbohydrate intake and physical activity predispose to wet beriberi.

The role of thiamin diphosphate in pyruvate dehydrogenase means that in deficiency there is impaired conversion of pyruvate to acetyl-CoA, and hence impaired entry of pyruvate into the citric acid cycle. Especially in subjects on a relatively high carbohydrate diet, this results in increased plasma concentrations of lactate and pyruvate, which may lead to life-threatening lactic acidosis. The increase in plasma lactate and pyruvate after a test dose of glucose has been used as a means of assessing thiamin nutritional status.

Dry beriberi

Chronic deficiency of thiamin, especially associated with a high carbohydrate diet, results in beriberi, which is a symmetrical ascending peripheral neuritis. Initially, the patient complains of weakness, stiffness and cramps in the legs, and is unable to walk more than a short distance. There may be numbness of the dorsum of the feet and ankles, and vibration sense may be diminished. As the disease progresses, the ankle jerk reflex is lost, and the muscular weakness spreads upwards, involving first the extensor muscles of the foot, then the muscles of the calf, and finally the extensors and flexors of the thigh. At this stage there is pronounced toe and foot drop: the patient is unable to keep either the toe or the whole foot extended off the ground. When the arms are affected there is a similar inability to keep the hand extended: wrist drop.

The affected muscles become tender, numb, and hyperesthetic. The hyperesthesia extends in the form of a band around the limb, the so-called stocking and glove distribution, and is followed by anesthesia. There is deep muscle pain, and in the terminal stages, when the patient is bed-ridden, even slight pressure, as from bedclothes, causes considerable pain.

Wet beriberi
The heart may also be affected in beriberi, with dilatation of arterioles, rapid blood flow, and increased pulse rate leading to right-sided heart failure and edema, so-called wet beriberi. The signs of chronic heart failure may be seen without peripheral neuritis. The arteriolar dilatation probably results from high circulating concentrations of lactate and pyruvate as a result of impaired activity of pyruvate dehydrogenase.

Acute pernicious (fulminating) beriberi: shoshin beriberi
Heart failure without increased cardiac output, and no peripheral edema, may also occur acutely, associated with severe lactic acidosis. This was a common presentation of deficiency in Japan, where it was called shoshin (meaning acute) beriberi; in the 1920s some 26 000 deaths a year were recorded.

With improved knowledge of the cause and improved nutritional status, the disease has become more or less unknown, although in the 1980s it reappeared among Japanese adolescents consuming a diet based largely on such high-carbohydrate, low-nutrient, foods as sweet carbonated drinks, "instant" noodles, and polished rice. It also occurs among alcoholics, when the lactic acidosis may be life-threatening, without clear signs of heart failure. Acute beriberi has also been reported when previously starved subjects are given intravenous glucose.

Wernicke–Korsakoff syndrome
Whereas peripheral neuritis, acute cardiac beriberi and lactic acidosis occur in thiamin deficiency associated with alcohol misuse, the more usual presentation is as the Wernicke–Korsakoff syndrome, due to central nervous system lesions.

Initially, there is a confused state, Korsakoff's psychosis, which is characterized by confabulation and loss of recent memory, although memory for past events may be unimpaired. Later, clear neurological signs develop: Wernicke's encephalopathy. This is characterized by nystagmus and extraocular palsy. Post-mortem examination shows characteristic brain lesions.

Like shoshin beriberi, Wernicke's encephalopathy can develop acutely, without the more gradual development of Korsakoff's psychosis, among previously starved patients given intravenous glucose and seriously ill patients given parenteral hyperalimentation.

Thiamin requirements
Because thiamin has a central role in energy-yielding, and especially carbohydrate, metabolism, requirements depend mainly on carbohydrate intake, and have been related to "non-fat calories." In practice, requirements and reference intakes are calculated on the basis of total energy intake, assuming that the average diet provides 40% of energy from fat. For diets that are lower in fat, and hence higher in carbohydrate, thiamin requirements may be somewhat higher.

From depletion/repletion studies, an intake of at least 0.2 mg of thiamin/1000 kcal is required to prevent the development of deficiency signs and maintain normal urinary excretion, but an intake of 0.23 mg/1000 kcal is required for a normal transketolase activation coefficient (see below).

Reference intakes are calculated on the basis of 100 μg/MJ (0.5 mg/1000 kcal) for adults consuming more than 2000 kcal/day, with a minimum requirement for people with a low energy intake of 0.8–1.0 mg/day to allow for metabolism of endogenous substrates.

Assessment of thiamin status
The impairment of pyruvate dehydrogenase in thiamin deficiency results in a considerable increase in the plasma concentrations of lactate and pyruvate. This has been exploited as a means of assessing thiamin status, by measuring changes in the plasma concentrations of lactate and pyruvate after an oral

dose of glucose and mild exercise. The test is not specific for thiamin deficiency since a variety of other conditions can also result in metabolic acidosis. Although it may be useful in depletion/repletion studies, it is little used nowadays in assessment of nutritional status.

Whole blood total thiamin below 150 nmol/l is considered to indicate deficiency. However, the changes observed in depletion studies are small. Even in patients with frank beriberi the total thiamin concentration in erythrocytes is only 20% lower than normal, so whole blood thiamin is not a sensitive index of status.

Although there are several urinary metabolites of thiamin, a significant proportion is excreted either unchanged or as thiochrome, and therefore the urinary excretion of the vitamin (measured as thiochrome) can provide information on nutritional status. Excretion decreases proportionally with intake in adequately nourished subjects, but at low intakes there is a threshold below which further reduction in intake has little effect on excretion.

The activation of apo-transketolase in erythrocyte lysate by thiamin diphosphate added *in vitro* has become the most widely used and accepted index of thiamin nutritional status. Apo-transketolase is unstable both *in vivo* and *in vitro*, so problems may arise in the interpretation of results, especially if samples have been stored for any appreciable time. An activation coefficient >1.25 is indicative of deficiency, and <1.15 is considered to reflect adequate thiamin status.

8.7 Vitamin B$_2$ (riboflavin)

Riboflavin deficiency is a significant public health problem in many areas of the world. The vitamin has a central role as a coenzyme in energy-yielding metabolism, yet deficiency is rarely, if ever, fatal, since there is very efficient conservation and recycling of riboflavin in deficiency.

The structures of riboflavin and the riboflavin-derived coenzymes are shown in Figure 8.9.

Milk and dairy products are important sources, providing 25% or more of total riboflavin intake in most diets, and it is noteworthy that average riboflavin status in different countries reflects milk consumption to a considerable extent. Other rich sources are eggs, meat, and fish. In addition, because of its

intense yellow color, riboflavin is widely used as a food color.

Photolytic destruction

Photolysis of riboflavin leads to the formation of lumiflavin (in alkaline solution) and lumichrome (in acidic or neutral solution), both of which are biologically inactive. Exposure of milk in clear glass bottles to sunlight or fluorescent light can result in the loss of significant amounts of riboflavin. This is potentially nutritionally important. Lumiflavin and lumichrome catalyze oxidation of lipids (to lipid peroxides) and methionine (to methional), resulting in the development of an unpleasant flavor, known as the "sunlight" flavor.

Absorption and metabolism

Apart from milk and eggs, which contain relatively large amounts of free riboflavin bound to specific binding proteins, most of the vitamin in foods is as flavin coenzymes bound to enzymes, which are released when the protein is hydrolyzed. Intestinal phosphatases then hydrolyze the coenzymes to liberate riboflavin, which is absorbed in the upper small intestine. The absorption of riboflavin is limited and after moderately high doses only a small proportion is absorbed.

Much of the absorbed riboflavin is phosphorylated in the intestinal mucosa and enters the bloodstream as riboflavin phosphate, although this does not seem to be essential for absorption of the vitamin.

About 50% of plasma riboflavin is free riboflavin, which is the main transport form, with 44% as flavin adenine dinucleotide (FAD) and the remainder as riboflavin phosphate. The vitamin is largely protein-bound in plasma; free riboflavin binds to both albumin and α- and β-globulins; both riboflavin and the coenzymes also bind to immunoglobulins.

Uptake into tissues is by passive carrier-mediated transport of free riboflavin, followed by metabolic trapping by phosphorylation to riboflavin phosphate, and onward metabolism to FAD.

Riboflavin phosphate and FAD that are not bound to proteins are rapidly hydrolyzed to riboflavin, which diffuses out of tissues into the bloodstream. Riboflavin and riboflavin phosphate that are not bound to plasma proteins are filtered at the glomerulus; renal tubular resorption is saturated at normal plasma concentrations. There is also active tubular secretion of

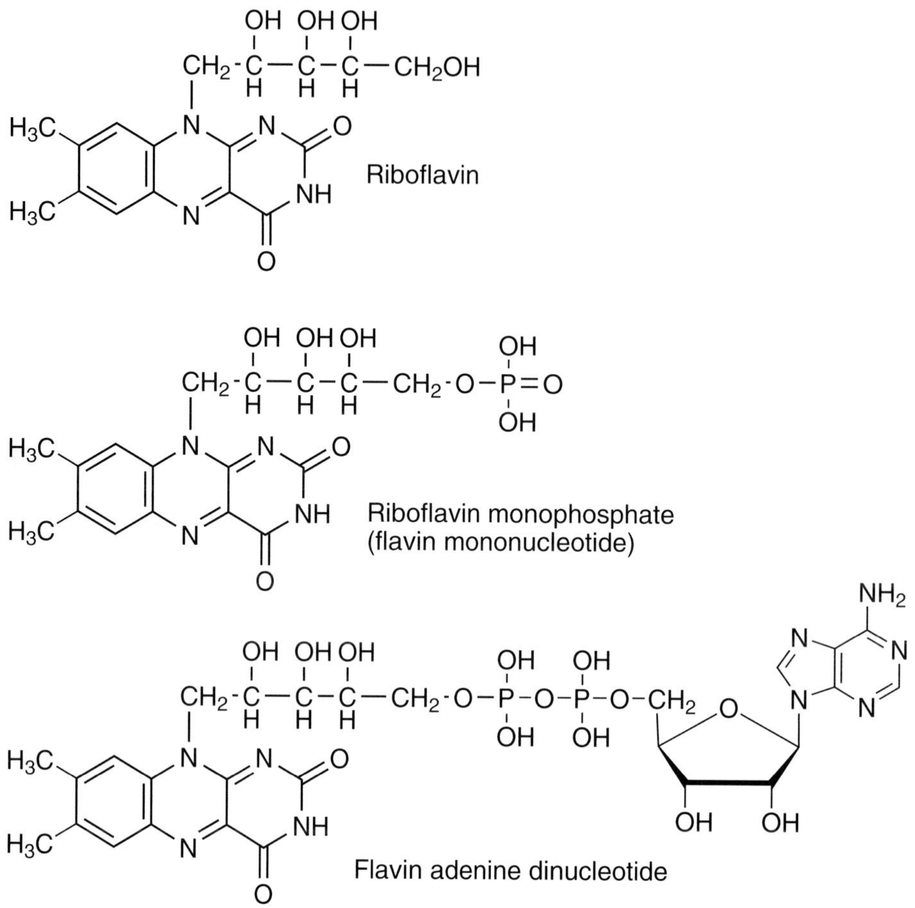

Figure 8.9 Riboflavin (vitamin B₂) and the flavin coenzymes, riboflavin monophosphate and flavin adenine dinucleotide.

the vitamin; urinary excretion of riboflavin after moderately high doses can be two- to threefold greater than the glomerular filtration rate.

Under normal conditions about 25% of the urinary excretion of riboflavin is as the unchanged vitamin, with a small amount as glycosides of riboflavin and its metabolites.

Riboflavin balance

There is no significant storage of riboflavin; apart from the limitation on absorption, any surplus intake is excreted rapidly, so that once metabolic requirements have been met urinary excretion of riboflavin and its metabolites reflects intake until intestinal absorption is saturated. In depleted animals, the maximum growth response is achieved with intakes that give about 75% saturation of tissues, and the intake to achieve tissue saturation is that

at which there is quantitative excretion of the vitamin.

There is very efficient conservation of riboflavin in deficiency, and almost the only loss from tissues will be the small amount that is covalently bound to enzymes and cannot be salvaged for reuse. There is only a fourfold difference between the minimum concentration of flavins in the liver in deficiency and the level at which saturation occurs. In the central nervous system there is only a 35% difference between deficiency and saturation.

Metabolic functions of the flavin coenzymes

The metabolic function of the flavin coenzymes is as electron carriers in a wide variety of oxidation and reduction reactions central to all metabolic processes, including the mitochondrial electron transport chain, and key enzymes in fatty acid and amino acid oxidation, and the citric acid cycle. The flavin coenzymes remain bound to the enzyme throughout the catalytic cycle. The majority of flavoproteins have FAD as the prosthetic group rather than riboflavin phosphate; some have both flavin coenzymes and some have other prosthetic groups as well.

Flavins can undergo a one-electron reduction to the semiquinone radical or a two-electron reduction to dihydroflavin. In some enzymes formation of dihydroflavin occurs by two single-electron steps, with intermediate formation of the semiquinone radical. Dihydroflavin can be oxidized by reaction with a substrate, $NAD(P)^+$, or cytochromes in a variety of dehydrogenases, or can react with molecular oxygen in oxygenases and mixed function oxidases (hydroxylases).

Flavins and oxidative stress

Reoxidation of the reduced flavin in oxygenases and mixed function oxidases proceeds by way of formation of the flavin radical and flavin hydroperoxide, with the intermediate generation of superoxide and perhydroxyl radicals and hydrogen peroxide. Because of this, flavin oxidases make a significant contribution to the total oxidant stress of the body. Overall, some 3–5% of the daily consumption of about 30 mol of oxygen by an adult is converted to singlet oxygen, hydrogen peroxide, and superoxide, perhydroxyl, and hydroxyl radicals, rather than undergoing complete reduction to water in the electron transport chain. There is thus a total production of some 1.5 mol of reactive oxygen species daily, potentially capable of causing damage to membrane lipids, proteins, and nucleic acids.

Riboflavin deficiency

Although riboflavin is involved in all areas of metabolism, and deficiency is widespread on a global scale, deficiency is not fatal. There seem to be two reasons for this. One is that, although deficiency is common, the vitamin is widespread in foods and most diets will provide minimally adequate amounts to permit maintenance of central metabolic pathways. The second, more important, reason is that in deficiency there is extremely efficient reutilization of the riboflavin that is released by the turnover of flavoproteins, so that only a very small amount is metabolized or excreted.

Riboflavin deficiency is characterized by lesions of the margin of the lips (cheilosis) and corners of the mouth (angular stomatitis), a painful desquamation of the tongue, so that it is red, dry, and atrophic (magenta tongue), and a seborrheic dermatitis, with filiform excrescences, affecting especially the nasolabial folds, eyelids, and ears.

There may also be conjunctivitis with vascularization of the cornea and opacity of the lens. This last is the only lesion of ariboflavinosis for which the biochemical basis is known: glutathione is important in maintaining the normal clarity of crystallin in the lens, and glutathione reductase is a flavoprotein that is particularly sensitive to riboflavin depletion.

The main metabolic effect of riboflavin deficiency is on lipid metabolism. Riboflavin-deficient animals have a lower metabolic rate than controls and require a 15–20% higher food intake to maintain body weight. Feeding a high-fat diet leads to more marked impairment of growth and a higher requirement for riboflavin to restore growth.

Resistance to malaria in riboflavin deficiency

Several studies have noted that in areas where malaria is endemic, riboflavin-deficient subjects are relatively resistant and have a lower parasite burden than adequately nourished subjects. The biochemical basis of this resistance to malaria in riboflavin deficiency is not known, but two possible mechanisms have been proposed.

- The malarial parasites may have a particularly high requirement for riboflavin. Some flavin analogues have antimalarial action.
- As a result of impaired antioxidant activity in erythrocytes, there may be increased fragility of erythrocyte membranes or reduced membrane fluidity. As in sickle cell trait, which also protects against malaria, this may result in exposure of the parasites to the host's immune system at a vulnerable stage in their development, resulting in the production of protective antibodies.

Riboflavin requirements

Estimates of riboflavin requirements are based on depletion/repletion studies to determine the minimum intake at which there is significant excretion of the vitamin. In deficiency there is virtually no excretion of the vitamin; as requirements are met, so any excess is excreted in the urine. On this basis the minimum adult requirement for riboflavin is 0.5–0.8 mg/day.

At intakes of 1.1–1.6 mg/day urinary excretion rises sharply, suggesting that tissue reserves are saturated.

A more generous estimate of requirements, and the basis of reference intakes, is the level of intake at which there is normalization of the activity of the red cell enzyme glutathione reductase; the activity of this flavoprotein is especially sensitive to riboflavin nutritional status. Normal values of the activation coefficient are seen in subjects whose habitual intake of riboflavin is between 1.2 mg/day and 1.5 mg/day.

Because of the central role of flavin coenzymes in energy-yielding metabolism, reference intakes are sometimes calculated on the basis of energy intake: 0.14–0.19 mg/MJ (0.6–0.8 mg/1000 kcal). However, in view of the wide range of riboflavin-dependent reactions, other than those of energy-yielding metabolism, it is difficult to justify this basis for the calculation of requirements.

Assessment of riboflavin nutritional status

The urinary excretion of riboflavin and its metabolites (either basal excretion or after a test dose) can be used as an index of status. However, riboflavin excretion is only correlated with intake in subjects who are in nitrogen balance. In subjects in negative nitrogen balance there may be more urinary excretion than would be expected, as a result of the catabolism of tissue flavoproteins, and loss of their prosthetic groups. Higher intakes of protein than are required to maintain nitrogen balance do not affect the requirement for riboflavin or indices of riboflavin nutritional status.

Glutathione reductase is especially sensitive to riboflavin depletion. The activity of the enzyme in erythrocytes can therefore be used as an index of riboflavin status. Interpretation of the results can be complicated by anemia, and it is more usual to use the activation of erythrocyte glutathione reductase (EGR) by FAD added *in vitro*. An activation coefficient of 1.0–1.4 reflects adequate nutritional status, whereas >1.7 indicates deficiency.

Interactions with drugs and other nutrients

The phenothiazines such as chlorpromazine, used in the treatment of schizophrenia, and the tricyclic antidepressant drugs such as imipramine, are structural analogues of riboflavin, and inhibit flavokinase. In experimental animals, administration of these drugs at doses equivalent to those used clinically results in an increase in the EGR activation coefficient and increased urinary excretion of riboflavin, with reduced tissue concentrations of riboflavin phosphate and FAD, despite feeding diets providing more riboflavin than is needed to meet requirements. Although there is no evidence that patients treated with these drugs for a prolonged period develop clinical signs of riboflavin deficiency, long-term use of chlorpromazine is associated with a reduction in metabolic rate.

Riboflavin deficiency is sometimes associated with hypochromic anemia as a result of impaired iron absorption. A greater proportion of a test dose of iron is retained in the intestinal mucosal cells bound to ferritin, and hence lost in the feces, rather than being absorbed, because the mobilization of iron bound to ferritin in mucosal cells for transfer to transferrin requires oxidation by a flavin-dependent enzyme.

Riboflavin depletion decreases the oxidation of dietary vitamin B_6 to pyridoxal; pyridoxine oxidase is a flavoprotein and is very sensitive to riboflavin depletion. It is not clear to what extent there is functional vitamin B_6 deficiency in riboflavin deficiency. This is partly because vitamin B_6 nutritional status is generally assessed by the metabolism of a test dose of tryptophan, and kynurenine hydroxylase in the tryptophan oxidative pathway is a flavoprotein; riboflavin deficiency can therefore disturb tryptophan metabolism quite separately from its effects on vitamin B_6 nutritional status.

The disturbance of tryptophan metabolism in riboflavin deficiency, due to impairment of kynurenine hydroxylase, can also result in reduced synthesis of NAD from tryptophan, and may therefore be a factor in the etiology of pellagra.

8.8 Niacin

Niacin is not strictly a vitamin, since it can be synthesized in the body from the essential amino acid tryptophan. Indeed, it is only when tryptophan metabolism is deranged that dietary preformed niacin becomes important. Nevertheless, niacin was discovered as a nutrient during studies of the deficiency disease pellagra, which was a major public health problem in the southern USA throughout the first half of the twentieth century, and continued to be a problem in parts of India and sub-Saharan Africa until the 1990s.

Vitamers and niacin equivalents

Two compounds, nicotinic acid and nicotinamide, have the biological activity of niacin. When nicotinic acid was discovered as the curative and preventive factor for pellagra, it was already known as a chemical compound, and was therefore never assigned a number among the B vitamins. The name niacin was coined in the USA when it was decided to enrich maize meal with the vitamin to prevent pellagra; it was considered that the name nicotinic acid was not desirable because of its similarity to nicotine. In the USA the term niacin is commonly used to mean specifically nicotinic acid, and nicotinamide is known as niacinamide; elsewhere "niacin" is used as a generic descriptor for both vitamers. Figure 8.10 shows the structures of nicotinic acid and niacin, as well as the nicotinamide nucleotide coenzymes, NAD and NADP.

The nicotinamide ring of NAD can be synthesized in the body from the essential amino acid tryptophan. In adults almost all of the dietary intake of tryptophan, apart from the small amount that is used for net new protein synthesis, and synthesis of the neurotransmitter serotonin, is metabolized by this pathway, and hence is potentially available for NAD synthesis.

Several studies have investigated the equivalence of dietary tryptophan and preformed niacin as precursors of the nicotinamide nucleotides, generally by determining the excretion of niacin metabolites in response to test doses of the precursors, in subjects maintained on deficient diets. The most extensive such study was that of Horwitt et al. in 1956. They found that there was a considerable variation between subjects in the response to tryptophan and niacin, and in order to allow for this individual variation they proposed the ratio of 60 mg of tryptophan equivalent to 1 mg of preformed niacin. Changes in hormonal status may result in considerable changes in this ratio, with between 7 and 30 mg of dietary tryptophan being equivalent to 1 mg of preformed niacin in late pregnancy.

The niacin content of foods is generally expressed as mg niacin equivalents; 1 mg niacin equivalent = mg preformed niacin + 1/60 × mg tryptophan. Because most of the niacin in cereals is biologically unavailable (see below), it is conventional to ignore preformed niacin in cereal products.

Because endogenous synthesis from tryptophan is more important than preformed dietary niacin, the main dietary sources of niacin are generally those that are also rich sources of protein. It is only when the dietary staple is a cereal such as maize, which is

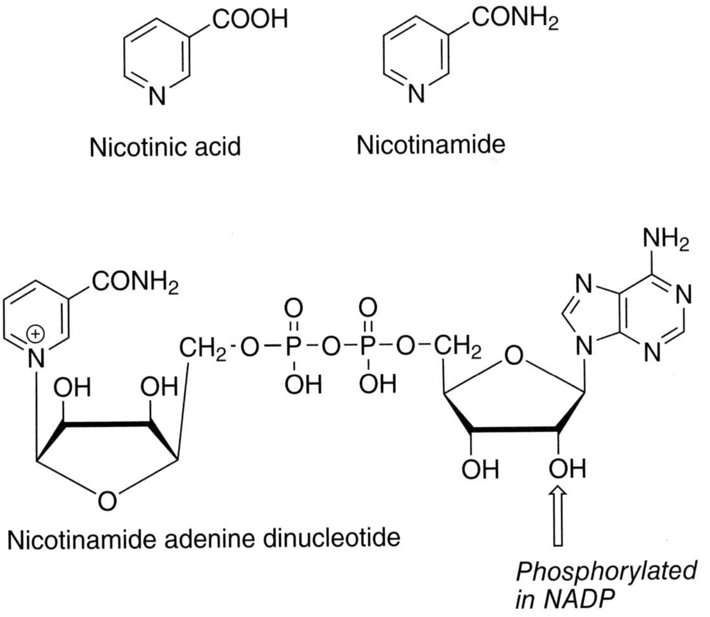

Figure 8.10 The niacin vitamers, nicotinic acid and nicotinamide, and the coenzyme nicotinamide adenine dinucleotide.

remarkably lacking in tryptophan, that problems of deficiency occur. Trigonelline in coffee beans is demethylated to nicotinic acid during roasting, and moderate coffee consumption may meet a significant proportion of niacin requirements.

Unavailable niacin in cereals

Chemical analysis reveals niacin in cereals (largely in the bran), but this is biologically unavailable, since it is bound as niacytin – nicotinoyl esters to a variety of macromolecules. In wheat bran some 60% is esterified to polysaccharides, and the remainder to polypeptides and glycopeptides.

Treatment of cereals with alkali (e.g., by soaking overnight in calcium hydroxide solution, as is the traditional method for the preparation of tortillas in Mexico) and baking with alkaline baking powder releases much of the nicotinic acid. This may explain why pellagra has always been rare in Mexico, despite the fact that maize is the dietary staple.

Up to 10% of the niacin in niacytin may be biologically available as a result of hydrolysis by gastric acid.

Absorption and metabolism

Niacin is present in tissues, and therefore in foods, largely as the nicotinamide nucleotides. The postmortem hydrolysis of NAD(P) is extremely rapid in animal tissues, so it is likely that much of the niacin of meat (a major dietary source of the preformed vitamin) is free nicotinamide.

Nicotinamide nucleotides present in the intestinal lumen are not absorbed as such, but are hydrolyzed to free nicotinamide. Many intestinal bacteria have high nicotinamide deamidase activity, and a significant proportion of dietary nicotinamide may be deamidated in the intestinal lumen. Both nicotinic acid and nicotinamide are absorbed from the small intestine by a sodium-dependent saturable process.

The nicotinamide nucleotide coenzymes can be synthesized from either of the niacin vitamers and from quinolinic acid, an intermediate in the metabolism of tryptophan. In the liver, synthesis of the coenzymes increases with increasing intake of tryptophan, but not preformed niacin. The liver exports nicotinamide, derived from turnover of coenzymes, for uptake by other tissues.

Catabolism of NAD(P)

The catabolism of NAD$^+$ is catalyzed by four enzymes:

- NAD glycohydrolase, which releases nicotinamide and ADP-ribose;
- NAD pyrophosphatase, which releases nicotinamide mononucleotide; this can be either hydrolyzed by NAD glycohydrolase to release nicotinamide, or reutilized to form NAD;
- ADP-ribosyltransferases;
- poly(ADP-ribose) polymerase.

The activation of ADP-ribosyltransferase and poly(ADP-ribose) polymerase by toxins, oxidative stress or DNA damage may result in considerable depletion of intracellular NAD(P), and may indeed provide a protective mechanism to ensure that cells that have suffered very severe DNA damage die as a result of NAD(P) depletion. The administration of DNA-breaking carcinogens to experimental animals results in the excretion of large amounts of nicotinamide metabolites and depletion of tissue NAD(P); addition of the compounds to cells in culture has a similar effect. Chronic exposure to such carcinogens and mycotoxins may be a contributory factor in the etiology of pellagra when dietary intakes of tryptophan and niacin are marginal.

Urinary excretion of niacin and metabolites

Under normal conditions there is little or no urinary excretion of either nicotinamide or nicotinic acid. This is because both vitamers are actively reabsorbed from the glomerular filtrate. It is only when the concentration is so high that the reabsorption mechanism is saturated that there is any significant excretion of niacin.

Nicotinamide in excess of requirements for NAD synthesis is methylated by nicotinamide N-methyltransferase. N^1-Methylnicotinamide is actively secreted into the urine by the proximal renal tubules. N^1-Methylnicotinamide can also be metabolized further, to yield methylpyridone-2- and 4-carboxamides.

Nicotinamide can also undergo oxidation to nicotinamide N-oxide when large amounts are ingested. Nicotinic acid can be conjugated with glycine to form nicotinuric acid (nicotinoyl-glycine) or may be methylated to trigonelline (N^1-methylnicotinic acid). It is not clear to what extent urinary excretion of trigonelline reflects endogenous methylation of nicotinic acid, since there is a significant amount of trigonelline in foods, which may be absorbed, but cannot be utilized as a source of niacin, and is excreted unchanged.

Metabolic functions of niacin

The best-defined role of niacin is in the metabolism of metabolic fuels, as the functional nicotinamide part of the coenzymes NAD and NADP, which play a major role in oxidation and reduction reactions. The oxidized coenzymes have a positive charge on the nicotinamide ring nitrogen and undergo a two-electron reduction. The oxidized forms are conventionally shown as $NAD(P)^+$ and the reduced forms either as $NAD(P)H_2$ or, more correctly, as $NAD(P)H + H^+$, since although it is a two-electron reduction, only one proton is incorporated into the ring, the other remaining associated with the coenzyme.

In general, NAD^+ acts as an electron acceptor in energy-yielding metabolism, being oxidized by the mitochondrial electron transport chain, while the major coenzyme for reductive synthetic reactions is NADPH. An exception to this general rule is the pentose phosphate pathway of glucose metabolism, which results in the reduction of $NADP^+$ to NADPH, and is the source of half the reductant for fatty acid synthesis.

In addition to its coenzyme role, NAD is the source of ADP-ribose for the ADP-ribosylation of a variety of proteins and poly(ADP-ribosylation) and hence activation of nucleoproteins involved in the DNA repair mechanism.

In the nucleus, poly(ADP-ribose)polymerase is activated by binding to breakage points in DNA. The enzyme is involved in activation of the DNA repair mechanism in response to strand breakage caused by radical attack or UV radiation. In cells that have suffered considerable DNA damage, the activation of poly (ADP-ribose) polymerase may deplete intracellular NAD to such an extent that ATP formation is impaired, leading to cell death.

ADP-ribose cyclase catalyzes the formation of cyclic ADP-ribose from NAD, and of nicotinic acid adenine dinucleotide phosphate from NADP (by catalyzing the exchange of nicotinamide for nicotinic acid). Both of these compounds act to raise cytosolic calcium concentrations by releasing calcium from intracellular stores, acting as second messengers in response to nitric oxide, acetylcholine, and other neurotransmitters.

Pellagra: a disease of tryptophan and niacin deficiency

Pellagra became common in Europe when maize was introduced from the New World as a convenient high-yielding dietary staple, and by the late nineteenth century it was widespread throughout southern Europe, north and south Africa, and the southern USA. The proteins of maize are particularly lacking in tryptophan, and as with other cereals little or none of the preformed niacin is biologically available.

Pellagra is characterized by a photosensitive dermatitis, like severe sunburn, typically with a butterfly-like pattern of distribution over the face, affecting all parts of the skin that are exposed to sunlight. Similar skin lesions may also occur in areas not exposed to sunlight, but subject to pressure, such as the knees, elbows, wrists, and ankles. Advanced pellagra is also accompanied by dementia (more correctly a depressive psychosis), and there may be diarrhea. Untreated pellagra is fatal.

The depressive psychosis is superficially similar to schizophrenia and the organic psychoses, but clinically distinguishable by sudden lucid phases that alternate with the most florid psychiatric signs. It is probable that these mental symptoms can be explained by a relative deficit of the essential amino acid tryptophan, and hence reduced synthesis of the neurotransmitter 5-hydroxytryptamine (serotonin), and not to a deficiency of niacin per se.

Additional factors in the etiology of pellagra

Pellagra also occurs in India among people whose dietary staple is jowar (Sorghum vulgare), even though the protein in this cereal contains enough tryptophan to permit adequate synthesis of NAD. Here the problem seems to be the relative excess of leucine in the protein, which can inhibit the synthesis of NAD from tryptophan. It is likely that leucine is a factor in the etiology of pellagra only when the dietary intakes of both tryptophan and niacin are low, a condition that may occur when sorghum is the dietary staple, especially at times of food shortage.

Although the nutritional etiology of pellagra is well established, and tryptophan or niacin will prevent or cure the disease, additional factors, including deficiency of riboflavin or vitamin B_6, both of which are required for synthesis of NAD from tryptophan, may be important when intakes of tryptophan and niacin are only marginally adequate.

During the first half of the twentieth century, of the 87 000 people who died from pellagra in the USA there were twice as many women as men. Reports of individual outbreaks of pellagra, both in the USA and more recently elsewhere, show a similar gender ratio. This may well be the result of inhibition of tryptophan metabolism by estrogen metabolites, and hence reduced synthesis of NAD from tryptophan.

Several bacterial, fungal and environmental toxins activate ADP-ribosyltransferase or poly(ADP-ribose) polymerase, and it is possible that chronic exposure to such toxins will deplete tissue NAD(P) and hence be a contributory factor in the development of pellagra when intakes of tryptophan and niacin are marginal.

Niacin requirements

On the basis of depletion/repletion studies in which the urinary excretion of niacin metabolites was measured after feeding tryptophan or preformed niacin, the average requirement for niacin is 1.3 mg of niacin equivalents/MJ energy expenditure, and reference intakes are based on 1.6 mg/MJ.

Average intakes of tryptophan in Western diets will more than meet requirements without the need for a dietary source of preformed niacin.

Assessment of niacin status

Although the nicotinamide nucleotide coenzymes function in a large number of oxidation and reduction reactions, this cannot be exploited as a means of assessing the state of the body's niacin reserves, because the coenzymes are not firmly attached to their apoenzymes, as are thiamin pyrophosphate, riboflavin, and pyridoxal phosphate, but act as cosubstrates of the reactions, binding to and leaving the enzyme as the reaction proceeds. No specific metabolic lesions associated with NAD(P) depletion have been identified.

The two methods of assessing niacin nutritional status are measurement of the ratio of NAD/NADP in red blood cells and the urinary excretion of niacin metabolites, neither of which is wholly satisfactory.

Niacin toxicity

Nicotinic acid has been used to lower blood triacylglycerol and cholesterol in patients with hyperlipidemia. However, relatively large amounts are required (of the order of 1–6 g/day, compared with reference intakes of 18–20 mg/day). At this level of intake, nicotinic acid causes dilatation of blood vessels and flushing, with skin irritation, itching, and a burning sensation. This effect wears off after a few days.

High intakes of both nicotinic acid and nicotinamide, in excess of 500 mg/day, also cause liver damage, and prolonged use can result in liver failure. This is especially a problem with sustained-release preparations of niacin, which permit a high blood level to be maintained for a relatively long time.

8.9 Vitamin B_6

Apart from a single outbreak in the 1950s, due to overheated infant milk formula, vitamin B_6 deficiency is unknown except under experimental conditions. Nevertheless, there is a considerable body of evidence that marginal status and biochemical deficiency may be relatively widespread in developed countries.

Vitamin B_6 is widely distributed in a variety of foods. However, a considerable proportion of the vitamin in plant foods may be present as glucosides, which are probably not biologically available, although a proportion may be hydrolyzed by intestinal bacteria.

When foods are heated, pyridoxal and pyridoxal phosphate can react with the ε-amino groups of lysine to form a Schiff base (aldimine). This renders both the vitamin B_6 and the lysine biologically unavailable; more importantly, the pyridoxyl-lysine released during digestion is absorbed and has antivitamin B_6 antimetabolic activity. Overall, it is estimated that some 70–80% of dietary vitamin B_6 is available.

Vitamers

The generic descriptor vitamin B_6 includes six vitamers: the alcohol pyridoxine, the aldehyde pyridoxal, the amine pyridoxamine, and their 5'-phosphates. There is some confusion in the older literature, because at one time "pyridoxine," which is now used specifically for the alcohol, was used as a generic descriptor, with "pyridoxol" as the specific name for the alcohol. The vitamers are metabolically interconvertible and, as far as is known, they have equal biological activity; they are all converted in the body to the metabolically active form, pyridoxal phosphate. 4-Pyridoxic acid is a biologically inactive end-product of vitamin B_6 metabolism.

Absorption and metabolism

The phosphorylated vitamers are dephosphorylated by membrane-bound alkaline phosphatase in the intestinal mucosa; pyridoxal, pyridoxamine, and pyridoxine are all absorbed rapidly by passive diffusion. Intestinal mucosal cells have pyridoxine kinase and pyridoxine phosphate oxidase (Figure 8.11), so that there is net accumulation of pyridoxal phosphate by metabolic trapping. Much of the ingested pyridoxine is released into the portal circulation as pyridoxal, after dephosphorylation at the serosal surface. Unlike other B vitamins, there seems to be no limit on the amount of vitamin B_6 that is absorbed.

Most of the absorbed vitamin is taken up by the liver by passive diffusion, followed by metabolic trapping as phosphate esters, which do not cross cell membranes, then oxidation to pyridoxal phosphate. The liver exports both pyridoxal phosphate (bound to albumin) and pyridoxal (which binds to both albumin and hemoglobin). Free pyridoxal remaining in the liver is rapidly oxidized to 4-pyridoxic acid, which is the main excretory product.

Extrahepatic tissues take up pyridoxal and pyridoxal phosphate from the plasma. The phosphate is

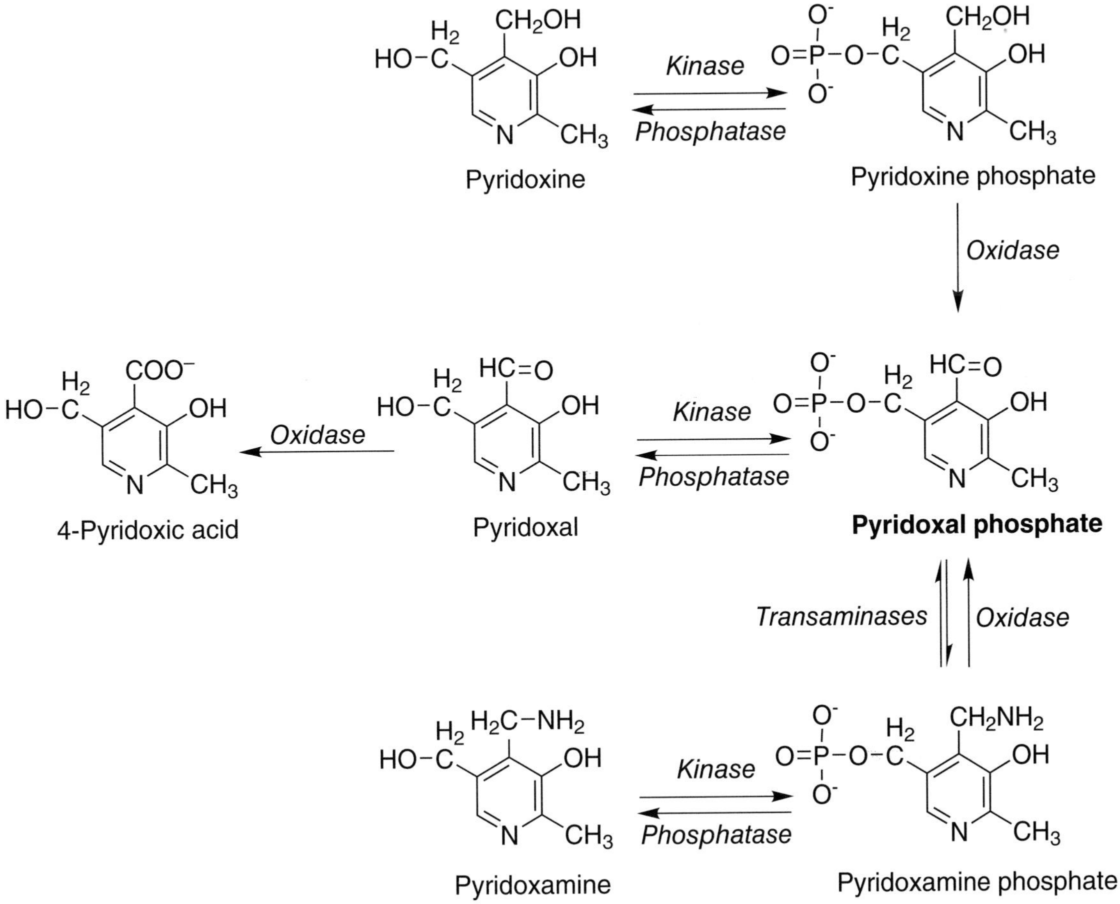

Figure 8.11 Interconversion of the vitamin B_6 vitamers. Pyridoxal kinase (EC 2.7.1.38), pyridoxine phosphate oxidase (EC 1.1.1.65), pyridoxamine phosphate oxidase (EC 1.4.3.5).

hydrolyzed to pyridoxal, which can cross cell membranes, by extracellular alkaline phosphatase, then trapped intracellularly by phosphorylation. Tissue concentrations of pyridoxal phosphate are controlled by the balance between phosphorylation and dephosphorylation.

Some 80% of the body's total vitamin B_6 is pyridoxal phosphate in muscle, mostly associated with glycogen phosphorylase. This does not function as a reserve of the vitamin and is not released from muscle in times of deficiency; it is released into the circulation (as pyridoxal) in starvation, when glycogen reserves are exhausted and there is less requirement for phosphorylase activity. Under these conditions it is available for redistribution to other tissues, and especially the liver and kidneys, to meet the increased need for transamination of amino acids to provide substrates for gluconeogenesis.

Metabolic functions of vitamin B_6

Pyridoxal phosphate is a coenzyme in three main areas of metabolism:

- in a wide variety of reactions of amino acids, especially transamination, in which it functions as the intermediate carrier of the amino group, and decarboxylation to form amines
- as the cofactor of glycogen phosphorylase in muscle and liver, where it is the phosphate group that is catalytically important
- in the regulation of the action of steroid hormones. Pyridoxal phosphate acts to remove the hormone–receptor complex from DNA binding, and so terminate the action of the hormones. In vitamin B_6 deficiency there is increased sensitivity and responsiveness of target tissues to low concentrations of steroid hormones, including estrogens, androgens, cortisol, and vitamin D.

Vitamin B_6 deficiency

Deficiency of vitamin B_6 severe enough to lead to clinical signs is extremely rare, and unequivocal deficiency has only been reported in one outbreak, during the 1950s, when babies were fed on a milk preparation that had been severely overheated during manufacture. Many of the affected infants suffered convulsions, which ceased rapidly following the administration of vitamin B_6.

The cause of the convulsions was severe impairment of the activity of the pyridoxal phosphate-dependent enzyme glutamate decarboxylase, which catalyzes the synthesis of the inhibitory neurotransmitter γ-aminobutyric acid (GABA), together with accumulation of hydroxykynurenine as a result of impaired activity of kynureninase, which is also pyridoxal phosphate dependent.

Moderate vitamin B_6 deficiency results in a number of abnormalities of amino acid metabolism, especially of tryptophan and methionine. In experimental animals, a moderate degree of deficiency leads to increased sensitivity of target tissues to steroid hormone action. This may be important in the development of hormone-dependent cancer of the breast, uterus, and prostate, and may therefore affect the prognosis. Vitamin B_6 supplementation may be a useful adjunct to other therapy in these common cancers; certainly, there is evidence that poor vitamin B_6 nutritional status is associated with a poor prognosis in women with breast cancer.

Vitamin B_6 requirements

Most studies of vitamin B_6 requirements have followed the development of abnormalities of tryptophan and methionine metabolism during depletion and normalization during repletion with graded intakes of the vitamin. Although the tryptophan load test is unreliable as an index of vitamin B_6 nutritional status in field studies, under the controlled conditions of depletion/repletion studies it gives a useful indication of the state of vitamin B_6 nutrition.

Since the major role of vitamin B_6 is in amino acid metabolism it is likely that protein intake will affect vitamin B_6 requirements. Adults maintained on vitamin B_6-deficient diets develop abnormalities of tryptophan and methionine metabolism more quickly, and their blood vitamin B_6 falls more rapidly, when their protein intake is relatively high (80–160 g/day in various studies) than on low protein intakes (30–50 g/day). Similarly, during repletion of deficient subjects, tryptophan and methionine metabolism and blood vitamin B_6 are normalized more rapidly at low than at high levels of protein intake.

From such studies the average requirement for vitamin B_6 is estimated to be 13 µg/g dietary protein, and reference intakes are based on 15–16 µg/g dietary protein.

Requirements of infants

Estimation of the vitamin B_6 requirements of infants presents a problem, and there is a clear need for further research. Human milk, which must be assumed to be adequate for infant nutrition, provides only some 2.5–3 µg of vitamin B_6/g protein. This is very much lower than the requirement for adults, although there is no reason why infants should have a lower requirement.

Based on the body content of 3.7 µg (15 nmol) of vitamin B_6/g body weight, and the rate of weight gain, a minimum requirement for infants over the first 6 months of life is 100 µg/day to establish tissue reserves, and an additional 20% to allow for metabolic turnover. Even if the mother receives daily supplements of 2.5 mg of vitamin B_6 throughout lactation, thus more than doubling her normal intake, the infant's intake ranges from 100 µg/day to 300 µg/day over the first 6 months of life. At 1 month this is only 8.5 µg/g protein, rising to 15 µg/g by 2 months.

Assessment of vitamin B_6 status

Fasting plasma total vitamin B_6 (measured microbiologically), or more specifically pyridoxal phosphate, is widely used as an index of vitamin B_6 nutritional status. Despite the fall in plasma pyridoxal phosphate in pregnancy, which has been widely interpreted as indicating vitamin B_6 depletion or an increased requirement, the plasma concentration of pyridoxal phosphate plus pyridoxal is unchanged. This suggests that determination of plasma pyridoxal phosphate alone may not be a reliable index of vitamin B_6 nutritional status.

About half of the normal dietary intake of vitamin B_6 is excreted as 4-pyridoxic acid. Urinary excretion of 4-pyridoxic acid will largely reflect the recent intake of the vitamin rather than the underlying nutritional status.

Coenzyme saturation of transaminases

The most widely used method of assessing vitamin B_6 status is by the activation of erythrocyte transaminases by pyridoxal phosphate added *in vitro*. An activation coefficient for alanine transaminase >1.25, or for aspartate transaminase >1.8, is considered to indicate deficiency.

The tryptophan load test

The tryptophan load test for vitamin B_6 nutritional status (the ability to metabolize a test dose of tryptophan) is one of the oldest metabolic tests for functional vitamin nutritional status. It was developed as a result of observation of the excretion of an abnormal colored compound, later identified as the tryptophan metabolite xanthurenic acid, in the urine of deficient animals.

Kynureninase (see Figure 8.12) is a pyridoxal phosphate-dependent enzyme, and its activity falls markedly in vitamin B_6 deficiency, at least partly because it undergoes a slow mechanism-dependent inactivation that leaves catalytically inactive pyridoxamine phosphate at the active site of the enzyme. The enzyme can only be reactivated if there is an adequate supply of pyridoxal phosphate. This means that in vitamin B_6 deficiency there is a considerable accumulation of both hydroxykynurenine and kynurenine, sufficient to permit greater metabolic flux than usual through kynurenine transaminase, resulting in increased formation of kynurenic and xanthurenic acids.

Xanthurenic and kynurenic acids, and kynurenine and hydroxykynurenine, are easy to measure in urine, so the tryptophan load test [the ability to metabolize a test dose of 2–5 g (150–380 µmol/kg body weight) of tryptophan] has been widely adopted as a convenient and very sensitive index of vitamin B_6 nutritional status. However, because glucocorticoid hormones increase tryptophan dioxygenase activity, abnormal results of the tryptophan load test must be regarded with caution, and cannot necessarily be interpreted as indicating vitamin B_6 deficiency. Increased entry of tryptophan into the pathway will overwhelm the capacity of kynureninase, leading to increased formation of xanthurenic and kynurenic acids. Similarly, estrogen metabolites inhibit kynureninase, leading to results that have been misinterpreted as vitamin B_6 deficiency.

The methionine load test

The metabolism of methionine includes two pyridoxal phosphate-dependent steps: cystathionine synthetase and cystathionase (see Figure 8.16). Cystathionase activity falls markedly in vitamin B_6 deficiency, and as a result there is an increase in the urinary excretion of homocysteine and cystathionine, both after a loading dose of methionine and under

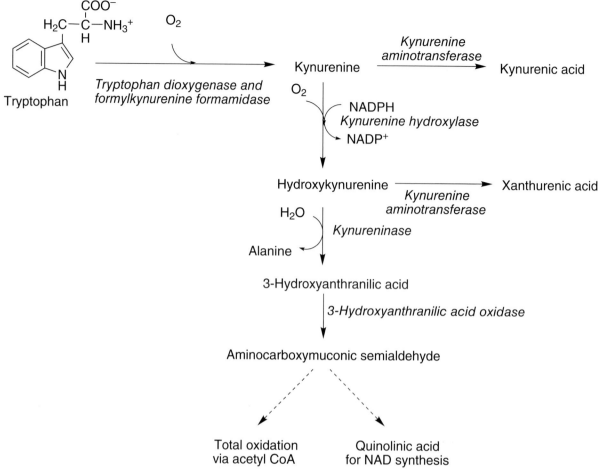

Figure 8.12 Oxidative pathway of tryptophan: the basis of the tryptophan load test. Tryptophan dioxygenase (EC 1.13.11.11), formylkynurenine formamidase (EC 3.5.1.9), kynurenine hydroxylase (EC 1.14.13.9), kynureninase (EC 3.7.1.3).

basal conditions. However, as discussed below, homocysteine metabolism is more affected by folate status than by vitamin B_6 status and, like the tryptophan load test, the methionine load test is probably not reliable as an index of vitamin B_6 status in field studies.

Non-nutritional uses of vitamin B_6

Several studies have suggested that oral contraceptives cause vitamin B_6 deficiency. As a result of this, supplements of vitamin B_6 of 50–100 mg/day, and sometimes higher, have been used to overcome the side-effects of oral contraceptives. Similar supplements have also been recommended for the treatment of the premenstrual syndrome, although there is little evidence of efficacy from placebo-controlled trials.

All of the studies that suggested that oral contraceptives cause vitamin B_6 deficiency used the metabolism of tryptophan as a means of assessing vitamin B_6 nutritional status. When other biochemical markers of status were also assessed, they were not affected by oral contraceptive use. Furthermore, most of these studies were performed using the now obsolete high-dose contraceptive pills.

Oral contraceptives do not cause vitamin B_6 deficiency. The problem is that estrogen metabolites inhibit kynureninase and reduce the activity of kynurenine hydroxylase. This results in the excretion of abnormal amounts of tryptophan metabolites, similar to what is seen in vitamin B_6 deficiency, but for a different reason.

Doses of 50–200 mg of vitamin B_6/day have an antiemetic effect, and the vitamin is widely used, alone or in conjunction with other antiemetics, to minimize the nausea associated with radiotherapy and to treat pregnancy sickness. There is no evidence that vitamin B_6 has any beneficial effect in pregnancy sickness, or that women who suffer from morning sickness have lower vitamin B_6 nutritional status than other pregnant women.

Doses of vitamin B_6 of 100 mg/day have been reported to be beneficial in the treatment of the carpal tunnel syndrome or tenosynovitis. However, most of the reports originate from one centre and there appears to be little independent confirmation of the usefulness of the vitamin in this condition.

Vitamin B_6 toxicity

In experimental animals, doses of vitamin B_6 of 50 mg/kg body weight cause histological damage to dorsal nerve roots, and doses of 200 mg/kg body weight lead to the development of signs of peripheral neuropathy, with ataxia, muscle weakness, and loss of balance. The clinical signs of vitamin B_6 toxicity in animals regress within 3 months after withdrawal of these massive doses, but sensory nerve conduction velocity, which decreases during the development of the neuropathy, does not recover fully.

Sensory neuropathy has been reported in seven patients taking 2–7 g of pyridoxine/day. Although there was some residual damage, withdrawal of these extremely high doses resulted in a considerable recovery of sensory nerve function. Other reports have suggested that intakes as low as 50 mg/day are associated with neurological damage, although these studies were based on patients reporting symptoms rather than objective neurological examination. There have been no reports of nerve damage in children with vitamin B_6-dependent homocystinuria, or other inborn errors of metabolism, who take 200–300 mg/day.

8.10 Vitamin B_{12}

Dietary deficiency of vitamin B_{12} occurs only in strict vegans, since the vitamin is found almost exclusively in animal foods. However, functional deficiency (pernicious anemia, with spinal cord degeneration) as a result of impaired absorption is relatively common, especially in older people with atrophic gastritis.

Structure and vitamers

The structure of vitamin B_{12} is shown in Figure 8.13. The term corrinoid is used as a generic descriptor for cobalt-containing compounds of this general structure that, depending on the substituents in the pyrrole rings, may or may not have vitamin activity. The term "vitamin B_{12}" is used as a generic descriptor for the cobalamins, that is, those corrinoids having the biological activity of the vitamin. Some of the corrinoids that are growth factors for microorganisms not only have no vitamin B_{12} activity, but may be antimetabolites of the vitamin.

Although cyanocobalamin was the first form in which vitamin B_{12} was isolated, it is not an important naturally occurring vitamer, but rather an artifact due to the presence of cyanide in the charcoal used in the extraction procedure. It is more stable to light than the other vitamers, and hence is used in pharmaceutical preparations. Photolysis of cyanocobalamin in solution leads to the formation of aquocobalamin or hydroxocobalamin, depending on pH. Hydroxocobalamin is also used in pharmaceutical preparations, and is better retained after parenteral administration than is cyanocobalamin.

Vitamin B_{12} is found only in foods of animal origin, although it is also formed by bacteria. There are no plant sources of this vitamin. This means that strict vegetarians (vegans), who eat no foods of animal origin, are at risk of developing dietary vitamin B_{12} deficiency, although the small amounts of vitamin B_{12} formed by bacteria on the surface of fruits may be adequate to meet requirements. Preparations of vitamin B_{12} made by bacterial fermentation that are ethically acceptable to vegans are readily available.

There are claims that yeast and some plants (especially some algae) contain vitamin B_{12}. This seems to be incorrect. The problem is that the officially recognized, and legally required, method of determining vitamin B_{12} in food analysis is a microbiological assay using organisms for which vitamin B_{12} is an essential growth factor. However, these organisms can also use some corrinoids that have no vitamin activity. Therefore, analysis reveals the presence of something that appears to be vitamin B_{12}, but in fact is not the active vitamin and is useless in human nutrition. Biologically active vitamin B_{12} has been identified in some preparations of algae, but this seems to be the result

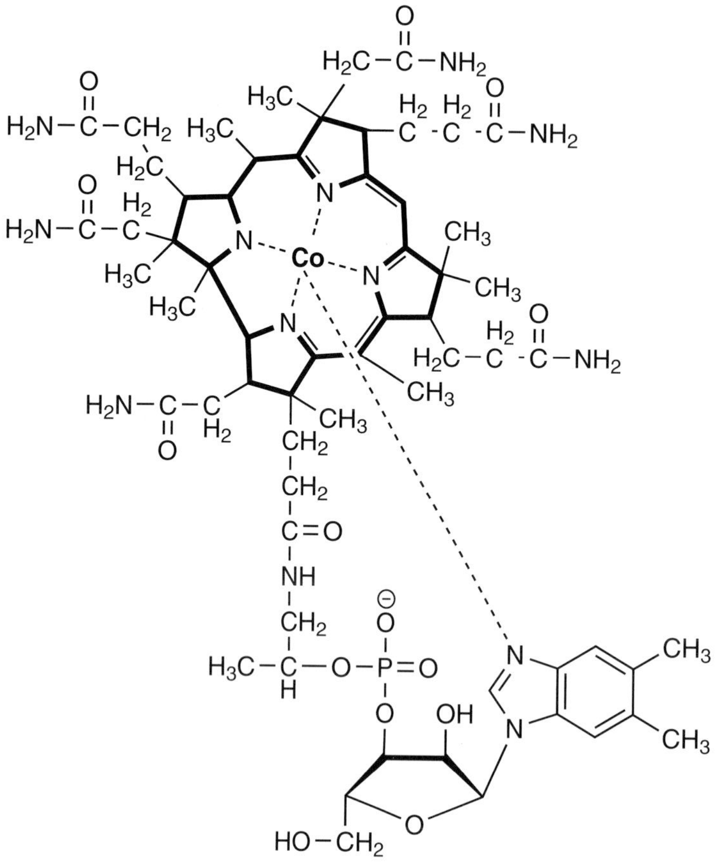

Figure 8.13 Vitamin B_{12}. Four coordination sites on the central cobalt atom are occupied by nitrogen atoms of the ring, and one by the nitrogen of the dimethylbenzimidazole side-chain. The sixth coordination site may be occupied by cyanide (cyanocobalamin), a hydroxyl ion (hydroxocobalamin), water (aquocobalamin), or a methyl group (methylcobalamin).

of bacterial contamination of the lakes where the algae were harvested.

Absorption and metabolism of vitamin B_{12}

Absorption

Very small amounts of vitamin B_{12} can be absorbed by passive diffusion across the intestinal mucosa, but under normal conditions this is insignificant; the major route of vitamin B_{12} absorption is by attachment to a specific binding protein in the intestinal lumen.

This binding protein is intrinsic factor, so called because in the early studies of pernicious anemia it was found that two curative factors were involved: an extrinsic or dietary factor, which is now known to be vitamin B_{12}, and an intrinsic or endogenously produced factor. Intrinsic factor is a small glycoprotein secreted by the parietal cells of the gastric mucosa, which also secrete hydrochloric acid.

Gastric acid and pepsin play a role in vitamin B_{12} nutrition, serving to release the vitamin from protein binding, so making it available. Atrophic gastritis is a relatively common problem of advancing age; in the early stages there is failure of acid secretion but more or less normal secretion of intrinsic factor. This can result in vitamin B_{12} depletion due to failure to release the vitamin from dietary proteins, although the absorption of free vitamin B_{12} (as in supplements or fortified foods) is unaffected. In the stomach, vitamin B_{12} binds to cobalophilin, a binding protein secreted in the saliva.

In the duodenum cobalophilin is hydrolyzed, releasing vitamin B_{12} to bind to intrinsic factor. Pancreatic insufficiency can therefore be a factor in the development of vitamin B_{12} deficiency, since failure to hydrolyze cobalophilin will result in the excretion of cobalophilin-bound vitamin B_{12} rather than transfer to intrinsic factor. Intrinsic factor binds the various vitamin B_{12} vitamers, but not other corrinoids.

Vitamin B_{12} is absorbed from the distal third of the ileum. There are intrinsic factor–vitamin B_{12} binding sites on the brush border of the mucosal cells in this region; neither free intrinsic factor nor free vitamin B_{12} interacts with these receptors.

In plasma, vitamin B_{12} circulates bound to transcobalamin I, which is required for tissue uptake of the vitamin, and transcobalamin II, which seems to be a storage form of the vitamin.

Enterohepatic circulation of vitamin B_{12}

There is a considerable enterohepatic circulation of vitamin B_{12}. A third plasma vitamin B_{12} binding protein, transcobalamin III, is rapidly cleared by the liver, with a plasma half-life of the order of 5 min. This provides a mechanism for returning vitamin B_{12} and its metabolites from peripheral tissues to the liver, as well as for clearance of other corrinoids without vitamin activity, which may arise from either foods or the products of intestinal bacterial action, and be absorbed passively across the lower gut.

These corrinoids are then secreted into the bile, bound to cobalophilins; 3–8 μg (2.25–6 nmol) of vitamin B_{12} may be secreted in the bile each day, about the same as the dietary intake. Like dietary vitamin B_{12} bound to salivary cobalophilin, the biliary cobalophilins are hydrolyzed in the duodenum, and the vitamin binds to intrinsic factor, so permitting reabsorption in the ileum. Although cobalophilins and transcorrin III have low specificity, and will bind a variety of corrinoids, intrinsic factor binds only cobalamins, and so only the biologically active vitamin is reabsorbed.

Metabolic functions of vitamin B_{12}

There are three vitamin B_{12}-dependent enzymes in human tissues: methylmalonyl-CoA mutase (discussed below under methylmalonic aciduria), leucine amino-mutase, and methionine synthetase (discussed in Section 8.11).

Vitamin B_{12} deficiency: pernicious anemia

Vitamin B_{12} deficiency causes pernicious anemia; the release into the bloodstream of immature precursors of red blood cells (megaloblastic anemia). As discussed below, vitamin B_{12} deficiency causes functional folate deficiency; this is what disturbs the rapid multiplication of red blood cells, causing immature precursors to be released into the circulation.

The other clinical feature of vitamin B_{12} deficiency, which is rarely seen in folic acid deficiency, is degeneration of the spinal cord; hence the name "pernicious" for the anemia of vitamin B_{12} deficiency. The spinal cord degeneration is due to a failure of the methylation of one arginine residue in myelin basic protein. About one-third of patients who present with megaloblastic anemia due to vitamin B_{12} deficiency also have spinal cord degeneration, and about one-third of deficient subjects present with neurological signs but no anemia.

The most common cause of pernicious anemia is failure of the absorption of vitamin B_{12}, rather than dietary deficiency. Classical pernicious anemia is due to failure of intrinsic factor secretion, commonly the result of autoimmune disease, with production of antibodies against either the gastric parietal cells or intrinsic factor. Atrophic gastritis with increasing age also leads to progressive failure of vitamin B_{12} absorption.

Dietary deficiency of vitamin B_{12} does occur, rarely, in strict vegetarians (vegans). The rarity of vitamin B_{12} deficiency among people who have no apparent dietary source of the vitamin suggests that bacterial contamination of water and foods with vitamin B_{12}-producing organisms will provide minimally adequate amounts of the vitamin. The fruit bat develops vitamin B_{12} deficiency when fed on washed fruit under laboratory conditions, but in the wild microbial contamination of the outside of the fruit provides an adequate intake of the vitamin.

Vitamin B_{12} requirements

Most estimates of vitamin B_{12} requirements are based on the amounts given parenterally to maintain normal health in patients with pernicious anemia due to a failure of vitamin B_{12} absorption. This overestimates normal requirements, because of the enterohepatic circulation of vitamin B_{12}; in people lacking intrinsic factor, or secreting anti-intrinsic factor antibodies, the vitamin that is excreted in the bile will be lost in the feces, whereas normally it is almost completely reabsorbed.

The total body pool of vitamin B_{12} is of the order of 2.5 mg (1.8 μmol), with a minimum desirable body pool of about 1 mg (0.3 μmol). The daily loss is about 0.1% of the body pool in subjects with normal enterohepatic circulation of the vitamin; on this basis requirements are about 1–2.5 μg/day and reference intakes for adults range between 1.4 μg and 2.0 μg.

Assessment of vitamin B_{12} status

Measurement of plasma concentrations of vitamin B_{12} is the method of choice, and several simple and reliable radioligand binding assays have been developed. A serum concentration of vitamin B_{12} below 110 pmol/l is associated with megaloblastic bone marrow, incipient anemia, and myelin damage. Below 150 pmol/l there are early bone marrow changes, abnormalities of the deoxyuridine monophosphate (dUMP) suppression test (see Section 8.11) and methylmalonic aciduria after a valine load.

The Schilling test for vitamin B_{12} absorption

The absorption of vitamin B_{12} can be determined by the Schilling test. An oral dose of $[^{57}Co]$ or $[^{58}Co]$-vitamin B_{12} is given with a parenteral flushing dose of 1 mg of non-radioactive vitamin to saturate body reserves, and the urinary excretion of radioactivity is followed as an index of absorption of the oral material. Normal subjects excrete 16–45% of the radioactivity over 24 h, whereas patients lacking the intrinsic factor excrete less than 5%.

The test can be repeated, giving the intrinsic factor orally together with the radioactive vitamin B_{12}; if the impaired absorption was due to a simple lack of intrinsic factor, and not to anti-intrinsic factor antibodies in the saliva or gastric juice, then a normal amount of the radioactive material should be absorbed and excreted.

Methylmalonic aciduria

Methylmalonyl-CoA is formed as an intermediate in the catabolism of valine and by the carboxylation of propionyl-CoA arising in the catabolism of isoleucine, cholesterol, and (rare) fatty acids with an odd number of carbon atoms. Normally, it undergoes vitamin B_{12}-dependent rearrangement to succinyl-CoA, catalyzed by methylmalonyl-CoA mutase. Vitamin B_{12} deficiency leads to an accumulation of methylmalonyl-CoA, which is hydrolyzed to methylmalonic acid, which is excreted in the urine. Urinary excretion of methylmalonic acid, especially after a loading dose of valine, provides a means of assessing vitamin B_{12} nutritional status.

8.11 Folic acid

Folic acid functions in the transfer of one-carbon fragments in a wide variety of biosynthetic and cata-bolic reactions; it is therefore metabolically closely related to vitamin B_{12}. Deficiency of either causes megaloblastic anemia, and the hematological effects of vitamin B_{12} deficiency are due to disturbance of folate metabolism.

Apart from liver, the main dietary sources of folate are fruits and vegetables. Although folate is widely distributed in foods, dietary deficiency is not uncommon, and a number of commonly used drugs can cause folate depletion. More importantly, there is good evidence that intakes of folate considerably higher than normal dietary levels reduce the risk of neural tube defects, and, where cereal products are not fortified with folate by law, pregnant women are recommended to take supplements. There is also evidence that high intakes of folate may be effective in reducing plasma homocysteine in subjects genetically at risk of hyperhomocystinemia (some 10–20% of the population), which may reduce the risk of ischemic heart disease and stroke.

Vitamers and dietary equivalence

As shown in Figure 8.14, folic acid consists of a reduced pterin linked to p-aminobenzoic acid, forming pteroic acid. The carboxyl group of the p-aminobenzoic acid moiety is linked by a peptide bond to the α-amino group of glutamate, forming pteroyl-glutamate (PteGlu). The coenzymes may have up to seven additional glutamate residues linked by γ-peptide bonds, forming pteroyldiglutamate (PteGlu$_2$), pteroyltriglutamate (PteGlu$_3$), etc., collectively known as folate or pteroyl polyglutamate conjugates (PteGlu$_n$).

"Folate" is the preferred trivial name for pteroyl-glutamate, although both "folate" and "folic acid" may be used as a generic descriptor to include various polyglutamates. PteGlu$_2$ is sometimes referred to as folic acid diglutamate, PteGlu$_3$ as folic acid triglutamate, and so on.

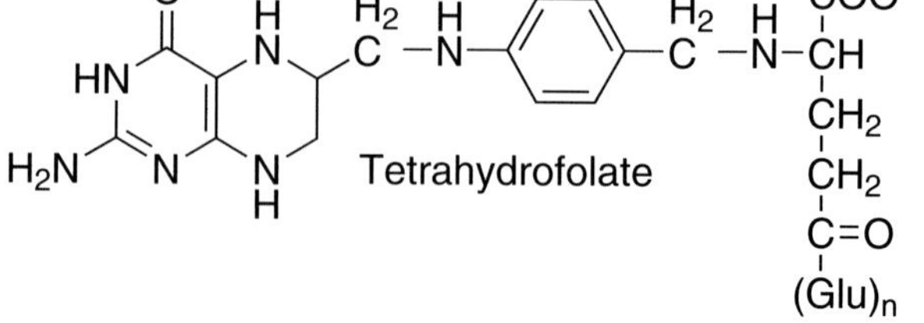

Figure 8.14 Tetrahydrofolate (folic acid).

Tetrahydrofolate can carry one-carbon fragments attached to N-5 (formyl, formimino, or methyl groups), N-10 (formyl), or bridging N-5–N-10 (methylene or methenyl groups). 5-Formyl-tetrahydrofolate is more stable to atmospheric oxidation than is folate, and is therefore commonly used in pharmaceutical preparations; it is also known as folinic acid, and the synthetic (racemic) compound as leucovorin.

The extent to which the different forms of folate can be absorbed varies; on average only about half of the folate in the diet is available, compared with more or less complete availability of the monoglutamate. To permit calculation of folate intakes, the dietary folate equivalent has been defined as 1 μg mixed food folates or 0.6 μg free folic acid. On this basis, total dietary folate equivalents = μg food folate + 1.7 × synthetic (free) folic acid.

Absorption and metabolism of folate

About 80% of dietary folate is as polyglutamates; a variable amount may be substituted with various one-carbon fragments or be present as dihydrofolate derivatives. Folate conjugates are hydrolyzed in the small intestine by conjugase (pteroylpolyglutamate hydrolase), a zinc-dependent enzyme of the pancreatic juice, bile, and mucosal brush border; zinc deficiency can impair folate absorption.

Free folate, released by conjugase action, is absorbed by active transport in the jejunum. The folate in milk is mainly bound to a specific binding protein; the protein–tetrahydrofolate complex is absorbed intact, mainly in the ileum, by a mechanism that is distinct from the active transport system for the absorption of free folate. The biological availability of folate from milk, or of folate from diets to which milk has been added, is considerably greater than that of unbound folate.

Much of the dietary folate undergoes methylation and reduction within the intestinal mucosa, so that what enters the portal bloodstream is largely 5-methyl-tetrahydrofolate. Other substituted and unsubstituted folate monoglutamates, and dihydrofolate, are also absorbed; they are reduced and methylated in the liver, then secreted in the bile. The liver also takes up various folates released by tissues; again, these are reduced, methylated and secreted in the bile.

The total daily enterohepatic circulation of folate is equivalent to about one-third of the dietary intake.

Despite this, there is very little fecal loss of folate; jejunal absorption of methyl-tetrahydrofolate is a very efficient process, and the fecal excretion of some 450 nmol (200 μg) of folates per day represents synthesis by intestinal flora and does not reflect intake to any significant extent.

Tissue uptake of folate

Methyl-tetrahydrofolate circulates bound to albumin, and is available for uptake by extrahepatic tissues, where it is trapped by formation of polyglutamates, which do not cross cell membranes.

The main circulating folate is methyl-tetrahydrofolate, which is a poor substrate for polyglutamylation; demethylation by the action of methionine synthetase (see below) is required for effective metabolic trapping of folate. In vitamin B_{12} deficiency, when methionine synthetase activity is impaired, there will therefore be impairment of the uptake of folate into tissues.

Folate excretion

There is very little urinary loss of folate, only some 5–10 nmol/day. Not only is most folate in plasma bound to proteins (either folate binding protein for unsubstituted folate or albumin for methyl-tetrahydrofolate), and thus protected from glomerular filtration, but the renal brush border has a high concentration of folate binding protein, which acts to reabsorb any filtered in the urine.

The catabolism of folate is largely by cleavage of the C-9–N-10 bond, catalyzed by carboxypeptidase G. The p-aminobenzoic acid moiety is amidated and excreted in the urine as p-acetamidobenzoate and p-acetamidobenzoyl-glutamate; pterin is excreted either unchanged or as a variety of biologically inactive compounds.

Metabolic functions of folate

The metabolic role of folate is as a carrier of one-carbon fragments, both in catabolism and in biosynthetic reactions. These may be carried as formyl, formimino, methyl or methylene residues. The major sources of these one-carbon fragments and their major uses, as well as the interconversions of the substituted folates, are shown in Figure 8.15.

The major point of entry for one-carbon fragments into substituted folates is methylene-tetrahydrofolate, which is formed by the catabolism of glycine, serine,

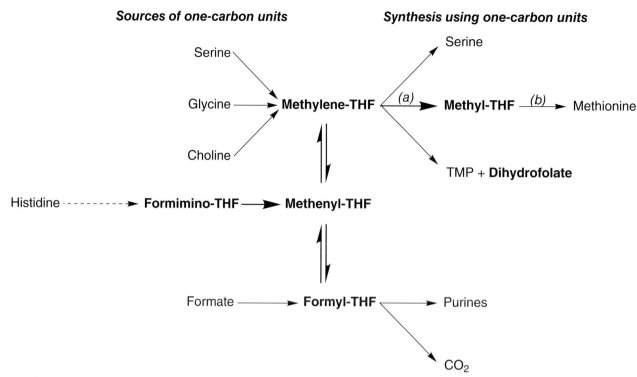

Figure 8.15 Interconversion of the principal one-carbon substituted folates; sources of one-carbon fragments are shown on the left, and pathways in which one-carbon units are used and free tetrahydrofolate is regenerated on the right. (a) Methylene-tetrahydrofolate reductase (EC 1.5.1.20); (b) methionine synthetase (EC 2.1.1.13).

and choline. Serine is the most important source of substituted folates for biosynthetic reactions, and the activity of serine hydroxymethyltransferase is regulated by the state of folate substitution and the availability of folate. The reaction is freely reversible, and under appropriate conditions in liver it functions to form serine from glycine as a substrate for gluconeogenesis.

Methylene-, methenyl-, and 10-formyl-tetrahydrofolates are freely interconvertible. This means that when one-carbon folates are not required for synthetic reactions, the oxidation of formyl-tetrahydrofolate to carbon dioxide and folate provides a means of maintaining an adequate tissue pool of free folate.

By contrast, the reduction of methylene-tetrahydrofolate to methyl-tetrahydrofolate is irreversible, and the only way in which free folate can be formed from methyl-tetrahydrofolate is by the reaction of methionine synthetase (see below).

Thymidylate synthetase and dihydrofolate reductase

The methylation of dUMP to thymidine monophosphate (TMP), catalyzed by thymidylate synthetase, is essential for the synthesis of DNA, although preformed TMP arising from the catabolism of DNA can be reutilized.

The methyl donor for thymidylate synthetase is methylene-tetrahydrofolate; the reaction involves reduction of the one-carbon fragment to a methyl group at the expense of the folate, which is oxidized to dihydrofolate. Dihydrofolate is then reduced to tetrahydrofolate by dihydrofolate reductase.

Thymidylate synthase and dihydrofolate reductase are especially active in tissues with a high rate of cell division, and hence a high rate of DNA replication and a high requirement for thymidylate. Because of this, inhibitors of dihydrofolate reductase have been exploited as anticancer drugs (e.g. methotrexate). Chemotherapy consists of alternating periods of administration of methotrexate to inhibit tumor growth, and folate (normally as 5-formyl-tetrahydrofolate, leucovorin) to replete tissues and avoid folate deficiency; this is known as leucovorin rescue.

Methionine synthetase and the methyl-folate trap

In addition to its role in the synthesis of proteins, methionine, as the S-adenosyl derivative, acts as a methyl donor in a wide variety of biosynthetic reactions. As shown in Figure 8.16, the resultant homocysteine may be either metabolized to yield cysteine or remethylated to yield methionine.

Two enzymes catalyze the methylation of homocysteine to methionine:

- Methionine synthetase is a vitamin B_{12}-dependent enzyme, for which the methyl donor is methyl-tetrahydrofolate.
- Homocysteine methyltransferase utilizes betaine (an intermediate in the catabolism of choline) as the methyl donor, and is not vitamin B_{12} dependent.

Both enzymes are found in most tissues, but only the vitamin B_{12}-dependent methionine synthetase is found in the central nervous system.

The reduction of methylene-tetrahydrofolate to methyl-tetrahydrofolate is irreversible, and the major source of folate for tissues is methyl-tetrahydrofolate. The only metabolic role of methyl-tetrahydrofolate is the methylation of homocysteine to methionine, and

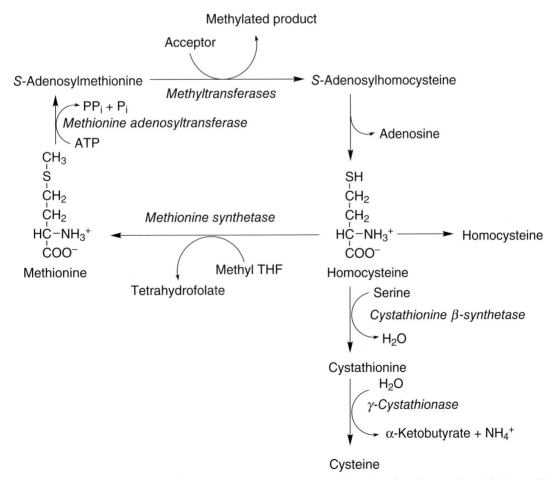

Figure 8.16 Methionine metabolism. Methionine synthetase (EC 2.1.1.13), methionine adenosyltransferase (EC 2.5.1.6), cystathionine synthetase (EC 4.2.1.22), cystathionase (EC 4.4.1.1).

this is the only way in which methyl-tetrahydrofolate can be demethylated to yield free folate in tissues. Methionine synthetase thus provides the link between the physiological functions of folate and vitamin B_{12}. Impairment of methionine synthetase activity in vitamin B_{12} deficiency will result in the accumulation of methyl-tetrahydrofolate, which can neither be utilized for any other one-carbon transfer reactions nor be demethylated to provide free folate.

This functional deficiency of folate is exacerbated by low tissue concentrations of methionine and an accumulation of homocysteine, since the transulfuration pathway to form cysteine from homocysteine is regulated by the availability of cysteine: it is a biosynthetic pathway rather than a pathway for disposal of methionine and homocysteine.

Methylene-tetrahydrofolate reductase and hyperhomocysteinemia

Elevated blood homocysteine is a significant risk factor for atherosclerosis, thrombosis, and hypertension, independent of factors such as dietary lipids and plasma lipoproteins. About 10–15% of the population, and almost 30% of people with ischemic heart disease, have an abnormal variant of methylene-tetrahydrofolate reductase, which is unstable, and loses activity more quickly than normal. As a result, people with the abnormal form of the enzyme have an impaired ability to form methyl-tetrahydrofolate (the main form in which folate is taken up by tissues) and suffer from functional folate deficiency. Therefore, they are unable to remethylate homocysteine to methionine adequately and develop hyperhomocysteinemia.

People with the abnormal variant of methylene-tetrahydrofolate reductase do not develop hyperhomocysteinemia if they have a relatively high intake of folate. This seems to be due to the methylation of folate in the intestinal mucosa during absorption; intestinal mucosal cells have a rapid turnover (some 48 h between proliferation in the crypts and shedding at the tip of the villus), and therefore it is not important that methylene-tetrahydrofolate reductase is less stable than normal, as there is still an adequate activity of the enzyme in the intestinal mucosa to maintain a normal circulating level of methyl-tetrahydrofolate.

This has led to the suggestion that supplements of folate will reduce the incidence of cardiovascular disease. However, a number of intervention trials with folate supplements have shown no reduction in death from myocardial infarction, nor any decrease in all-cause mortality, despite a significant decrease in plasma homocysteine. Similarly, in countries where there has been mandatory enrichment of flour with folate for some years, there is no evidence of reduced mortality from cardiovascular disease. It is possible that elevated plasma homocysteine is not so much a cause of atherosclerosis (although there are good mechanisms to explain why it might be atherogenic) as the result of impaired kidney function due to early atherosclerosis. If this is so, the lowering of plasma homocysteine by increasing folate intake would not be expected to affect the development of atherosclerosis.

Folate in pregnancy

During the 1980s a considerable body of evidence accumulated that spina bifida and other neural tube defects (which occur in about 0.75–1% of pregnancies) were associated with low intakes of folate, and that increased intake during pregnancy might be protective. It is now established that supplements of folate begun periconceptually result in a significant reduction in the incidence of neural tube defects, and it is recommended that intakes be increased by 400 μg/day before conception. (Closure of the neural tube occurs by day 28 of pregnancy, which is before the woman knows she is pregnant.) The studies were conducted using folate monoglutamate and it is unlikely that an equivalent increase in intake could be achieved from unfortified foods. In many countries there is mandatory enrichment of flour with folate, and there has been a 25–50% decrease in the number of infants born with neural tube defects since the introduction of fortification. The true benefit is greater than this, since some affected fetuses abort spontaneously and there are few data on the number of therapeutic terminations of pregnancy for neural tube defects detected by antenatal screening; therefore, supplements are recommended. Where folate enrichment is not mandatory, the advice is that all women who are, or may be about to become, pregnant, should take supplements of 400 μg/day.

Folate and cancer

Much of the regulation and silencing of gene expression that underlies tissue differentiation involves methylation of CpG islands in DNA, and there is evidence that some cancers (and especially colorectal cancer) are associated with under-methylation of CpG islands as a result of low folate status. A number of small studies have suggested that folate supplements may be protective against colorectal cancer, but no results from large-scale randomized controlled trials have yet been reported, and to date there is no evidence of a decrease in colorectal cancer in countries where folate enrichment of flour is mandatory.

Folate deficiency: megaloblastic anemia

Dietary deficiency of folic acid is not uncommon and, as noted above, deficiency of vitamin B_{12} also leads to functional folic acid deficiency. In either case, it is cells that are dividing rapidly, and therefore have a large requirement for thymidine for DNA synthesis, that are most severely affected. These are the cells of the bone marrow that form red blood cells, the cells of the intestinal mucosa and the hair follicles. Clinically, folate deficiency leads to megaloblastic anemia, the release into the circulation of immature precursors of red blood cells.

Megaloblastic anemia is also seen in vitamin B_{12} deficiency, where it is due to functional folate deficiency as a result of trapping folate as methyl-tetrahydrofolate. However, the neurological degeneration of pernicious anemia is rarely seen in folate deficiency, and indeed a high intake of folate can mask the development of megaloblastic anemia in vitamin B_{12} deficiency, so that the presenting sign is irreversible nerve damage.

Folate requirements

Depletion/repletion studies to determine folate requirements using folate monoglutamate suggest a requirement of the order of 80–100 μg (170–220 nmol)/day. The total body pool of folate in adults is some 17 μmol (7.5 mg), with a biological half-life of 101 days. This suggests a minimum requirement for replacement of 37 μg (85 nmol)/day. Studies of the urinary excretion of folate metabolites in subjects maintained on folate-free diets suggest that there is catabolism of some 80 μg (170 nmol) of folate/day.

Because of the problems in determining the biological availability of the various folate polyglutamate conjugates found in foods, reference intakes allow a wide margin of safety, and are based on an allowance of 3 μg (6.8 nmol)/kg body weight.

Assessment of folate status

Measurement of the serum or red blood cell concentration of folate is the method of choice, and several simple and reliable radioligand binding assays have been developed. There are problems involved in radioligand binding assays for folate, and in some centers microbiological determination of plasma or whole blood folates is the preferred technique. Serum folate below 7 nmol/l or erythrocyte folate below 320 nmol/l indicates negative folate balance and early depletion of body reserves. At this stage the first bone marrow changes are detectable.

Histidine metabolism: the formiminoglutamate test

The ability to metabolize a test dose of histidine provides a sensitive functional test of folate nutritional status; formiminoglutamate (FIGLU) is an intermediate in histidine catabolism, and is metabolized by the folate-dependent enzyme formiminoglutamate formiminotransferase. In folate deficiency the activity of this enzyme is impaired, and FIGLU accumulates and is excreted in the urine, especially after a test dose of histidine: the so-called FIGLU test.

Although the FIGLU test depends on folate nutritional status, the metabolism of histidine will also be impaired, and hence a positive result obtained, in vitamin B_{12} deficiency, because of the secondary deficiency of free folate. About 60% of vitamin B_{12}-deficient subjects show increased FIGLU excretion after a histidine load.

The dUMP suppression test

Rapidly dividing cells can either use preformed TMP for DNA synthesis, or synthesize it *de novo* from dUMP. Stimulated lymphocytes incubated with [³H]-TMP will incorporate the label into DNA. In the presence of adequate amounts of methylene-tetrahydrofolate, the addition of dUMP as a substrate for thymidylate synthetase reduces the incorporation of [³H]-TMP as a result of dilution of the pool of labeled material by newly synthesized TMP and inhibition of thymidylate kinase by thymidine triphosphate.

In normal cells the incorporation of [³H]-thymidine into DNA after preincubation with dUMP is 1.4–1.8% of that without preincubation. By contrast, cells that are deficient in folate form little or no thymidine from dUMP, and hence incorporate nearly as much of the [^{3}H]-thymidine after incubation with dUMP as they do without preincubation.

Either a primary deficiency of folic acid or functional deficiency secondary to vitamin B$_{12}$ deficiency will have the same effect. In folate deficiency, addition of any biologically active form of folate, but not vitamin B$_{12}$, will normalize the dUMP suppression of [^{3}H]-thymidine incorporation. In vitamin B$_{12}$ deficiency, addition of vitamin B$_{12}$ or methylene-tetrahydrofolate, but not methyl-tetrahydrofolate, will normalize dUMP suppression.

Drug–nutrient interactions of folate

Several folate antimetabolites are used clinically, as cancer chemotherapy (e.g., methotrexate), and as antibacterial (trimethoprim) and antimalarial (pyrimethamine) agents. Drugs such as trimethoprim and pyrimethamine act by inhibiting dihydrofolate reductase, and they owe their clinical usefulness to a considerably higher affinity for the dihydrofolate reductase of the target organism than the human enzyme; nevertheless, prolonged use can result in folate deficiency.

A number of anticonvulsants used in the treatment of epilepsy, including diphenylhydantoin (phenytoin), and sometimes phenobarbital and primidone, can also cause folate deficiency. Although overt megaloblastic anemia affects only some 0.75% of treated epileptics, there is some degree of macrocytosis in 40%. The megaloblastosis responds to folic acid supplements, but in about 50% of such patients treated with relatively high supplements for 1–3 years there is an increase in the frequency of epileptic attacks.

Folate toxicity

There is some evidence that folate supplements in excess of 400 μg/day may impair zinc absorption. In addition, there are two potential problems that have to be considered when advocating either widespread use of folate supplements or enrichment of foods with folate for protection against neural tube defect and possibly cardiovascular disease and cancer.

- Folate supplements will mask the megaloblastic anemia of vitamin B$_{12}$ deficiency, so that the presenting sign is irreversible nerve damage. This is especially a problem for older people, who may suffer impaired absorption of vitamin B$_{12}$ as a result of atrophic gastritis. This problem might be over-

come by adding vitamin B$_{12}$ to foods as well as folate. Whereas gastric acid is essential for the release of vitamin B$_{12}$ bound to dietary proteins, crystalline vitamin B$_{12}$ used in food enrichment is free to bind to cobalophilin without the need for gastric acid.
- Antagonism between folic acid and the anticonvulsants used in the treatment of epilepsy is part of their mechanism of action; about 2% of the population have (drug-controlled) epilepsy. Relatively large supplements of folic acid (in excess of 1000 μg/day) may antagonize the beneficial effects of some anticonvulsants and may lead to an increase in the frequency of epileptic attacks. If enrichment of a food such as bread with folate is to provide 400 μg/day to those who eat little bread, those who eat a relatively large amount may well have an intake in excess of 1000 μg/day. There is, however, no evidence of a significant problem in countries where enrichment of flour has been mandatory for some years.

8.12 Biotin

Biotin was originally discovered as part of the complex called *bios*, which promoted the growth of yeast and, separately, as vitamin H, the protective or curative factor in "egg white injury," the disease caused in humans and experimental animals being fed diets containing large amounts of uncooked egg white. The structures of biotin, biocytin, and carboxy-biocytin (the active metabolic intermediate) are shown in Figure 8.17.

Biotin is widely distributed in many foods. It is synthesized by intestinal flora, and in balance studies the total output of biotin in urine plus feces is three to six times greater than the intake, reflecting bacterial synthesis. It is not known to what extent this is available to the host.

Absorption and metabolism of biotin

Most biotin in foods is present as biocytin (ε-amino-biotinyllysine), which is released on proteolysis, then hydrolyzed by biotinidase in the pancreatic juice and intestinal mucosal secretions, to yield free biotin. The extent to which bound biotin in foods is biologically available is not known.

Free biotin is absorbed from the small intestine by active transport. Biotin circulates in the bloodstream

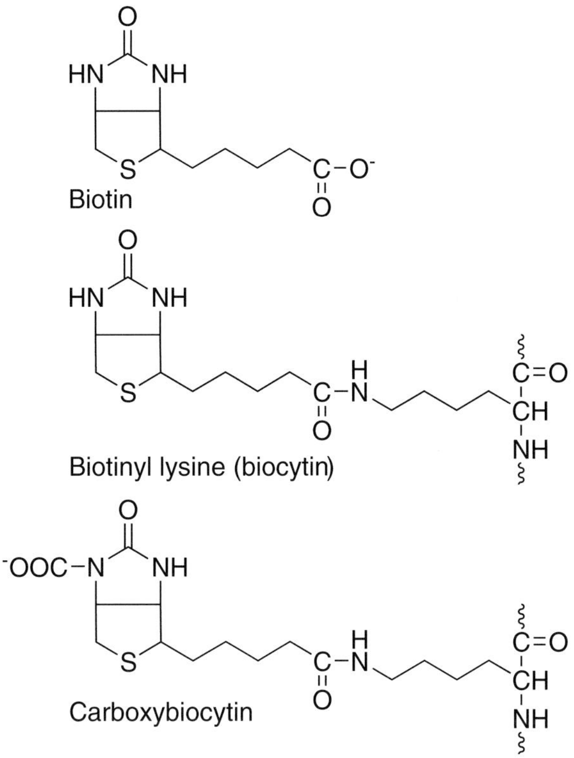

Figure 8.17 Biotin, biotinyl-lysine (biocytin) and the role of biocytin as a carbon dioxide carrier.

both free and bound to a serum glycoprotein that has biotinidase activity, catalyzing the hydrolysis of biocytin.

Biotin enters tissues by a saturable transport system and is then incorporated into biotin-dependent enzymes as the ε-amino-lysine peptide, biocytin. Unlike other B vitamins, where concentrative uptake into tissues can be achieved by facilitated diffusion followed by metabolic trapping, the incorporation of biotin into enzymes is relatively slow, and cannot be considered part of the uptake process. On catabolism of the enzymes, biocytin is hydrolyzed by biotinidase, permitting reutilization.

Metabolic functions of biotin

Biotin functions to transfer carbon dioxide in a small number of carboxylation reactions. The reactive intermediate is 1-*N*-carboxy-biocytin (Figure 8.17), formed from bicarbonate in an ATP-dependent reaction. A single enzyme acts on the apoenzymes of acetyl-CoA carboxylase, pyruvate carboxylase, propi-

onyl-CoA carboxylase, and methylcrotonyl-CoA carboxylase to form the active holoenzymes from (inactive) apoenzymes and free biotin.

Biotin also has a role in the control of the cell cycle, and acts via cell surface receptors to regulate the expression of key enzymes involved in glucose metabolism. In response to mitogenic stimuli there is a considerable increase in the tissue uptake of biotin, much of which is used to biotinylate histones and other nuclear proteins.

Biotin deficiency and requirements

Biotin is widely distributed in foods and deficiency is unknown, except among people maintained for many months on total parenteral nutrition, and a very small number of people who eat large amounts of uncooked egg. Avidin, a protein in egg white, binds biotin extremely tightly and renders it unavailable for absorption. Avidin is denatured by cooking and then loses its ability to bind biotin. The amount of avidin in uncooked egg white is relatively small, and problems of biotin deficiency have only occurred in people eating a dozen or more raw eggs a day, for some years.

The few early reports of human biotin deficiency are all of people who consumed large amounts of uncooked eggs. They developed a fine scaly dermatitis and hair loss (alopecia). Histology of the skin showed an absence of sebaceous glands and atrophy of the hair follicles. Provision of biotin supplements of 200–1000 μg/day resulted in cure of the skin lesions and regrowth of hair, despite continuing the abnormal diet providing large amounts of avidin. There have been no studies of providing modest doses of biotin to such patients, and none in which their high intake of uncooked eggs was not either replaced by an equivalent intake of cooked eggs (in which avidin has been denatured by heat, and the yolks of which are a good source of biotin) or continued unchanged, so there is no information from these case reports of the amounts of biotin required for normal health. More recently, similar signs of biotin deficiency have been observed in patients receiving total parenteral nutrition for prolonged periods after major resection of the gut. The signs resolve following the provision of biotin, but again there have been no studies of the amounts of biotin required; intakes have ranged between 60 μg/day and 200 μg/day.

Glucose metabolism in biotin deficiency

Biotin is the coenzyme for one of the key enzymes of gluconeogenesis, pyruvate carboxylase, and deficiency can lead to fasting hypoglycemia. In addition, biotin acts via cell surface receptors to induce the synthesis of phosphofructokinase and pyruvate kinase (key enzymes of glycolysis), phospho-enolpyruvate carboxykinase (a key enzyme of gluconeogenesis) and glucokinase.

Rather than the expected hypoglycemia, biotin deficiency may sometimes be associated with hyperglycemia as a result of the reduced synthesis of glucokinase. Glucokinase is the high K_m isoenzyme of hexokinase that is responsible for uptake of glucose into the liver for glycogen synthesis when blood concentrations are high. It also acts as the sensor for hyperglycemia in the β-islet cells of the pancreas; metabolism of the increased glucose 6-phosphate formed by glucokinase leads to the secretion of insulin. There is some evidence that biotin supplements can improve glucose tolerance in diabetes.

Lipid metabolism in biotin deficiency

The skin lesions of biotin deficiency are similar to those seen in deficiency of essential fatty acids, and serum linoleic acid is lower than normal in biotin-deficient patients owing to impairment of the elongation of PUFAs as a result of reduced activity of acetyl-CoA carboxylase.

The impairment of lipogenesis also affects the tissue fatty acid composition, with an increase in the proportion of palmitoleic acid, mainly at the expense of stearic acid, apparently as a result of increased fatty acid desaturase activity in biotin deficiency. Although dietary protein and fat intake also affect tissue fatty acid composition, the ratio of palmitoleic to stearic acid may provide a useful index of biotin nutritional status in some circumstances.

Biotin deficiency also results in an increase in the normally small amounts of odd-chain fatty acids (mainly C15:0 and C17:0) in triacylglycerols, phospholipids, and cholesterol esters. This is a result of impaired activity of propionyl-CoA carboxylase, leading to an accumulation of propionyl-CoA, which can be incorporated into lipids in competition with acetyl-CoA.

Safe and adequate levels of intake

There is no evidence on which to estimate requirements for biotin. Average intakes are between 10 μg/day and 200 μg/day. Since dietary deficiency does not occur, such intakes are obviously more than adequate to meet requirements.

8.13 Pantothenic acid

Pantothenic acid (sometimes known as vitamin B_5, and at one time called vitamin B_3) has a central role in energy-yielding metabolism as the functional moiety of coenzyme A (CoA) and in the biosynthesis of fatty acids as the prosthetic group of acyl carrier protein. The structures of pantothenic acid and CoA are shown in Figure 8.18.

Pantothenic acid is widely distributed in all foodstuffs; the name derives from the Greek for "from everywhere," as opposed to other vitamins that were originally isolated from individual especially rich sources. As a result, deficiency has not been unequivocally reported in human beings except in specific depletion studies, most of which have used the antagonist ω-methyl-pantothenic acid.

Absorption, metabolism, and metabolic functions of pantothenic acid

About 85% of dietary pantothenic acid is as CoA and phosphopantetheine. In the intestinal lumen these are hydrolyzed to pantetheine; intestinal mucosal cells have a high pantetheinase activity and rapidly hydrolyze pantetheine to pantothenic acid. The intestinal absorption of pantothenic acid seems to be by simple diffusion and occurs at a constant rate throughout the length of the small intestine; bacterial synthesis may contribute to pantothenic acid nutrition.

The first step in pantothenic acid utilization is phosphorylation. Pantothenate kinase is rate limiting, so that, unlike vitamins that are accumulated by metabolic trapping, there can be significant accumulation of free pantothenic acid in tissues. It is then used for synthesis of CoA and the prosthetic group of acyl carrier protein. Pantothenic acid arising from the turnover of CoA and acyl carrier protein may be either reused or excreted unchanged in the urine.

Coenzyme A and acyl carrier protein

All tissues are capable of forming CoA from pantothenic acid. CoA functions as the carrier of fatty acids, as thioesters, in mitochondrial β-oxidation. The resultant two-carbon fragments, as acetyl-CoA, then undergo oxidation in the citric acid cycle. CoA also functions as a carrier in the transfer of acetyl (and

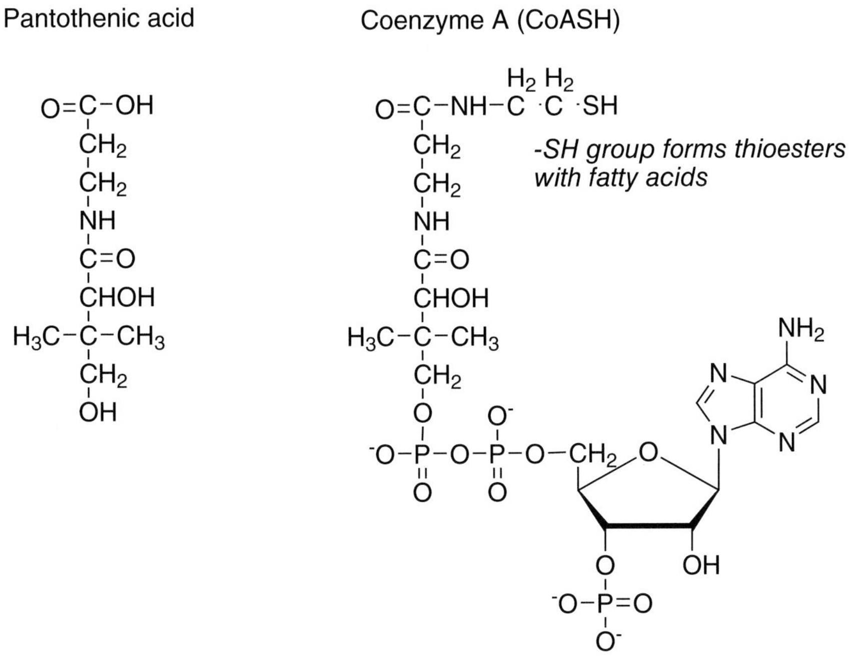

Pantothenic acid   Coenzyme A (CoASH)

$$O=C-OH$$
$$CH_2$$
$$CH_2$$
$$NH$$
$$C=O$$
$$CHOH$$
$$H_3C-C-CH_3$$
$$CH_2$$
$$OH$$

$$O=C-NH-\overset{H_2}{C}\cdot\overset{H_2}{C}\cdot SH$$

-SH group forms thioesters with fatty acids

$$CH_2$$
$$CH_2$$
$$NH$$
$$C=O$$
$$CHOH$$
$$H_3C-C-CH_3$$
$$CH_2$$

Figure 8.18 Pantothenic acid and coenzyme A.

other fatty acyl) moieties in a variety of biosynthetic and catabolic reactions, including:

- cholesterol and steroid hormone synthesis
- long-chain fatty acid synthesis from palmitate and elongation of PUFAs in mitochondria
- acylation of serine, threonine and cysteine residues on proteolipids, and acetylation of neuraminic acid.

Fatty acid synthesis is catalyzed by a cytosolic multi-enzyme complex in which the growing fatty acyl chain is bound by thioester linkage to an enzyme-bound 4′-phosphopantetheine residue, rather than to free CoA, as in β-oxidation. This component of the fatty acid synthetase complex is the acyl carrier protein.

Pantothenic acid deficiency and safe and adequate levels of intake

Prisoners of war in the Far East in the 1940s, who were severely malnourished, showed, among other signs and symptoms of vitamin deficiency diseases, a new condition of paresthesia and severe pain in the feet and toes, which was called the "burning foot syndrome" or nutritional melalgia. Although it was tentatively attributed to pantothenic acid deficiency, no specific trials of pantothenic acid were conducted, rather the subjects were given yeast extract and other rich sources of all vitamins as part of an urgent program of nutritional rehabilitation.

Experimental pantothenic acid depletion, together with the administration of ω-methyl-pantothenic acid, results in the following signs and symptoms after 2–3 weeks:

- neuromotor disorders, including paresthesia of the hands and feet, hyperactive deep tendon reflexes, and muscle weakness. These can be explained by the role of acetyl-CoA in the synthesis of the neurotransmitter acetylcholine, and impaired formation of threonine acyl esters in myelin. Dysmyelination may explain the persistence and recurrence of neurological problems many years after nutritional rehabilitation in people who had suffered from burning foot syndrome
- mental depression, which again may be related to either acetylcholine deficit or impaired myelin synthesis
- gastrointestinal complaints, including severe vomiting and pain, with depressed gastric acid secretion in response to gastrin
- increased insulin sensitivity and a flattened glucose tolerance curve, which may reflect decreased antagonism by glucocorticoids

- decreased serum cholesterol and decreased urinary excretion of 17-ketosteroids, reflecting the impairment of steroidogenesis
- decreased acetylation of *p*-aminobenzoic acid, sulfonamides and other drugs, reflecting reduced availability of acetyl-CoA for these reactions
- increased susceptibility to upper respiratory tract infections.

There is no evidence on which to estimate pantothenic acid requirements. Average intakes are between 3 mg/day and 7 mg/day, and since deficiency does not occur, such intakes are obviously more than adequate to meet requirements.

Non-nutritional uses of pantothenic acid

Blood levels of pantothenic acid have been reported to be low in patients with rheumatoid arthritis; some workers have reported apparently beneficial effects of supplementation, but these reports remain unconfirmed and there are no established pharmacological uses of the vitamin.

Pantothenic acid deficiency in rats leads to a loss of fur color and at one time pantothenic acid was known as the "anti-grey hair factor." There is no evidence that the normal graying of hair with age is related to pantothenic acid nutrition, or that pantothenic acid supplements have any effect on hair color. Its use in shampoo is not based on any evidence of efficacy.

Pantothenic acid has very low toxicity; intakes of up to 10 g/day of calcium pantothenate (compared with a normal dietary intake of 2–7 mg/day) have been given for up to 6 weeks with no apparent ill-effects.

8.14 Vitamin C (ascorbic acid)

Vitamin C is a vitamin for only a limited number of vertebrate species: humans and the other primates, the guinea pig, bats, the passeriform birds, and most fishes. Ascorbate is synthesized as an intermediate in the gulonolactone pathway of glucose metabolism; in those vertebrate species for which it is a vitamin, one enzyme of the pathway, gulonolactone oxidase, is absent.

The vitamin C deficiency disease, scurvy, has been known for many centuries and was described in the Ebers papyrus of 1500 BC and by Hippocrates. The Crusaders are said to have lost more men through scurvy than were killed in battle, while in some of the long voyages of exploration of the fourteenth and fifteenth centuries up to 90% of the crew died from scurvy. Cartier's expedition to Quebec in 1535 was struck by scurvy; the local native Americans taught him to use an infusion of swamp spruce leaves to prevent or cure the condition.

Recognition that scurvy was due to a dietary deficiency came relatively early. James Lind demonstrated in 1757 that orange juice and lemon juice were protective, and Cook kept his crew in good health during his circumnavigation of the globe (1772–1775) by stopping frequently to take on fresh fruit and vegetables. In 1804 the British Navy decreed a daily ration of lemon or lime juice for all ratings, a requirement that was extended to the merchant navy in 1865.

The structure of vitamin C is shown in Figure 8.19; both ascorbic acid and dehydroascorbic acid have vitamin activity. Monodehydroascorbate is a stable radical formed by reaction of ascorbate with reactive oxygen species, and can be reduced back to ascorbate by monodehydroascorbate reductase. Alternatively, 2 mol of monodehydroascorbate can react together to yield 1 mol each of ascorbate and dehydroascorbate. Dehydroascorbate may either be reduced to ascorbate or undergo hydration to diketogulonate and onward metabolism.

Vitamin C is found in fruits and vegetables. Very significant losses occur as vegetables wilt, or when

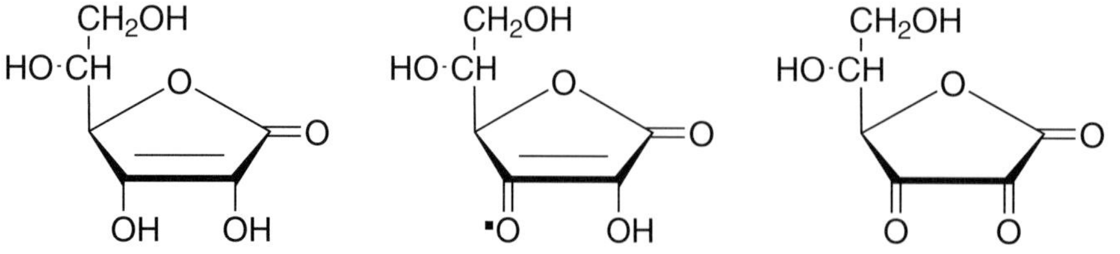

Figure 8.19 Vitamin C (ascorbic acid, monodehydroascorbate and dehydroascorbate).

they are cut, as a result of the release of ascorbate oxidase from the plant tissue. Significant losses of the vitamin also occur in cooking, both through leaching into the cooking water and also atmospheric oxidation, which continues when foods are left to stand before serving.

Absorption and metabolism of vitamin C

There is active transport of the vitamin at the intestinal mucosal brush border membrane. Both ascorbate and dehydroascorbate are absorbed across the buccal mucosa by carrier-mediated passive processes. Intestinal absorption of dehydroascorbate is carrier mediated, followed by reduction to ascorbate before transport across the basolateral membrane.

Some 80–95% of dietary ascorbate is absorbed at usual intakes (up to about 100 mg/day). The fractional absorption of larger amounts of the vitamin is lower, and unabsorbed ascorbate from very high doses is a substrate for intestinal bacterial metabolism, causing gastrointestinal discomfort and diarrhea.

About 70% of blood ascorbate is in plasma and erythrocytes, which do not concentrate the vitamin from plasma. The remainder is in white cells, which have a marked ability to concentrate it.

Both ascorbate and dehydroascorbate circulate in free solution, and also bound to albumin. About 5% of plasma vitamin C is normally dehydroascorbate. Both vitamers are transported into cells by glucose transporters, and concentrations of glucose of the order of those seen in diabetic hyperglycemia inhibit tissue uptake of ascorbate.

There is no specific storage organ for ascorbate; apart from leukocytes (which account for only 10% of total blood ascorbate), the only tissues showing a significant concentration of the vitamin are the adrenal and pituitary glands. Although the concentration of ascorbate in muscle is relatively low, skeletal muscle contains much of the body's pool of 900–1500 mg (5–8.5 mmol).

Diketogulonate arising from dehydroascorbate can undergo metabolism to xylose, thus providing a route for entry into central carbohydrate metabolic pathways via the pentose phosphate pathway. However, oxidation to carbon dioxide is only a minor fate of ascorbate in humans. At usual intakes of the vitamin, less than 1% of the radioactivity from [^{14}C]-ascorbate is recovered as carbon dioxide. Although more $^{14}CO_2$ is recovered from subjects receiving high intakes of the vitamin, this is the result of bacterial metabolism of unabsorbed vitamin in the intestinal lumen.

The fate of the greater part of ascorbic acid is excretion in the urine, either unchanged or as dehydroascorbate and diketogulonate. Both ascorbate and dehydroascorbate are filtered at the glomerulus then reabsorbed. When glomerular filtration of ascorbate and dehydroascorbate exceeds the capacity of the transport systems, at a plasma concentration of ascorbate between 70 and 85 μmol/l, the vitamin is excreted in the urine in amounts proportional to intake.

Metabolic functions of vitamin C

Ascorbic acid has specific roles in two groups of enzymes: the copper-containing hydroxylases and the 2-oxoglutarate-linked iron-containing hydroxylases. It also increases the activity of a number of other enzymes *in vitro*, although this is a non-specific reducing action rather than reflecting any metabolic function of the vitamin. In addition, it has a number of non-enzymic effects due to its action as a reducing agent and oxygen radical quencher.

Copper-containing hydroxylases

Dopamine β-hydroxylase is a copper-containing enzyme involved in the synthesis of the catecholamines norepinephrine (noradrenaline) and epinephrine (adrenaline) from tyrosine in the adrenal medulla and central nervous system. The enzyme contains Cu^+, which is oxidized to Cu^{2+} during the hydroxylation of the substrate; reduction back to Cu^+ specifically requires ascorbate, which is oxidized to monodehydroascorbate.

Some peptide hormones have a carboxy-terminal amide that is hydroxylated on the α-carbon by a copper-containing enzyme, peptidylglycine hydroxylase. The α-hydroxyglycine residue then decomposes non-enzymically to yield the amidated peptide and glyoxylate. The copper prosthetic group is oxidized in the reaction, and, as in dopamine β-hydroxylase, ascorbate is specifically required for reduction back to Cu^+.

Oxoglutarate-linked iron-containing hydroxylases

Several iron-containing hydroxylases share a common reaction mechanism, in which hydroxylation of the substrate is linked to decarboxylation of 2-oxoglutarate. Many of these enzymes are involved in the modification of precursor proteins to yield the final, mature, protein. This is a process of postsynthetic modification of an amino acid residue after it has been incorporated into the protein during synthesis on the ribosome.

- Proline and lysine hydroxylases are required for the postsynthetic modification of procollagen in the formation of mature, insoluble, collagen, and proline hydroxylase is also required for the postsynthetic modification of the precursor proteins of osteocalcin and the C1q component of complement.
- Aspartate β-hydroxylase is required for the postsynthetic modification of the precursor of protein C, the vitamin K-dependent protease that hydrolyzes activated factor V in the blood-clotting cascade.
- Trimethyl-lysine and γ-butyrobetaine hydroxylases are required for the synthesis of carnitine.

Ascorbate is oxidized during the reaction of these enzymes, but not stoichiometrically with the decarboxylation of 2-oxoglutarate and hydroxylation of the substrate. The purified enzyme is active in the absence of ascorbate, but after some 5–10 s (about 15–30 cycles of enzyme action) the rate of reaction begins to fall. At this stage the iron in the catalytic site has been oxidized to Fe^{3+}, which is catalytically inactive; activity is restored only by ascorbate, which reduces it back to Fe^{2+}. The oxidation of Fe^{2+} is the consequence of a side-reaction rather than the main reaction of the enzyme, which explains how 15–30 cycles of enzyme activity can occur before there is significant loss of activity in the absence of ascorbate, and why the consumption of ascorbate is not stoichiometric.

Pro-oxidant and antioxidant roles of ascorbate

Ascorbate can act as a radical-trapping antioxidant, reacting with superoxide and a proton to yield hydrogen peroxide, or with the hydroxy radical to yield water. In each instance the product is the monodehydroascorbate radical. Thus, as well as reducing the tocopheroxyl radical formed by interaction of α-tocopherol in membranes with lipid peroxides, ascorbate acts to trap the oxygen radicals that would otherwise react to form lipid peroxides.

At high concentrations, ascorbate can reduce molecular oxygen to superoxide, being oxidized to

monodehydroascorbate. At physiological concentrations of ascorbate, both Fe^{3+} and Cu^{2+} ions are reduced by ascorbate, yielding monodehydroascorbate. Fe^{2+} and Cu^+ are readily reoxidized by reaction with hydrogen peroxide to yield hydroxide ions and hydroxyl radicals. Cu^+ also reacts with molecular oxygen to yield superoxide. Thus, as well as its antioxidant role, ascorbate has potential pro-oxidant activity. However, because at high levels of intake the vitamin is excreted quantitatively, is it unlikely that tissue concentrations will rise high enough for there to be significant formation of oxygen radicals.

Vitamin C deficiency: scurvy

The vitamin C deficiency disease scurvy was formerly a common problem at the end of winter, when there had been no fresh fruit and vegetables for many months.

Although there is no specific organ for storage of vitamin C in the body, signs of deficiency do not develop in previously adequately nourished subjects until they have been deprived of the vitamin for 4–6 months, by which time plasma and tissue concentrations have fallen considerably. The earliest signs of scurvy in volunteers maintained on a vitamin C-free diet are skin changes, beginning with plugging of hair follicles by horny material, followed by enlargement of the hyperkeratotic follicles, and petechial hemorrhage with significant extravasation of red cells, presumably as a result of the increased fragility of blood capillaries.

At a later stage there is also hemorrhage of the gums, beginning in the interdental papillae and progressing to generalized sponginess and bleeding. This is frequently accompanied by secondary bacterial infection and considerable withdrawal of the gum from the necks of the teeth. As the condition progresses, there is loss of dental cement, and the teeth become loose in the alveolar bone and may be lost.

Wounds show only superficial healing in scurvy, with little or no formation of (collagen-rich) scar tissue, so that healing is delayed and wounds can readily be reopened. The scorbutic scar tissue has only about half the tensile strength of that normally formed.

Advanced scurvy is accompanied by intense pain in the bones, which can be attributed to changes in bone mineralization as a result of abnormal collagen synthesis. Bone formation ceases and the existing bone becomes rarefied, so that the bones fracture with minimal trauma.

The name scurvy is derived from the Italian *scorbutico*, meaning an irritable, neurotic, discontented, whining, and cranky person. The disease is associated with listlessness and general malaise, and sometimes changes in personality and psychomotor performance and a lowering of the general level of arousal. These behavioral effects can be attributed to impaired synthesis of catecholamine neurotransmitters, as a result of low activity of dopamine β-hydroxylase.

Most of the other clinical signs of scurvy can be accounted for by the effects of ascorbate deficiency on collagen synthesis, as a result of impaired proline and lysine hydroxylase activity. Depletion of muscle carnitine, due to impaired activity of trimethyllysine and γ-butyrobetaine hydroxylases, may account for the lassitude and fatigue that precede clinical signs of scurvy.

Anemia in scurvy

Anemia is frequently associated with scurvy, and may be either macrocytic, indicative of folate deficiency, or hypochromic, indicative of iron deficiency.

Folate deficiency may be epiphenomenal, since the major dietary sources of folate are the same as those of ascorbate. However, some patients with clear megaloblastic anemia respond to the administration of vitamin C alone, suggesting that there may be a role of ascorbate in the maintenance of normal pools of reduced folates, although there is no evidence that any of the reactions of folate is ascorbate dependent.

Iron deficiency in scurvy may well be secondary to reduced absorption of inorganic iron and impaired mobilization of tissue iron reserves (see below). At the same time, the hemorrhages of advanced scurvy will cause a significant loss of blood.

There is also evidence that erythrocytes have a shorter half-life than normal in scurvy, possibly as a result of peroxidative damage to membrane lipids owing to impairment of the reduction of tocopheroxyl radical by ascorbate.

Vitamin C requirements

Vitamin C illustrates extremely well how different criteria of adequacy, and different interpretations of experimental data, can lead to different estimates of requirements, and to reference intakes ranging between 30 and 90 mg/day for adults.

The requirement for vitamin C to prevent clinical scurvy is less than 10 mg/day. However, at this level of intake wounds do not heal properly because of the requirement for vitamin C for the synthesis of collagen in connective tissue. An intake of 20 mg/day is required for optimum wound healing. Allowing for individual variation in requirements, this gives a reference intake for adults of 30 mg/day, which was the British recommended daily allowance (RDA) until 1991.

The 1991 British reference nutrient intake (RNI) for vitamin C is based on the level of intake at which the plasma concentration rises sharply, showing that requirements have now been met, tissues are saturated and there is spare vitamin C being transported between tissues, available for excretion. This criterion of adequacy gives an RNI of 40 mg/day for adults.

The alternative approach to determining requirements is to estimate the total body content of vitamin C, then measure the rate at which it is metabolized, by giving a test dose of radioactive vitamin. This is the basis of both the former US RDA of 60 mg/day for adults and the Netherlands RDA of 80 mg/day. Indeed, it also provides an alternative basis for the RNI of 40 mg/day.

The problem lies in deciding what is an appropriate body content of vitamin C. The studies were performed on subjects whose total body vitamin C was estimated to be 1500 mg at the beginning of a depletion study. However, there is no evidence that this is a necessary, or even a desirable, body content of the vitamin. It is simply the body content of the vitamin of a small group of people eating a self-selected diet rich in fruit. There is good evidence that a total body content of 900 mg is more than adequate. It is three times larger than the body content at which the first signs of deficiency are observed, and will protect against the development of any signs of deficiency for several months on a completely vitamin C-free diet.

There is a further problem in interpreting the results. The rate at which vitamin C is metabolized varies with the amount consumed. This means that as the experimental subjects become depleted, so the rate at which they metabolize the vitamin decreases. Thus, calculation of the amount that is required to maintain the body content depends on both the way in which the results obtained during depletion studies are extrapolated to the rate in subjects consuming a normal diet and the amount of vitamin C in that diet.

An intake of 40 mg/day is more than adequate to maintain a total body content of 900 mg of vitamin C (the British RNI). At a higher level of habitual intake, 60 mg/day is adequate to maintain a total body content of 1500 mg (the former US RDA). Making allowances for changes in the rate of metabolism with different levels of intake, and allowing for incomplete absorption of the vitamin gives the Netherlands RDA of 80 mg/day.

The current US reference intake (75 mg for women and 90 mg for men) is based on intakes required to saturate leukocytes with vitamin C.

Assessment of vitamin C status

Urinary excretion and saturation testing
Urinary excretion of ascorbate falls to undetectably low levels in deficiency, and therefore very low excretion will indicate deficiency. However, no guidelines for the interpretation of urinary ascorbate have been established.

It is relatively easy to assess the state of body reserves of vitamin C by measuring the excretion after a test dose. A subject who is saturated will excrete more or less the whole of a test dose of 500 mg of ascorbate over 6 h. A more precise method involves repeating the loading test daily until more or less complete recovery is achieved, thus giving an indication of how depleted the body stores were.

Blood concentrations of ascorbate
The plasma concentration of vitamin C falls relatively rapidly during experimental depletion studies to undetectably low levels within 4 weeks of initiating a vitamin C-free diet, although clinical signs of scurvy may not develop for a further 3–4 months, and tissue concentrations of the vitamin may be as high as 50% of saturation. In field studies and surveys, subjects with plasma ascorbate below 11 μmol/l are considered to be at risk of developing scurvy, and anyone with a plasma concentration below 6 μmol/l would be expected to show clinical signs.

The concentration of ascorbate in leukocytes is correlated with the concentrations in other tissues, and falls more slowly than plasma concentration in depletion studies. The reference range of leukocyte ascorbate is 1.1–2.8 mol/10^6 cells; a significant loss of leukocyte ascorbate coincides with the development of clear clinical signs of scurvy.

Without a differential white cell count, leukocyte ascorbate concentration cannot be considered to give a meaningful reflection of vitamin C status. The different types of leukocyte have different capacities to accumulate ascorbate. This means that a change in the proportion of granulocytes, platelets, and mononuclear leukocytes will result in a change in the total concentration of ascorbate/10^6 cells, although there may well be no change in vitamin nutritional status. Stress, myocardial infarction, infection, burns, and surgical trauma all result in changes in leukocyte distribution, with an increase in the proportion of granulocytes, and hence an apparent change in leukocyte ascorbate. This has been widely misinterpreted to indicate an increased requirement for vitamin C in these conditions.

Possible benefits of high intakes of vitamin C

There is evidence from a variety of studies that high vitamin C status and a high plasma concentration of the vitamin is associated with reduced all-cause mortality.

At intakes above about 100–120 mg/day the body's capacity to metabolize vitamin C is saturated, and any further intake is excreted in the urine unchanged. Therefore, it would not seem justifiable to recommend higher levels of intake. However, in addition to its antioxidant role and its role in reducing the tocopheroxyl radical, and thus sparing vitamin E, vitamin C is important in the absorption of iron, and in preventing the formation of nitrosamines. Both of these actions depend on the presence of the vitamin in the gut together with food, and intakes totaling more than 100 mg/day may be beneficial.

Iron absorption
Inorganic dietary iron is absorbed as Fe^{2+} and not as Fe^{3+}; ascorbic acid in the intestinal lumen will both maintain iron in the reduced state and chelate it, thus increasing the amount absorbed. A dose of 25 mg of vitamin C taken together with a meal increases the absorption of iron by around 65%, while a 1 g dose gives a ninefold increase. This occurs only when ascorbic acid is present together with the test meal; neither intravenous administration of vitamin C nor intake several hours before the test meal has any effect on iron absorption. Optimum iron absorption may

therefore require significantly more than 100 mg of vitamin C/day.

Inhibition of nitrosamine formation

The safety of nitrates and nitrites used in curing meat, a traditional method of preservation, has been questioned because of the formation of nitrosamines by reaction between nitrite and amines naturally present in foods under the acid conditions in the stomach. In experimental animals nitrosamines are potent carcinogens, and some authorities have limited the amounts of these salts that are permitted, although there is no evidence of any hazard to humans from endogenous nitrosamine formation. Ascorbate can prevent the formation of nitrosamines by reacting non-enzymatically with nitrite and other nitrosating reagents, forming NO, NO_2, and N_2. Again, this is an effect of ascorbate present in the stomach at the same time as the dietary nitrites and amines, rather than an effect of vitamin C nutritional status.

Pharmacological uses of vitamin C

Several studies have reported low ascorbate status in patients with advanced cancer, which is perhaps an unsurprising finding in seriously ill patients. With very little experimental evidence, it has been suggested that very high intakes of vitamin C (of the order of 10 g/day or more) may be beneficial in enhancing host resistance to cancer and preventing the development of the acquired immunodeficiency syndrome (AIDS) in people who are human immunodeficiency virus (HIV) positive. In controlled studies with patients matched for age, gender, site and stage of primary tumors and metastases, and previous chemotherapy, there was no beneficial effect of high-dose ascorbic acid in the treatment of advanced cancer.

High doses of vitamin C have been recommended for the prevention and treatment of the common cold, with some evidence that the vitamin reduces the duration of symptoms. However, the evidence from controlled trials is unconvincing.

Toxicity of vitamin C

Regardless of whether or not high intakes of ascorbate have any beneficial effects, large numbers of people habitually take between 1 and 5 g/day of vitamin C supplements (compared with reference intakes of 40–90 mg/day) and some take considerably more.

There is little evidence of significant toxicity from these high intakes. Once the plasma concentration of ascorbate reaches the renal threshold, it is excreted more or less quantitatively with increasing intake, and there is no evidence that higher intakes increase the body pool above about 110 μmol/kg body weight. Unabsorbed ascorbate in the intestinal lumen is a substrate for bacterial fermentation, and may cause diarrhea and intestinal discomfort.

Ascorbate can react non-enzymatically with amino groups in proteins to glycate the proteins, in the same way as occurs in poorly controlled diabetes mellitus, and there is some evidence of increased cardiovascular mortality associated with vitamin C supplements in diabetics.

Up to 5% of the population are at risk from the development of renal oxalate stones. The risk is from both ingested oxalate and that formed endogenously, mainly from the metabolism of glycine. Some reports have suggested that people consuming high intakes of vitamin C excrete more oxalate in the urine. However, no pathway for the formation of oxalate from ascorbate is known, and it seems that the oxalate is formed non-enzymatically under alkaline conditions either in the bladder or after collection, and hence high vitamin C intake is not a risk factor for renal stone formation.

8.15 Perspectives on the future

Current estimates of requirements and reference intakes of vitamins are based on the amounts required to prevent or reverse subtle indices of deficiency, and can thus be considered to be amounts required to prevent deficiency, but possibly not to promote optimum nutritional status and health. There is currently very little evidence on which to base reference intakes above those required to prevent (subtle biochemical) deficiency, but indices of enhanced immune system function and whole-body oxidative stress and other biomarkers may do so in due course.

There are several compounds that have clearly defined functions in the body but can be synthesized in apparently adequate amounts, so that they are not considered to be dietary essentials. These substances have been receiving increasing attention, and these, in addition to other compounds, are likely to continue to stimulate interest and discussion in the future.

Bioflavonoids

The most studied flavonoids are hesperitin and quercitin. Because they are biologically active, they are commonly called bioflavonoids. Most fruits and green leafy vegetables contain relatively large amounts of flavonoids; altogether some 2000 have been identified, and average intakes of flavonoids from a mixed diet are of the order of 1 g/day.

There is no evidence that bioflavonoids are dietary essentials, but they have potentially useful antioxidant actions. Oxidation of flavonoids may serve to protect susceptible nutrients from damage in foods and the intestinal lumen, and they may also act as antioxidants in plasma and tissues. Epidemiological evidence suggests that the intake of flavonoids is inversely correlated with mortality from coronary heart disease.

Carnitine

Carnitine has a central role in the transport of fatty acids across the mitochondrial membrane. It is synthesized in both liver and skeletal muscle by methylation of lysine, followed by two vitamin C-dependent hydroxylations. In experimental animals, deficiency of lysine has little effect on plasma and tissue concentrations, but methionine deficiency can lead to carnitine depletion, and carnitine has a methionine-sparing effect in methionine-deficient animals.

Deficiency of vitamin C may result in impaired synthesis of carnitine in species for which ascorbate is a vitamin.

The administration of the anticonvulsant valproic acid can lead to carnitine depletion. This results in impaired β-oxidation of fatty acids and ketogenesis, and hence a nonketotic hypoglycemia, with elevated plasma nonesterified fatty acids and triacylglycerols. There may also be signs of liver dysfunction, with hyperammonemia and encephalopathy. The administration of carnitine supplements in these conditions has a beneficial effect.

Although carnitine is not generally nutritionally important, it may be required for premature infants, since they have a limited capacity to synthesize it. There is some evidence that full-term infants may also have a greater requirement for carnitine than can be met by endogenous synthesis; infants fed on carnitine-free soya-milk formula have higher plasma concentrations of nonesterified fatty acids and triacylglycerols than those receiving carnitine supplements. Carnitine depletion, with disturbed lipid metabolism, has also been reported in adults maintained for prolonged periods on total parenteral nutrition. There is some evidence that supplements of carnitine may increase the ability of muscle to oxidize fatty acids, and so increase physical work capacity, although other studies have shown no effect.

Choline

Choline is important as a base in phospholipids: both phosphatidylcholine (lecithin) in all cell membranes and sphingomyelin in the nervous system. In addition, acetylcholine is a transmitter in the central and parasympathetic nervous systems and at neuromuscular junctions. There is some evidence that the availability of choline may be limiting for the synthesis of acetylcholine in the central nervous system under some conditions. In animals, deficiency of choline results in fatty infiltration of the liver, apparently as a result of impairment of the export of lipoproteins from hepatocytes; prolonged deficiency may result in cirrhosis. The kidney can also be affected, with tubular necrosis and interstitial hemorrhage, probably as a result of lysosomal membrane disruption.

There is no evidence that choline is a dietary essential for humans, and no condition similar to the effects of choline deficiency in experimental animals has been reported. Since phosphatidylcholine is found in all biological membranes, dietary deficiency is unlikely to occur except when people are maintained on defined diets free from phospholipids. Plasma concentrations fall during long-term total parenteral nutrition, and it is possible that the impaired liver function seen in such patients is partly the result of choline depletion.

Inositol

The main function of inositol is in phospholipids; phosphatidylinositol constitutes some 5–10% of the total membrane phospholipids. In addition to its structural role in membranes, phosphatidylinositol has a major function in the intracellular responses to hormones and neurotransmitters, yielding two intracellular second messengers, inositol trisphosphate, and diacylglycerol.

There is no evidence that inositol is a dietary essential. Infants may have a higher requirement than can be met by endogenous synthesis. Untreated diabetics have high plasma concentrations of free inositol and high urinary excretion of inositol, associated with relatively low intracellular concentrations of inositol, suggesting that elevated plasma glucose may inhibit tissue uptake of inositol. There is some evidence that impaired nerve conduction velocity in diabetic neuropathy in both patients and experimental animals is associated with low intracellular concentrations of inositol, and inositol supplements may improve nerve conduction velocity. However, high intracellular concentrations of inositol also impair nerve conduction velocity, and supplements may have a deleterious effect.

Taurine

Until about 1976 it was assumed that taurine was a metabolic end-product, the only function of which was the conjugation of bile acids. The occurrence of changes in the electrical activity of the retina in children maintained on long-term total parenteral nutrition without added taurine has shown that it has physiological functions, and has raised the question of whether or not it should be regarded as a dietary essential.

Ubiquinone (coenzyme Q, "vitamin Q")

Ubiquinone is one of the electron carriers in mitochondria. Therefore, it has an essential function in all energy-yielding metabolism and may also have a general antioxidant role in membranes. Like vitamin E, it can be anchored in membranes by the hydrophobic tail, with the reactive quinone group at the membrane surface. Ubiquinone is readily synthesized in the body, and there is no evidence that it is a dietary essential, or that supplements serve any useful purpose, although they may have non-specific antioxidant actions and so spare vitamin E.

"Phytoceuticals"

In addition to the compounds with clearly defined metabolic functions discussed above, various compounds naturally present in foods, and especially in foods of plant origin, have potentially beneficial effects, although they are not nutrients. Collectively, they are known as phytoceuticals (substances of plant origin with potential pharmaceutical action) or nutraceuticals. The following compounds are examples of phytoceuticals:

- Many glucosinolates and glycosides either inhibit the enzymes of phase I metabolism of foreign compounds (the reactions that activate many potential carcinogens) or induce the reactions leading to conjugation and excretion of foreign compounds.
- Terpenes that are found in the volatile (essential) oils of herbs and spices are potentially active as lipid-soluble antioxidants, as are many of the carotenoids that are not active as precursors of vitamin A.
- Compounds such as squalene, which are precursors of cholesterol synthesis, may have a hypocholesterolemic action, by reducing the activity of the rate-limiting enzyme of cholesterol synthesis, hydroxymethylglutaryl-CoA reductase.
- Various water-soluble compounds, including polyphenols, anthocyanins, and flavonoids, have antioxidant action.
- Several plants (especially soyabeans) contain compounds with estrogenic action (phytoestrogens) that also have antiestrogenic action and appear to be protective against the development of hormone-dependent cancer of the breast and uterus.

Reference

Horwitt MK. *J Nutr* 1956; **60** (Suppl 1): 1–43.

Further reading

Bender DA. *Nutritional Biochemistry of the Vitamins*, 2nd edn. Cambridge University Press, Cambridge, 2003.

9
Minerals and Trace Elements

JJ (Sean) Strain and Kevin D Cashman

Key messages

- This chapter defines the essential minerals and trace elements.
- It describes the functions and routes of metabolism within the body of each of the minerals and trace elements in turn.
- Dietary requirements and dietary sources are discussed for each mineral.

- Health effects and symptoms of both inadequate and toxic intakes are described.
- Methods of assessing the body status of each mineral and trace element are reviewed.

9.1 Introduction

Essential minerals, including the trace elements, are inorganic elements (see Figure 9.1) that have a physiological function within the body. These must be supplied in the diet (food and fluids) and vary from grams per day for the major (macro) minerals through milligrams to micrograms per day for the trace elements.

It has been proposed that the environment (most probably in the primordial sea around hydrothermal vents) in which living organisms evolved was a primary determinant of which elements became essential for life by providing structural integrity and catalytic ability to the first complex organic molecules. As life evolved from the oceans on to land, a natural selection process may have resulted in some elements becoming relatively more important because of superior catalytic abilities over other elements. In any event, the uneven distribution of elements in a land-based environment meant that efficient homeostatic mechanisms had to be in place to conserve essential elements and to eliminate excesses of essential and nonessential elements. The processes of absorption from the gastrointestinal tract and excretion with body fluids, therefore, are major ways in which the concentration and amount of an element

can be controlled in the body. In addition, storage in inactive sites or in an unreactive form can prevent an element from causing adverse effects in the body, and release from storage can be important in times of dietary insufficiency.

All elements have the potential to cause toxic symptoms, whereas some, the known essential elements in Figure 9.1, have the potential to cause deficiency symptoms. Even so, deficiencies of only four of these inorganic elements are known to be prevalent in human populations. Two of these deficiencies, iodine and iron, are widespread in human populations whereas the other two, zinc and selenium, only occur in some population groups under specially defined conditions. Overt clinical signs of deficiency of any of the other inorganic elements are exceptional in humans and mainly occur secondary to other clinical conditions. Such observations do not preclude the possibility that suboptimum status of the great majority of the elements indicated in Figure 9.1 is important in human nutrition. Indeed, there is an increasing awareness of the potential role of suboptimal as well as supraoptimal nutritional status of minerals and trace elements in the development of degenerative age-related diseases, such as coronary heart disease, cancer, and osteoporosis. Moreover, other elements, which currently have no published dietary recom-

1a	2a	3a	4a	5a	6a	7a	8			1b	2b	3b	4b	5b	6b	7b	8b
1 H																	2 He
3 Li	4 Be											5 B	6 C	7 N	8 O	9 F	10 Ne
11 Na	12 Mg											13 Al	14 Si	15 P	16 S	17 Cl	18 Ar
19 K	20 Ca	21 Sc	22 Ti	23 V	24 Cr	25 Mn	26 Fe	27 Co	28 Ni	29 Cu	30 Zn	31 Ga	32 Ge	33 As	34 Se	35 Br	36 Kr
37 Rb	38 Sr	39 Y	40 Zr	41 Nb	42 Mo	43 Tc	44 Ru	45 Rh	46 Pd	47 Ag	48 Cd	49 In	50 Sn	51 Sb	52 Te	53 I	54 Xe
55 Cs	56 Ba	57 La	72 Hf	73 Ta	74 W	75 Re	76 Os	77 Ir	78 Pt	79 Au	80 Hg	81 Tl	82 Pb	83 Bi	84 Po	85 At	86 Rn
87 Fr	88 Ra	89 Ac	104	105	106												

Lanthanides	58 Ce	59 Pr	60 Nd	61 Pm	62 Sm	63 Eu	64 Gd	65 Tb	66 Dy	67 Ho	68 Er	69 Tm	70 Yb	71 Lu
Actinides	90 Th	91 Pa	92 U	93 Np	94 Pu	95 Am	96 Cm	97 Bk	98 Cf	99 Es	100 Fm	101 Md	102 No	103 Lr

Figure 9.1 The periodic table of the elements. The widely accepted or putative essential elements are encircled.

mendations but are highlighted in Figure 9.1, might prove to be essential for the optimum health and well-being of humans.

Major constraints to the elucidation of the potential roles of minerals and trace elements in the onset of degenerative diseases include difficulties in assessing status, and thereby defining requirements, and myriad interactions among minerals and other nutrient and nonnutrients in the diet. Sometimes, natural experiments of genetic disorders can throw light on the potential roles of minerals in disease processes and these will also be discussed as appropriate in the following sections.

9.2 Calcium

Calcium is a metallic element, fifth in abundance in the Earth's crust, of which it forms more than 3%. Calcium is never found in nature uncombined; it occurs abundantly as chalk, granite, eggshell, seashells, "hard" water, bone, and limestone. The metal is used as a reducing agent in preparing other metals such as thorium, uranium, and zirconium, and is used as a deoxidizer, disulfurizer, or decarburizer for various ferrous and nonferrous alloys. It is also used as an alloying agent for aluminum, beryllium, copper, lead, and magnesium alloys. Calcium was among the first materials known to be essential in the diet. All foods of vegetable origin contain small but useful amounts of calcium. Animals concentrate calcium in milk, and milk and dairy products are the most important food sources of calcium for many human populations.

Absorption, transport, and tissue distribution

The adult human body contains about 1200 g of calcium, which amounts to about 1–2% of body weight. Of this, 99% is found in mineralized tissues, such as bones and teeth, where it is present as calcium phosphate (together with a small component of calcium carbonate), providing rigidity and structure. The remaining 1% is found in blood, extracellular fluid (ECF), muscle, and other tissues.

Calcium is under close homeostatic control, with processes such as absorption, excretion and secretion, and storage in bone being involved in maintaining the concentration of ionized calcium in the plasma within a tightly regulated range. This tight regulation of plasma calcium concentration is achieved through a complex physiological system comprising the interaction of the calcitropic hormones, such as parathyroid hormone (PTH), 1,25-dihydroxycholecalciferol [1,25(OH)$_2$D$_3$] and calcitonin, with specific target tissues (kidney, bone, and intestine) that serve to increase or to decrease the entry of calcium into the extracellular space (plasma) (Figure 9.2). Only in extreme circumstances, such as severe malnutrition or hyperparathyroidism, is the serum ionized calcium concentration below or above the normal range. The secretion of these hormones is governed wholly, or in part, by the plasma concentration of ionized calcium, thus forming a negative feedback system. PTH and 1,25(OH)$_2$D$_3$ are secreted when plasma calcium is low, whereas calcitonin is secreted when plasma calcium is high.

Calcium in food occurs as salts or associated with other dietary constituents in the form of complexes of calcium ions. Calcium must be released in a soluble, and probably ionized, form before it can be absorbed.

Calcium is absorbed in the intestine by two routes, transcellular and paracellular (Figure 9.3). The transcellular route involves active transport of calcium by the mucosal calcium transport protein, calbindin, and is saturable and subject to physiological and nutritional regulation via vitamin D. The paracellular route involves passive calcium transport through the tight junctions between mucosal cells; it is nonsaturable, essentially independent of nutritional and physiological regulation, and concentration dependent. Most calcium absorption in humans occurs in the small intestine, but there is some evidence for a small colonic component. Transcellular calcium absorption responds to calcium needs, as reflected by changes in plasma calcium concentration, by hormone-mediated up- or down-regulation of calbindin in mucosal cells; for example, reduced plasma calcium evokes a PTH-mediated increase in plasma 1,25(OH)$_2$D$_3$, which stimulates increased calbindin synthesis in intestinal mucosal cells.

On average, between 10% and 30% of the calcium is absorbed from a mixed diet by healthy adults.

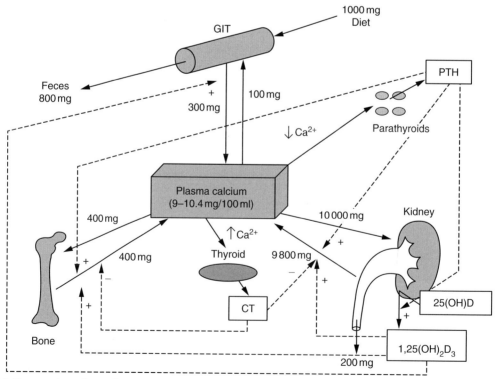

Figure 9.2 Homeostatic regulation of serum calcium, showing the integration of hormone action at the tissue level. CT, calcitonin; PTH, parathyroid hormone; 1,25(OH)$_2$D$_3$, 1,25-dihydroxycholecalciferol (to convert from mg/day to mmol/day multiply by 40).

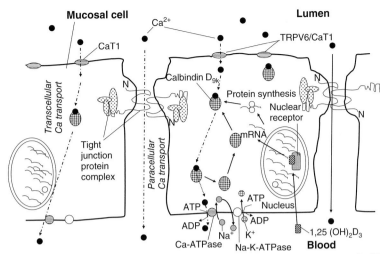

Figure 9.3 Calcium transport across the intestinal mucosal lining: paracellular calcium transport (between mucosal cells) and transcellular calcium transport (across the mucosal cell).

However, the efficiency of intestinal calcium absorption is influenced by a variety of physiological factors (Table 9.1). Calcium absorption may also be influenced by a number of dietary factors (Table 9.1).

Metabolic function and essentiality

Calcium is required for normal growth and development of the skeleton. During skeletal growth and maturation, i.e., until the early twenties in humans, calcium accumulates in the skeleton at an average rate of 150 mg/day. During maturity, the body, and therefore the skeleton, is more or less in calcium equilibrium. From the age of about 50 years in men and from the menopause in women, bone balance becomes negative and bone is lost from all skeletal sites. This bone loss is associated with a marked rise in fracture rates in both sexes, but particularly in women. Adequate calcium intake is critical to achieving optimal peak bone mass (PBM) and modifies the rate of bone loss associated with aging. Extraskeletal calcium (representing around 1% of total body calcium) plays a role in mediating vascular contraction and vasodilatation, muscle contraction, nerve transmission, glandular secretion, and as an important second messenger molecule.

Deficiency symptoms

Because of the small metabolic pool of calcium (less than 0.1% in the ECF compartment) relative to the large skeletal reserve, for all practical purposes meta-

Table 9.1 Factors affecting calcium absorption

Increased absorption	Decreased absorption
Physiological factors	
Vitamin D adequacy	Vitamin D deficiency
Increased mucosal mass	Decreased mucosal mass
Calcium deficiency	Menopause
Phosphorus deficiency	Old age
Pregnancy	Decreased gastric acid (without a meal)
Lactation	Rapid intestinal transit time
Disease states (e.g., hyperparathyroidism, sarcoidosis, idiopathic hypercalciuria)	Disease states (e.g., malabsorption syndrome, celiac disease, Crohn's disease, chronic renal failure, diabetes, hypoparathyroidism, primary biliary cirrhosis)
Dietary factors	
Lactose (in infants)	Phytate
Casein phosphopeptides (?)[a]	Oxalate
Nondigestible oligosaccharides	Large calcium load
Small calcium load	High habitual calcium intake
Low habitual calcium intake	Ingestion without a meal
Ingestion with a meal	

[a] Conflicting data in the literature.

bolic calcium deficiency probably never exists, at least not as a nutritional disorder. An inadequate intake or poor intestinal absorption of calcium causes the circulating ionized calcium concentration to decline acutely, which triggers an increase in PTH synthesis and release. PTH acts on three target organs (either directly or indirectly) to restore the circulating calcium concentration to normal (Figure 9.2). At the kidney, PTH promotes the reabsorption of calcium in the distal tubule. PTH affects the intestine indirectly by stimulating the production of $1,25(OH)_2D_3$ (in the kidney), which, in turn, leads to increased calcium absorption. PTH also induces bone resorption (by signaling osteoclasts), thereby releasing calcium into blood. Owing to the action of PTH and $1,25(OH)_2D_3$ on the target tissues, plasma calcium concentrations are restored within minutes to hours.

If, however, there is a continual inadequate intake or poor intestinal absorption of calcium (e.g., because of vitamin D deficiency), circulating calcium concentration is maintained largely at the expense of skeletal mass, that is, from an increased rate of bone resorption. This PTH-mediated increase in bone resorption is one of several important causes of reduced bone mass and osteoporosis. The cumulative effect of calcium depletion (by whatever mechanism) on the skeleton over many years contributes to the increasing frequency of osteoporotic fractures with age. Prolonged inadequate calcium intake in younger people reduces the rate of accretion of the skeleton and may prevent the attainment of the genetically determined maximal PBM. This may increase the risk of osteoporosis as the PBM in adulthood is predictive of bone mass in later life. Chronic inadequate intake or poor intestinal absorption of calcium may also play some role in the etiologies of hypertension, including pre-eclampsia and colon cancer. Calcium intake may also play a role in body weight regulation; however, this requires further investigation.

Toxicity

The available data on the adverse effects of high calcium intakes in humans are primarily from the intake of calcium from nutrient supplements. The three most widely studied and biologically important are:

- kidney stone formation (nephrolithiasis);
- the syndrome of hypercalcemia and renal insufficiency, with or without alkalosis (referred to historically as milk alkali syndrome associated with peptic ulcer treatments);
- the effect on absorption of other essential minerals, e.g., iron, zinc, magnesium and phosphorus.

Based largely on the data concerning the association of high calcium intakes with hypercalcemia and renal

insufficiency in adults, the US Food and Nutrition Board established a tolerable upper intake level (UL) of calcium of 2500 mg/day for children, adolescents, and adults, as well as pregnant and lactating women.

Genetic diseases

Two rare inborn errors of vitamin D metabolism, vitamin D-dependent rickets types I and II, have an associated hypocalcemia that can impair the bone calcification process. Type I vitamin D-dependent rickets appears to be caused by mutations in the enzyme $25(OH)D_3$-1-α-hydroxylase [responsible for the synthesis of $1,25(OH)_2D_3$ from $25(OH)D_3$], leading to defective activity of this enzyme, whereas type II vitamin D-dependent rickets, which is associated with normal or elevated levels of $1,25(OH)_2D_3$, is thought to result from target tissue resistance to the action of $1,25(OH)_2D_3$. This resistance arises owing to changes in the vitamin D receptor molecule. Daily vitamin D_3 administration seems to be an effective therapy for both disorders.

A hypercalcemia has been noted in familial benign hypercalcemia (types I and III). Type I familial benign hypercalcemia, a renal tubular defect in calcium reabsorption, is caused by a mutation in the gene encoding the calcium-sensing receptor. Type III familial benign hypercalcemia represents a distinct genetic entity. However, the gene(s) responsible for this type of hypocalciuric hypercalcemia is still being mapped.

Assessing status

There is, as yet, no biochemical indicator that reflects calcium nutritional status. Blood calcium concentration, for example, is not a good indicator because it is tightly regulated. There are, however, some potential indicators of nutritional calcium adequacy, which are related to content or metabolism of the skeletal calcium reserve. Measures of bone mass may be used as indicators of body calcium status. These include bone mineral content (BMC, which is the amount of mineral at a particular skeletal site such as the femoral neck, lumbar spine, or total body) and bone mineral density (BMD, which is BMC divided by the area of the scanned region). Besides their relationship to bone mass and strength, BMD and BMC are strong predictors of fracture risk and are thus functional indicators of calcium status. The US Food and Nutrition Board used data relating dietary calcium intake to BMD and BMC to establish the estimates of calcium intake requirements for pregnancy and lactation. Desirable calcium retention, which is based on balance data, may be considered a functional indicator of nutritional adequacy of calcium in population groups and was used by the US Food and Nutrition Board in 1997 to establish recommendations for daily calcium intakes. This is based on the concept that to maximize skeletal strength, optimum bone mass must be attained through a maximum skeletal calcium reserve. Finally, recent research suggests that biochemical markers of bone turnover that predict bone mass changes and fracture risk may be functional indicators of the adequacy of calcium intake. This requires more investigation.

Requirements and dietary sources

Milk and milk products are the most important dietary sources of calcium for most people in Western countries, with cereal products and fruits and vegetables each making a much smaller contribution (Table 9.2). For example, the contribution of dairy products to total calcium intake has been estimated as 73% in the Netherlands, 51–52% in Germany, 51–52% in the USA, 57% in the UK and 44% in Ireland. Tinned fish, such as sardines, are rich sources of calcium but do not make a significant contribution to intake for most people. In general, foods of plant origin are not very rich sources of calcium. However, owing to the level of consumption, foods of plant origin make a significant contribution to total calcium intake. For example, in the USA, cereals contribute about 25–27% of total calcium intake, whereas in the UK cereals contribute about 25% of total calcium intake with about 14% from bread because of calcium fortification of white flour. Increased availability of calcium-fortified foods and dietary supplements containing calcium salts is leading to a wider range of rich dietary sources of calcium. Contributions from nutritional supplements or medicines may be significant for some people. Given the high proportion of body calcium which is present in bone, and the importance of bone as the major reservoir for calcium, development and maintenance of bone is the major determinant of calcium needs. Thus, unlike other nutrients, the requirement for calcium is considered to relate not to the maintenance of the metabolic function of the nutrient but to the maintenance of an optimal reserve and the support of the reserve's function (i.e., bone integrity).

Table 9.2 Calcium and phosphorus contents of some common foods

Food source	Description	Range (mg/100 g) Ca	P
Cheese	Hard, from milk	400–1200	400–810
Cheese	Soft, from milk	60–700	100–790
Sardines	Tinned, in oil	550	520
Milk	Cow's (3.9, 1.6 and 0.1% fat)	115–120	92–94
Yoghurt	Whole milk	160–200	130–170
Ice cream	Dairy	110–130	99–110
Eggs	Chicken, raw, whole	57	200
Chicken, duck, turkey	Raw	9–12	190–200
Beef, mutton, pork	Raw	7–10	60–200
Cod, plaice, whiting	Raw	16–51	170–180
Wheat flour	Whole flour	38	320
Wheat flour	White flour	15–140	110–120
Bread	White	100–180	79–120
Bread	Brown	100–140	150–180
Spinach	Raw	170	45
Watercress	Raw	170	52
Broccoli	Green, raw	56	87
Peas	Processed, canned	33	89
Rice	Raw, white, polished	18–25	54–67
Potatoes	Raw	5–6	34–37
Tofu	Soyabean, steamed, or fried	510–1480	95–270

Data from Holland *et al.* (1995). Reproduced with permission from HMSO.

Calcium requirements, therefore, vary throughout an individual's life, with greater needs during the periods of rapid growth in childhood and adolescence, during pregnancy and lactation, and in later life. There are important genetic and environmental influences of calcium requirements. Genetic influences include such factors as bone architecture and geometry, and responsiveness of bone to hormones that mediate the function of bone as the body's calcium reserve. Environmental influences include factors such as dietary constituents and the degree of mechanical loading imposed on the skeleton in everyday life. Because of their effects on urinary calcium losses, high intakes of both sodium and protein increase dietary calcium requirements.

There is considerable disagreement over human calcium requirements, and this is reflected in the wide variation in estimates of daily calcium requirements made by different expert authorities. For example, expert committees in the USA and the EU have

Table 9.3 Recommended calcium intakes in the USA and UK

UK RNI (1998)[a]		US AI (1997)[b]	
Age group (years)	mg/day	Age group (years)	mg/day
0–1	525	0–0.5	210
1–3	350	0.5–1	270
4–6	450	1–3	500
7–10	550	4–8	800
11–14 M	1000	9–13	1300
15–18 M	1000	14–18	1300
11–14 F	800	19–30	1000
15–18 F	800	31–50	1000
19–50	700	51–70	1200
>50	700	>70	1200
		Pregnancy	
Pregnancy	NI	≤18	1300
		19–50	1000
Lactation	+550	Lactation	
		≤18	1300
		19–50	1000

[a] Reference nutrient intake (RNI); UK Department of Health (1991).
[b] Adequate intake (AI); US Institute of Medicine (1997).
Estimates of Ca requirements refer to both males and females unless stated otherwise.
M, requirements for males; F, requirements for females; NI, no increment.

established very different recommendations for calcium intake (Table 9.3). Much of this divergence arises because of different interpretations of available human calcium balance data. The higher recommendations in the USA derive from defining calcium requirements based on desirable calcium retention estimated from human calcium balance studies, i.e., that which results in the maximum skeletal calcium reserve.

Micronutrient interactions

There is considerable evidence from studies on experimental animals that excessive calcium intake can impair the nutritional status of other nutrients, particularly iron, zinc, and magnesium, but data on humans are not clear. While calcium interacts with magnesium and phosphorus, and reduces their absorption, there is no evidence that high calcium intakes are associated with depletion of the affected nutrient. Calcium inhibits the absorption of iron in a dose-dependent and dose-saturable fashion. However, the available human data fail to show cases of iron deficiency or even decreased iron stores as a result of high calcium intake. There is some evidence that high dietary calcium intakes reduce zinc absorption and

balance in humans and may increase the zinc requirement. Overall, the available data on the interaction of calcium with these nutrients do not show any clinically or functionally significant depletion of the affected nutrient in humans and, in the context of risk assessment, these interactions should probably not be considered adverse effects of calcium. However, such interactions deserve further investigation. It is well established that a deficiency of vitamin D (arising from a lack of exposure to sunlight, inadequate dietary intake, or both) can result in a reduced efficiency of intestinal calcium absorption that, in turn, can lead to a decrease in serum ionized calcium.

9.3 Magnesium

Like calcium, magnesium is an alkaline earth metal. Magnesium is the eighth most abundant element in the Earth's crust. It does not occur uncombined, but is found in large deposits in the form of magnesite, dolomite, and other minerals. The metal is used in flashlight photography, flares, and pyrotechnics. It is one-third lighter than aluminum, and in alloys is essential for airplane and missile construction. Magnesium is used in producing nodular graphite in cast iron and as an additive to conventional propellants. The hydroxide (milk of magnesia), chloride, sulfate (Epsom salts), and citrate are used in medicine.

Magnesium was first shown to be an essential dietary component for rats in 1932 and later for humans. This essentiality is a reflection of the role that magnesium plays in the stabilization of ATP and other molecules. Since then, nutritionists have come to realize that frank magnesium deficiency is rare and that it only occurs in clinical settings as a secondary consequence of another disease. More recently, moderate or marginal deficiency has been proposed as a risk factor for chronic diseases such as osteoporosis, cardiovascular disease, and diabetes. These associations are controversial.

Absorption, transport and tissue distribution

Magnesium is the second most common cation found in the body (about 25 g). It is evenly distributed between the skeleton (50–60% of total) and the soft tissues (40–50% of total). In the skeleton, about one-third of the magnesium is on the surface of bone. This magnesium pool is thought to be exchangeable and thus may serve to maintain serum or soft-tissue magnesium concentrations in times of need. Body magnesium is most closely associated with cells; only 1% of total body magnesium is extracellular. Within the cell, magnesium is found in all of the compartments.

Magnesium homeostasis is maintained by controlling the efficiency of intestinal absorption and magnesium losses through the urine. The latter process is a stronger regulatory control mechanism for magnesium. Magnesium absorption is presumed to occur throughout the small intestine of humans. In normal, healthy individuals, magnesium absorption is between 20% and 70% of magnesium in a meal. Magnesium crosses the intestinal epithelium by three different mechanisms: passive diffusion, solvent drag (i.e., following water movement) and active transport. Regulation of intestinal nutrient absorption is generally thought to occur only for the active component of absorption. The mechanisms controlling intestinal magnesium absorption are unclear at this time. Because of the chemical similarity of magnesium to calcium, scientists have examined whether vitamin D status regulates magnesium absorption. It appears that only large changes in vitamin D status lead to alterations in magnesium absorption. Only limited information is available on the influence of dietary components on magnesium in humans. Phosphate may be an inhibitor of magnesium absorption. Free phosphate may form insoluble salt complexes with magnesium; phosphate groups in phytate may also inhibit magnesium absorption. Fiber-rich foods have been shown to lower magnesium bioavailability. However, it is not clear whether this was an independent effect of fiber or a reflection of the phytate content of these foods. Protein and fructose may enhance magnesium absorption.

As mentioned above, the kidney is the principal organ involved in magnesium homeostasis. The renal handling of magnesium in humans is a filtration–reabsorption process. Approximately 70% of serum magnesium is ultrafiltrable, and the normal healthy kidney reabsorbs about 95% of filtered magnesium. When an individual is fed a low-magnesium diet, renal output of magnesium is reduced. Excessive magnesium loss via urine is a clinical condition contributing to magnesium depletion in patients with renal dysfunction.

Metabolic function and essentiality

Magnesium is essential for a wide range of fundamental cellular reactions, and is involved in at least 300 enzymic steps in intermediary metabolism, for example in the glycolytic cycle converting glucose to pyruvate, in β-oxidation of fatty acids, and in protein synthesis. Magnesium plays an important role in the development and maintenance of bone; about 60% of total body magnesium is present in bone. Magnesium has also been demonstrated to enhance the condensation of chromatin, and given the role of chromosomal condensation in the regulation of gene activity, magnesium depletion could indirectly affect gene transcription.

Deficiency symptoms

Magnesium homeostasis can be maintained over a wide range of intakes in normal, healthy individuals. Thus, magnesium deficiency does not appear to be a problem in healthy people. Frank magnesium deficiency is only seen in humans under two conditions: as a secondary complication of a primary disease state (diseases of cardiovascular and neuromuscular function, endocrine disorders, malabsorption syndromes, muscle wasting) and resulting from rare genetic abnormalities of magnesium homeostasis. Symptoms of frank magnesium deficiency include:

- progressive reduction in plasma magnesium (10–30% below controls) and red blood cell magnesium (slower and less extreme than the fall in plasma magnesium)
- hypocalcemia and hypocalciuria
- hypokalemia resulting from excess potassium excretion and leading to negative potassium balance
- abnormal neuromuscular function.

All of these symptoms are reversible with dietary magnesium repletion. Disrupted calcium metabolism is also evident from the effect of magnesium depletion on serum PTH and $1,25(OH)_2D_3$ concentrations.

Scientists have attempted to demonstrate that suboptimal intake of magnesium [e.g., below the recommended dietary allowance (RDA) but not frank deficiency] is a contributor to the development of chronic maladies such as cardiovascular disease, diabetes mellitus, hypertension, eclampsia and pre-eclampsia, and osteoporosis. However, the results of studies in this area are ambiguous. The lack of positive findings may reflect the lack of sensitive and reliable tools for assessing magnesium status, the failure to account for magnesium intake from water (in dietary studies), or the difficulty in attributing causality to a single nutrient owing to the apparent heterogeneity of causes arising from epidemiological data relating to most chronic diseases. The fact that in 1997 the US RDA for magnesium was raised for most groups is a reflection that nutrition scientists believe that there is a negative consequence to sub-optimal magnesium intake. Additional research is needed to justify this concern.

Toxicity

Magnesium, when ingested as a naturally occurring substance in foods, has not been demonstrated to exert any adverse effects in people with normal renal function. However, adverse effects of excess magnesium intake (e.g., diarrhea, nausea, abdominal cramping) have been observed with intakes from nonfood sources such as various magnesium salts used for pharmacological purposes. For this reason the US Food and Nutrition Board established the tolerable UL for adolescents and adults as 350 mg of nonfood magnesium.

Genetic diseases

Several disease states are associated with magnesium deficiency, some of which have genetic roots, for example hypomagnesemia with secondary hypocalcemia, primary hypomagnesemia with hypercalciuria, renal hypomagnesemia 2, Bartter's syndrome, and Gitelman's syndrome.

Primary hypomagnesemia with hypercalciuria is caused by a mutation in the paracellin-1 (*PCLN1*) gene on chromosome 3. *PCLN1* is a component of the tight junction complex in nephrons and, therefore, has a role in renal magnesium ion reabsorption. Hypomagnesemia with secondary hypocalcemia is an autosomal recessive disorder and is determined by a mutation in a gene located on 9q12–q22.2.

Renal hypomagnesemia 2 is believed to be due to an autosomal dominant isolated renal magnesium loss, which is caused by misrouting of the $Na^+/K^{(+)}$-ATPase gamma-subunit. This small, type I membrane protein is localized on the basolateral membranes of nephron epithelial cells and is expressed in the distal convoluted tubule, the main site of active renal magnesium reabsorption.

It has been proposed that Bartter's syndrome is a heterogeneous entity with at least two subsets, Gitelman's syndrome and "true" Bartter's syndrome. True Bartter's syndrome, a hypokalemic alkalosis with hypercalciuria, is caused by mutation in the NaK_2Cl cotransporter gene *SLC12A1* on chromosome 15. Bartter's syndrome is also caused by mutations in the $K^{(+)}$ channel gene *ROMK* on chromosome 11. Gitelman's syndrome, a hypokalemic alkalosis with hypocalciuria and hypomagnesemia, is caused by mutations in the thiazibesensitive NaCl cotransporter gene on 16q13.

Assessing status

Estimating magnesium requirements and establishing magnesium–disease relationships depend on accurate and specific indicators of magnesium status. Several such indicators have been described. All of these are based on measurement of the magnesium content in various body pools. Analysis of total magnesium in serum is often used as an indicator of magnesium status, although only about 1% of total body magnesium is present in ECF. It has been suggested that the concentration of ionized magnesium in serum may be a more reliable and relevant determinant of magnesium deficiency. In addition, intracellular magnesium concentration (usually measured in accessible tissues such as erythrocytes and lymphocytes) provides a more accurate assessment of body magnesium status than does the concentration of magnesium in serum. The dietary balance approach is considered to be the best available method for estimating magnesium requirements. Although this method is a powerful research tool for the study of magnesium homeostasis, it is time, resource, and labor intensive, and these limit its application to large populations. None of the currently available procedures is perfect for all circumstances.

Requirements and dietary sources

In 1997, the US RDA [the nutrient intake value that is sufficient to meet the requirement of nearly all (97–98%) individuals in a life-stage and sex group] for magnesium was revised upwards for most groups. The current RDA for adult women is now 320 mg/day and for adult men is 420 mg/day. An additional value is now part of the US Food and Nutrition Board's dietary reference intakes, the estimated average requirement (EAR; the nutrient intake value that is estimated to meet the requirement of 50% of the individuals in a life-stage and sex group). This estimate was set to 265 and 350 mg/day for adult women and men, respectively. This value is similar to the mean magnesium intake reported for women and men in the USA (228 and 323 mg/day). Collectively, these data suggest that most Americans are not consuming enough magnesium in their diet and this also appears to be the case for several European populations. However, while the public health relevance of this observation is currently being debated, the fact that there is not a universally accepted reliable magnesium status assessment tool makes it difficult to determine the actual consequence of this apparent low intake.

For those who want to increase their magnesium intake, a number of high magnesium foods and dietary practices will lead to adequate intake. Foods with a high magnesium content include whole grains, legumes, green leafy vegetables, and tofu; meat, fruits, and dairy products have an intermediate magnesium content (Table 9.4). The poorest sources of magnesium are refined foods. Although high levels of calcium, phosphate, or fiber may lead to reduced bioavailability of magnesium, differences in bioavailability of magnesium from various food sources does not

Table 9.4 Magnesium content of some common foods

Food source	Description	Mg content (mg/100 g)
Beef	Lean (from six different cuts)	20
Lamb	Lean (from six different cuts)	24
Pork	Lean (from three different cuts)	22
Chicken	Raw, meat only	25
Cod, plaice, whiting	Raw	22–28
Eggs	Chicken, whole, raw	12
Cheese	Soft and hard varieties	8–45
Pulses	Raw	17–250
Wheat flour	Whole flour	120
Wheat flour	White flour	20–31
Milk	Cow's (3.9, 1.6 and 0.1% fat)	11–12
Yoghurt	Whole milk	19
Tofu	Soyabean, steamed	23–59
Green leafy vegetables	Raw	8–34
Rice	Raw, white, polished	32
Potatoes	Raw	14–17

Data from Holland *et al.* (1995). Reproduced with permission from HMSO.

appear to be a significant barrier to achieving adequate magnesium status. Thus, the current recommendations for a healthy diet based on the food pyramid are consistent with the goals of reaching the US RDA for magnesium.

Micronutrient interactions

As mentioned above, phosphorus as phosphate, especially in phytate, may decrease intestinal magnesium absorption. In general, calcium intake in the usual dietary range does not affect magnesium absorption, but calcium intakes in excess of 2.6 g have been reported to reduce magnesium balance. Magnesium intake in the usual dietary range does not appear to alter calcium balance.

9.4 Phosphorus

Phosphorus is never found free in nature, but is widely distributed in combination with minerals. Phosphate rock, which contains the mineral apatite, an impure tricalcium phosphate, is an important source of the element. Phosphorus is most commonly found in nature in its pentavalent form in combination with oxygen as phosphate (PO_4^{3-}). Phosphorus (as phosphate) is an essential constituent of all known protoplasm and is uniform across most plant and animal tissues. A practical consequence is that, as organisms consume other organisms lower in the food chain (whether animal or plant), they automatically obtain their phosphorus.

Absorption, transport, and tissue distribution

Phosphorus makes up about 0.65–1.1% of the adult body (~600 g). In the adult body 85% of phosphorus is in bone and the remaining 15% is distributed in soft tissues. Total phosphorus concentration in whole blood is 13 mmol/l, most of which is in the phospholipids of erythrocytes and plasma lipoproteins, with approximately 1 mmol/l present as inorganic phosphate. This inorganic component, while constituting only a minute percentage of body phosphorus (<0.1%), is of critical importance. In adults, this component makes up about 15 mmol in total and is located mainly in the blood and ECF. It is into the inorganic compartment that phosphate is inserted on absorption from the diet and resorption from bone, and from this compartment that most urinary phosphorus and hydroxyapatite mineral phosphorus are derived (Figure 9.4). This compartment is also the primary source from which the cells of all tissues derive both structural and high-energy phosphate.

Food phosphorus is a mixture of inorganic and organic forms. Intestinal phosphatases hydrolyze the organic forms contained in ingested protoplasm and, thus, most phosphorus absorption occurs as inorganic phosphate. On a mixed diet, absorption of total phosphorus ranges from 55% to 70% in adults. There is no evidence that this absorption varies with dietary intake. Furthermore, there appears to be no apparent adaptive mechanism that improves phosphorus absorption at low intakes. This situation is in sharp contrast to calcium, for which absorption efficiency increases as dietary intake decreases and for which adaptive mechanisms exist that improve absorption still further at habitual low intakes. While a portion of phosphorus absorption is by way of a saturable, active transport facilitated by $1,25(OH)_2D_3$ the fact that fractional phosphorus absorption is virtually constant across a broad range of intakes suggests that the bulk of phosphorus absorption occurs by passive, concentration-dependent processes. Phosphorus absorption is reduced by ingestion of aluminum-containing antacids and by pharmacological doses of calcium carbonate. There is, however, no significant interference with phosphorus absorption by calcium at intakes within the typical adult range. Excretion of endogenous phosphorus is mainly through the kidneys. Inorganic serum phosphate is filtered at the glomerulus and reabsorbed in the proximal tubule. In the healthy adult, urine phosphorus is essentially equal to absorbed dietary phosphorus, minus small amounts of phosphorus lost in shed cells of skin and intestinal mucosa.

Metabolic function and essentiality

Structurally, phosphorus occurs as hydroxyapatite in calcified tissues and as phospholipids, which are a major component of most biological membranes, and as nucleotides and nucleic acid. Other functional roles of phosphorus include:

- buffering of acid or alkali excesses, hence helping to maintain normal pH
- the temporary storage and transfer of the energy derived from metabolic fuels

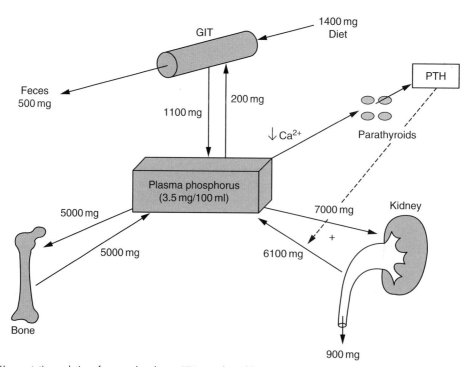

Figure 9.4 Homeostatic regulation of serum phosphorus. PTH, parathyroid hormone.

- by phosphorylation, and hence activation of many catalytic proteins.

As phosphorus is not irreversibly consumed in these processes and can be recycled indefinitely, the actual functions of dietary phosphorus are first to support tissue growth (either during individual development or through pregnancy and lactation), and second to replace excretory and dermal levels. In both processes, it is necessary to maintain a normal level of inorganic phosphate in the ECF, which would otherwise be depleted of phosphorus by growth and excretion.

Deficiency symptoms

Inadequate phosphorus intake is expressed as hypophosphatemia. Only limited quantities of phosphate are stored within cells, and most tissues depend on ECF inorganic phosphate for their metabolic phosphate. When ECF inorganic phosphate levels are low, cellular dysfunction follows. At a whole organism level, the effects of hypophosphatemia include anorexia, anemia, muscle weakness, bone pain, rickets and osteomalacia, general debility, increased susceptibility to infection, paresthesia, ataxia, confusion, and even death. The skeleton will exhibit either rickets in children or osteomalacia in adults. In both groups, the disorder consists of a failure to mineralize forming growth plate cartilage or bone matrix, together with impairment of chrondroblast and osteoblast function. These severe manifestations are usually confined to situations in which ECF phosphate falls below approximately 0.3 mmol/l. Phosphorus is so ubiquitous in various foods that near total starvation is required to produce dietary phosphorus deficiency.

Toxicity

Serum inorganic phosphate rises as total phosphorus intake increases. Excess phosphorus intake from any source is expressed as hyperphosphatemia and, essentially, all the adverse effects of phosphorus excess are owing to the elevated inorganic phosphate in the ECF. The principal effects that have been attributed to hyperphosphatemia are:

- adjustments in the hormonal control system regulating the calcium economy
- ectopic (metastatic) calcification, particularly of the kidney
- in some animal models, increased porosity of the skeleton

- a suggestion that high phosphorus intakes could decrease calcium absorption by complexing calcium in the chyme.

Concern about high phosphorus intake has been raised in recent years because of a probable population level increase in phosphorus intake through such sources as cola beverages and food phosphate additives.

Genetic diseases

Several disease states are associated with phosphorus deficiency, some of which have genetic roots, for example X-linked hypophosphatemia, hypophosphatemic bone disease, and Fanconi's syndrome.

X-linked hypophosphatemia is, as the name implies, inherited as an X-linked dominant trait with the mutant gene located in Xp22.2–p.22.1. The classical triad, fully expressed in hemizygous male patients, consists of:

- hypophosphatemia
- lower limb deformities
- stunted growth rate.

Although low serum phosphate is evident early after birth, it is only at the time of weight bearing that leg deformities and progressive departure from the normal growth rate become sufficiently striking to attract attention and make parents seek medical opinion. It is generally accepted that hypophosphatemia is the consequence of a primary inborn error of phosphate transport, probably located in the proximal nephron.

Hypophosphatemic bone disease is characterized clinically by modest shortening of stature, bowing of the lower limbs, and nonrachitic bone changes (somewhat resembling metaphyseal chondrodysplasia) and biochemically by hypophosphatemia. Although a defect in renal transport of phosphate was demonstrated, the defect appeared to be different from that of X-linked hypophosphatemia.

Fanconi's syndrome is an autosomal dominant disorder. It is characterized by lactic aciduria and tubular proteinuria in childhood, with glycosuria and aminoaciduria developing in the second decade and osteomalacia from the start of the fourth decade. Glomerular function deteriorates slowly but is compatible with a normal lifespan. There has been reported linkage of the disorder to chromosome 15q15.3.

Assessing status, requirements and dietary sources

Previously, dietary phosphorus recommendations have been tied to those for calcium, usually on an equimass or equimolar basis, and this approach was used in the USA, EU, and UK in establishing recommended dietary allowances, population reference intakes, and reference nutrient intakes, respectively, for phosphorus. However, in 1997 the US Food and Nutrition Board suggested that a calcium–phosphorus concept of defining phosphorus requirements is of severely limited value, in that there is little merit in having the ratio "correct" if the absolute quantities of both nutrients are insufficient to support optimal growth. Therefore, because the phosphorus intake directly affects serum inorganic phosphate, and because both hypophosphatemia and hyperphosphatemia directly result in dysfunction or disease, the US Food and Nutrition Board considered that the most logical indicator of nutritional adequacy of phosphorus intake in adults is inorganic phosphate. If serum inorganic phosphate is above the lower limits of normal for age, the phosphorus intake may be considered adequate to meet cellular and bone formation needs of healthy individuals. Current US RDAs for phosphorus are infants 100 mg (first 6 months), 275 mg (7–12 months), children 460 mg (1–3 years), 500 mg (4–8 years), 1250 mg (9–18 years), adults 700 mg, pregnant women 1250 mg (<18 years), 700 mg (19–50 years), and lactating women 1250 mg (<18 years), 700 mg (19–50 years).

Phosphates are found in foods as naturally occurring components of biological molecules and as food additives in the form of various phosphate salts. The phosphorus density of cow's milk and other dairy produce is higher than that of most other foods in a typical diet (Table 9.2). The same is true for diets high in colas and a few other soft drinks that use phosphoric acid as an acidulant.

Micronutrient interactions

It has been reported that intakes of polyphosphates, such as are found in food additives, can interfere with the absorption of iron, copper, and zinc.

9.5 Sodium and chloride

Sodium is the sixth most abundant element in the Earth's crust and salt (sodium chloride) makes up about 80% of the dissolved matter in seawater. Although there is a wide variety of sodium salts, many of which are used as additives in food processing (e.g., sodium nitrate and monosodium glutamate), sodium chloride is the major source of sodium in foods. As sodium and chloride intakes in humans are so closely matched, both will be considered together in this text.

Salt was of major importance in early civilizations and in prehistory. Humans have special taste and salt appetite systems, which led to special culinary uses for salt and made it a much sought-after commodity. Nowadays, salt is still used widely to modify flavor, to alter the texture and consistency of food, and to control microbial growth (Table 9.5).

Absorption, transport and tissue distribution

Sodium is the major extracellular electrolyte and exists as the fully water-soluble cation. Chloride is also mainly found in ECF and is fully water soluble as the chloride anion. Both ions are readily absorbed from the digestive tract. Glucose and anions such as citrate, propionates, and bicarbonate enhance the uptake of sodium. The "average" 70 kg male has about 90 g of sodium with up to 75% contained in the mineral apatite of bone. Plasma sodium is tightly regulated through a hormone system, which also regulates water balance, pH, and osmotic pressure.

Table 9.5 Sodium-containing additives used in food processing

Additive	Use
Sodium citrate	Flavoring, preservative
Sodium chloride	Flavoring, texture, preservative
Sodium nitrate	Preservative, color fixative
Sodium nitrite	Preservative, color fixative
Sodium tripoliphosphate	Binder
Sodium benzoate	Preservative
Sodium eritrobate	Antioxidant
Sodium propionate	Preservative
Monosodium glutamate	Flavor enhancer
Sodium aluminosilicate	Anticaking agent
Sodium aluminum phosphate acidic	Acidity regulatory, emulsifier
Sodium cyclamate	Artificial sweetener
Sodium alginate	Thickener and vegetable gum
Sodium caseinate	Emulsifier
Sodium bicarbonate	Yeast substitute

Angiotensin and aldosterone both act to conserve sodium by increasing sodium reabsorption by the kidney. Sodium depletion stimulates the renal production of renin, which generates active angiotensin in the circulation. The latter stimulates vasoconstriction, which increases blood pressure, decreases water loss, and stimulates aldosterone release from the adrenal cortex. Atrial natriuretic hormone counteracts the sodium retention mechanisms by suppressing renin and aldosterone release and by inducing water and sodium excretion. It also decreases blood pressure and antagonizes angiotensin. A raised plasma sodium concentration stimulates the renal reabsorption of water and decreases urinary output via antidiuretic hormone from the posterior pituitary. In contrast to sodium, chloride is passively distributed throughout the body and moves to replace anions lost to cells via other processes.

The main excretory route for both sodium and chloride is the urine. Sweat loss of these ions tends to be very low except with severe exertion in hot climates. Fecal losses are also low in healthy individuals.

Metabolic function and essentiality

The sodium cation is an active participant in the regulation of osmotic and electrolyte balances, whereas the chloride anion is a passive participant in this regulatory system. Each ion, however, has other functions within the body.

Sodium is involved in nerve conduction, active cellular transport and the formation of mineral apatite of bone. Central to its role in water balance, nerve conduction, and active transport is the plasma membrane enzyme sodium–potassium-ATPase (Na^+/K^+-ATPase). This enzyme pumps sodium out of the cell and at the same time returns potassium to the intracellular environment while ATP is hydrolyzed. Signal transmission along nerve cells, active transport of nutrients into the enterocyte and muscle contraction/relaxation all depend on the Na^+/K^+-ATPase pump. In the muscle there is an additional pump, the sodium–calcium system. The ATP utilized by the sodium pump makes up a substantial part of the total metabolic activity and thermogenesis.

Among the main functions of the chloride anion are as dissociated hydrochloric acid in the stomach and in the chloride shift in the erythrocyte plasma membrane, where it exchanges with the bicarbonate ion.

Deficiency symptoms

Obligatory losses of sodium are very low, and low plasma sodium or chloride depletion is difficult to induce. Low plasma sodium or chloride is not diet related but rather caused by a variety of clinical conditions, including major trauma and cachexia and overuse of diuretics. Loss of sodium can also ensue as a result of excessive water intake, anorexia nervosa, ulcerative colitis, liver disease, congestive heart failure with edema, and severe infection and diarrhea. Acute diarrhea is the most common cause of sodium deficiency, and oral rehydration depends on the efficient enteric uptake of sodium from isotonic glucose/saline solutions and saves many lives worldwide. Vomiting, chronic renal disease, renal failure, and chronic respiratory acidosis can result in chloride depletion.

Toxicity

Excessive salt intakes are usually excreted efficiently in healthy individuals, whereas high plasma sodium and chloride are commonly caused by diabetes insipidus, brainstem injury, and dehydration through either excessive sweating or deficient water intake. Excessive salt intake may have roles in the degenerative diseases of coronary heart disease, stroke, gastric cancer, osteoporosis, and bronchial hyperactivity. There are accumulating data from epidemiological studies and controlled clinical trials to indicate an adverse effect of sodium intake on blood pressure, and that most people are sodium sensitive. It now appears that lowering this intermediate or surrogate measure (blood pressure) of disease can be translated into reduced morbidity and mortality of cardiovascular disease from long-term follow-up assessed 10–15 years after the original dietary sodium reduction trials. The mechanism linking salt intake with blood pressure is unclear but probably relates to sodium homeostasis. It has been suggested that extracellular sodium concentrations may adversely affect vascular reactivity and growth and stimulate myocordial fibrosis. Low-sodium diets differ in nutrient composition from the prevailing diet, and animal experimentation indicates that low potassium or calcium intake encourages a salt-induced increase in blood pressure, as does feeding simple carbohydrates (sucrose, glucose, or fructose). Copper deficiency in rats has been demonstrated to increase blood pressure independently of sodium intake. Epidemiological and other studies indicate that heavy metals, such as lead and mercury, may also contribute to increased blood pressure.

Efficient sodium conservation mechanisms mean that current sodium intakes in many populations are unnecessarily high and are probably much higher than the generally lower sodium diets eaten during the long period of human evolution. Clinical studies indicate that a high-sodium diet increases calcium excretion and measures of bone resorption, thereby suggesting a possible role for high salt intakes in osteoporosis.

Cross-cultural epidemiology suggests that high salt intakes are associated with gastric cancer, whereas a low-salt diet is regarded as having a potentially favorable effect in asthma patients.

Genetic diseases

A number of rare genetic disorders have thrown some light on the pathological mechanisms linking sodium balance and hypertension (pathologically elevated blood pressure). A number of candidate genes have been identified in monogenic forms of low renin salt-sensitive hypertension. These encode for enzymes involved in aldosterone biosynthesis or cortisol metabolism and for the epithelial sodium channel. These genetic defects decrease the ability of the renal tubules to excrete sodium. It is possible that similar genetic mechanisms operate in more common forms of hypertension such as essential hypertension and especially salt-sensitive hypertension. Moreover, molecular mechanisms associated with renin–angiotensin–aldosterone are central to the pathophysiology of this condition. Common essential hypertension, however, is complex and heterogeneous and has a genetic heritability of about 30%.

Assessing status

The tight regulation of plasma sodium and, in turn, chloride ensures that fluctuations in the plasma concentration of these ions are minimized and changes only occur in certain pathological circumstances. Measurements of plasma sodium, therefore, are of little consequence as far as nutritional status is concerned. Total body (excluding bone) sodium, however, is increased in malnutrition and trauma and this total exchangeable sodium can be measured, with some technical difficulty, using radioisotopes.

Salt intakes are notoriously difficult to measure, and urinary sodium excretion is considered to be a valid measure of sodium intake under circumstances where little sodium is lost in sweat. Sodium in urine is easily measured, but the collection of complete 24 h urinary samples is difficult because of subject compliance, and the completeness of these collections should be validated using a marker such as para-amino benzoic acid. Lithium (as carbonate) fused with sodium chloride can act as a reliable tracer to estimate discretionary salt (cooking and table) intakes.

Requirements and dietary sources

Average requirements for sodium and chloride are estimated to be about 500 and 750 mg/day, respectively. Normal sodium (mostly from salt) intake varies from about 2 g/day to 14 g/day, with chloride (mostly from salt) intakes generally slightly in excess of sodium (Table 9.6). Snack and processed foods have more added salt than unprocessed foods. The amount of discretionary salt added in cooking or at the table appears to vary greatly among individuals and among countries. Discretionary salt intakes can vary from less than 10% to 20–30% of total salt intake and these figures emphasize the major effect of processed foods on total salt intakes in most populations (Table 9.7).

Micronutrient interactions

The major interactions between sodium (and chloride) and other micronutrients are with respect to potassium and calcium. Data from animals (and some clinical studies) indicate that dietary potassium and calcium potentiate increases in blood pressure in salt-sensitive experimental models. There is evidence to suggest that the sodium to potassium ratio correlates more strongly with blood pressure than does either nutrient alone. As indicated previously, the metabolism of sodium, chloride, and potassium is closely related, and sodium and calcium ions have a close metabolic relationship within cells.

9.6 Potassium

Potassium, sodium, and chloride make up the principal electrolytes within the body. In contrast to sodium and chloride, nutritional concerns with potassium are mainly concerned with the possibility of underconsumption.

Table 9.6 Salt intake as NaCl (g/day)

Before 1982	Year	Intake	From 1988	Year	Intake
Communities not using added salt					
Brazil (Yanomamo Indian)	1975	0.06			
New Guinea (Chimbus)	1967	0.40			
Solomon Islands (Kwaio)		1.20			
Botswana (Kung bushmen)		1.80			
Polynesia (Pukapuka)		3.60			
Alaska (Eskimos)	1961	4.00			
Marshall Islands in the Pacific		7.00			
Salt-using communities					
Kenya (Sambura nomads)		5–8	Mexico (Tarahumsa Indian)		3–10
Mexico (Tarahumsa Indian)	1978	5–8	Mexico, rural (Nalinalco)	1992	5.7
			Mexico, urban (Tlaplan)	1991	7.18
Denmark		9.8	Denmark	1988	8.00
Canada (Newfoundland)		9.9	Canada		8–10
New Zealand		10.1			
Sweden (Göteborg)		10.2			
USA (Evans Country, Georgia)		10.6	USA (Chicago)		7.7
Iran		10.9			
Belgium	1966	11.4	Belgium	1988	8.4
UK (Scotland)		11.5			
Australia		12.0			
India (north)		12–15	India		9–11.4
Federal Republic of Germany		13.1			
Finland (east)		14.3	Finland		10.6
Bahamas		15–30			
Kenya (Samburus, army)	1969	18.6			
Korea		19.9			
Japan					
Japan (farmers)	1955	60.3	Japan	1988	8–15
Japan (Akita)		27–30			
Japan	1964	20.9			

Absorption, transport, and tissue distribution

Potassium is the major intracellular electrolyte and exists as the fully water-soluble cation. More than 90% of dietary potassium is absorbed from the digestive tract.

Few dietary components affect absorption of potassium, although olive oil can increase and dietary fiber decrease absorption to some extent. The "average" 70 kg man contains about 120 g of potassium, depending on muscle mass, with men having proportionally greater muscle mass, and hence potassium, than women. Almost all of the body potassium is exchangeable, intracellular concentration being more than 30 times the concentration of the ECF. Potassium is distributed within the body in response to energy-dependent sodium redistribution. Various hormonal and other factors regulate potassium homeostasis, both within cells and with the external environment. Hyperkalemia (too much potassium in the ECF) stimulates insulin, aldosterone, and epinephrine (adrenaline) secretions, which promote the uptake of potassium by body cells. The aldosterone hormone also stimulates potassium excretion by the kidney and, at the same time, conserves sodium. Hypokalemia has opposite effects, such that more potassium is released from cells. As with sodium, the kidney regulates potassium balance. Urine is the major excretory route in healthy people, with only small amounts lost in the feces and minimal amounts in sweat.

Metabolic function and essentiality

Potassium, sodium, and chloride are the major determinants of osmotic pressure and electrolyte balance.

Table 9.7 Salting (mg/100 g fresh weight) of foods in Western societies

	Na	K	Ca	Mg
Maize-based products				
Corn	4	284	55	41
Tortilla, rural	11	192	177	65
Breakfast cereals	866	101	3	11
Processed snacks	838	197	102	56
Wheat-based products				
Natural cereals	39	1166	94	343
Tortillas, wheat	622	73	11	17
Breakfast cereals	855	869	81	236
Processed bread (urban)	573	126	47	31
Salted bread, made locally (rural)	410	92	10	74
Sweet bread, made locally (rural)	97	93	87	18
Processed bread (rural)	344	79	213	18
Processed biscuits	582	80	16	17
Pulses				
Unprocessed, cooked	53	373	50	41
Processed, canned	354	371	27	79

Reproduced from Sánchez-Castillo and James in Sadler *et al. Encyclopedia of Human Nutrition*, copyright 1999 with permission of Elsevier.

The concentration difference of potassium and sodium across cell membranes is maintained by the Na^+/K^+-ATPase pump and is critical for nerve transmission and muscle function. The physiological importance of potassium in the body covers many systems including cardiovascular, respiratory, digestive, renal, and endocrine. In addition, potassium is a cofactor for enzymes involved in *inter alia* energy metabolism, glycogenesis, and cellular growth and division.

Deficiency symptoms

The low concentration of potassium in plasma is tightly regulated. Hypokalemia, however, can result from either excessive uptake of potassium by cells or potassium depletion from the body. Insulin excess, catecholamine increases, Cushing's disease (excess steroids), diuretics that enhance potassium loss, chronic renal disease, diarrhea, vomiting, and laxative abuse can result in hypokalemia. Low potassium intakes are unlikely to lead to clinical potassium depletion and hypokalemia except during starvation and anorexia nervosa.

The activity of nerves and muscles is affected in potassium depletion, and other clinical sequelae involve cardiac (including cardiac arrest), renal, and

metabolic alterations. Potassium supplementation may have a role to play in treating chronic heart failure, and increased potassium intakes can decrease blood pressure via antagonistic metabolic interactions with sodium, resulting in increased sodium excretion, and also via a direct vasodilatory effect. Oral administration of potassium salts has been shown to improve calcium and phosphorus balance, reduce bone resorption and increase the rate of bone formation.

Toxicity

Hyperkalemia, as a result of either a shift of potassium from cells to the ECF or excessive potassium retention, can be caused by major trauma and infection, metabolic acidosis, Addison's disease (aldosterone insufficiency) and chronic renal failure. Overuse of potassium supplements can also result in potassium excess. As with potassium depletion, the most important clinical consequence of potassium excess is cardiac arrest.

Assessing status

The plasma concentration of potassium is not a reliable index of whole-body potassium status. Total body potassium can be measured by ^{42}K dilution or by whole body counting of the naturally abundant ^{40}K to determine the amount of lean body tissue. More direct measures of tissue potassium can be obtained by muscle biopsies.

Requirement and dietary sources

Adult requirements for potassium are estimated to be about 2 g/day. Because of potential beneficial antagonistic effects against high salt intakes, higher intakes (around 3.5 g/day) of potassium are considered to be optimal, although chronic intakes above 5.9 g/day may be dangerous for individuals with impaired renal function. Potassium, like sodium and chloride, is naturally widely distributed in foods (Table 9.8). Food processing (through leaching) may decrease potassium content as well as increasing salt content. Legumes, nuts, dried fruit, and fresh fruit, especially bananas, melons, avocados, and kiwi fruit, are rich sources of potassium. Major vegetable sources of potassium are potatoes and spinach, although cereal and dairy products, which have a lower potassium content but are consumed in large quantities, are also important dietary sources. In addition, meat and fish contain appreciable quantities of potassium. People who eat large quantities of fruit and vegetables

Table 9.8 Sodium and potassium content of various foods (mg/100 g edible portion)

Food	Na	K
Legumes		
Red kidney beans	18	1370
Soyabeans	5	1730
Lentils	12	940
Dried fruit		
Raisins	60	1020
Figs	62	970
Nuts		
Walnuts	7	450
Almonds	14	780
Fruit and vegetables		
Banana	1	400
Melon	5–32	100–210
Potato	11	320
Spinach	140	500
Meat and fish		
Beef, veal, lamb	52–110	230–260
Chicken	81	320
Herring	120	320
Halibut	60	410
Tuna	47	400
Mussels	290	320
Miscellaneous		
Cow's milk	55	140
Chocolate	11	300

Reproduced from Sánchez-Castillo and James in Sadler *et al. Encyclopedia of Human Nutrition*, copyright 1999 with permission of Elsevier.

may have dietary intakes of potassium exceeding 6 g/day.

Micronutrient interactions

As might be expected from the close metabolic interactions among the major electrolytes, potassium and sodium dietary interactions may be important in determining the risk of coronary heart disease and stroke. Another potentially important interaction concerns calcium. Potassium appears to have positive effects on calcium balance by regulating the acid–base balance and ameliorating any effects of sodium on calcium depletion.

9.7 Iron

Iron is a relatively abundant element in the universe. It is found in the sun and many types of stars in con-

siderable quantity. The core of the Earth is thought to be largely composed of iron and it makes up 4.7% of the Earth's crust. The most common ore is hematite, which is frequently seen as black sands along beaches and streams. Taconite is becoming increasingly important as a commercial ore. Because iron is easy to obtain, its discovery is lost in the history of man, many thousands of years ago. The early Greeks were aware of the health-giving properties of iron. Iron has been used for centuries as a health tonic. It is therefore paradoxical that although the need for iron was discovered long ago and although it is the most common and cheapest of all metals, iron deficiency is probably the most frequent deficiency disorder in the world and the main remaining nutritional deficiency in Europe. Iron can exist in oxidation states ranging from -2 to $+6$. In biological systems, these oxidation states occur primarily as the ferrous (Fe^{2+}) and ferric (Fe^{3+}) forms and these are interchangeable.

Absorption, transport, and tissue distribution

The iron content of a typical 70 kg adult man is approximately 4–5 g. Of this content, approximately two-thirds is utilized as functional iron such as hemoglobin (60%), myoglobin (5%), and various heme (cytochromes and catalase) and nonheme (NADH hydrogenase, succinic dehydrogenase, aconitase) enzymes (5%). The remaining iron is found in body storage as ferritin (20%) and hemosiderin (10%), the two major iron storage proteins. Only very minor quantities of iron (<0.1%) are found as a transit chelate with transferrin, the main iron transport protein in the body.

The metabolism of iron differs from that of other minerals in one important respect: there is no physiological mechanism for iron excretion. The body has three unique mechanisms for maintaining iron balance and preventing iron deficiency and iron overload:

- storage of iron (with ferritin being an important reversible storage protein for iron)
- reutilization of iron (especially of iron in erythrocytes)
- regulation of iron absorption.

In theory, therefore, when the body needs more iron, absorption is increased, and when the body is iron sufficient, absorption is restricted. This control is not perfect but is still of great importance for the prevention of iron deficiency and excess. Iron from food is absorbed mainly in the duodenum by an active process that transports iron from the gut lumen into the mucosal cell. When required by the body for metabolic processes, iron passes directly through the mucosal cell into the bloodstream, where it is transported by transferrin, together with the iron released from old blood cells (i.e., the efficient iron recycling system, Figure 9.5), to the bone marrow (80%) and other tissues (20%). If iron is not required by the body, iron in the mucosal cell is stored as ferritin and is excreted in feces when the mucosal cell is exfoliated. Any absorbed iron in excess of needs is stored as ferritin or hemosiderin in the liver, spleen, or bone marrow. Iron can be released from these iron stores for utilization in times of high need, such as during pregnancy.

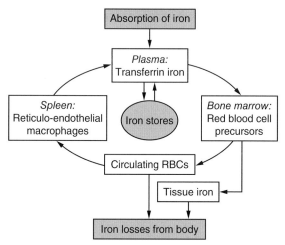

Figure 9.5 Metabolism of iron. There is a main internal loop with a continuous reutilization of iron and an external loop represented by iron losses from the body and absorption from the diet. Adapted from Hallberg *et al.* (1993) with permission of Elsevier.

Heme iron is absorbed by a different mechanism from nonheme iron. The heme molecule is absorbed intact into the mucosal cell, where iron is released by the enzyme heme oxygenase. Its absorption is little influenced by the composition of the meal, and varies from 15% to 35% depending on the iron status of the consumer. Although heme iron represents only 10–15% of dietary iron intake in populations with a high meat intake, it could contribute 40% or more of the total absorbed iron (Figure 9.6). Many poorer regions of the world consume little animal tissue and rely entirely on nonheme iron. The absorption of nonheme iron is strongly influenced by dietary components, which bind iron in the intestinal lumen. The complexes formed can be either insoluble or so tightly bound that the iron is prevented from being absorbed. Alternatively, the complexes can be soluble and iron absorption is facilitated. Under experimental conditions, nonheme iron absorption can vary widely from less than 1% to more than 90%, but under more typical dietary conditions it is usually in the region of 1–20%. The main inhibitory substances and enhancers of iron absorption are shown in Table 9.9.

Metabolic function and essentiality

Iron acts as a catalytic center for a broad spectrum of metabolic functions. As present in hemoglobin, iron is required for the transport of oxygen, critical for cell respiration. As myoglobin, iron is required for oxygen storage in muscle. Iron is also a component of various tissue enzymes, such as the cytochromes, that are critical for energy production, and enzymes necessary for immune system functioning. Therefore, these iron-containing molecules ensure that body fuels, such as carbohydrate, fat, and protein are oxidized to

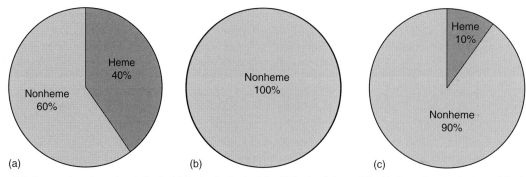

Figure 9.6 Heme and nonheme iron in foods: (a) foods of animal origin; (b) foods of plant origin; (c) dietary iron intake from all foods, daily average.

Table 9.9 Factors affecting (a) heme and (b) nonheme iron absorption

Increased absorption	Decreased absorption
(a) Heme	
Physiological factors	
Low iron status	High iron status
Dietary factors	
Low heme iron intake	High heme iron intake
Meat	Calcium
(b) Nonheme	
Physiological factors	
Depleted iron status	Replete iron status
Pregnancy	Achlorhydria (low gastric acid)
Disease states (aplastic anemia, hemolytic anemia, hemochromatosis)	
Dietary factors	
Ascorbic acid	Phytate
Meat, fish, seafood	Iron-binding phenolic compounds
Certain organic acids	Calcium

provide the energy necessary for all physiological processes and movement. The importance of iron as an element necessary for life derives from its redox reactivity as it exists in two stable, interchangeable forms, ferrous (Fe^{2+}) and ferric (Fe^{3+}) iron. This reaction is an essential part of the electron transport chain, responsible for the generation of ATP during the oxidation of substances in intermediary metabolism and for the reductions necessary in the synthesis of larger molecules from their components.

Deficiency symptoms

The progression from adequate iron status to iron-deficiency anemia develops in three overlapping stages. The first stage consists of depletion of storage iron, which is characterized by a decrease in serum ferritin, which, in turn, reflects the size of the iron stores in the liver, bone marrow, and spleen. The second stage is a decrease in transported iron and is characterized by a decline in serum iron and an increase in the total iron-binding capacity, as transferrin has more free binding sites than in normal iron status. The third stage develops when the supply of iron is insufficient to provide for enough hemoglobin for new erythrocytes and insufficient to fulfill other physiological functions. During the last stage, free protoporphyrin, destined for hemoglobin, increases in plasma two- to fivefold, indicating a lack of tissue iron. The harmful consequences of iron deficiency occur mainly in conjunction with anemia. Iron deficiency anemia is most common in infants, preschool children, adolescents, and women of child-bearing age, particularly in developing countries.

The functional effects of iron deficiency anemia result from both a reduction in circulating hemoglobin and a reduction in iron-containing enzymes and myoglobin. Both factors presumably play a role in the fatigue, restlessness, and impaired work performance associated with iron deficiency anemia. Other functional defects include disturbances in normal thermoregulation and impairment of certain key steps in the immune response. For example, there is evidence that iron deficiency anemia is associated with lower T- and B-lymphocyte, macrophage, and neutrophil function. Although the phagocytic uptake of neutrophils is usually normal, the intracellular killing mechanism is usually defective. This abnormality is thought to be owing to a defect in the generation of reactive oxygen intermediates resulting from a decrease in the iron-containing enzyme myeloperoxidase. Iron deficiency anemia can also have an adverse effect on psychomotor and mental development in children, and the mortality and morbidity of mother and infant during pregnancy.

Toxicity

The very effective regulation of iron absorption prevents overload of the tissues by iron from a normal diet, except in individuals with genetic defects, as in idiopathic hemochromatosis (see below). Excess iron via overuse of iron supplements could pose a possible health risk. The mechanism of cellular and tissue injury resulting from excess iron is not fully understood. Liabilities may include increased risks for bacterial infection, neoplasia, arthropathy, cardiomyopathy, and endocrine dysfunctions. However, there is still much debate as to the strength of evidence to support a relationship between dietary iron intake and cancer or cardiovascular disease.

Gastrointestinal distress does not occur from consuming a diet containing naturally occurring or fortified iron. Individuals taking iron at high levels (>45 mg/day) may encounter gastrointestinal side-effects (constipation, nausea, vomiting, and diarrhea), especially when taken on an empty stomach. Based largely on the data on gastrointestinal effects following supplemental elemental iron intake in apparently healthy adults, the US Food and Nutrition Board established a tolerable UL of iron of 45 mg/day.

Genetic diseases

Primary idiopathic hemochromatosis is a hereditary disorder of iron metabolism characterized by an abnormally high iron absorption owing to a failure of the iron absorption control mechanism at the intestinal level. High deposits of iron in the liver and the heart can lead to cirrhosis, hepatocellular cancer, congestive heart failure, and eventual death. Sufferers of this disorder can develop iron overload through consumption of a normal diet, but would be at much higher risk if consuming iron-fortified foods. Thus, early detection of the disease via genetic screening followed by regular blood removal has proven to be a successful treatment.

Assessing status

Several different laboratory methods must be used in combination to diagnose iron deficiency anemia correctly. The most commonly used methods to assess iron status include:

- serum ferritin
- transferrin saturation
- erythrocyte protoporphyrin
- mean corpuscular volume
- serum transferrin receptor
- hemoglobin or packed cell volume.

Iron deficiency anemia is usually defined as a hemoglobin level below the cut-off value for age and sex plus at least two other abnormal iron status measurements. The most commonly used are probably low serum ferritin, high protoporphyrin, and, more recently, high serum transferrin receptor.

Requirements and dietary sources

Daily (absorbed or physiological) iron requirements are calculated from the amount of dietary iron necessary to cover basal iron losses, menstrual losses, and growth needs. They vary according to age and sex,

and, in relation to body weight, they are highest for the young infant. An adult man has obligatory iron losses of around 1 mg of iron/day, largely from the gastrointestinal tract (exfoliation of epithelial cells and secretions), skin, and urinary tract. Thus, to remain replete with regard to iron, an average adult man needs to absorb only 1 mg of iron from the diet on a daily basis. Similar obligatory iron losses for women amount to around 0.8 mg/day. However, adult women experience additional iron loss owing to menstruation, which raises the median daily iron requirement for absorption to 1.4 mg (this covers 90% of menstruating women; 10% will require daily absorption of at least 2.4 mg iron to compensate for their very high menstrual losses). Pregnancy creates an additional demand for iron, especially during the second and third trimesters, leading to daily requirements of 4–6 mg. Growing children and adolescents require 0.5 mg iron/day in excess of body losses to support growth. Physiological iron needs can be translated into dietary requirements by taking into account the efficiency at which iron is absorbed from the diet (typically around 10%). Current RDAs for iron (recommended by the US Food and Nutrition Board in 2001) are infants 0.27 mg (first 6 months; this is an adequate intake value), 11 mg (7–12 months), children 7 and 10 mg (1–3 and 4–8 years, respectively), teenage boys 8 and 11 mg (9–13 and 14–18 years, respectively), adult men 8 mg (19 years and older), teenage girls 8 and 15 mg (9–13 and 14–18 years, respectively), adult women 18 and 8 mg (19–50 years and 51 years and older, respectively), pregnant women 27 mg and lactating women 10 and 9 mg (younger than 18 years and 19–50 years, respectively).

Iron is widely distributed in meat, eggs, vegetables, and cereals, but the concentrations in milk, fruit, and vegetables are low (Table 9.10). The iron content per se of individual foods has little meaning as iron absorption varies considerably. There are two types of food iron: nonheme iron, which is present in both plant foods and animal tissues, and heme iron, coming from the hemoglobin and myoglobin in animal products. Heme iron represents 30–70% of the total iron in lean meat and is always well absorbed. Nonheme iron from meat and vegetable foods enters a common nonheme iron pool in the gastric juice, from which the amount of iron absorbed depends to a large extent on the presence of enhancing and inhibiting sub-

Table 9.10 Iron content of some common foods

Food source	Description	Fe content (mg/100 g)
Liver	Raw, calf	8.0
Beef	Lean (from six different cuts)	2.1
Black (blood) sausage	Fried	20.0
Chicken	Raw, meat only	0.7
Cod, plaice, whiting	Raw	0.3–1.0
Eggs	Chicken, whole, raw	1.9
Pulses	Raw	0.6–11.1
Wheat flour	Whole flour	3.9
Wheat flour	White flour	1.5–2.0
Milk	Cow's (3.9, 1.6 and 0.1% fat)	0.05–0.06
Green leafy vegetables	Raw	0.7–2.2
Rice	Raw, white, polished	0.5
Potatoes	Raw	0.3–0.4

Data from Holland *et al.* (1995). Reproduced with permission from HMSO.

Table 9.11 Approximate zinc content of major organs and tissues in the adult man

Tissue	Total Zn content (g)	Percentage of body Zn (%)
Skeletal muscle	1.53	~57
Bone	0.77	29
Skin	0.16	6
Liver	0.13	5
Brain	0.04	1.5
Kidneys	0.02	0.7
Heart	0.01	0.4
Hair	<0.01	~0.1
Blood (plasma)	<0.01	~0.1

Modified from Mills CF, ed, *Zinc in Human Biology*, copyright 1998 with kind permission of Springer Science + Business Media.

stances in the meal and on the iron status of the individual.

Micronutrient interactions

The fact that serum copper has been found to be low in some cases of iron deficiency anemia suggests that iron status has an effect on copper metabolism. Copper deficiency impinges on iron metabolism, causing an anemia that does not respond to iron supplementation. Interactions between iron and copper seem to be owing to impaired utilization of one in the absence of the other. As mentioned above, calcium can inhibit iron absorption under certain circumstances. In aqueous solutions iron impairs zinc absorption, but this interaction does not take place when iron is added to an animal protein meal, indicating different uptake mechanisms for solutions and solid foods.

9.8 Zinc

The natural abundance of zinc in the Earth's crust is 0.02%. The principal ores of zinc are sphalerite or blende (sulfide), smithsonite (carbonate), calamine (silicate), and franklinite (zinc iron oxide). Zinc is used to form numerous alloys with other metals.

Brass, nickel, silver, typewriter metal, commercial bronze, spring brass, German silver, soft solder, and aluminum solder are some of the more important alloys. Large quantities of zinc are used to produce die castings, used extensively by the automotive, electrical, and hardware industries. Zinc is also extensively used to galvanize other metals, such as iron to prevent corrosion. Zinc oxide is widely used in the manufacture of paints, rubber products, cosmetics, pharmaceuticals, floor coverings, plastics, printing inks, soap, storage batteries, textiles, electrical equipment, and other products. Zinc sulfide is used in making luminous dials, X-ray and television screens, and fluorescent lights. The chloride and chromate are also important compounds. In biological systems zinc is virtually always in the divalent (+2) state. Unlike iron, zinc does not exhibit any direct redox chemistry.

Absorption, transport, and tissue distribution

Zinc is ubiquitous in the body. It is the most abundant intracellular trace element, with >95% of the body zinc intracellular. An adult human contains about 2 g of zinc, of which about 60% and 30% are in skeletal muscle and bone, respectively, and 4–6% is present in skin (Table 9.11). Zinc turnover in these tissues is slow and, therefore, the zinc in these tissues is not accessible at times of deprivation. Because zinc is essential for the synthesis of lean tissue, it is while this is occurring that it may become a limiting nutrient. Although some zinc may be available in short-term zinc deprivation from a mobile hepatic pool, it is generally assumed that the body has no specific zinc reserve and is dependent on a regular supply of the element.

With essential roles in many fundamental cellular processes (see below), it is not surprising that whole-body zinc content is tightly controlled. Zinc in foods is absorbed via a carrier-mediated transport process, which under normal physiological conditions appears not to be saturated. Zinc is absorbed throughout the small intestine. Proximal intestinal absorption is efficient, but it has a large enteropancreatic circulation; the net intestinal absorption of zinc is achieved by the distal small intestine. Zinc is transported in the plasma by albumin and α_2-macroglobulin, but only 0.1% of body zinc is found in plasma. Body zinc content is regulated by homeostatic mechanisms over a wide range of intakes by changes in fractional absorption (normally 20–40%) and urinary (0.5 mg/day) and intestinal (1–3 mg/day) excretion. For example, during periods of low zinc intake, absorption is enhanced and secretion of endogenous zinc into the gastrointestinal lumen is suppressed. In contrast, high zinc intake is associated with decreased absorption and enhanced secretion of endogenous zinc. Within cells, fluctuations in zinc content are modulated by changes in the amount of the metal associated with the storage protein metallothionein but there is a large number and variety of zinc homeostatic proteins found throughout cells. Although zinc transporters are very important for generating and maintaining zinc gradients across membranes and within cellular compartments, little is known about many aspects of their functions and regulatory modes of action.

The bioavailability of dietary zinc depends on dietary enhancers and inhibitors and host-related factors (Table 9.12). Diets can be roughly classified as having a low, medium, or high bioavailability, according to the content of zinc, phytate, and animal protein. From a mixed animal and plant product diet, 20–30% zinc absorption can be expected. The lowest absorption, 10–15%, is seen from diets prevalent in developing countries that are based on cereals and legumes with a high phytate content and with negligible amounts of animal protein.

Metabolic function and essentiality

Zinc has three major groups of functions in the human body: catalytic, structural, and regulatory. Most biochemical roles of zinc reflect its involvement in the folding and activity of a large number (up to 10%) of proteins and over 100 different zinc metal-loenzymes have been identified, including RNA nucleotide polymerase I and II, alkaline phosphatase and carbonic anhydrases. Important structural roles for zinc are in the zinc finger motif in proteins, but also in metalloenzymes [e.g., copper/zinc superoxide dismutase (Cu/Zn-SOD)]. Zinc is also required by protein kinases that participate in signal transduction processes and as a stimulator of transacting factors responsible for regulating gene expression. Zinc plays an important role in the immune system and, though not a redox-active transition metal, is an antioxidant *in vivo*.

Deficiency symptoms

The clinical manifestations of severe zinc deficiency in humans are growth retardation, sexual and skeletal immaturity, neuropsychiatric disturbances, dermatitis, alopecia, diarrhea, increased susceptibility to infections, and loss of appetite. Many of these features, by and large, represent the dependence on zinc of tissues with a high rate of turnover. However, severe zinc deficiency in humans is rare, and more interest has been focused on marginal zinc deficiency. This is more difficult to diagnose and often occurs with other micronutrient deficiencies including iron. The current understanding of zinc deficiency is largely based on responses to zinc supplementation. Zinc supplementation has been reported to stimulate growth and development in infants and young children, and reduce morbidity (diarrhea and respiratory infections) in children, particularly in developing countries and can increase both innate and adaptive immunity. In women, low serum zinc concentration during pregnancy was found to be a significant

Table 9.12 Factors affecting zinc absorption

Increased absorption	Decreased absorption
Physiological factors	
Depleted zinc status	Replete zinc status
	Disease state (acrodermatitis enteropathica)
Dietary factors	
Low zinc intake	High zinc intake
Certain organic acids	Phytate
Certain amino acids	Certain metals
Human milk	

predictor of low birth weight, and low maternal zinc intake has been associated with an approximately twofold increased risk of low birth weight and increased risk of preterm delivery in poor urban women.

Toxicity

Gross acute zinc toxicity has been described following the drinking of water that has been stored in galvanized containers or the use of such water for renal dialysis. Symptoms include nausea, vomiting, and fever, and are apparent after acute ingestion of 2 g or more. The more subtle effects of moderately elevated intakes, not uncommon in some populations, are of greater concern, because they are not easily detected. Prolonged intakes of supraphysiological intakes of zinc (75–300 mg/day) have been associated with impaired copper utilization (producing features such as microcytic anemia and neutropenia), impaired immune responses and a decline of high-density lipoproteins, but some have argued that even short-term intakes of about 25–50 mg zinc/day may interfere with the metabolism of both iron and copper. The US Food and Nutrition Board reported that there was no evidence of adverse effects from intake of naturally occurring zinc in food; however, they derived a tolerable UL of 40 mg/day for adults older than 19 years, which applies to total zinc intake from food, water, and supplements (including fortified foods). Data on reduced copper status in humans were used to derive this UL for zinc. Using similar data but different uncertainty factors, the UL for total zinc intake was set at 25 mg/day in the EU.

Genetic diseases

Acrodermatitis enteropathica, a rare, inborn, autosomal recessive disease, is a disorder of primary zinc malabsorption. It is characterized by alopecia; vesicular, pustular and/or eczematoid skin lesions, specifically of the mouth, face, hands, feet and groin; growth retardation; mental apathy; diarrhea and secondary malabsorption, defects in cellular and phagocytic immune function; and intercurrent infections. The disorder responds very well to zinc therapy.

Assessing status

Measurement of zinc in plasma or activities of zinc metalloenzymes or peptides in blood are frequently used to measure zinc status. They are not ideal indices, however, as they are relatively resistant to changes in dietary zinc and, moreover, metabolic conditions unrelated to zinc status cause them to decline. The development of zinc deficiency is different from that of many other nutrients because a functional reserve or store of zinc does not seem to be available when zinc intake is inadequate. Tissue zinc is conserved by reduction or cessation of growth in growing organisms or by decreased excretion in nongrowing organisms. Depending on the degree of deficiency, zinc homeostasis can be re-established by adjusting growth and excretion or, with a more severe deficiency, further metabolic changes occur, resulting in a negative zinc balance and loss of tissue zinc.

Requirements and dietary sources

The US RDA for zinc was based primarily on data derived from metabolic balance studies. Such studies are technically difficult to perform and it is uncertain whether information from these studies reflects true requirements. A different approach, using the factorial method, was proposed for estimates of zinc requirements and future RDAs. Factorial calculations to estimate zinc requirements require knowledge of obligatory losses, tissue composition, and needs for growth and tissue repair. Current RDAs for zinc (recommended by the US Food and Nutrition Board in 2001) are infants 2 mg [first 6 months; this is an adequate intake (AI) value], 3 mg (7–12 months), children 3 and 5 mg (1–3 and 4–8 years, respectively), teenage boys 8 and 11 mg (9–13 and 14–18 years, respectively), adult men 11 mg (19 years and more), teenage girls 8 and 9 mg (9–13 and 14–18 years, respectively), adult women 8 mg (19 years and older), pregnant women 13 and 11 mg (younger than 18 years and 19–50 years, respectively) and lactating women 14 and 12 mg (younger than 18 years and 19–50 years, respectively).

The zinc content of some common foods is given in Table 9.13, whereas Table 9.14 classifies foods based on zinc energy density. The bioavailability of zinc in different foods varies widely, from 5% to 50%. Meat, seafood (in particular oysters) and liver are good sources of bioavailable zinc. It has been estimated that approximately 70% of dietary zinc in the US diet is provided by animal products. In meat products, the zinc content to some extent follows the color of the meat, so that the highest content, approximately 50 mg/kg, is found in lean red meat, at least twice that

Table 9.13 Zinc content of some common foods

Food source	Description	Zn content (mg/100 g)
Liver	Raw, calf	7.8
Beef	Lean (from six different cuts)	4.3
Lamb	Lean (from six different cuts)	4.0
Pork	Lean (from three different cuts)	2.4
Chicken	Raw, meat only	1.1
Cod, plaice, whiting	Raw	0.3–0.5
Muscles	Boiled	2.1
Oysters	Raw	90–200
Crab	Boiled	5.5
Eggs	Chicken, whole, raw	1.3
Cheese	Soft and hard varieties	0.5–5.3
Pulses	Raw	0.2–5.0
Wheat flour	Whole flour	2.9
Wheat flour	White flour	0.6–0.9
Milk	Cow's (3.9, 1.6 and 0.1% fat)	0.4
Yoghurt	Whole milk	0.5–0.7
Green leafy vegetables	Raw	0.2–0.6
Rice	Raw, white, polished	1.8
Potatoes	Raw	0.2–0.3

Data from Holland *et al.* (1995). Reproduced with permission from HMSO.

Table 9.14 Classification of foods based on zinc energy density

Zinc energy	mg Zn/1000 kcal	Foods
Very poor	0–2	Fats, oils, butter, cream cheese, confectionery, soft/alcoholic drinks, sugar, preserves
Poor	1–5	Fish, fruit, refined cereal products, biscuits, cakes, tubers, sausage
Rich	4–12	Whole grains, pork, poultry, milk, low-fat cheese, yoghurt, eggs, nuts
Very rich	12–882	Lamb, leafy and root vegetables, crustaceans, beef kidney, liver, heart, molluscs

Adapted from Solomons, N.W. (2001) Dietary sources of zinc and factors affecting its bioavailability. *Food and Nutrition Bulletin*, **22**, 138–54.

in chicken. However, in many parts of the world, most zinc is provided by cereals. In cereals, most of the zinc is found in the outer fiber-rich part of the kernel. The degree of refinement, therefore, determines the total zinc content. Wholegrain products provide 30–50 mg/kg, but a low extraction rate wheat flour contains 8–10 mg/kg. The bioavailability of zinc can be low from plant-based diets, in particular from wholegrain cereals and legumes, owing to the high content of phytic acid, a potent inhibitor of zinc absorption.

Micronutrient interactions

A decrease in copper absorption has been reported in the presence of excessive zinc. Data indicate that the level necessary to impair bioavailability is >40–50 mg/day; therapeutic levels (150 mg/day) over extended periods produce symptoms of copper deficiency. As mentioned above, iron under certain circumstances impairs zinc absorption. Animal studies have suggested an interaction between calcium and zinc in phytate-rich diets, but this has not been confirmed in human studies.

9.9 Copper

Copper occurs in the environment in three oxidation states. Copper (0) metal is used widely in the building industry (e.g., water pipes, electrical wires) because of its properties of malleability, ductibility, and high thermal and electrical conductivity. Brass, an alloy of copper and zinc, is used for cooking utensils and musical instruments, and bronze, an alloy of copper and tin, has been used in castings since early times. Copper-based alloys and amalgams are used in dental bridges and crowns, and copper is a constituent of intrauterine contraceptive devices. Copper compounds are widely used in the environment as fertilizers and nutritional supplements and, because of their microbicidal properties, as fungicides, algicides, insecticides, and wood preservatives. Other industrial uses include dye manufacturing, petroleum refining, water treatment, and metal finishing. Copper compounds in the cuprous (1) state are easily oxidized to the more stable cupric (2) state, which is found most often in biological systems.

The most important copper ores are chalcocite (Cu_2S), chalcopyrite ($CuFeS_2$), and malachite [$CuCO_3 \cdot Cu(OH)_2$]. Copper concentrations in soil vary from 5 to 50 mg Cu/kg and in natural water from 4 to 10 µg Cu/l. Concentrations of copper in water, however, depend on acidity, softness, and the extent of copper pipes, and municipal water supplies can contain appreciably higher concentrations. The taste threshold of copper ranges from 1 to 5 mg Cu/l, producing a slight blue–green color at concentrations >5 mg/l copper. Acute copper toxicity symptoms, mainly nausea and gastrointestinal irritation, can occur at concentrations of >4 mg/l copper.

Absorption, transport, and tissue distribution

About 50–75% of dietary copper is absorbed, mostly via the intestinal mucosa, from a typical diet. The amount of dietary copper appears to be the primary factor influencing absorption, with decreases in the percentage absorption as the amount of copper ingested increases. High intakes of several nutrients can also influence copper bioavailability. These include antagonistic effects of zinc, iron, molybdenum, ascorbic acid, sucrose, and fructose, although evidence for some of these is mainly from animal studies. Drugs and medication, such as penicillamine and thiomolybdates, restrict copper accumulation in the body and excessive use of antacids can inhibit copper absorption. Although high intakes of sulfur amino acids can limit copper absorption, absorption of copper is promoted from high-protein diets.

Ionic copper can be released from partially digested food particles in the stomach, but immediately forms complexes with amino acids, organic acids, or other chelators. Soluble complexes of these and other highly soluble species of the metal, such as the sulfate or nitrate, are readily absorbed. Regulation of absorption at low levels of copper intake is probably by a saturable active transport mechanism, while passive diffusion plays a role at high levels of copper intake. Regulation of copper absorption is also effected via metallothionein, a metal-binding protein found in the intestine and other tissues. Metallothionein-bound copper in mucosal cells will be lost when these cells are removed by intestinal flow. The major regulator of copper elimination from the body, however, is biliary excretion. Most biliary copper is not reabsorbed and is eliminated in the feces. The overall effect of these regulatory mechanisms is a tight homeostasis of body copper status. Little copper is lost from the urine, skin, nails, and hair.

After absorption from the intestinal tract, ionic copper (2) is transported tightly bound to albumin and transcuprein to the liver via the portal bloodstream, with some going directly to other tissues, especially the kidney. Hepatic copper is mostly incorporated into ceruloplasmin, which is then released into the blood and delivered to other tissues. Uptake of copper by tissues can occur from various sources, including ceruloplasmin, albumin, transcuprein, and low molecular weight copper compounds. Chaperone proteins are then thought to bind the copper and transfer bound copper across the cell membrane to the intracellular target proteins, for example cytochrome c oxidase. The ATPase proteins may form part of the transfer process.

The body of a healthy 70 kg adult contains a little over 0.1 g of copper, with the highest concentrations found in the liver, brain, heart, bone, hair, and nails. Over 25% of body copper resides in the muscle, which forms a large part of the total body tissue. Much of the copper in the body is functional. Storage of copper, however, is very important to the neonate. At birth, infant liver concentrations are some five to 10 times the adult concentration and these stores are used during early life when copper intakes from milk are low.

Metabolic functions and essentiality

Copper is a component of several enzymes, cofactors, and proteins in the body. These enzymes and proteins have important functions in processes fundamental to human health (Table 9.15). These include a requirement for copper in the proper functioning of the immune, nervous and cardiovascular systems, for bone health, for iron metabolism and formation of red blood cells, and in the regulation of mitochondrial and other gene expression. In particular, copper functions as an electron transfer intermediate in redox reactions and as a cofactor in several copper-containing metalloenzymes. As well as a direct role in maintaining cuproenzyme activity, changes in copper status may have indirect effects on other enzyme systems that do not contain copper.

Deficiency symptoms

Owing to remarkable homeostatic mechanisms, clinical symptoms of copper deficiency occur in humans only under exceptional circumstances. Infants are more susceptible to overt symptoms of copper deficiency than are any other population group. Among the predisposing factors of copper deficiency are prematurity, low birth weight, and malnutrition,

Table 9.15 Human enzymes and proteins that contain copper

Enzyme or protein	Function
Cytochrome c oxidase	Mitochondrial enzyme involved in the electron transport chain; reduces oxygen to water and allows formation of ATP; activity is highest in the heart and also high in the brain, liver, and kidney
Ceruloplasmin (ferroxidase I)	Glycoprotein with six or seven copper atoms; four copper atoms involved in oxidation/reduction reactions; role of other copper atoms not fully known; scavenges free radicals; quencher of superoxide radicals generated in the circulation; oxidizes some aromatic amines and phenols; catalyzes oxidation of ferrous iron to ferric iron; assists with iron transport from storage to sites of hemoglobin synthesis; about 60% of plasma copper bound to ceruloplasmin; primarily extracellular; activity will be low during severe copper restriction
Ferroxidase II	Catalyzes oxidation of iron; no other functions known; in human plasma is only about 5% of ferroxidase activity
Hephaestin	Membrane-bound ceruloplasmin homologue; probably a multicopper oxidase required for iron export from the intestine
Monoamine oxidase	Inactivates catecholamines; reacts with serotonin, norepinephrine (noradrenaline), tyramine, and dopamine; activity inhibited by some antidepressant medications
Diamine oxidase	Inactivates histamine and polyamines; highest activity in small intestine; also high activity in kidney and placenta
Lysyl oxidase	Acts on lysine and hydroxylysine found in immature collagen and elastin; important for integrity of skeletal and vascular tissue; use of estrogen increases activity
Dopamine β-hydroxylase	Catalyzes conversion of dopamine to norepinephrine (noradrenaline), a neurotransmitter; contains two to eight copper atoms; important in brain and adrenal glands
Copper, zinc superoxide dismutase	Contains two copper atoms; primarily in cytosol, protects against oxidative damage by converting superoxide ion to hydrogen peroxide; erythrocyte concentrations are somewhat responsive to changes in copper intake
Extracellular superoxide dismutase	Protects against oxidative damage by scavenging superoxide ion radicals and converting them to hydrogen peroxide; small amounts in plasma; larger amounts in lungs, thyroid, and uterus
Tyrosinase	Involved in melanin synthesis; deficiency of this enzyme in skin leads to albinism; catalyzes conversion of tyrosine to dopamine and oxidation of dopamine to dopaquinone; present in eye and skin and forms color in hair, skin, and eyes
Metallothionein	Cysteine-rich protein that binds zinc, cadmium, and copper; important for sequestering metal ions and preventing toxicity
Albumin	Binds and transports copper in plasma and interstitial fluids; about 10–15% of copper in plasma is bound to albumin
Transcuprein	Binds copper in human plasma; may transport copper
Blood clotting factors V and VIII	Role in clotting and thrombogenesis; part of structure homologous with ceruloplasmin

especially when combined with feeding practices such as cow's milk or total parenteral nutrition. The most frequent symptoms of copper deficiency are anemia, neutropenia, and bone fractures, while less frequent symptoms are hypopigmentation, impaired growth, increased incidence of infections, and abnormalities of glucose and cholesterol metabolism and of electrocardiograms. Various attempts have been made to relate these symptoms to alterations in copper metalloenzymes (see Table 9.15) and noncopper enzymes that may be copper responsive, and to identify the role of copper as an antioxidant, in carbohydrate metabolism, immune function, bone health, and cardiovascular mechanisms. Notwithstanding the rarity of

frank copper deficiency in human populations, some have speculated that suboptimal copper intakes over long periods may be involved in the precipitation of chronic diseases, such as cardiovascular disease and osteoporosis. The pathological significance of subtle changes, in the longer term, in those systems that respond to copper deficiency have yet to be defined for humans.

Toxicity

Acute copper toxicity in humans is rare and usually occurs from contamination of drinking water, beverages, and foodstuffs from copper pipes or containers, or from accidental or deliberate ingestion of large amounts of copper salts. Symptoms include vomiting, diarrhea, hemolytic anemia, renal and liver damage, sometimes (at about 100 g or more) followed by coma and death. Clinical symptoms of chronic copper toxicity appear when the capacity for protective copper binding in the liver is exceeded. These symptoms include hepatitis, liver cirrhosis, and jaundice.

Consumption of formula milks, heavily contaminated with copper after boiling or storage in brass vessels, is usually a feature of Indian childhood cirrhosis, which occurs in early-weaned infants between the ages of 6 months and 5 years. Symptoms include abdominal distension, irregular fever, excessive crying, and altered appetite, followed by jaundice and often death. Some believe that a genetic disorder enhances susceptibility to this toxicity syndrome, associated with excessive dietary exposure to copper and massive accumulation of liver copper.

Genetic diseases

There are several disorders that result in deficiency or toxicity from exposure to copper intakes that are adequate or tolerated by the general population. The most important of these are Menkes' syndrome, an X-linked copper deficiency that is usually fatal in early childhood; Wilson's disease, an autosomal recessive disorder resulting in copper overload; and aceruloplasminemia, an autosomal recessive disorder of iron metabolism. All three disorders are characterized by low serum copper and ceruloplasmin.

Menkes' syndrome, which affects 1 in 300 000 in most populations, is caused by mutations in the gene that encodes a novel member of the family of cation-transporting p-type ATPases. The gene is expressed in extrahepatic tissues, and symptoms result from an inability to export copper from cells, particularly from intestinal cells and across the placenta. The syndrome has three forms, classic, mild, and occipital horn. Among the symptoms of the classic (most severe) Menkes' syndrome are abnormal myelination with cerebellar neurodegeneration (giving progressive mental retardation), abnormal (steely, kinky) hair, hypothermia, hypopigmentation, seizures, convulsions, failure to thrive, and connective tissue abnormalities resulting in deformities in the skull, long bones and ribs, and twisted, tortuous arteries. Death usually occurs in the severe forms before 3 years of age.

Wilson's disease, which affects 1 in 30 000 in most populations, is caused by numerous (over 100 recognized) mutations in the gene for a copper-transporting ATPase. The defect results in impaired biliary excretion of copper and accumulation of copper in the liver and brain of homozygous individuals or compound heterozygotes. Abnormalities in copper homeostatis, however, may also occur in heterozygous carriers, who may make up 1–2% of the population. The age of onset is from childhood onwards and patients may present in three different ways: with hepatic symptoms (liver cirrhosis and fatty infiltration in the latter stages), with neurological symptoms (degeneration of the basal ganglia resulting in defective movement, slurred speech, difficulty swallowing, face and muscle spasms, dystonia, and poor motor control), or with psychiatric and behavioral problems (including depression and schizophrenia, loss of emotional control, temper tantrums, and insomnia). Kayser–Fleischer rings (corneal copper deposits) in the eyes are generally present in neurological or psychiatric presentations. The phenotypic differences between Wilson's disease and Menkes' syndrome are probably owing to the tissue-specific expression of the ATPase genes.

If Wilson's disease is diagnosed early, copper chelation therapy, usually with D-penicillamine, can be beneficial, although neurological symptoms are often irreversible and liver disease may be advanced at the time of diagnosis. Zinc supplements limit copper absorption and subsequent accumulation, and this is the treatment of choice for maintenance therapy.

Aceruloplasminemia, which affects about 1 in 2 million individuals, is caused by mutations in the ceruloplasmin gene. Ceruloplasmin is involved in iron metabolism and, in the disease, there is an accumulation of ferrous iron within the recticuloendothelial system with pathogenesis mainly linked to the slow accumulation of iron in the brain, rather than other tissues. Symptoms include dementia, speech problems, retinal degeneration, poor muscle tone, and diabetes. Early therapy with the high-affinity iron chelator desferoxamine can relieve some of the symptoms.

Disruption of copper metabolism may be involved in other neurodegenerative diseases such as the accumulation of amyloid β-protein in Alzheimer's disease and the accumulation of modified prion protein in human prion disease.

About 10% of motor neuron disease cases are familial and 20% of these are owing to autosomal dominant inheritance of mutations in the Cu/Zn-SOD (*SODI*) gene. It is unclear how changes in activity of this copper enzyme might be involved in the progressive muscle weakness and atrophy of motor neuron disease or in Down's syndrome, where additional Cu/Zn-SOD activity results from the *SODI* gene being present in the extra chromosome 21.

Assessing status

It is possible to diagnose severe copper deficiency in infants from plasma or serum copper, ceruloplasmin protein, and neutrophils. These measures, however, cannot be used to detect suboptimal copper status in individuals, as such measures are insensitive to small changes in copper status and there are intractable problems in interpretation. Ceruloplasmin, the major copper protein in plasma or serum, is an acute-phase reactant and is raised by cigarette smoking, oral contraceptives, estrogens, pregnancy, infections, inflammation, hematological diseases, hypertension, diabetes, cardiovascular diseases, cancer, and cirrhosis, and after surgery and exercise.

Currently, there is no adequate measure of suboptimal (or supraoptimal) copper status and this is a major barrier to determining precise dietary requirements for copper and the possible role of suboptimal or supraoptimal copper status in the etiology of chronic disease. Table 9.16 gives some of the functional indices (classified as molecular, biochemical, and physiological) that might be used to define suboptimal or supraoptimal status in humans. A valid functional index of copper status in humans must respond sensitively, specifically, and predictably to changes in the concentration and supply of dietary copper or copper stores, be accessible for measurement and measurable, and impact directly on health. As such, indices in Table 9.16 have not been validated and many lack sensitivity and specificity. Perhaps, the best way forward is to use a combination of measures. Among the more promising are erythrocyte super-oxide dismutase activity, platelet cytochrome c oxidase, plasma diamine oxidase, plasma peptidyl glycine α-amidating mono-oxygenase, urinary pyridinium cross-links of collagen (may indicate lowered activity of the cuproenzyme, lysyl oxidase), and various immunological measures.

Table 9.16 Putative functional indices of copper status

Molecular indices
Changes in activity/concentration of Cu-metalloproteins
Ceruloplasmin oxidase
Ceruloplasmin protein
Superoxide dismutase
Cytochrome c oxidase
Lysyl oxidase
Diamine oxidase
Dopamine β-monooxygenase
Peptidylglycine α-amidating monooxygenase
Tyrosinase
Factor V
Factor VIII
Transcuprein

Biochemical indices
Pyridinium cross-links of collagen
Various measures of oxidative stress (TBARS)
Catecholamines
Encephalins
Polyamines

Physiological indices
Immune function
Hemostasis
Cholesterol metabolism
Glucose tolerance
Blood pressure
Arterial compliance
Arterial plaque
DNA damage and repair
Bone density

Requirements and dietary sources

Although copper is the third most abundant trace element, after iron and zinc, in the body, precise dietary requirements for copper are still subject to conjecture because of the difficulty in assessing copper status. Current estimates suggest that the requirements for copper for the great majority of adults are below about 1.5 mg copper/day, while most people can tolerate 3 mg copper/day or more over the long term and 8–10 mg copper/day or more in the shorter term (over several months). Using similar data from copper supplementation trials where there was an absence of any adverse effects on liver function, UL for copper was derived to be 10 mg/day in the US and 5 mg/day in the EU; the difference owing to the use of different uncertainty factors in the derivation.

Estimates of average intakes of copper are about 1.5 and 1.2 mg copper/day for men and women, respectively, on mixed diets, with higher intakes for those on vegetarian diets or those consuming water with appreciable concentrations of copper. Particularly rich food sources of copper include offal, seafood, nuts, seeds, legumes, wholegrain cereals, and chocolate. Milk and dairy products are very low in copper and infants are at risk of copper deficiency if they are fed exclusively on cow's milk.

Micronutrient interactions

The major micronutrient interactions with copper are those involving zinc and iron, high intakes of which can restrict copper utilization in infants and adults. The mechanism by which zinc appears to exert on antagonistic effect on copper status is through the induction of metallothionein synthesis by zinc in mucosal cells in the intestine. Metallothionein has a particularly strong affinity for copper. Metallothionein-bound copper is not available for transport into the circulation and is eventually lost in the feces when the mucosal cells are sloughed off. Molybdenum also has a strong interaction with copper and thiomolybdates are potent systemic copper antagonists. Although both cadmium and lead can inhibit copper utilization, this inhibition only occurs at dietary intakes of these heavy metals above those normally consumed by humans. Vitamin E, selenium, and manganese have metabolic interactions with copper as antioxidants, but data on beneficial interactions of these on symptoms of copper deficiency are largely confined to animal studies. Copper deficiency exerts an effect on iodine metabolism resulting in hypothyroidism, at least in animal models.

9.10 Selenium

Selenium is a nonmetallic element that has similar chemical properties to sulfur and has four natural oxidation states $(0, -2, +4, +6)$. It combines with other elements to form inorganic selenides [sodium selenide (-2) Na_2Se], selenites [sodium selenite $(+4)$ Na_2SeO_3] and selenates [sodium selenate $(+6)$ Na_2SeO_4], and with oxygen to form oxides [selenium $(+4)$ dioxide SeO_2] and oxyacids [selenic $(+6)$ acid H_2SeO_4]. Selenium replaces sulfur to form a large number of organic selenium compounds, particularly as selenocysteine, the twenty-first amino acid. Selenium is a component of selenoproteins, where it also occurs as selenides on the side-chains of selenocysteine at physiological pH. Selenium also displaces sulfur to form the amino acid selenomethionine.

Elemental selenium is stable and has three allotropic forms, deep red crystals, red amorphous powder, and the black vitreous form.

Selenium has many industrial uses, e.g., in electronics, glass, ceramics, pigments, as alloys in steel, as catalysts in pharmaceutical production, in rubber vulcanization and in agriculture, as feed supplements and fertilizers. Because of its increasing use, selenium has become a potential health and environmental hazard. The primary pathway of exposure to selenium for the general population is food, followed by water (predominantly inorganic selenate and selenite), and air (mainly as elemental particulate selenium from combustion of fossil fuels and from volcanic gas).

Absorption, transport and tissue distribution

Absorption of dietary selenium takes place mainly in the small intestine, where some 50–80% is absorbed. Organic forms of selenium are more readily absorbed than inorganic forms and selenium compounds from plants are generally more bioavailable than those from animals, and particularly from fish. Some naturally occurring inorganic and organic compounds of selenium are given in Table 9.17.

The bioavailability of selenium from water (mainly inorganic selenates) and supplements is lower than from food. The overall bioavailability of selenium from the diet depends on a number of factors, including selenium status, lipid composition, and metals.

Inorganic forms of selenium are passively transported across the intestinal brush border, whereas organic forms (selenomethionine and probably selenocysteine) are actively transported. On reaching the bloodstream, selenium is transported largely bound to protein (mainly very low-density β-lipoprotein with a small amount bound to albumin) for

Table 9.17 Some naturally occurring inorganic and organic compounds of selenium

Selenite $\{SeO_3^{2-}\}$
Selenate $\{SeO_4^{2-}\}$
Methylselenol (CH_3SH)
Dimethylselenide (CH_3-Se-CH_3)
Trimethyselenonium ion [($CH_3)_3$-Se^+]
Selenocysteine
Selenomethionine
Se-Methyl-selenocysteine

deposition in various organs. Liver and kidney are the major target organs when selenium intake is high but, at lower intakes, the selenium content of the liver is decreased. Heart and muscle tissue are other target organs, with the latter, because of its total bulk, accounting for the greatest proportion of body selenium. The total body content of selenium can vary from about 3 mg to 15 mg depending on dietary intakes.

In the body, dietary selenium can be bound to selenium binding proteins but can also be directly incorporated into selenoproteins during translation at the ribosome complex using a transfer RNA specific for the amino acid selenocysteine; thus, selenocysteine can be considered as the twenty-first amino acid in terms of ribosome-mediated protein synthesis.

The major excretion routes of selenium are in urine (mainly as trimethylselenonium ion), in feces (via biliary pancreatic and intestinal secretions, together with unabsorbed dietary selenium), and in breath (as volatile dimethylselenide). Unlike copper, and particularly iron, which have inefficient excretion mechanisms, selenium is rapidly excreted in the urine. Figure 9.7 gives an overall view of selenium metabolism and excretion.

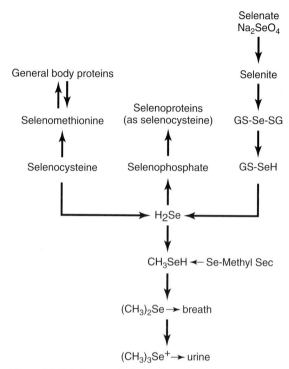

Figure 9.7 Selenium metabolism and excretion.

Metabolic function and essentiality

Selenocysteine is a component of at least 30 selenoproteins, some of which have important enzymic functions (Table 9.18). Selenocysteine is generally at the active site of those selenoproteins with catalytic activity, and functions as a redox center for the selenium-dependent glutathione peroxidases (cystolic, phospholipid hydroperoxide, extracellular, and gastrointestinal), iodothyronine deiodinases (types I, II, and III), and thioredoxin reductases. The glutathione peroxidase isozymes, which account for about 36% of total body selenium, differ in their tissue expression and map to different chromosomes.

Deficiency symptoms

Keshan's disease is a cardiomyopathy that affects children and women of child-bearing age and occurs in areas of China where the soil is deficient in selenium. Despite the strong evidence for an etiological role for selenium in Keshan's disease (i.e., the occurrence of the disease only in those regions of China with low selenium soils and, hence, low amounts of selenium in the food chain, and only in those individuals with

poor selenium status together with the prevention of the disease in an at-risk population by supplementation with selenium), there are certain epidemiological features of the disease that are not readily explained solely on the basis of selenium deficiency. A similar situation occurs with Kashin–Beck disease, a chronic osteoarthropathy that most commonly affects growing children and occurs in parts of Siberian Russia and in China, where it overlaps with Keshan's disease. Although oral supplementation with selenium is effective in preventing the disease, it is likely that other factors, apart from selenium deficiency, are involved in the etiology of Kashin–Beck disease. There are also some selenium-responsive conditions with symptoms similar to Keshan's disease that occur in patients receiving total parenteral nutrition.

One explanation for the complex etiology of selenium-responsive diseases in humans is that low selenium status may predispose to other deleterious conditions, most notably the increased incidence, virulence, or disease progression of a number of viral infections. For example, in a selenium-deficient animal model, harmless coxsackie virus can become virulent and cause myocarditis, not only in the

Table 9.18 Selenoproteins

Selenoprotein	Function
Glutathione peroxidases (GPx1, GPx2, GPx3, GPx4; cystolic, gastrointestinal, extracellular and phospholipid hydroperoxide, respectively)	Antioxidant enzymes: remove hydrogen peroxide, and lipid and phospholipid hydroperoxides (thereby maintaining membrane integrity, modulating eiconsanoid synthesis, modifying inflammation, and likelihood of propagation of further oxidative damage to biomolecules, such as lipids, lipoproteins and DNA)
(Sperm) mitochondrial capsule selenoprotein	Form of glutathione peroxidase (GPx4): shields developing sperm cells from oxidative damage and later polymerizes into structural protein required for stability/motility of mature sperm
Iodothyronine deiodinases (three isoforms)	Production and regulation of level of active thyroid hormone, T_3, from thryoxine T_4
Thioredoxin reductases (three isoforms)	Reduction of nucleotides in DNA synthesis; regeneration of antioxidant systems; maintenance of intracellular redox state, critical for cell viability and proliferation; regulation of gene expression by redox control of binding of transcription factors to DNA
Selenophosphate synthetase, SPS2	Required for biosynthesis of selenophosphate, the precursor of selenocysteine, and therefore for selenoprotein synthesis
Selenoprotein P	Found in plasma and associated with endothelial cells; appears to protect endothelial cells against damage from peroxynitrite
Selenoprotein W	Needed for muscle function
Prostate epithelial selenoprotein (15 kDa)	Found in epithelial cells of ventral prostate; seems to have redox function (resembles GPx4), perhaps protecting secretory cells against development of carcinoma
DNA-bound spermatid selenoprotein (34 kDa)	Glutathione peroxidase-like activity; found in stomach and in nuclei of spermatoza; may protect developing sperm
18 kDa selenoprotein	Important selenoprotein, found in kidney and large number of other tissues; preserved in selenium deficiency

Reprinted with permission from Elsevier (Rayman, MP *Lancet*, 2000, **356**, pp. 233–241).

selenium-deficient host, but also when isolated and injected into selenium-replete animals. A coxsackie virus has been isolated from the blood and tissues of patients with Keshan's disease and the infection may be responsible for the cardiomyopathy of that disease. It has been speculated that similar events linked with other RNA viruses may explain the emergence of new strains of influenza virus in China and the postulated crossing-over of the human immunodeficiency virus (HIV) to humans in the selenium-deficient population of Zaire. Many human viral pathogens (e.g., HIV, coxsackie, hepatitis, and measles viruses) can synthesize viral selenoproteins and, thereby, lower the selenium available to the host. In any event, selenium deficiency is accompanied by loss of immunocompetence, with the impairment of both cell-mediated immunity and B-cell function. Covert suboptimal selenium status may be widespread in human populations, as selenium supplementation in subjects considered to be selenium replete had marked immunostimulant effects, including increased proliferation of activated T-cells. Such immunostimulant effects or the production of antitumorigenic metabolites may explain the lowering of cancer incidence, particularly prostate cancer, after selenium supplementation in selenium-replete subjects (those who already had maximized selenoenzyme activity). Other proposed mechanisms for a cancer chemoprotective effect of selenium include antioxidant protection and reduction of inflammation; inactivation of protein kinase C; altered carcinogen metabolism; reduction in DNA damage, stimulation of DNA repair (p53), and alteration in DNA methylation; cell cycle effects; enhanced apoptosis and inhibition of angiogenesis. Further evidence for any chemoprotective effect of selenium against cancer should arise from the Selenium and Vitamin E cancer Prevention Trial (SELECT), which is a large randomized controlled trial investigating the efficacy of selenium (200 μg of L-selenomethionine) and vitamin E (400 IU, dl-α-tocopherol acetate) alone and in combination for the prevention of prostate cancer in over 35 000 healthy men in 435 sites in the USA, Puerto Rico, and Canada and which should report sometime after 2008.

The evidence for suboptimal selenium status increasing the risk of cardiovascular disease is more fragmentary, but it has been proposed that optimizing the activity of the seleno-dependent glutathione peroxidases and, thereby, increasing antioxidant activity may be a factor. As selenium has well-recognized antioxidant and anti-inflammatory roles, other oxidative stress or inflammatory conditions (e.g., rheumatoid arthritis, ulcerative colitis, pancreatitis, and asthma) may benefit from selenium supplementation. In addition, some, but certainly not all, studies have suggested beneficial (possibly antioxidant) effects of selenium on mood and reproduction in humans. The evidence, however, supporting a role for optimum selenium status preventing or ameliorating most inflammatory conditions is not strong and may be confounded by other dietary antioxidants, particularly vitamin E, compensating for low selenium status.

Toxicity

There is a narrow margin, perhaps not much more than three- or fourfold, between beneficial and harmful intakes of selenium. The dose necessary to cause chronic selenosis in humans is not well defined, but the threshold for toxicity appears to lie somewhere in the range of 850–900 mg/day. Symptoms of chronic selenium toxicity include brittle hair and nails, skin lesions with secondary infections, and garlic odor on the breath, resulting from the expiration of dimethyl selenide. Toxicity depends on the chemical form of selenium, with most forms having low toxicity. Data from animal studies indicate that selenite and selenocysteine are a little more toxic than selenomethionine and much more toxic than other organic selenium compounds (dimethyl selenide, trimethyselenonium ion, selenoethers, selenobetaine). Methylation in the body is important for detoxification of the element.

Genetic diseases

Although no important genetic diseases affecting selenium status are apparent, polymorphisms in gene sequences of some selenoenzymes may determine selenium utilization and metabolic needs, and hence dietary requirements. These polymorphisms may explain the signifi-cant variation among individuals in the extent of the response to supplementation of selenoenzyme activities.

Assessing status

Plasma or whole blood, hair, and toenail selenium concentrations can indicate changes in selenium status in humans. Plasma and serum selenium concentrations respond rapidly to changes in selenium intakes, whereas erythrocyte selenium is an index of longer term or chronic intake. Dietary intake data, however, are insufficient to determine selenium status in individuals because of uncertainties about bioavailability and variations in the content and form of selenium in foodstuffs. Although plasma (or preferably platelet) glutathione peroxidase activities have been used as functional indices to estimate selenium requirements, it has not been established how these measurements relate to other biochemical functions of selenium, such as thyroid metabolism, or immune function and their health sequelae. For example, at higher levels of selenium intake, glutathione peroxidase activities plateau but immunoenhancement may be evident at supplementation levels higher than those needed to optimize the selenoenzyme activity. Perhaps the best way forward is to select from a battery of functional indices, such as selenoenzyme activity, plasma thyroid hormone concentrations, and immune measures, according to the function or disease under investigation.

Requirements and dietary sources

Dietary intakes of selenium vary widely with geographical spread (Table 9.19). Requirements for selenium have been estimated at intakes required to saturate plasma glutathione peroxidase activity

Table 9.19 Dietary selenium intakes worldwide

Country (region)	Range (µg/day)
Australia	57–87
Canada	98–224
China (Keshan county)	3–22
China (Enshi county)	3200–6690
Greece	110–220
Mexico	10–223
New Zealand (Dunedin)	6–70
Portugal	10–100
Russia	60–80
UK	30–60
USA	62–216

After Reilly, *Selenium in Food and Health,* copyright 1996 with kind permission of Springer Science + Business Media.

(which corresponds to lower status and intake than that needed to saturate platelet glutathione peroxidase activity) in the vast majority (97.5%) of all individuals in a population. The RDAs for both men and women is 55 μg/day in the USA. In the UK, the reference nutrient intake (RNI) has thus been set at 75 and 60 μg/day selenium for men and women, respectively. Blood selenium concentrations in the UK population have declined by approximately 50% over the past 30 years and current UK intakes are only about 50% of the RNI. As explained previously, however, there is uncertainty as to what constitutes optimum selenium status and the intakes of selenium in various dietary regimens needed to achieve optimum status. Optimum status may not necessarily be reflected in saturated glutathione peroxidase activity. The UL for adults is set at 400 μg/day in the USA and at 300 μg/day in the EU.

Selenium enters the food chain through plants that, in general, largely reflect concentrations of the element in the soil on which the plants were grown. The absorption of selenium by plants, however, is dependent not only on soil selenium content but also on pH, microbial activity, rainfall, and the chemical form of selenium. Higher plants absorb selenium preferentially as selenate and can synthesize organic selenium compounds, e.g., selenomethionine, and to a lesser extent selenocysteine. Brazil nuts contain high concentrations of selenium because of the seleniferous soils in the Andes mountains but also the efficiency of accumulation of selenium by the plants species. Selenium concentrations of cereals and staples are much lower, but the content and bioavailability of selenium in wheat usually make this a major contributor to overall selenium intakes because of the high quantities of wheat consumed as bread and other baked products. Wheat is the most efficient accumulator of selenium within the common cereal crops (wheat > rice > maize > barley > oats). There are major varietal differences in selenium uptake and for wheat, tomatoes, soybean, and onions, there are up to fourfold differences in uptake of selenium from soils amongst cultivars. The ability of plants to accumulate selenium has been useful for agronomic biofortification, which differs from food fortification where the nutrient is added during food processing. The Finnish Policy (1984) has led to a 10-fold increase in cereal grain selenium concentration as well as marked increases in fruit and vegetables and meat concentrations as a result of adding selenium to fertilizers used for grain production and horticulture and fodder crop and hay production. The resulting increase in the selenium status of the population is largely owing to wheat (bread) consumption but the biofortification of vegetables may also have an impact on public health as, in contrast to wheat, where the major selenocompound is selenomethionine, selenomethylselenocysteine is the predominant form in vegetables; the last compound may have important cancer chemoprotective effects (see also Figure 9.8) Fish, shellfish, and offal (liver, kidney) are rich sources of selenium, followed by meat and eggs. Animal sources, however, have lower bioavailability of selenium than do plant sources.

Micronutrient interactions

Selenium is an antioxidant nutrient and has important interactions with other antioxidant micronutrients, especially vitamin E (Figure 9.8). Vitamin E, as an antioxidant, can ameliorate some of the symptoms of selenium deficiencies in animals. Copper deficiency also increases oxidative stress, and the expression of glutathione peroxidase genes is decreased in the copper-deficient animal.

The metabolic interactions between selenium and other micronutrients, however, extend beyond those between selenium, vitamin E, and other antioxidants. Peripheral deiodination of thyroxine (T_4), the predominant hormone secreted by the thyroid, to the more biologically active triiodothyronine (T_3) in extrathyroidal tissues is accomplished through the selenium-dependent deiodinase enzymes. Selenium deficiency, therefore, can contribute to iodine deficiency disorders, and goiter complications have been noted in up to 80% of Keshan's disease casualties after autopsy. Moreover, higher serum T_4 concentrations were found in patients with subacute Keshan's disease and in children with latent Keshan's disease compared with the respective controls. All thyroid hormone concentrations in these studies were within normal ranges, suggesting that selenium deficiency, or even suboptimal selenium status, was blocking optimum thyroid and iodine metabolism.

Excess selenium intake interferes with zinc bioavailability, decreases tissue iron stores, and increases copper concentrations in the heart, liver, and kidney. Vitamins C and E, sulfur amino acids and sulfate, arsenic, and heavy metals can decrease the toxicity of

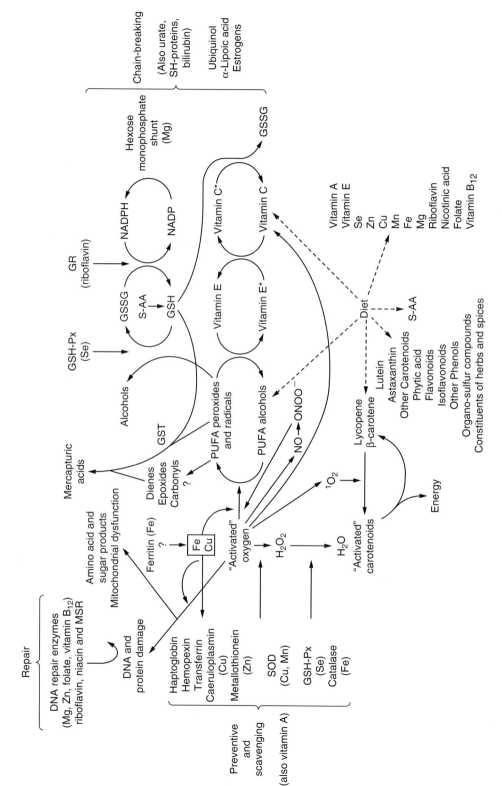

GR, glutathione reductase (EC1.6.4.2); GSH, reduced glutathione; GSH-Px glutathione peroxidase (EC1.11.1.9); GSSG, oxidized glutathione; GST, glutathione-S-transferase (EC 2.5.1.18); MSR, methionine sulfoxide reductase (EC1.8.4.5); PUFA, polyunsaturated fatty acids; S-AA, sulfur amino acids; SH-proteins, sulfydryl proteins; SOD, superoxide dismutase (EC1.15.1.1); $\boxed{\substack{\text{Fe}\\\text{Cu}}}$, transition metal-catalyzed oxidant damage to biomolecules. ? Biological relevance.

Figure 9.8 Antioxidant defense system (from Strain and Benzie, 1999).

selenium. Conversely, selenium modifies the toxicity of many heavy metals. In seafoods, selenium is combined with mercury or methyl mercury and this interaction may be one of the factors that decreases the bioavailability of selenium in these foods. Indeed, well-known antagonistic interactions of selenium with both mercury and arsenic suggest that selenium can promote detoxification effects with respect to these toxins.

9.11 Iodine

Iodine is a nonmetallic element of the halogen group with common oxidation states of −1 (iodides), +5 (iodates), and +7 (periodates), and less common states of +1 (iodine monochloride) and +3 (iodine trichloride). Elemental iodine (0) is a soft blue–black solid, which sublimes readily to form a violet gas.

The principal industrial uses of iodine are in the pharmaceutical industry, medical and sanitary uses (e.g., iodized salt, water treatment, protection from radioactive iodine, and disinfectants), as catalysts (synthetic rubber, acetic acid synthesis), and in animal feeds, herbicides, dyes, inks, colorants, photographic equipment, lasers, metallurgy, conductive polymers, and stabilizers (nylon). Naturally occurring iodine minerals are rare and occur usually in the form of calcium iodates. Commercial production of iodine is largely restricted to extraction from Chilean deposits of nitrates (saltpeter) and iodine in caliche (soluble salts precipitated by evaporation), and from concentrated salt brine in Japan. Iodine is the least abundant halogen in the Earth's crust, at concentrations of 0.005%. The content of iodine in soils varies and much of the original content has been leached out in areas of high rainfall, previous glaciation, and soil erosion.

The concentration of iodine (as iodide and iodate) in the oceans is higher, at about 0.06 mg/l. Iodine volatilizes from the surface of the oceans and sea spray as salt particles, iodine vapor or methyl iodide vapor. Some iodine can then return to land in rainwater (0.0018–0.0085 mg iodine/l). There is a large variation of iodine content in drinking water (0.0001–0.1 mg iodine/l).

Absorption, transport, and tissue distribution

Iodine, usually as an iodide or iodate compound in food and water, is rapidly absorbed in the intestine and circulates in the blood to all tissues in the body. The thyroid gland traps most (about 80%) of the ingested iodine, but salivary glands, the gastric mucosa, choroid plexus, and the lactating mammary gland also concentrate the element by a similar active transport mechanism. Several sulfur-containing compounds, thiocyanate, isothiocyanate, and goitrin inhibit this active transport by competing for uptake with iodide, and their goitrogenic activity can be overcome by iodine supplementation. These active goitrogens are released by plant enzymes from thioglucosides or cyanogenic glucosides found in cassava, kale, cabbage, sprouts, broccoli, kohlrabi, turnips, swedes, rapeseed, and mustard. The most important of these goitrogen-containing foods is cassava, which can be detoxified by soaking in water. Tobacco smoke also contributes thiocyanate and other antithyroid compounds to the circulation.

Metabolic functions and essentiality

Iodine is an essential constituent of the thyroid hormones, thyroxine (T_4) and triiodothyronine (T_3), which have key modifying or permissive roles in development and growth. Although T_4 is quantitatively predominant, T_3 is the more active. The mechanism of action of thyroid hormones appears to involve binding to nuclear receptors that, in turn, alter gene expression in the pituitary, liver, heart, kidney, and, most crucially, brain cells. Overall, thyroid hormones stimulate enzyme synthesis, oxygen consumption and basal metabolic rate and, thereby, affect the heart rate, respiratory rate, mobilization, and metabolism of carbohydrates, lipogenesis and a wide variety of other physiological activities. It is probable that iodine has additional roles to those of thyroid hormone activity, for example in antibiotic and anticancer activity, but these are poorly understood.

Once iodide (−1) is trapped from the circulation and actively transported to the lumen of the thyroid gland, it is oxidized to I_2 (0) and reacts with tyrosine in thyroglobulin protein to form monoiodotyrosine or diiodotyrosine. These reactions are catalyzed by thyroid peroxidase. The iodinated compounds, in turn, couple to form T_3 and T_4, which are secreted from the thyroid into the circulation.

Flavonoids, found in many plants, including pearl millet, and phenol derivatives, released into water from soil humus, inhibit thyroid peroxidase and the organification of iodide. The concentration of iodine in the thyroid gland also affects the uptake of iodide into the follicle, the ratio of T_3 to T_4, and the rate of release of these hormones into the circulation. This process is also under hormonal control by the hypothalamus of the brain, which produces thyroid-releasing hormone, which then stimulates the pituitary gland to secrete thyroid-stimulating hormone (TSH), which, in turn, acts on the thyroid gland to produce more thyroid hormones.

Almost all of the thyroid hormones released from the thyroid are bound to transport proteins, mainly thyroxine-binding globulin. The longer half-life of T_4 ensures that there is a reservoir for conversion to the more active T_3 with a much shorter half-life of 1 day. The deiodination of T_4 to T_3 takes place in extrathyroidal tissues (mainly the liver). Excretion of iodine is predominantly in the urine.

Deficiency symptoms

A deficiency of iodine causes a wide spectrum of disorders from mild goiter (a larger thyroid gland than normal) to the most severe forms of endemic congenital hypothyroidism (cretinism) (severe, irreversible mental, and growth retardation). Collectively, these manifestations of iodine deficiency are termed iodine deficiency disorders (IDDs) and symptoms differ depending on the life stage at which iodine deficiency occurs. The most severe disorders (congenital hypothyroidism) arise if the fetus suffers from iodine deficiency. The clinical features of endemic congenital hypothyroidism are either a predominant neurological syndrome with severe to profound mental retardation, including defects of hearing and speech (often deaf–mutism), squint, and disorders of stance and gait of varying degrees (neurological congenital hypothyroidism), or predominant features of hypothyroidism and stunted growth with less severe mental retardation (myxedematous congenital hypothyroidism). Profound hypothyroidism is biochemically defined as high serum TSH and very low T_4 and T_3, and is accompanied by a low basal metabolic rate, apathy, slow reflex relaxation time with slow movements, cold intolerance, and myxedema (skin and subcutaneous tissue are thickened because of an accumulation of mucin, and become dry and swollen). Although congenital hypothyroidism is the severest form of IDD, varying degrees of intellectual or growth retardation are apparent when iodine deficiency occurs in the fetus, infancy or childhood and adolescence. In adulthood, the consequences of iodine deficiency are more serious in women, especially during pregnancy, than in men.

The mildest form of IDD, goiters, range from those only detectable by touch (palpation) to very large goiters that can cause breathing problems. The enlargement of the thyroid gland to produce goiter arises from stimulation of the thyroid cells by TSH and, without the ability to increase hormone production owing to iodine deficiency, the gland becomes hyperplastic.

Apart from congenital hypothyroidism, hypothyroidism, and goiter, other features linked to IDDs are decreased fertility rates, increased stillbirth and spontaneous abortion rates, and increased perinatal and infant mortality. The public health significance of iodine deficiency cannot be underestimated, with over 1 billion people (worldwide, but mostly in Asia and Africa) estimated to be living in iodine-deficient areas and, therefore, at risk of IDDs. Estimates of those with IDDs demonstrate the scale of the problem, with 200–300 million goitrous people, over 40 million affected by some degree of mental impairment and some 7 million people with congenital hypothyroidism. Fortunately, these figures should decrease as public health programs using preventive interventions with iodized oil (oral or intramuscular injection) salt, bread, water, or even sugar have an impact. Treatment with iodine supplementation in older children and adults can reverse many of the clinical manifestations of IDDs, including mental deficiency, hypothyroidism and goiter. Although iodine deficiency is the primary cause of IDDs, goitrogenic factors limiting bioavailability appear to be superimposed on the primary cause. In addition, genetic variation, immunological factors, sex, age, and growth factors seem to modify expression of the conditions, producing a wide range of symptoms and severity of IDDs with similar iodine intakes.

Toxicity

A wide range of iodine intakes is tolerated by most individuals, owing to the ability of the thyroid to regulate total body iodine. Over 2 mg iodine/day for long periods should be regarded as excessive or potentially harmful to most people. Such high intakes are unlikely to arise from natural foods, except for diets that are very high in seafood and/or seaweed or comprising foods contaminated with iodine. In contrast to iodine-replete individuals, those with IDDs or previously exposed to iodine-deficient diets may react to sudden moderate increases in iodine intake, such as from iodized salt. Iodine-induced thyrotoxicosis (hyperthyroidism) and toxic nodular goiter may result from excess iodine exposure in these individuals. Hyperthyroidism is largely confined to those over 40 years of age and symptoms are rapid heart rate, trembling, excessive sweating, lack of sleep, and loss of weight and strength.

Individuals who are sensitive to iodine, usually have mild skin symptoms, but very rarely fever, salivary gland enlargement, visual problems, and skin problems, and, in severe cases, cardiovascular collapse, convulsions, and death may occur. The occurrence of allergic symptoms, for example to iodine medications or antiseptics, however, is rare.

Genetic diseases

Pendred's syndrome is an autosomal recessive inherited disorder with a frequency of 100 or less per 100 000. It is characterized by goiter and profound deafness in childhood and is caused by mutations in the Pendrin gene located on chromosome 7. The gene codes for pendrin, a transporter protein for chloride/iodine transport across the thyroid apical membrane. This results in defective iodination of thyroglobulin. Mutations in another gene, the sodium/iodide symporter (*NIS*) gene, occasionally cause defective iodide transport and goiter, whereas single nucleotide polymorphisms in the TSH receptor gene may predispose individuals to the hyperthyroidism of toxic multinodular goiter and Graves' disease.

Assessing status

The critical importance of iodine for the thyroid indicates that iodine status is assessed by thyroid function. A standard set of indicators (goiter by palpation, thyroid volume by ultrasound, median urinary iodine, and whole blood TSH) is used to determine prevalence in countries with endemic deficiency. Measurement of plasma thyroid hormones (TSH, T_4, and T_3) provides useful indicators of functional iodine status in the individual. Of these, TSH is the most sensitive functional indicator of suboptimal iodine status. Concentrations of T_4 decline in more severe iodine deficiency whereas T_3 concentrations decline only in the most severe of iodine deficiencies.

Dietary intakes and requirements

Requirements in infancy and childhood range from 40 to 150 µg iodine/day. Adult requirements are estimated at 150 µg iodine/day, increasing to 175 and 200 µg/day for pregnancy and lactation. The UL for adults is set at 600 µg/day (EU) and at 1.1 mg/day (USA).

Under normal circumstances, about 90% of iodine intake is from food, with about 10% from water. The concentration of iodine in most foods is low and, in general, reflects the iodine content of the soil, water, and fertilizers used in plant and animal production. In most countries other sources, such as iodized salts or foods, are required. Seafoods and seaweed concentrate iodine from seawater and are particularly rich sources. In some populations, milk has become a major source of iodine, owing to the use of iodized salt licks and iodine-enriched cattle feed for dairy herds. Minor amounts may come from adventitious contamination from iodophor disinfectants (teat-dip). Iodine-enriched cattle feed will also increase the iodine content of meat for beef herds raised on concentrated feedstuffs. Processed foods contribute some additional iodine from food additives, such as calcium iodate used in the baking industry.

Micronutrient interactions

From a public health viewpoint, the most important metabolic interaction of iodine with other micronutrients is with selenium. Adequate selenium status is essential for thyroid hormone metabolism and, therefore, normal growth development, by ensuring sufficient T_3 supply to extrathyroidal tissues. Most T_3 is formed from T_4 by the selenium-dependent deiodinases. Iodine and selenium deficiencies overlap in various parts of the world and concurrent deficiencies of both may contribute to the etiologies of Kashin–Beck disease in Russia, China, and Tibet, and myxedematous congenital hypothyroidism in Zaire. In addition, both nutrients are required for normal reproduction, normal gene expression, synthesis of zenobiotic and metabolizing enzymes in the liver, and normal tolerance against cold stress. It is possible that hypothyroidism associated with suboptimal selenium status may explain some of the etiology of cardiovascular disease and certain cancers.

Hypothyroidism is associated with deficiencies of other trace elements, including zinc, iron, and copper, while there are close metabolic relationships at the molecular and transport levels between iodine and vitamin A. Conversely, the widespread disruption of metabolism in IDDs can affect the proper utilization of a host of other nutrients.

9.12 Manganese

Manganese is widely distributed in the biosphere: it constitutes approximately 0.085% of the Earth's crust, making it the twelfth most abundant element. Manganese is a component of numerous complex minerals, including pyroluosite, rhodochrosite, rhodanite, braunite, pyrochite, and manganite. Chemical forms of manganese in their natural deposits include oxides, sulfides, carbonates, and silicates. Anthropogenic sources of manganese are predominantly from the manufacturing of steel, alloys, and iron products. Manganese is also widely used as an oxidizing agent, as a component of fertilizers and fungicides, and in dry cell batteries. The permanganate is a powerful oxidizing agent and is used in quantitative analysis and medicine.

Manganese is a transition element. It can exist in 11 oxidation states from -3 to $+7$, with the most common valences being $+2$, $+4$, and $+7$. The $+2$ valence is the predominant form in biological systems, the $+4$ valence occurs in MnO_2, and the $+7$ valence is found in permanganate.

Absorption, transport, and tissue distribution

The total amount of manganese in the adult human is approximately 15 mg. Up to 25% of the total body stores of manganese may be located in the skeleton and may not be readily accessible for use in metabolic pathways. Relatively high concentrations have been reported in the liver, pancreas, intestine, and bone.

Intestinal absorption of manganese occurs throughout the length of the small intestine. Mucosal uptake appears to be mediated by two types of mucosal binding, one that is saturable with a finite capacity and one that is nonsaturable. Manganese absorption, probably as Mn^{2+}, is relatively inefficient, generally less than 5%, but there is some evidence of improvement at low intakes. High levels of dietary calcium, phosphorus, and phytate impair the intestinal uptake of the element but are probably of limited significance because, as yet, no well-documented

case of human manganese deficiency has been reported.

Systemic homeostatic regulation of manganese is brought about primarily through hepatobiliary excretion rather than through regulation of absorption (e.g., the efficiency of manganese retention does not appear to be dose dependent within normal dietary levels). Manganese is taken up from blood by the liver and transported to extrahepatic tissues by transferrin and possibly α_2-macroglobulin and albumin. Manganese is excreted primarily in feces. Urinary excretion of manganese is low and has not been found to be sensitive to dietary manganese intake.

Metabolic function and essentiality

Manganese is required as a catalytic cofactor for mitochondrial superoxide dismutase, arginase, and pyruvate carboxylase. It is also an activator of glycosyltransferases, phosphoenolpyruvate carboxylase, and glutamine synthetase.

Deficiency symptoms

Signs of manganese deficiency have been demonstrated in several animal species. Symptoms include impaired growth, skeletal abnormalities, depressed reproductive function, and defects in lipid and carbohydrate metabolism. Evidence of manganese deficiency in humans is poor. It has been suggested that manganese deficiency has never been observed in noninstitutionalized human populations because of the abundant supply of manganese in edible plant materials compared with the relatively low requirements of mammals. There is only one report of apparent human manganese deficiency. A male subject was fed a purified diet deficient in vitamin K, which was accidentally also deficient in manganese. Feeding this diet caused weight loss, dermatitis, growth retardation of hair and nails, reddening of black hair, and a decline in concentrations of blood lipids. Manganese deficiency may be more frequent in infants owing to the low concentration of manganese in human breast milk and varying levels in infant formulae.

Toxicity

Manganese toxicity of dietary origin has not been well documented. Toxicity has been observed only in workers exposed to high concentrations of manganese dust or fumes in air. For example, mine-workers in Chile exposed to manganese ore dust developed, possibly as a result of inhalation rather than ingestion, "manganic madness," manifested by psychosis, hallucinations, and extrapyramidal damage with features of parkinsonism.

In 2001, the US Food and Nutrition Board set the tolerable UL for manganese at 11 mg/day for adults (19 years and older). Elevated blood manganese concentrations and neurotoxicity were selected as the critical adverse effects on which to base their UL for manganese.

Assessing status

Progress in the field of manganese nutrition has been hampered because of the lack of a practical method for assessing manganese status. Blood manganese concentrations appear to reflect the body manganese status of rats fed deficient or adequate amounts of manganese, but consistent changes in blood or plasma manganese have not been observed in depleted or repleted human subjects. Researchers are actively investigating whether the activities of manganese-dependent enzymes, such as manganese-SOD in blood lymphocytes and blood arginase, may be of use in detecting low manganese intake; however, there is evidence that these enzymes can be influenced by certain disease states.

Requirements and dietary sources

Relatively high concentrations of manganese have been reported in cereals (20–30 mg/kg), brown bread (100–150 mg/kg), nuts (10–20 mg/kg), ginger (280 mg/kg), and tea (350–900 mg/kg dry tea). Concentrations of manganese in crops are dependent on soil factors such as pH, whereby increasing soil pH decreases plant uptake of manganese. Products of animal origin such as eggs, milk, fish, poultry, and red meat contain low amounts of manganese (Table 9.20). Many multivitamin and mineral supplements for adults provide 2.5–5.0 mg of manganese.

Table 9.20 Dietary sources of manganese

Rich sources (>20 mg/kg)	Intermediate sources (1–5 mg/kg)	Poor sources (<1 mg/kg)
Nuts	Green leafy vegetables	Animal tissue
Wholegrain cereals	Dried fruits	Poultry
Dried legumes	Fresh fruits	Dairy products
Tea	Nonleafy vegetables	Seafood

There is currently no RDA set for dietary manganese; instead, there is an AI value [these values were established by the US Food and Nutrition Board in 2001]: infants 0.003 mg (first 6 months), 0.6 mg (7–12 months), children 1.2 and 1.5 mg (1–3 and 4–8 years, respectively), teenage boys 1.9 and 2.2 mg (9–13 and 14–18 years, respectively), adult men 2.3 mg (19 years and older), teenage girls 1.6 mg (9–18 years), adult women 1.8 mg (19 years and older), pregnant women 2.0 mg, and lactating women 2.6 mg. The AI was set based on median intakes reported from the US Food and Drug Administration Total Diet Study.

Micronutrient interactions

Iron–manganese interactions have been demonstrated whereby iron deficiency increased manganese absorption, and high amounts of dietary iron inhibit manganese absorption, possibly by competition for similar binding and absorption sites between nonheme iron and manganese.

9.13 Molybdenum

Molybdenum does not exist naturally in the pure metallic state but rather in association with other elements, or predominantly in solution as the molybdate anion. Insoluble molybdenum compounds include molybdenum dioxide and molybdenum disulfide. The metal has five oxidation states (2–6), of which +4 and +6 are the predominant species. Major molybdenum-containing ores are molybdenum sulfites and ferric molybdenum ores, usually produced as by-products of copper mining operations, while other molybdenum salts are by-products of uranium mining. Molybdenum is used mostly in metallurgical applications such as stainless steel and cast iron alloys, and in metal–ceramic composites. Molybdenum compounds have anticorrosive and lubricant properties and can act as chemical catalysts.

Molybdenum uptake into plants and hence into the food chain occurs mostly from alkaline or neutral soils. Water usually contains little molybdenum except near major mining operations.

Absorption, transport, and tissue distribution

Molybdenum is readily absorbed (40–100%) from foods and is widely distributed in cells and in the ECF. Some accumulation can occur in liver, kidneys, bones, and skin. The major excretory route of molybdenum after ingestion is the urine, with significant amounts also excreted in bile.

Metabolic functions and essentiality

Molybdenum functions as a cofactor for the iron- and flavin-containing enzymes that catalyze the hydroxylation of various substrates. The molybdenum cofactor in the enzymes aldehyde oxidase (oxidizes and detoxifies purines and pyrimidines), xanthine oxidase/hydrogenase (production of uric acid from hypoxanthine and xanthine), and sulfite oxidase (conversion of sulfite to sulfate) has molybdenum incorporated as part of the molecule.

Deficiency symptoms

Although there is a clear biochemical basis for the essentiality of molybdenum, deficiency signs in humans and animals are difficult to induce. Naturally occurring deficiency, uncomplicated by molybdenum antagonists, is not known with certainty. In animal experiments, where large amounts of the molybdenum antagonist tungsten have been fed, deficiency signs are depressed food consumption and growth, impaired reproduction, and elevated copper concentrations in the liver and brain.

Toxicity

In 2001, the US Food and Nutrition Board set the tolerable UL for molybdenum at 2 mg/day for adults (aged 19 years and older). Impaired reproduction and growth in animals were selected as the critical adverse effects on which to base their UL for molybdenum.

Genetic diseases

A rare unborn error of metabolism, resulting in the absence of the molybdenum pterin cofactor, may give some clue to the essentiality of molybdenum. These patients have severe neurological dysfunction, dislocated ocular lenses, mental retardation, and biochemical abnormalities, including increased urinary excretion of xanthine and sulfite and decreased urinary excretion of uric acid and sulfate.

Assessing status

Determining the body status of molybdenum is difficult. Homeostatic control of molybdenum ensures that plasma concentrations are not elevated, except after extremely high dietary intakes. Decreased urinary concentrations of sulfite, hypoxanthine, zorithine, and other sulfur metabolites, however, are generally indicative of impaired activities of the molybdoenzymes. Adult requirements for molybdenum have been estimated at about 45 μg/day (Institute of Medicine, USA, 2001). Average intakes tend to be considerably above this value. Milk, beans, bread, and cereals (especially the germ) are good sources of molybdenum, and water also contributes small amounts to the total dietary intakes.

Micronutrient interactions

The major micronutrient interactions with molybdenum are those involving tungsten and copper. Molybdenum supplementation depletes body levels of the essential trace element, copper, and has been used as a chelating agent for conditions such as Wilson's disease, which cause elevated concentrations of copper in the body.

9.14 Fluoride

Fluorine occurs chiefly in fluorspar and cryolite, but is widely distributed in other minerals. Fluoride is the ionic form of fluorine, a halogen, and the most electronegative of the elements in the periodic table; the two terms are often used interchangeably. Fluorine and its compounds are used in producing uranium and more than 100 commercial fluorochemicals, including many well-known high-temperature plastics. Hydrofluoric acid is extensively used for etching the glass of light bulbs, etc. Fluorochlorohydrocarbons are extensively used in air conditioning and refrigeration. Fluorine is present in small but widely varying concentrations in practically all soils, water supplies, plants and animals, and is a constituent of all diets.

Absorption, transport and tissue distribution

Fluoride appears to be soluble and rapidly absorbed, and is distributed throughout the ECF in a manner similar to chloride. The concentrations of fluorine in blood, where it is bound to albumin, and tissues are small. The elimination of absorbed fluoride occurs almost exclusively via the kidneys. Fluoride is freely filtered through the glomerular capillaries and undergoes tubular reabsorption in varying degrees.

Fifty percent of orally ingested fluoride is absorbed from the gastrointestinal tract after approximately 30 minutes. In the absence of high dietary concentrations of calcium and certain other cations with which fluoride may form insoluble and poorly absorbed compounds, 80% or more is typically absorbed. Body fluid and tissue fluoride concentrations are proportional to the long-term level of intake; they are not homeostatically regulated. About 99% of the body's fluoride is found in calcified tissues (bone and teeth), to which it is strongly but not irreversibly bound.

In general, the bioavailability of fluoride is high, but it can be influenced to some extent by the vehicle with which it is ingested. When a soluble compound such as sodium fluoride is ingested with water, absorption is nearly complete. If it is ingested with milk, baby formula, or foods, especially those with high concentrations of calcium and certain other divalent or trivalent ions that form insoluble compounds, absorption may be reduced by 10–25%. Fluoride is absorbed passively from the stomach, but protein-bound organic fluoride is less readily absorbed.

The fractional retention (or balance) of fluoride at any age depends on the amount absorbed and the amount excreted. In healthy, young, or middle-aged adults, approximately 50% of absorbed fluoride is retained by uptake in calcified tissues and 50% is excreted in urine. In young children, as much as 80% can be retained owing to the increased uptake by the developing skeleton and teeth. In later life, it is likely that the fraction excreted is greater than the fraction retained. However, this possibility needs to be confirmed.

Metabolic function and essentiality

Although there is no known metabolic role in the body for fluorine, it is known to activate certain enzymes and to inhibit others. While the status of fluorine (fluoride) as an essential nutrient has been debated, the US Food and Nutrition Board in 1997 established a dietary reference intake for the ion that might suggest their willingness to consider fluorine to be a beneficial element for humans, if not an "essential nutrient."

The function of fluoride appears to be in the crystalline structure of bones; fluoride forms calcium fluorapatite in teeth and bone. The incorporation of fluoride in these tissues is proportional to its total intake. There is an overall acceptance of a role for fluoride in the care of teeth. The cariostatic action (reduction in the risk of dental caries) of fluoride on erupted teeth of children and adults is owing to its

effect in the metabolism of bacteria in dental plaque (i.e., reduced acid production) and on the dynamics of enamel demineralization and remineralization during an acidogenic challenge. The ingestion of fluoride during the pre-eruptive development of the teeth also has a cariostatic effect because of the uptake of fluoride by enamel crystallite and formation of fluorhydroxyapatite, which is less acid soluble than hydroxyapatite. When drinking water contains 1 mg/l there is a coincidental 50% reduction in tooth decay in children. Fluoride (at relatively high intakes) also has the unique ability to stimulate new bone formation and, as such, it has been used as an experimental drug for the treatment of osteoporosis. Recent evidence has shown an especially positive clinical effect on bone when fluoride (23 mg/day) is administered in a sustained-release form rather than in forms that are quickly absorbed from the gastrointestinal tract.

Deficiency symptoms

The lack of exposure to fluoride, or the ingestion of inadequate amounts of fluoride at any age, places the individual at increased risk for dental caries. Many studies conducted before the availability of fluoride-containing dental products demonstrated that dietary fluoride exposure is beneficial, owing to its ability to inhibit the development of dental caries in both children and adults. This was particularly evident in the past when the prevalence of dental caries in communities without water fluoridation was shown to be much higher than that in communities who had their water fluoridated. Both the intercommunity transport of foods and beverages and the use of fluoridated dental products have blurred the historical difference in the prevalence of dental caries between communities with and without water fluoridation. This is referred to as a halo or diffusion effect. The overall difference in caries prevalence between fluoridated and nonfluoridated area regions in the USA was reported to be 18% (data from a 1986–1987 national survey), whereas the majority of earlier studies reported differences of approximately 50%. Therefore, ingestion of adequate amounts of fluoride is of importance in the control of dental caries.

Toxicity

Fluorine, like other trace elements, is toxic when consumed in excessive amounts. The primary adverse effects associated with chronic, excessive fluoride intake are enamel and skeletal fluorosis. Enamel fluorosis is a dose-related effect caused by fluoride ingestion during the pre-eruptive development of the teeth. After the enamel has completed its pre-eruptive maturation, it is no longer susceptible. Inasmuch as enamel fluorosis is regarded as a cosmetic effect, it is the anterior teeth that are of most concern. The pre-eruptive maturation of the crowns of the anterior permanent teeth is finished and the risk of fluorosis is over by 8 years of age. Therefore, fluoride intake up to the age of 8 years is of most interest. Mild fluorosis (which is not readily apparent) has no effect on tooth function and may render the enamel more resistant to caries. In contrast, the moderate and severe forms of enamel fluorosis are generally characterized by esthetically objectionable changes in tooth color and surface irregularities.

Skeletal fluorosis has been regarded as having three stages. Stage 1 is characterized by occasional stiffness or pain in joints and some osteosclerosis of the pelvis and vertebrae, whereas the clinical signs in stages 2 and 3, which may be crippling, include dose-related calcification of ligaments, osteosclerosis, exostoses, and possibly osteoporosis of long bones, muscle wasting, and neurological defects owing to hypercalcification of vertebrae. The development of skeletal fluorosis and its severity are directly related to the level and duration of exposure. Most epidemiological research has indicated that an intake of at least 10 mg/day for 10 or more years is needed to produce the clinical signs of the milder form of the condition. Crippling skeletal fluorosis is extremely rare. For example, only five cases have been confirmed in the USA since the mid-1960s.

Based largely on the data on the association of high fluoride intakes with risk of skeletal fluorosis in children (>8 years) and adults, the US Food and Nutrition Board has established a tolerable UL of fluoride of 10 mg/day for children (>8 years), adolescents, and adults, as well as pregnant and lactating women.

Assessing status

A high proportion of the dietary intake of fluoride appears in urine. Urinary output in general reflects the dietary intake.

Requirements and dietary sources

Most foods have fluoride concentrations well below 0.05 mg/100 g. Exceptions to this observation include fluoridated water, beverages, and some infant formulae that are made or reconstituted with fluoridated water, teas, and some marine fish. Because of the ability of tea leaves to accumulate fluoride to concentrations exceeding 10 mg/100 g dry weight, brewed tea contains fluoride concentrations ranging from 1 to 6 mg/l depending on the amount of dry tea used, the water fluoride concentration and brewing time.

Intake from fluoridated dental products adds considerable fluoride, often approaching or exceeding intake from the diet, particularly in young children who have poor control of the swallowing reflex. The major contributors to nondietary fluoride intake are toothpastes, mouth rinses, and dietary fluoride supplements.

In 1997 the US Food and Nutrition Board established AI values for fluoride: infants 0.01 mg (first 6 months), 0.5 mg (7–12 months), children and adolescents 0.7, 1.0, and 2.0 mg (1–3, 4–8, and 9–13 years, respectively), male adolescents and adults 3 and 4 mg (14–18 and 19 years and older, respectively), female adolescents and adults 3 mg (over 14 years, including pregnancy and lactation). The AI is the intake value of fluoride (from all sources) that reduces the occurrence of dental caries maximally in a group of individuals without causing unwanted side-effects. With fluoride, the data are strong on caries risk reduction but the evidence upon which to base an actual requirement is scant, thus driving the decision to adopt an AI as the reference value.

Micronutrient interactions

The rate and extent of fluoride absorption from the gastrointestinal tract are reduced by the ingestion of foods particularly rich in calcium (such as milk or infant formulae).

9.15 Chromium

Chromium has an abundance of 0.033% in the Earth's crust. It is a transition element that can occur in a number of valence states, with 0, +2, +3, and +6 being the most common. Trivalent chromium is the most stable form in biological systems. The principal ore is chromite. Chromium is used to harden steel, to manufacture stainless steel, and to form many useful alloys. It finds wide use as a catalyst. Hexavalent chromium is a strong oxidizing agent that comes primarily from industrial sources.

Absorption, transport, and tissue distribution

The human body contains only a small amount of chromium, less than 6 mg. The kidney, followed by the spleen, liver, lungs, heart, and skeletal muscle are the tissues with the greatest chromium concentrations.

Absorbed chromium is excreted primarily in urine and only small amounts of chromium are lost in the hair, sweat, and bile. Therefore, urinary chromium excretion can be used as an accurate estimation of absorbed chromium. At normal dietary chromium intakes (10–40 μg/day), chromium absorption is inversely related to dietary intake. Chromium intake is approximately 0.5% at a daily intake of 40 μg/day and increases to 2% when the intake drops to 10 μg/day. The inverse relationship between chromium intake and absorption appears to be a basal control mechanism to maintain a minimal level of absorbed chromium. It is absorbed in the small intestine, primarily in the jejunum in humans. The mechanism is not well understood, but a nonsaturable passive diffusion process seems likely. Ascorbic acid promotes chromium absorption.

Chromium absorption in young and old subjects is similar, but insulin-dependent diabetic patients absorb two to four times more chromium than other apparently healthy subjects. Diabetic subjects appear to have an impaired ability to convert inorganic chromium to a usable form. Therefore, diabetic subjects require additional chromium and the body responds with increased absorption, but the absorbed chromium cannot be utilized effectively and is excreted in the urine. The chromium content of tissues of these patients is also lower.

Chromium is transported to the tissues primarily bound to transferrin, the same protein that transports iron. It has been hypothesized that iron interferes with the transport of chromium in hemochromatosis and that this may explain the high incidence of diabetes in hemochromatosis patients, and which may be induced by chromium deficiency.

Metabolic function and essentiality

Chromium in the trivalent form is an essential nutrient that functions in carbohydrate, lipid, and nucleic acid metabolism. The essentiality of chromium was documented in 1977 when the diabetic signs and symptoms of a patient on total parenteral nutrition were reversed by supplemental chromium. Chromium functions primarily through its role in the regulation of insulin. Adequate dietary chromium leads to a normalization of insulin, with reductions in blood glucose concentration in subjects with elevated blood glucose levels, increases in subjects with low blood glucose levels, and no effect on subjects with near-optimal glucose tolerance. Improved insulin function is also associated with an improved lipid profile. Supplemental chromium also leads to increased insulin binding and increased insulin receptor numbers, and recent evidence suggests that chromium may be involved in the phosphorylation and dephosphorylation of the insulin receptor proteins.

Deficiency symptoms

The hallmark of marginal chromium deficiency is impaired glucose tolerance. In studies of patients whose total parenteral nutrition solutions contained no chromium or were supplemented with inadequate amounts of chromium, insulin requirements were reduced and glucose intolerance was reversed with chromium chloride supplementation. Two of these patients had weight loss that was restored with chromium supplementation. Peripheral neuropathy was seen in one of the patients and it too was reversed with chromium supplementation.

Toxicity

Trivalent chromium, the form of chromium found in foods and nutrient supplements, is one of the least toxic nutrients. The chromium often found in paints, welding fumes, and other industrial settings is hexavalent and is several times more toxic than the trivalent form. Because trivalent chromium is poorly absorbed, high oral intakes would be necessary to attain toxic levels. In 2001, the US Food and Nutrition Board concluded that there are insufficient data to establish a tolerable UL for trivalent chromium. However, because of the current widespread use of chromium supplements, more research is needed to assess the safety of high-dose chromium intake from supplements.

Assessing status

There is no accurate method for reliable detection of marginal chromium deficiency. Chromium concentrations in hair, urine, blood, and tissues can be used to assess recent chromium exposure, but are not long-term measures of chromium status. The only reliable indicator of chromium status is to monitor blood levels of glucose, insulin, lipid, and/or related variables before and after chromium supplementation. A response in blood glucose can often be seen in 2 weeks or less, whereas effects on blood lipids may take longer.

Requirements and dietary sources

The dietary chromium content of foods varies widely. The richest dietary sources of chromium are spices such as black pepper, brewer's yeast, mushrooms, prunes, raisins, nuts, asparagus, beer, and wine. Refining of cereals and sugar removes most of the native chromium, but stainless-steel vessels in contact with acidic foods may contribute additional chromium.

There is currently no RDA set for dietary chromium, instead there are AI values [which were established by the US Food and Nutrition Board in 2001]: infants 0.2 μg (first 6 months), 5.5 μg (7–12 months), children 11 and 15 μg (1–3 and 4–8 years, respectively), teenage boys 25 and 35 μg (9–13 and 14–18 years, respectively), adult men 35 and 30 μg (19–50 years and 50 years and older, respectively), teenage girls 21 and 24 μg (9–13 and 14–18 years, respectively), adult women 25 and 20 μg (19–50 years and 51 years and older, respectively), pregnant women 29 and 30 μg (less than 18 years and 19–50 years, respectively), and lactating women 44 and 45 μg (less than 18 and 19–50 years, respectively). An AI was set based on representative dietary intake data from healthy individuals from the Third Nutrition and Health Examination Survey (NHANES III).

9.16 Other elements

In addition to the essential elements discussed in this chapter, other elements in the periodic table may emerge as being essential for human nutrition. For 15 elements, aluminum, arsenic, boron, bromine, cadmium, chromium, fluorine, germanium, lead, lithium, nickel, rubidium, silicon, tin, and vanadium, specific biochemical reactions have not been defined and their suspected essentiality is based on circumstantial evidence from data emanating from animal models, from essential functions in lower forms of life, or from biochemical actions consistent with

a biological role or beneficial action in humans. Two elements, fluorine and lithium, have beneficial actions when ingested in high (pharmacological) amounts. Lithium is used to treat bipolar disorder, and fluorine (as fluoride) is discussed in Section 9.14 because of its important beneficial actions in preventing dental caries in susceptible population groups. Some consider that the circumstantial evidence for chromium is sufficiently substantial to warrant special attention in dietary requirement recommendations, and this element is discussed in Section 9.15. The estimated or suspected requirement of all of these elements (including the essential trace elements, iodine, selenium, and molybdenum) is usually less than 1 mg/day and they are defined as ultratrace elements. Cobalt is not included in the list of ultratrace elements because the only requirement for cobalt is as a constituent of preformed vitamin B_{12}.

These elements are not discussed at length in this chapter and the reader is referred to other reading material. For completeness, three tables, on absorption, transport, and storage characteristics (Table 9.21), excretion, retention, and possible biological roles of the ultratrace elements (Table 9.22), and human body content and food sources (Table 9.23) are included here.

9.17 Perspectives on the future

The preceding parts of this chapter have highlighted some issues in the area of minerals and trace elements for which we have an incomplete understanding. In the future, nutritional scientists, dieticians, and other health care professionals will have to:

- obtain a greater understanding of the molecular and cellular processes involved in the intestinal absorption and tissue uptake of certain minerals and trace elements
- identify functional markers of mineral and trace element status. These markers could be defined as a physiological/biochemical factor that (1) is related to function or effect of the nutrient in target tissue(s) and (2) is affected by dietary intake or stores of the nutrient (which may include markers of disease risk). Examples of such indicators or markers are those related to risk of chronic diseases, such as osteoporosis, coronary heart disease,

Table 9.21 Absorption, transport and storage characteristics of the ultratrace elements

Element	Major mechanism(s) for homeostasis	Means of absorption	Percentage of ingested absorbed	Transport and storage vehicles
Aluminum	Absorption	Uncertain; some evidence for passive diffusion through the paracellular pathway; also, evidence for active absorption through processes shared with active processes of calcium; probably occurs in proximal duodenum; citrate combined with aluminum enhances absorption	<1%	Transferrin carries aluminum in plasma; bone a possible storage site
Arsenic	Urinary excretion; inorganic arsenic as mostly dimethylarsinic acid and organic arsenic as mostly arsenobetaine	Inorganic arsenate becomes sequestered in or on mucosal tissue, then absorption involves a simple movement down a concentration gradient; organic arsenic absorbed mainly by simple diffusion through lipid regions of the intestinal boundary	Soluble inorganic forms, >90%; slightly soluble inorganic forms, 20–30%; inorganic forms with foods, 60–75%; methylated forms, 45–90%	Before excretion inorganic arsenic is converted into monomethylarsonic acid and dimethylarsinic acid; arsenobetaine not biotransformed; arsenocholine transformed to arsenobetaine
Boron	Urinary excretion	Ingested boron is converted into $B(OH)_3$ and absorbed in this form, probably by passive diffusion	>90%	Boron transported through the body as undissociated $B(OH)_3$; bone a possible storage site
Cadmium	Absorption	May share a common absorption mechanism with other metals (e.g. zinc) but mechanism is less efficient for cadmium	5%	Incorporated into metallothionein which probably is both a storage and transport vehicle
Germanium	Urinary excretion	Has not been conclusively determined but probably is by passive diffusion	>90%	None identified
Lead	Absorption	Uncertain; thought to be by passive diffusion in small intestine but evidence has been presented for an active transport perhaps involving the system for calcium	Adults 5–15%, children 40–50%	Bone is a repository for lead
Lithium	Urinary excretion	Passive diffusion by paracellular transport via the tight junctions and pericellular spaces	Lithium chloride highly absorbed: >90%	Bone can serve as a store for lithium
Nickel	Both absorption and urinary excretion	Uncertain, evidence for both passive diffusion (perhaps as an amino acid or other low molecular weight complex) and energy-driven transport; occurs in the small intestine	<10% with food	Transported in blood principally bound to serum albumin with small amounts bound to L-histidine and α_2-macroglobulin; no organ accumulates physiological amounts of nickel
Rubidium	Excretion through kidney and intestine	Resembles potassium in its pattern of absorption; rubidium and potassium thought to share a transport system	Highly absorbed	None identified
Silicon	Both absorption and urinary excretion	Mechanisms involved in intestinal absorption have not been described	Food silicon near 50%; insoluble or poorly soluble silicates ~1%	Silicon in plasma believed to exist as undissasociated monomeric silicic acid
Tin	Absorption	Mechanisms involved in intestinal absorption have not been described	~3%; percentage increases when very low amounts are ingested	None identified; bone might be a repository
Vanadium	Absorption	Vanadate has been suggested to be absorbed through phosphate or other anion transport systems; vanadyl has been suggested to use iron transport systems; absorption occurs in the duodenum	<10%	Converted into vanadyltransferrin and vanadyl-ferritin; whether transferrin is the transport vehicle and ferritin is the storage vehicle for vanadium remains to be determined; bone is a repository for excess vanadium

Reproduced from Nielsen (1999) in Sadler et al. *Encyclopaedia of Human Nutrition*, copyright 1999 with permission of Elsevier.

Table 9.22 Excretion, retention, and possible biological roles of the ultratrace elements

Element	Organs of high content (typical concentration)	Major excretory route after ingestion	Molecules of biological importance	Possible biological role
Aluminum	Bone (1–12 μg/g) Lung (35 μg/g)	Urine; also significant amounts in bile	Aluminum binds to proteins, nucleotides and phospholipids; aluminum-bound transferrin apparently is a transport molecule	Enzyme activator
Arsenic	Hair (0.65 μg/g) Nails (0.35 μg/g) Skin (0.10 μg/g)	Urine	Methylation of inorganic oxyarsenic anions occurs in organisms ranging from microbial to mammalian; methylated end-products include arsenocholine, arsenobetaine, dimethylarsinic acid and methylarsonic acid; arsenite methyltransferase and monomethylarsonic acid methyltransferase use S-adenosylmethionine for the methyl donor	Metabolism of methionine, or involved in labile methyl metabolism; regulation of gene expression
Boron	Bone (1.6 μg/g) Fingernails (15 μg/g) Hair (1 μg/g) Teeth (5 μg/g)	Urine	Boron biochemistry essentially that of boric acid, which forms ester complexes with hydroxyl groups, preferably those adjacent and *cis*, in organic compounds; five naturally occurring boron esters (all antibiotics) synthesized by various bacteria have been characterized	Cell membrane function or stability such that it influences the response to hormone action, transmembrane signaling or transmembrane movement of regulatory cations or anions
Bromine	Hair (30 μg/g) Liver (40 μg/g) Lung (6.0 μg/g) Testis (5.0 μg/g)	Urine	Exists as Br⁻ ion *in vivo*, binds to proteins and amino acids	Electrolyte balance
Cadmium	Kidney (14 μg/g) Liver (4 μg/g)	Urine and gastrointestinal tract	Metallothionein, a high sulfhydryl-containing protein involved in regulating cadmium distribution	Involved in metallathionein metabolism and utilization
Germanium	Bone (9 μg/g) Liver (0.3 μg/g) Pancreas (0.2 μg/g) Testis (0.5 μg/g)	Urine	None identified	Role in immune function
Lead	Aorta (1–2 μg/g) Bone (25 μg/g) Kidney (1–2 μg/g) Liver (1–2 μg/g)	Urine; also significant amounts in bile	Plasma lead mostly bound to albumin; blood lead binds mostly to hemoglobin but some binds a low molecular weight protein in erythrocytes	Facilitates iron absorption and/or utilization
Lithium	Adrenal gland (60 ng/g) Bone (100 ng/g) Lymph nodes (200 ng/g) Pituitary gland (135 ng/g)	Urine	None identified	Regulation of some endocrine function

Element	Tissue concentrations	Excretion	Chemical forms	Biological function
Nickel	Adrenal glands (25 ng/g), Bone (33 ng/g), Kidney (10 ng/g), Thyroid (30 ng/g)	Urine as low molecular weight complexes	Binding of Ni^{2-} by various ligands including amino acids (especially histidine and cysteine), proteins (especially albumin) and a macroglobulin called nickeloplasmin important in transport and excretion; Ni^{2+} component of urease; Ni^{3+} essential for enzymic hydrogenation, desulfurization and carboxylation reactions in mostly anaerobic microorganisms	Cofactor or structural component in specific metalloenzymes; role in a metabolic pathway involving vitamin B_{12} and folic acid; role similar to potassium; neurophysiological function
Rubidium	Brain (4 µg/g), Kidney (5 µg/g), Liver (6.5 µg/g), Testis (20 µg/g)	Urine; also significant amounts excreted through intestinal tract	None identified	Role similar to potassium; neurophysiological function
Silicon	Aorta (16 µg/g), Bone (18 µg/g), Skin (4 µg/g), Tendon (12 µg/g)	Urine	Silicic acid ($SiOH_4$) is the form believed to exist in plasma; magnesium orthosilicate is probably the form of silicon in urine. The bound form of silicon has never been rigorously identified	Structural role in some mucopolysaccharides or collagen; role in the initiation of calcification and in collagen formation
Tin	Bone (0.8 µg/g), Kidney (0.2 µg/g), Liver (0.4 µg/g)	Urine; also significant amounts in bile	Sn^{2+} is absorbed and excreted more readily than Sn^{4+}	Role in some redox reactions
Vanadium	Bone (120 ng/g), Kidney (120 ng/g), Liver (120 ng/g), Spleen (120 ng/g), Testis (200 ng/g)	Urine; also significant amounts in bile	Vanadyl (VO^{2+}), vanaclate ($H_2VO_4^-$ or VO_3^-) and peroxovanadyl [V-OO]; VO^{2+} complexes with proteins, especially those associated with iron (e.g. transferrin, hemoglobin)	Lower forms of life have haloperoxidases that require vanadium for activity; a similar role may exist in higher forms of life

Reproduced from Nielsen (1999) in Sadler et al. *Encyclopaedia of Human Nutrition*, copyright 1999 with permission of Elsevier.
None of the suggested biological functions or roles of any of the ultratrace elements has been conclusively or unequivocally identified in higher forms of life.

Table 9.23 Human body content and deficient, typical, and rich sources of intakes of ultratrace elements

Element	Apparent deficient intake (species)	Human body content	Typical human daily dietary intake	Rich sources
Aluminum	160 µg/kg (goat)	30–50 mg	2–10 mg	Baked goods prepared with chemical leavening agents (e.g. baking powder), processed cheese, grains, vegetables, herbs, tea, antacids, buffered analgesics
Arsenic	<25 µg/kg (chicks) <35 µg/kg (goat) <15 µg/kg (hamster) <30 µg/kg (rat)	1–2 mg	12–60 µg	Shellfish, fish, grain, cereal products
Boron	<0.3 mg/kg (chick) 0.25–0.35 mg/day (human) <0.3 mg/kg (rat)	10–20 mg	0.5–3.5 mg	Food and drink of plant origin, especially noncitrus fruits, leafy vegetables, nuts, pulses, legumes, wine, cider, beer
Bromine	0.8 mg/kg (goat)	200–350 mg	2–8 mg	Grain, nuts, fish
Cadmium	<5 µg/kg (goat) <4 µg/kg (rat)	5–20 mg	10–20 µg	Shellfish, grains, especially those grown on high-cadmium soils, leafy vegetables
Germanium	0.7 mg/kg (rat)	3 mg	0.4–3.4 mg	Wheat bran, vegetables, leguminous seeds
Lead	<32 µg/kg (pig) <45 µg/kg (rat)	Children less than 10 years old 2 mg, Adults 120 mg	15–100 µg	Seafood, plant foodstuffs grown under high-lead conditions
Lithium	<1.5 mg/kg (goat) <15 µg/kg (rat)	350 µg	200–600 µg	Eggs, meat, processed meat, fish, milk, milk products, potatoes, vegetables (content varies with geological origin)
Nickel	<100 µg/kg (goat) <20 µg/kg (rat)	1–2 mg	70–260 µg	Chocolate, nuts, dried beans and peas, grains
Rubidium	180 µg/kg (goat)	360 mg	1–5 mg	Coffee, black tea, fruits and vegetables (especially asparagus), poultry, fish
Silicon	<20 mg kg (chick) <4.5 mg/kg (rat)	2–3 g	20–50 mg	Unrefined grains of high fiber content, cereal products
Tin	<20 µg/kg (rat)	7–14 mg	1–40 mg	Canned foods
Vanadium	<10 µg/kg (goat)	100 µg	10–30 µg	Shellfish, mushrooms, parsley, dill, seed, black pepper, some prepared foods

Reproduced from Nielsen (1999) in Sadler *et al. Encyclopaedia of Human Nutrition,* copyright 1999 with permission of Elsevier..

hypertension or diabetes. However, for many nutrients there are as yet no functional indicators that respond to dietary intake and, in such cases, nutrient requirements are established using more traditional approaches, such as balance data. The lack of functional markers of mineral and trace element status is a significant disadvantage for studies relating their intake or status to health outcomes such as hypertension, cardiovascular disease, osteoporosis, diabetes, and other disorders. For example, widely used biochemical indicators of essential trace element status generally lack both the sensitivity and the specificity that are required to define optimal intake at various stages of the life cycle. Recent efforts have provided a number of potential "sensors" of cellular copper, zinc, and manganese status that merit further evaluation. The judicious application of methods in molecular biology (including genomics and proteomics) and noninvasive imaging techniques is likely to provide new breakthroughs and rapid advances in the nutrition and biology of trace elements

- evaluate further the specific health risks associated with marginal deficiencies of various minerals and trace elements. There is a need to determine reliable relationships between mineral status and disease and then to demonstrate that the incidence or severity of specific diseases is reversible by repletion of mineral status. The development and validation of reliable assessment tools and functional markers of mineral status are the utmost priority for this field

- define the adverse effects of acute and chronic high intakes of some minerals and trace elements. Interest in mineral fortification of foods is higher than ever before. Governments worldwide are increasingly tackling the common deficiencies of iron and iodine by adding these minerals to widely consumed staple foods such as cereal flours, sugar, or soy sauce. The food industry in industrialized countries is manufacturing an increasing number of functional foods designed to provide the consumer with protection against diseases of major public health significance, such as osteoporosis, cancer, and heart disease, and fortified with minerals such as calcium, selenium, zinc, magnesium, and copper. The same minerals are added to dietetic products, including infant foods, foods for pregnant and lactating women, and enteral feeds for hospital patients, all designed to cover the nutritional requirements of specific consumers. This raises the issues not only of the possible health benefits of fortification but also of possible toxicity. Therefore, there is an ever-increasing emphasis placed on upper safe levels of mineral intake and on fortification legislation

- elucidate the impact of single nucleotide polymorphisms in the human genome on mineral and trace element dietary requirements. The key to future applications of the DNA polymorphisms will be to mine the human genome for DNA sequence information that can be used to define biovariation in nutrient absorption and use. However, before this can be accomplished, a vast amount of nutritional biology research is needed to correlate gene polymorphism with nutritional outcomes.

References

Committee on Medical Aspects of Food Policy. *Report on Health and Social Subjects 41. Dietary Reference Values for Food Energy and Nutrients in the UK.* HMSO, Department of Health, London, 1991.

Hallberg L, Sandstrom B, Aggett PJ. In: JS Garrow, WPT James, A Ralph, eds. *Human Nutrition and Dietetics*, 9th edn. Churchill Livingstone, London, 1993.

Holland B, Welch AA, Unwin ID, Buss DH, Paul AA, Southgate DAT, eds. *McCance & Widdowson's The Composition of Foods*, 5th edn. Royal Society of Chemistry and Ministry of Agriculture, Fisheries and Food. London: HMSO, 1995.

Institute of Medicine (USA). *Dietary Reference Intakes for Calcium, Phosphorus, Magnesium, Vitamin D, and Fluoride.* National Academy Press, Washington DC, 1997.

Institute of Medicine (USA). *Dietary Reference Intakes for Vitamin A, Vitamin K, Arsenic, Boron, Chromium, Copper, Iodine, Iron, Manganese, Molybdenum, Nickel, Silicon, Vanadium, and Zinc.* National Academy Press, Washington DC, 2001.

Mills CF, ed. *Zinc in Human Biology.* Springer-Verlag, London, 1989.

Nielsen F. In: MJ Sadler, JJ Strain, B Caballero, eds. *Encyclopedia of Human Nutrition.* Academic Press, London, 1999.

Rayman MP. The importance of selenium to human health. 2000; *Lancet* **356**: 233–241.

Reilly C. *Selenium in Food and Health.* Blackie, London, 1996.

Reilly C. *The Nutritional Trace Metals.* Blackwell Publishing, Oxford, 2006

Sánchez-Castillo CP, James WPT. In: MJ Sadler, JJ Strain & B Caballero, eds. *Encyclopedia of Human Nutrition.* Academic Press, London, 1999.

Strain JJ, Benzie IFF. In: MJ Sadler, JJ Strain & B Caballero, eds. *Encyclopedia of Human Nutrition.* London: Academic Press, 1999.

Further reading

Bowman B, Russel R, eds. *Present Knowledge in Nutrition*, 8th edn. ILSI Press, Washington DC, 2001.

Passmore R, Eastwood MA, eds. *Davidsons and Passmore Human Nutrition and Dietetics*, 8th edn. Churchill Livingstone, London, 1986.

Optimal Nutrition Symposium. A series of papers. *Proceedings of the Nutrition Society* 1999; **58**: 395–512.

Sadler MJ, Strain JJ, Caballero B, eds. *Encyclopedia of Human Nutrition*, Vol. 3, Parts 1–3. Academic Press, London, 1999.

Website

Online Mendelian Genetics in Man (OMIM) website at the National Institute for Biotechnology Information: http://www.ncbi.nlm.nih.gov/Omim

10
Measuring Food Intake

Una E MacIntyre

Key messages

- Measuring the food intake in free-living individuals is a complex task.
- All measurements of food intake are subject to sources of error.
- The dietary assessment method used depends on the purpose of the study.
- The existence of error means that it is always important to be aware of and, whenever possible, to assess the nature and magnitude of the error.
- To increase our understanding of the error associated with measurements of food intake it is also necessary to develop and use physiological and biochemical markers of food intake.
- To evaluate food intake data effectively it is important to collect sufficient additional data to allow individuals to be identified not only by age and gender, but also by body mass index, physical activity, and supplement use.

10.1 Introduction

The purpose of this chapter is to describe the various ways in which one can determine what people eat. The task may be to find out about the national food supply, the usual intake of a group or a household, or the intake of a given individual over a specified period.

The many reasons for finding out about the food that people eat fall into three broad categories:

1 Public Health: to evaluate the adequacy and safety of the food that people eat at national or community level and to identify the need for or to evaluate nutrition-based intervention programs.
2 Clinical: to assist with the prevention, diagnosis, and treatment of diet-related conditions.
3 Research: to study the interrelationships between food intake and physiological function or disease conditions under controlled conditions or in field conditions.

The kind and amount of food intake data required differ in each situation and may require data at the national, community, household, or individual level.

Assessment of nutritional status

Nutritional health is maintained by a state of equilibrium in which nutrient intake is balanced by nutritional requirements. Malnutrition occurs when net nutrient intake is less than requirements (undernutrition) or exceeds requirements (overnutrition). Both under- and overnutrition lead to metabolic changes which have acute and chronic consequences for health.

There is no ideal tool to measure a person's nutritional status accurately. Attempts to predict the influence of malnutrition based on single measurements fail to consider the many interacting factors between nutrition and disease state. For this reason, it is necessary to look at several different measurements in order to assess a person's nutritional status. This process is known as the A, B, C, D of nutritional assessment:

- Anthropometry (discussed in detail in Chapter 2)
- Biochemical and hematological variables
- Clinical and physical assessment
- Dietary intake.

The rest of this chapter will concentrate on the measurement of food (dietary) intake, but more detailed descriptions of the assessment of nutritional status, at the individual and population level, can be found in the *Public Health Nutrition* and *Clinical Nutrition* textbooks in this series.

Obtaining data on food intake is probably the most difficult aspect of nutritional assessment and is associated with several problems:

- "Food intake" is not a simple measure of one variable, such as weight or height, but requires data on the intake of many different food items.
- Food intake data are subject to many sources of variability, since even the same individuals eat different foods, at different times, in different places, in many different combinations, and with many different preparation methods. The net effect of all these sources of variability is that more data are needed to generate reliable results than would be the case with a less variable measure.
- We are rarely in a position to know the truth about food intake. With many biological measurements it is possible to check the results obtained against a reference method that is known to give accurate results or by means of an independent measure. For example, we can check an infant's birth weight by checking the accuracy of the weighing equipment used to measure it by means of a standard weight or, if the information was obtained by means of a questionnaire, we may be able to check the data from official records. With food intake data we have to rely on the individuals who eat the food to provide us with the answers to our questions. We ask individuals to remember what and how much they ate, to estimate how often they eat particular foods, or, even, in some situations, to weigh or measure their food intake for a number of days. For this reason one of the most important considerations, when obtaining information on food intake from individuals, is to take all possible steps to obtain their full cooperation. It is also extremely important that individuals understand the purpose of the process and what is expected of them. This may well involve much time and effort on the part of the investigator(s), but is essential for high-quality data.
- There are a number of different methods to obtain dietary intake data. Each method has its purposes,

advantages, and disadvantages. It is, therefore, essential that the purpose of collecting dietary data is clearly defined, so that the most appropriate dietary assessment method is used.

It is also essential to recognize that finding out what people eat requires adequate resources. Appropriately trained personnel must be employed not only for the period of data collection but also for the time it takes to review, enter, and analyze the data. It may not always be necessary to obtain detailed data on food intake in order to answer a particular question. When resources are limited it is probably more useful to collect limited data of high quality than to attempt to collect comprehensive dietary data with inadequate resources. Being able to recognize this situation is important for maximizing available resources. Table 10.1 lists the different approaches to measurement of food intake that are described in this chapter.

Finally, it is important that the interpretation and application of data derived from food intake studies take into account the limitations of the data. This clearly does not improve the quality of the data per se, but maximizes their usefulness for the purpose for which they were originally collected. Recognition of the limitations of dietary data involves more than simply stating the limitations. External comparisons to check whether the data are consistent with independent sources of information on food intake and to determine the likely direction and magnitude of any bias are an integral part of the interpretation of dietary data. Relevant sources of comparative information may include food supply and expenditure data and physiological or biochemical measures related to nutrient intake.

10.2 Indirect measurement of food intake

Indirect measurements of food intake make use of information on the availability of food at national, regional, or household levels to estimate food intakes, rather than using information obtained directly from individuals who consume the food. Indirect methods are most useful at the population and household levels for determining the amount and types of foods:

- available for consumption at national level (commodity-level food supply data)

Table 10.1 Approaches to the measurement of food intake in population groups, households, and individuals

Type and nature of data	Name of method	Used for assessing differences between
Commodity-level food supply data, e.g., production, imports, and exports (indirect)	Food balance sheets	Countries and regions of the world
Product-level food supply data, e.g., retail and wholesale sales data (indirect)	Food disappearance data	Country, locality, and season
Household food expenditure, e.g., money spent on food (indirect)	Household expenditure surveys	Country, locality, season, and type of household
Household food acquisition, e.g., amount of food entering the household (indirect)	Household budget surveys Household food account Household food procurement Household food inventory	Country, locality, season, and type of household
Household food consumption (direct)	Household food records	Country, locality, season, and type of household
Qualitative record of foods (but not amounts) eaten over the course of 1–7 days by individuals (direct)	Menu records	Geographical, seasonal, and demographic subgroups and individuals
Quantitative record of food intake, e.g., record of foods eaten over the course of 1–7 days by individuals (direct)	Weighed records and records estimated in household measures	Geographical, seasonal, and demographic subgroups and individuals
Qualitative or semiquantitative recall, usually of a specified list of foods, eaten in the previous month or year by individuals (direct)	Food frequency questionnaires	Geographical, seasonal, and demographic subgroups and individuals
Quantitative recall of foods eaten on the previous day, usually obtained from individuals by interview (direct)	Single or multiple 24 hour recalls	Geographical, seasonal, and demographic subgroups and individuals (if multiple recalls obtained)
Quantitative recall of habitual intake in the immediate past obtained from individuals by interview (direct)	Diet history	Temporal and demographic subgroups and individuals

- traded at wholesale or retail levels (product-level food supply data)
- purchased at household level (household-based budget/expenditure data).

Commodity level food supply data

Food supply data are usually produced at national level from compilations of data from multiple sources. The primary sources of data are records of agricultural production and food exports and imports adjusted for changes in stocks and for agricultural and industrial use of food crops and food products. National food supply data are usually referred to as "food balance sheets" or as "apparent consumption data." Food balance sheets give the total production and utilization of reported food items and show the sources (production, stocks, and imports) and utilization (exports, industrial use, wastage, and human consumption) of food items available for human consumption in a country for a given reference period. The amount of each food item is usually expressed per caput (per person) in grams or kilograms per year by dividing the total amount of food available for

human consumption by relevant population statistics. An analysis of the energy, protein, and fat provided by the food item may also be given.

The Food and Agriculture Organization (FAO) has compiled and published food balance sheet data for most countries in the world since 1949. Regularly updated food balance sheet data are available online at www.fao.org for most countries for about 100 primary crop, livestock, and fishery commodities and some products such as sugar, oils, and fats derived from them. Table 10.2 shows an extract from the food balance sheet for the Southern African Development Community for 2003.

The accuracy of food balance sheets and apparent consumption data depends on the reliability of the basic statistics used to derive them, i.e., population, supply, utilization, and food composition data. These can vary markedly between countries not only in terms of coverage but also in terms of accuracy.

Several internal and external consistency checks are built into the preparation of the FAO food balance sheets, but users still need to evaluate the data for themselves in the context of the purpose for which

Table 10.2 Extract from the food balance sheet for the Southern African Development Community, 2003

Items	Production quantity (1000 tonnes)	Import quantity (1000 tonnes)	Stock variation (1000 tonnes)	Export quantity (1000 tonnes)	Domestic supply (1000 tonnes)	Feed quantity (1000 tonnes)	Seed quantity (1000 tonnes)	Food manufacture (1000 tonnes)	Waste quantity (1000 tonnes)	Other uses quantity (1000 tonnes)	Food quantity (1000 tonnes)	Food/ capita/year (kg)	Calories/ capita/ day	Proteins/ capita/ day (g)	Fat/capita/ day (g)
Cereals, excluding beer	24862.65	8500.95	1847.63	1622.89	33588.34	4823.37	473.57	1634	1317.2	356.34	24984.3	118.4	960.06	24.82	7.11
Wheat	2041.13	4256.29	183.54	381.07	6099.89	22.68	68.04	19.05	105.43	2.47	5882.29	27.88	171.31	5.18	0.68
Rice (milled equivalent)	857.34	1432.74	70.97	38.06	2322.99	1.2	42.84	2.57	58.87	4.67	2213.09	10.49	103.23	1.98	0.15
Barley	277.4	355.47	18.64	20.39	631.12	18.17	6.54	559.87	10	26.33	10.22	0.05	0.34	0.01	0
Maize	19463.18	2271.36	1348.92	1164.19	21919.27	4485.34	309.62	400.67	961.91	322.87	15438.9	73.16	627.56	16.05	5.79
Rye	0.23	13.39	0	0.48	13.14	5.93	0.08	0	0.01	0	7.12	0.03	0.26	0.01	0
Oats	33.91	34.63	31.07	1.08	98.52	44.7	2.04	0	1.67	0	50.17	0.24	1.49	0.05	0.03
Millet	629.77	11.22	9	1.91	648.09	16.2	16.67	156.42	48.45	0	410.35	1.95	16.46	0.38	0.12
Sorghum	1521.78	81.1	180.5	4.11	1779.27	216.22	27.69	495.46	130.45	0	909.45	4.31	37.21	1.1	0.33
Cereals, other	37.9	44.75	5.01	11.61	76.05	12.92	0.07	0	0.39	0	62.76	0.3	2.2	0.06	0.01

Reproduced with permission of FAO (http://fao.org).

they are being used. One of the crucial factors in using the data appropriately is to understand the terminology used. Box 10.1 provides "in principle" definitions of the key terms.

Food balance sheets provide important data on food supply and availability in a country and show whether the food supply of the country as a whole is adequate for the nutritional needs of its population.

Box 10.1

Commodity coverage: all potentially edible commodities whether used for human consumption or used for nonfood purposes.

Exports: all movements out of the country during the reference period.

Feed: the quantity of the commodity available for feeding livestock and poultry.

Food quantity: the amounts of the commodity and any commodity derived therefrom available for human consumption during the reference period, e.g., for maize includes maize, maize meal, and any other products derived from maize that are available for human consumption.

Imports: all movements of the commodity into the country, e.g., commercial trade, food aid, donated quantities, and estimates of unrecorded trade.

Industrial uses: commodities used for manufacture for nonfood purposes, e.g., oils for soap.

Per caput supply: adjustments are made when possible to the resident population for temporary migrants, refugees, and tourists. The figures represent only the average supply available for the population as a whole and not what is actually consumed by individuals. Many commodities are not consumed in the primary form in which they are reported in food balance sheets. To take this into account the protein and fat content shown against primary commodities are derived by applying appropriate food composition factors to the relevant amounts of processed foods, and not by multiplying the quantities shown in the food balance sheet by food composition factors relating to the primary commodity.

Production: total domestic production whether produced inside or outside the agricultural sector, i.e., includes noncommercial production and production from home gardens.

Seed: quantity of the commodity set aside for sowing or planting or any other form of reproduction for animal or human consumption.

Stock variation: changes in stocks occurring during the reference period at all levels between the production and retail levels, i.e., stocks held by the government, manufacturers, importers, exporters, wholesale and retail merchants, and distributors. In practice, the available information often only relates to government stocks.

Waste: commodities lost through all stages between postharvest production and the household, i.e., waste in processing, storage, and transportation, but not domestic waste. Losses occurring during the manufacture of processed products are taken into account by means of extraction/conversion rates.

Over a period of years, food balance sheets show trends in national food supply and food consumption patterns. They may be used for population comparisons such as comparing population estimates of fat intake with cardiovascular disease rates.

In practice, the data needed to compile food balance sheets are not always available and imputations or estimates may have to be used at each stage in the calculation of per caput food and nutrient availability. In most industrialized countries reliable data are usually available on primary commodities, but this is not necessarily the case for the major processed products. For example, data may be available on flour but not on products such as bread and other cereal products made from flour that may have quite different nutrient characteristics. The overall impact of incomplete data will vary from country to country, but it has been suggested that in general underestimation of per caput availability of nutrients is more likely in less developed countries and overestimation in countries where most of the food supply is consumed in the form of processed products.

It is also very important to keep in mind that food balance sheets show only data on foods available for consumption, not the actual consumption of foods; nor do they show the distribution of foods within the population, for example among different regions or among different socioeconomic, age, and gender groups within the population. Food balance sheets also do not provide information on seasonal variations in food supply.

Product-level food supply data

In some countries (e.g., Canada and the USA) data on per caput food availability are prepared from information on raw and processed foods available at the retail or wholesale level. Such data are derived mainly from food industry organizations and firms engaged in food production and marketing such supermarkets. Errors arise mainly from inappropriate conversion factors for processing, the absence of data for some processed products, and the lack of data on food obtained from noncommercial sources such as home gardens, fishing, and hunting.

Commercial databases such as those produced by the AC Neilsen Company and the electronic stock-control records from individual supermarkets, from which they are compiled, have the potential for monitoring national-, regional-, and local-level trends in the food supply, at a product-specific level. Their principal disadvantage at present lies in the costs associated with processing or otherwise accessing, on a regular basis, the very large amounts of data that are involved.

FAO food balance sheets and similar sources of information are primarily useful for formulating agricultural and health policy, for monitoring changes in national food supplies over time, and as a basis for forecasting food consumption patterns. They can also be used to make intercountry comparisons of food and nutrient supplies, provided that potential differences in data coverage and accuracy are taken into account.

Household-based surveys

Household-based surveys determine the foods and beverages available for consumption at family, household, or institutional levels. Some surveys such as household expenditure or household budget surveys determine the amount of money spent on food for a given period, while others, such as the food account, food inventory, and food record methods, attempt to describe the food available and/or consumed by a household or institution.

Household food expenditure surveys

Household food expenditure surveys determine the amount of money spent on food by a household over a given period. Household food expenditure data can provide useful information for nutritionists on food expenditure patterns of different types of households, but without quantitative information this cannot be translated into nutrient patterns.

Household budget surveys (HBSs) are conducted at regular intervals in many European countries and many also collect data on food quantities as well as cost. HBSs have several advantages:

- they are usually conducted at regular intervals of between 1 and 5 years
- they are conducted on representative samples of households
- the food supply information collected can be classified by sociodemographic characteristics, geographical location, and season.

The large amount of nutrition-related information collected by these surveys offers the potential to assess the nutritional patterns of different population groups, to identify high-risk groups for nutrition-related conditions, to monitor trends in food patterns over time, and for developing nutrition policy. A modification of the HBS, known as the list recall method, includes quantities of items purchased, which strengthens the information. The information available from HBSs, however, also needs to be considered in the context of their limitations.

- Information provided by HBSs differs from country to country both in the number of food items recorded and in the type of information collected.
- Most surveys do not include expenditure information on food consumed outside the home.
- Most surveys do not collect information on foods acquired by means other than purchase. For example, food obtained as gifts, produced by the household itself, or harvested from the wild.
- Most surveys do not collect information on domestic wastage, i.e., food given to pets, spoiled food and plate waste, or food provided for guests.
- It is often difficult to estimate the nutrient content of the food available to the household because data are reported only at food group and not individual food level.
- Differences in food coding systems between countries make it difficult to compare data between countries.

Three conclusions emerge from this list. First, the data obtained from HBSs are not necessarily comparable between countries. Second, most HBSs do not collect all of the information needed to provide an accurate assessment of the total food supply available at household level. Third, provided that the HBS methodology remains consistent, HBSs can provide a great deal of valuable information about food patterns over time, in different sociodemographic groups, and in different parts of the country, and how these relate to social, economic, and technological changes in the food supply.

Household food account method

In the food account method, the household member responsible for the household's food keeps a record of the types and amounts of all food entering the household including purchases, gifts, foods produced by the household itself such as from vegetable and fruit gardens, foods obtained from the wild, or from other sources. Amounts are usually recorded in retail units (if applicable) or in household measures. Information may also be collected on brand names and costs. The recording period is usually 1 week but may be as long as 4 weeks.

This method is used to obtain food selection patterns from populations or subgroups within a population. It has the advantage of being fairly cost-effective and is particularly useful for collecting data from large samples. It may also be repeated at different times of the year to identify seasonal variations in food procurement.

The food account method does not measure food consumption, wastage, or other uses, nor does it account for foods consumed outside the home. It assumes that household food stocks stay constant throughout the recording period, which may not necessarily be the case. For example, food purchases may be done once a month and therefore stocks may be depleted in the days preceding the purchase. It also does not reflect the distribution of food within the household and therefore cannot be used to determine food consumption by individuals within the household. Since the method relies on the respondents being literate and cooperative, bias may be introduced in populations with high levels of illiteracy. The fact of having to record the acquisition may lead to respondents changing their procurement patterns either to simplify recording or to impress the investigator.

Household food procurement questionnaire/interview

A food procurement questionnaire or interview may be used as an alternative method to the food account method. In this method, the respondent indicates, from a list of foods, which are used, where these are obtained, the frequency of purchase, and the quantities acquired for a given period. The uses of the food procurement method are similar to those of the food account: to describe food acquisition patterns of populations or subpopulations. In contrast to the food account method, it does not require the respondent to be literate as it may be administered as an interview and it does not influence purchasing or other procurement patterns.

The food procurement questionnaire/interview does not provide information on actual food consumption or distribution within the household. As the method relies on recalled information, errors may

be introduced by inaccurate memory or expression of answers.

Household food inventory method

The food inventory method uses direct observation to describe all foods in the household on the day of the survey. The investigator records the types and amounts of foods present in a household, whether raw, processed, or cooked, at the time of the study. Information may also be collected on how and where food is stored.

A food inventory may be combined with the food account to determine the changes of food stocks during the survey period. It may also be used together with a food procurement questionnaire to describe the acquisition of foods in the household. This method is time-consuming for the investigator and very intrusive for the respondent, but is useful when foods are procured by means other than purchase and when levels of food security in vulnerable households need to be assessed.

Household food record

All foods available for consumption by the household are weighed or estimated by household measures prior to serving. Detailed information such as brand names, ingredients, and preparation methods are also recorded over a specific period, usually 1 week. This method provides detailed information on the food consumption patterns of the household, but it is very time-consuming and intrusive and relies heavily on the cooperation of the household. As for the other household methods, it does not provide information on distribution of food within the household or on individual consumption. When details of the household composition are given, estimates of individual intakes may be calculated. The method also does not determine foods eaten away from the home nor does it take into account food eaten by guests to the home.

10.3 Direct measures of food intake

Information on food intake can be obtained directly from consumers in a number of different ways. Direct measures are usually used to obtain food intake data from individuals but may also be used to obtain data from households. For example, in societies where it is usual for members of the household to eat out of the same pot this may be the only practical approach because it does not disrupt the normal pattern of food intake. Unlike the indirect measures of food intake, direct measures provide sufficient information on food consumption to convert the food intake into energy and nutrient intakes.

Irrespective of the method used, the process of obtaining food intake information and converting this to energy and nutrient data is the same. The procedure for measuring food and nutrient intake involves five steps (Figure 10.1).

1 obtaining a report of all the foods consumed by each individual
2 identifying these foods in sufficient detail to choose an appropriate item in the food tables
3 quantifying the portion sizes
4 measuring or estimating the frequency with which each food is eaten
5 calculation of nutrient intake from food tables.

To convert the information on food intake into nutrient intake, the nutrient content of each food eaten is calculated from food tables as:

$$\text{Portion size (g)} \times \text{Frequency} \times \text{Nutrient content per g}$$

and summed for all foods eaten by each individual during the study period.

Direct measurement of food intake can be divided into two basic approaches:

1 reports of foods consumed on specified days: menu records, weighed records, estimated records, and 24 hour recalls
2 reports of food intake over a period in the past, which are used to construct typical food patterns: food frequency questionnaires and diet histories.

Records are usually limited to fairly short periods, usually not longer than 7 consecutive days, while recalls may relate to a single period of 24 hours or occasionally 48 hours. Diet histories and food frequency questionnaires relate to longer periods and their purpose is to obtain an assessment of habitual intake over the period in question and not a detailed day-to-day recall of what was eaten during that time. When records are kept portions may be either weighed

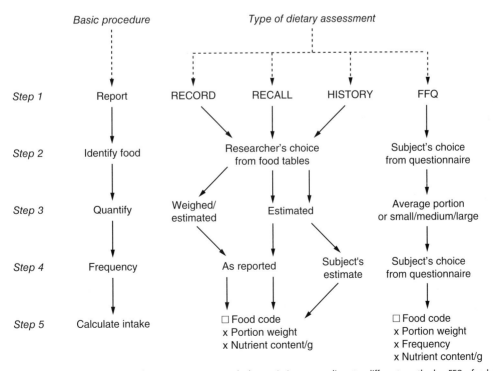

Figure 10.1 The five basic steps in a dietary assessment and the variations according to different methods. FFQ, food frequency questionnaire.

or estimated in terms of standard household measures. In recalls and questionnaires quantities always have to be estimated. Dimensions, photographs of foods, food models, and, sometimes, actual foods may be used to assist in this process. Each of these approaches has specific advantages and disadvantages and no single method of measuring food intake can be regarded as the ideal method for all situations.

Until recently, weighed intake recorded over a 7 day period was taken as the reference method against which less detailed methods were compared. It has, however, been realized that this method has its limitations and that it is not only desirable but also necessary to use physiological and biochemical measures to determine whether any method of measuring food intake is actually measuring what it sets out to measure. This will be discussed in more detail in Section 10.6.

Basic concepts

Before describing the most commonly used direct dietary assessment methods it is appropriate to introduce four fundamental concepts relevant to the process of dietary assessment and evaluation. A brief definition of terms related to these concepts is given in Box 10.2. Terms are listed in the box in alphabetical order for ease of reference.

Habitual intake

The objective of virtually all dietary assessments is to obtain an estimate of the habitual or average long-term intake for the group or the individual of interest. Habitual intake represents what is "usual" in the long term and not simply at a specific moment in time. It is this level of intake that is relevant for maintenance of energy balance and nutrient status, and for the assessment of relationships between nutrient intake and health in the long term. Habitual intake, however, is difficult to measure because food intake varies widely from day to day and, to a lesser extent, from week to week and month to month. Figure 10.2 illustrates the energy intake of one individual who maintained a weighed record every sixth day for 1 year. The horizontal line indicates the overall average intake over the year in MJ per day. The open circles show the intake on individual days and the solid circles the average intake over 7 day periods. It is obvious that intake on a single day does not provide a reliable estimate of habitual intake and that even average

Box 10.2

Accuracy: the extent to which an estimate approximates the true value.

Bias: the extent by which an estimate differs from the true value.

Coefficient of variation: the standard deviation of a set of observations expressed as a percentage of their mean.

Habitual intake: an estimate of the long-term average intake of an individual.

Precision: the extent to which a method is repeatable. Usually expressed in terms of the coefficient of variation, i.e., the standard deviation of the results of repeated analyses of the same parameter expressed as a percentage of their mean.

Random errors: errors that are randomly distributed about the true value. Random errors increase the variability of a set of observations but do not affect their mean.

Repeatability (reproducibility): a method is repeatable or reproducible when it gives the same result on repeated measurement.

Systematic errors: errors that are not randomly distributed about the true value. Systematic errors can increase or decrease the variability of a set of observations and also affect the estimate of their mean. The effect on the mean is referred to as bias.

Validity: a method is valid if it measures what it is intended to measure, i.e., the true value:

- **Absolute validity or accuracy:** terms used to describe the extent to which a method measures the true value. It is not possible to determine the absolute accuracy of a dietary method by comparison with another dietary method.
- **Face or content validity:** a method which gives results that are consistent with other data related to the parameter they are intended to measure.
- **Relative (comparative) validity:** the extent to which a test method performs in relation to a criterion or reference method, i.e., the dietary method judged to provide the "best" available measure of the true value.
- **Validity at group level:** a method is valid at the group level if it provides an unbiased estimate of mean intake for the group.
- **Validity at individual level:** a method is valid at the individual level if it is able to rank respondents correctly (usually evaluated in terms of the same proportion in the same quintile or tertile of the distribution compared with the "true" or more usually a "reference" value).

Variance: statistical term to describe the variation that occurs in a set of observations. It is equal to the square of the standard deviation of the individual observations:

- **Between-person variance:** the variance arising from differences between individuals.
- **Within-person variance:** the variance arising from differences within individuals.

intake over 7 days can differ by as much as 20% from the overall mean.

The nature of error

There is not, and probably never will be, a method that can estimate dietary intake without error. This

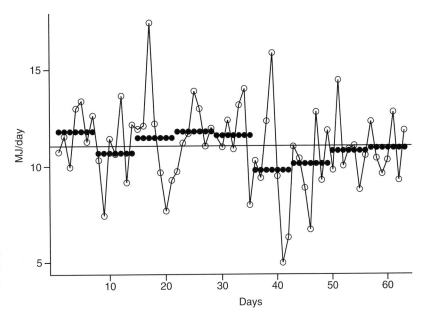

Figure 10.2 Energy intake of one individual from weighed records obtained for 1 day every sixth day over 1 year. —, overall mean; ●●●, weekly mean; ∞∞, intake on individual days.

does not mean that we should stop collecting dietary data but rather that dietary data need independent validation. Methods need to be developed to assess the error structure of dietary datasets so that it can be taken into account in analyzing and evaluating the data. Basically, there are two types of error: random error and systematic error.

Random error increases the variance of the estimates obtained and consequently reduces their precision (see below). The effects of random error can be reduced by increasing the number of observations. Day-to-day variation in food intake in individuals is one example of a random error that can be reduced by increasing the number of days of observation (Figure 10.2).

In contrast, the effects of systematic error cannot be reduced by increasing the number of observations. Systematic error arises from errors that are not randomly distributed in the group or in the data from a given individual. Inappropriate nutrient data for some food items will not affect the food intake data for all individuals in the same way. For example, inappropriate nutrient data will have a greater effect on nutrient intake data of individuals who consume the food in large amounts than on the data of those who consume only small amounts of the food. Systematic error leads to bias in the estimates of intake obtained.

Precision/repeatability

In the laboratory the precision of a method is given by the coefficient of variation (CV) of repeated determinations on the same sample made under the same conditions (see Box 10.2). In the context of dietary studies we determine whether the same method gives the same answer when repeated in the same individuals, and the terms repeatability and reproducibility are commonly used to describe the precision of a method. It is important to note that it is possible for a method to have high precision (good repeatability) yet not provide an accurate (valid) estimate of intake.

Accuracy/validity

An accurate method is one that measures what the method intends to measure, i.e., the "truth." In the context of dietary studies the truth represents the actual intake over the period of the study. For example, a valid diet record is a complete and accurate record of all the food and drink consumed over the period that the record is kept. To be a valid record of habitual intake it also needs to reflect what would have been consumed had the individual not been keeping a record. If the process of recording influenced what was eaten then the record is not a valid record of habitual intake, although it may be a true record of actual intake over the period. Similarly, a valid 24 hour recall is a complete and accurate account of all food and drink consumed during the specified period if it reflects all foods and drinks consumed in the amounts that they were actually consumed. It may not, however, be a valid reflection of habitual intake if the items consumed were not typical of the individual's usual intake.

Determining the validity of a dietary technique has been impossible in the absence of external markers of intake, except for the 24 hour recall or for individual meals.

Methods for measuring intake on specified days

Menu records

Menu records are the simplest way of recording information on food intake. They only require the respondent to write down descriptions of the food and drink consumed at each meal and snack throughout the day for the specified days without quantifying the portions. A menu record is useful when information on food patterns rather than intake is required over a longer period or when respondents have difficulty in providing quantitative information. For example, elderly people may have difficulty in reading the divisions on household scales or in measuring out food portions. To derive information on nutrient intake from menu records investigators also need to obtain information on portion sizes of commonly eaten foods. Information on portion sizes may be derived from existing data or collected in a preliminary study.

Menu records work well when the diet is relatively consistent and does not contain a great variety of foods. The method can be used to distinguish differences in the frequency of use of specific foods over time, to determine whether quantitative short-term intake records are likely to be representative of habitual intake and as a way of assessing compliance with special diets.

Weighed records

Weighed records require the respondent, or a fieldworker, to weigh each item of food or drink at the time it is consumed and to write down a description of this item and its weight in a booklet specially designed for this purpose (sometimes referred to as a food diary). Weighed records are usually kept for 3, 4, 5, or 7 consecutive days. To obtain accurate information it is necessary to use trained fieldworkers to collect the data or to demonstrate the procedures and

to provide clear instructions to the respondents not only on how to weigh foods but also on how to describe and record foods and recipes. When respondents are responsible for weighing, the investigator needs to make regular visits to the respondent during the recording period to ensure that the equipment is being used correctly and that information is recorded accurately and in sufficient detail.

Weighing can be carried out in two different ways:

1 The ingredients used in the preparation of each meal or snack, as well as the individual portions of prepared food, must be weighed. Any food waste occurring during preparation and serving or food not consumed is also weighed.
2 All food and beverage items are weighed, in the form in which they are consumed, immediately before they are eaten, and any previously weighed food that is not consumed is also weighed.

The first approach is sometimes referred to as the precise weighing technique and is usually carried out by trained fieldworkers rather than the respondents themselves. It is thus very labor intensive, time-consuming, and expensive to carry out. It is most appropriate when the food composition tables available contain few data on cooked and mixed dishes or if exposure to contaminants is being assessed. It should be noted, however, that the precise weighing technique does not allow for nutrient losses in cooking. To take these into account information on cooking losses for the most commonly used cooking methods must also be available.

The second procedure, which is more widely used, involves weighing all food eaten in the form in which it is consumed. It is sometimes referred to as the weighed inventory method. Using this method the nutrient content of the diet can be determined either by chemical analysis of duplicate portions of individual foods or aliquots of the total food consumed or, most often, from tables of food composition. Scales used for weighing food need to be robust and able to weigh up to 2 kg, accurate to at most 5 g and preferably to 1–2 g. Digital scales are preferred as these are more accurate and easier to read than spring-balance scales. Record books must have clear instructions, be easy to use, and of a convenient size. They should contain guidelines for weighing and examples illustrating the level of detail required. Figure 10.3 shows an extract from the instructions and record

Seven day food diary

instructions

1. Please use this booklet to write down everything you eat or drink for the following seven days.

   As you will see, each day is marked into sections, beginning with first thing in the morning and ending with bedtime. For each part of the day write down everything that you eat or drink, how much you eat or drink, and a description if necessary. If you do not eat or drink anything during that part of the day, draw a line through the section.

2. You have been provided with: a scale to weigh food, a measuring jug to measure liquids, and a set of measuring spoons to measure small amounts of foods and liquids.

3. Write down everything at the time you eat or drink it. Do not try to remember what you have eaten at the end of the day.

4. Before eating or drinking, the **prepared** food or drink must be weighed or measured and written in the record book. If you do not consume all the food or drink, what is left must also be weighed or measured and recorded in the book.

5. Please prepare foods and drinks as you always do. Also eat and drink in the same way as normal: eat the foods and drink in the amounts and at the times that you always eat and drink. Try not to change the way you eat and drink at all.

6. We need to know **ALL** the food and drink you take during these 7 days. So if you eat away from home (e.g., at work, with friends, at a cafe or restaurant) please take your measuring equipment with you so you can still measure your food. Also do not forget to measure food bought at take-aways.

7. Please write down the recipes of homemade dishes such as stews, soups, cakes, biscuits, or puddings. Also say how many people can eat from them or how many biscuits or cakes you get from the recipe.

8. On the next page is a list of popular foods and drinks. Next to each item is the sort of thing we need to know so that we can tell how it is made and how much you had. This list does not contain all foods, so if a food that you have eaten is missing, try to find a food that is similar to it. Please tell us as much about the food as you can.

9. Please tell us the amount and type of oil or fat that you use for cooking, frying, or baking.

Figure 10.3 Extract of instructions and record sheets from a 7 day weighed food record (MacIntyre, 1998)

10. Most packet and tinned foods, like Simba chips, Niknaks, corned meat, tinned pilchards, have weights printed on them. Tins, bottles, and boxes of cold drinks and alcoholic drinks also have weights printed on them. Please use these to show us how much you ate or drank. When possible, please keep the empty packets, bottles, or tins.

    Please note: we need to know the amount **you** eat or drink. So, if you do not eat the whole packet or tin of food, or drink the whole bottle of cold drink, please **measure** the amount you eat or drink.

11. At the end of each day there is a list of snacks and drinks that can easily be forgotten. Please write any extra items in here if you have not already written them down in some part of the day.

12. The research assistant will visit you during the record days to help you if you have any questions or problems. She will collect the equipment and record book after the 7 days.

    All the information you give us is strictly confidential. It will only be used for research purposes. Only your subject number appears on the record book. Nobody will be able to identify you from the record book.

EXAMPLE

Breakfast					
Food/drink	Description and preparation	Amount served	Amount left	Amount eaten	Code
Mealie meal porridge	Iwiza. Soft, 1 cup meal and 3 cups water	300g			
Milk	Fresh, full cream Clover	300ml			
Bread	Brown	1 × 60g			
Margarine	Rama, soft	10 ml			
Tea	Glenn tea bags	1 cup			
Milk	Fresh full cream	25 ml			
Sugar	White	2 heaped teaspoons			

Figure 10.3 *Continued*

Day no. 1

Date ___/___/ ____   Day of week_____

Early morning – Before breakfast

Food/drink	Description and preparation	Amount served	Amount left	Amount eaten	Code

Breakfast

Food/drink	Description and preparation	Amount served	Amount left	Amount eaten	Code

Mid-morning – Between breakfast and lunch time

Food/drink	Description and preparation	Amount served	Amount left	Amount eaten	Code

Lunch time

Food/drink	Description and preparation	Amount served	Amount left	Amount eaten	Code

Mid-afternoon – Between lunch and dinner

Food/drink	Description and preparation	Amount served	Amount left	Amount eaten	Code

Figure 10.3 *Continued*

Dinner time					
Food/drink	Description and preparation	Amount served	Amount left	Amount eaten	Code
Late night — up to last thing at night					
Food/drink	Description and preparation	Amount served	Amount left	Amount eaten	Code

Between meals, snacks and drinks if not already written in before					
Food/drink	Description and preparation	Amount served	Amount left	Amount eaten	Code
Sweets and chocolates					
Biscuits or cakes					
Simba chips					
Peanuts					
Other snacks					
Cold drinks					
Beer					
Tea					
Coffee					
Milk					

Figure 10.3 *Continued*

sheets of a 7 day weighed record used in a dietary intake study in South Africa.

The strengths of the weighed record are that it provides the most accurate measurement of portion sizes, as food is recorded as it is consumed, it does not rely on memory, and it gives an indication of food habits such as the number and times of meals and snacks. Weighed records kept for 3 or more days and including a weekend day are usually considered to represent habitual intake.

Limitations are that weighed records are time-consuming and require a high level of motivation and commitment from both the investigator/fieldworkers and respondents. Respondents may change their food habits to simplify measuring and recording or may not measure and record food items accurately. Samples of respondents who keep weighed records may not be representative of the population for three reasons:

1 because of the high respondent burden, respondents must be volunteers and thus random sampling cannot be used
2 respondents are limited to those who are literate and who are willing to participate
3 those who volunteer may have a specific interest in food intake, e.g., being very health conscious, and thus may not be representative of the population.

Metabolic studies carried out to determine absorption and retention of specific nutrients from measurements of intake and excretion are a specialized application of the weighed food intake record. In metabolic studies all foods consumed by the respondents are usually either preweighed or weighed by the investigators at the time of consumption. The foods consumed are usually also analyzed for the nutrient constituents of interest or prepared from previously analyzed ingredients.

Estimated records

This method of recording food intake is essentially similar to weighed records except that the amounts of food and beverages consumed are assessed by volume rather than by weight, i.e., they are described in terms of cups, teaspoons, or other commonly used household measures, dimensions, or units. Food photographs, models, or household utensils may be used to assist quantification. These descriptive terms have then to be converted to weights by the investigator,

using appropriate conversion data when available, or by obtaining the necessary information when not. For example, the investigator can determine the volume of the measures commonly used in a given household and then convert these to weights by weighing food portions of appropriate size or using information about the density (g/ml) of different kinds of foods. A record book for this kind of study is similar to that for a weighed record study. In some situations a precoded record form that lists the commonly eaten foods in terms of typical portion sizes may be appropriate, but an open record form is generally preferred.

Since there is no need for weighing scales to be provided the record forms can be distributed by mail rather than by interviewers. This is convenient if a large number of respondents located over a large geographical area is involved. In this situation the follow-up interview, after completion of the record, could be conducted by telephone. In situations in which respondents may not be familiar with measuring foods, the investigator needs to train and provide clear instructions to the respondents and to check that respondents are performing measurements and recording correctly during the record period.

The strengths and limitations of estimated records are similar to those of the weighed record, but the method has a lower respondent burden and thus a higher degree of cooperation. Loss of accuracy may occur during the conversion of household measures to weights, especially if the investigator is not familiar with the utensils used in the household.

Weighed records are used in countries where kitchen scales are a common household item and quantities in recipes are given by weight, e.g., the UK. Estimated records are favored in countries where it is customary for recipe books to give quantities by standard spoons and cups, e.g., the USA and Canada. The dietary literature frequently uses the phrase "diet record" without specifying how portions were quantified. In these instances, estimated records are most likely to have been used.

Recalled intake

Information on dietary intake over a specified period can also be obtained by asking individuals to recollect the types and amounts of food they have eaten. This approach therefore does not influence the type of food actually consumed in the way that a food record may do. However, it is open to misrepresentation of the dietary pattern, with respondents either reporting a "good" dietary pattern in order to project a good self-image or reporting a "poor" dietary pattern in the hope of receiving hand-outs or other assistance. Response rates in short-term recall studies tend to range from 65% to 95% and depend largely on how, under what conditions, and from whom the information is obtained. A recall may consist of a face-to-face or telephone interview or of a self-completed questionnaire.

The 24 hour recall is probably the most widely used method of obtaining information on food intake from individuals. It is often used in national surveys because it has a relatively high response rate and can provide the detailed information required by regulatory authorities for representative samples of different population subgroups.

The 24 hour recall is an attempt to reconstruct quantitatively the amount of food consumed either in the previous 24 hours or on the previous day. This period is considered to provide the most reliable recall of information. With longer periods memory becomes an increasing limitation. Incomplete recalls are more likely with self-completed records unless these records are subsequently checked with the respondent by the investigator. An example of a 24 hour recall sheet is shown in Figure 10.4.

Traditionally, the food intake has been reviewed chronologically, i.e., starting from the time the respondent wakes up and going through the day until the following morning. Recalling daily activities often assists the respondent to remember food intakes. Problems encountered in estimating the amounts of foods consumed are similar to those encountered with estimated records. Recalls conducted by means of a face-to-face interview often use aids such as photographs, food models, and household utensils to help the respondent to describe how much food was eaten. In telephone recalls respondents may be provided with pictures or other two-dimensional aids prior to the interview to help them to describe the amounts consumed. There is, however, very little information on how effective these aids are. For this type of study a standardized interview protocol, which is based on a thorough knowledge of local food habits and commonly used foods, is essential when more than one interviewer is involved.

In its simplest form, the 24 hour recall consists of foods and the amounts consumed over a 24 hour period. In order to obtain sufficient information to quantitatively analyze food intakes from a 24 hour recall, a skilled interviewer will use several "passes" or stages in questioning the respondent. This procedure has become known as the multiple-pass 24 hour recall. This is an interviewing technique consisting of three to five steps which take the respondent through the previous day's food consumption at different levels of detail. All multiple-pass 24 hour recalls commence with the respondent simply listing all foods and beverages consumed during the previous 24 hours. The content and number of further steps differ from study to study. The US Department of Agriculture (USDA) has developed a five-step multiple pass method comprising the following passes (steps) (Conway et al., 2003).

Pass 1 Quick list: the respondent lists all food and beverages consumed during the preceding 24 hours in any order without any prompting or interruptions from the interviewer.

Pass 2 Forgotten foods list: the interviewer asks about categories of foods, such as snacks and sweets, which are frequently forgotten.

Pass 3 Time and occasion: the interviewer asks for details of the times and names of the eating occasions at which foods were consumed.

Pass 4 Detail: the interviewer asks for details, such as descriptions and preparation methods, and amounts of foods consumed.

Pass 5 Review: the interviewer goes through the information probing for any foods which may have been omitted.

A simplified version of the multiple-pass 24 hour recall consists of three steps:

Pass 1 the respondents provide a list of all foods eaten on the previous day using any recall strategy they desire, not necessarily chronological.

Pass 2 the interviewer obtains more detailed information by probing for amounts consumed, descriptions of mixed dishes and preparation methods, additions to foods such as cream in coffee, and giving respondents an opportunity to recall food items that were initially forgotten.

Pass 3 in a third pass the interviewer reviews the list of foods to stimulate reports of more foods and eating occasions.

Place (home, work, friends, etc.)	Food/drink and preparation method	Amount (HHM)	Amount (g) (office use only)	Code (office use only)
	Did you eat or drink anything when you got up yesterday? What did you have?			
	Did you eat or drink anything during the morning (before about midday/lunch time)? What did you have?			
	Did you eat or drink anything in the middle of the day (lunch time)? What did you have?			
	Did you eat or drink anything during the afternoon (between lunch and dinner time)? What did you have?			
	Did you eat or drink anything at dinner time? What did you have?			
	Did you eat or drink anything during the night (after dinner and before you went to sleep)? What did you have?			
	Is there anything else that you ate or drank yesterday that you haven't told me already?			

Figure 10.4 Example of a 24-hour recall record sheet (Reproduced from Kruger, 2003, with permission of the author). HHM, household measure.

The multiple-pass approach is thought to assist recall more effectively than chronological cues and thus provide more accurate and complete information. This approach, however, is more time-consuming than the traditional 24 hour recall and may irritate respondents by seemingly asking about the food intake over and over again. Irrespective of the approach used, it is essential that all interviewers are thoroughly trained, that the approach is tested in the target population prior to the study, and that the same procedure is used by all interviewers with all respondents throughout the study.

A major drawback of the 24 hour recall is that it provides information for only a single day and therefore does not take account of day-to-day variation in the diet. In large cross-sectional studies in which the aim is to determine average intakes of a group of individuals, a single 24 hour recall may be sufficient. When the diets of individuals are assessed or when sample sizes are small, repeated 24 hour recalls are required. This method is known as multiple 24 hour recalls. The number of recalls depends on the aim of the study, the nutrients of interest, and the degree of precision needed. For example, when diets consist of a limited variety of foods two 24 hour recalls may be sufficient whereas four or more recalls may be required when diets are complex. Recalls may also be repeated during different seasons to take account of seasonal variations. (Note that multiple 24 hour recalls must not be confused with the multiple-pass 24 hour recall technique. The multiple-pass 24 hour recall refers to an interviewing technique, whereas the multiple 24 hour recall method refers to repeated 24 hour recalls conducted per respondent.)

The strengths of the 24 hour recall method are that it has a low respondent burden in comparison with food records and thus compliance is high, it does not require respondents to be literate, it does not alter usual food intake, and it is relatively quick and inexpensive to administer and therefore is cost-effective when large numbers of respondents are involved. It is most successful in populations with limited dietary variety and when respondents are able to accurately recall and express the types and amounts of foods consumed and when interviewers are skilled in the interview technique.

As already stated a major drawback of the 24 hour recall is that it does not give an accurate reflection of habitual dietary intake if only a single 24 hour recall is conducted. This may be overcome to some extent by conducting repeated 24 hour recalls. Another difficulty is that the 24 hour recall relies on the respondent to accurately recall and report the types and amounts of foods consumed. There is a tendency for respondents to overestimate low intakes and underestimate high intakes. This is known as the flat slope syndrome. Respondents may omit certain foods that are considered "bad" or include foods not consumed but considered "good" (phantom foods) in order to impress the interviewer.

Of the methods so far described weighed records should contain the least error as they report all food consumed on specified days with weighed portions. Estimating the size of portions increases error and, if menu records are quantified with average portions, then the error at the individual level is further increased. If food that has already been eaten has to be recalled then poor memory can introduce an additional source of error. All methods that report intake on specified days are also subject, in individuals, to the error associated with day-to-day variation in intake, but this error can be reduced by increasing the number of days studied.

Methods for measuring intake over the longer term

Food frequency questionnaires

Food frequency questionnaires consist of a list of foods and options to indicate how frequently each food is consumed. Respondents indicate the frequency of consumption during a specified period by marking the appropriate option column. The food lists may contain only a few food items or may contain up to 200 foods. The type and number of foods included is determined by the purpose of the study and the target population. For example, a food frequency questionnaire designed to determine calcium intake would contain only foods which provide calcium, while a questionnaire to measure overall dietary adequacy would need to contain all foods known to be consumed by the target population. Likewise, a food frequency questionnaire designed to assess dietary intakes of a homogeneous target population with a diet of limited variety will be shorter than one designed to assess food intakes of a heterogeneous population with a variety of food intake patterns. There are several types of food frequency question-

Box 10.3

Food frequency questionnaire (FFQ) (simple/nonquantitative): respondents report usual consumption of foods and beverages from a set list of items for a specific period. Portion sizes are not determined.

Semiquantitative food frequency questionnaire: a FFQ which includes estimation of portion sizes as small, medium, or large. A reference portion (usually medium) may be provided as a guide.

Quantitative food frequency questionnaire: more precise estimates of portion sizes are given by reference to portion size measurement aids (PSMAs) such as food models and photographs of known weight, household measures, or by direct weighing.

List-based food frequency questionnaire: food items are listed according to groups or categories of similar foods or foods usually eaten together.

Meal-based food frequency questionnaire: foods are asked about according to meals or the time of day at which they are consumed.

Culture-sensitive food frequency questionnaire: a FFQ that takes account of the food values, beliefs, and behaviors of a specific population or cultural group.

- 1–2 times per week
- 1–2 times per month
- occasionally
- never.

This type of response format requires only that the appropriate columns be marked and is most suitable for self-administered questionnaires. When appropriately designed, such questionnaires can be optically scanned, which saves time on data entry and checking procedures (Figure 10.5).

Closed response options, however, treat the frequency of consumption as a categorical variable and assume that frequency of consumption is constant throughout the recall period. The choice of categories may bias the results: too few categories may underestimate frequencies whereas too many may overestimate frequencies. Respondents may have difficulty in matching their food intake to the available categories. For example, when food is purchased on a monthly basis food items such as fresh fruit and vegetables may be consumed every day while the stocks last, but, once used up, will not be consumed until purchased in the following month.

An alternative method for recording responses is to provide columns headed as the number of times per day, per week and per month, seldom, and never. From this, the average frequency of consumption and the amount of food consumed per day can be calculated. Table 10.3 shows an extract from such a food frequency questionnaire. The advantage of this response format is that it allows the respondent to describe the frequency of consumption in detail. Responses such as consumption of a food twice a day for 6 days of the week can be recorded. The disadvantages are that clear instructions must be given, making this method more appropriate for interviewer-administered questionnaires than self-administered questionnaires, and the interview takes longer and requires more writing and calculations than the closed format, making more room for errors.

naires, which are defined in Box 10.3. The type of food frequency questionnaire used depends on the purpose of the study, the target population, and the required level of accuracy of food portion estimation.

The period of recall depends on the study objectives. In the past, most food frequency questionnaires used the preceding year or 6 months as the reference period. Theoretically, this should eliminate the effects of season. In practice, however, respondents tend to answer according to what is in season or available at the time of the study. For example, intake of oranges was found to be higher when interviews were carried out during the citrus season than at other times of the year. Information may be more reliable when recall period is shorter. Recent recommendations are that recall periods should not be longer than 1 month. If annual intakes are required, the food frequency questionnaire must be repeated in different seasons. It is very important that the respondent understands what the recall period is and that only this period should be considered when giving frequencies of intake.

The frequency of consumption is usually indicated by options such as:

- more than once a day
- daily
- 3–4 times per week

Most food frequency questionnaires obtain information only on the frequency of consumption of a food over a given period and not on the context in which the foods were eaten, i.e., on meal patterns. Meal-based food frequency questionnaires have been used on the basis that it may be easier for respondents to provide the information in the context of meals.

Please completely fill one oval in every line. Please MARK LIKE THIS: ⊙ ● ⊙ ⊙	N E V E R	1 time	2 times	3 or more times	1 time	2 times	3 or 4 times	5 or 6 times	Less than once	1–3 times
		per month			per week				per day	
Flavoured milk drink (cocoa, Milo™ etc.)	⊙	⊙	⊙	⊙	⊙	⊙	⊙	⊙	⊙	⊙
Nuts	⊙	⊙	⊙	⊙	⊙	⊙	⊙	⊙	⊙	⊙
Peanut butter or peanut paste	⊙	⊙	⊙	⊙	⊙	⊙	⊙	⊙	⊙	⊙
Corn chips, potato crisps, Twisties™ etc.	⊙	⊙	⊙	⊙	⊙	⊙	⊙	⊙	⊙	⊙
Jam, marmalade, honey or syrups	⊙	⊙	⊙	⊙	⊙	⊙	⊙	⊙	⊙	⊙
Vegemite™, Marmite™ or Promite™	⊙	⊙	⊙	⊙	⊙	⊙	⊙	⊙	⊙	⊙
Dairy products, meats and fish										
Cheese	⊙	⊙	⊙	⊙	⊙	⊙	⊙	⊙	⊙	⊙
Ice cream	⊙	⊙	⊙	⊙	⊙	⊙	⊙	⊙	⊙	⊙
Yoghurt	⊙	⊙	⊙	⊙	⊙	⊙	⊙	⊙	⊙	⊙
Beef	⊙	⊙	⊙	⊙	⊙	⊙	⊙	⊙	⊙	⊙
Veal	⊙	⊙	⊙	⊙	⊙	⊙	⊙	⊙	⊙	⊙
Chicken	⊙	⊙	⊙	⊙	⊙	⊙	⊙	⊙	⊙	⊙
Lamb	⊙	⊙	⊙	⊙	⊙	⊙	⊙	⊙	⊙	⊙
Pork	⊙	⊙	⊙	⊙	⊙	⊙	⊙	⊙	⊙	⊙
Bacon	⊙	⊙	⊙	⊙	⊙	⊙	⊙	⊙	⊙	⊙

Figure 10.5 Typical layout of a food frequency questionnaire suitable for optical scanning (reproduced with permission of Anti Cancer Council of Victoria, Melbourne, Australia).

The information on meal patterns obtained from such questionnaires is, however, more limited than that which can be obtained from a dietary history. Additional questions, if included, can provide some information on cooking methods.

Some food frequency questionnaires also attempt to quantify the frequency information by obtaining data on portion size. Information on the quantity of each food consumed may be obtained by asking respondents to indicate on the questionnaire whether their usual portions are small, medium, or large relative to those eaten by others, by asking subjects to describe their usual portion size in terms of a standard portion size described on the questionnaire (semiquantitative food frequency questionnaire), or by reference to a picture atlas of food portions, food models, or actual food portions (quantitative food frequency questionnaire). When portion sizes are used, it is important that these reflect the consumption patterns of the population.

Food frequency questionnaires are mainly used in studies designed to look for associations between food intake and disease or risk of disease, particularly when specific foods rather than the level of consumption of a nutrient are thought to be the important factor. Since the cost of administration and respondent burden are relatively low, they are suitable for use when sample sizes are large, particularly if a postal method is used.

The success of a food frequency questionnaire depends on how closely the food list and portion size descriptions reflect the food patterns of the target population. This is sometimes referred to as being culture sensitive. Much time and care must be put into the development of a food frequency questionnaire in order to ensure that it provides an accurate reflection of the dietary intakes of a population. Preliminary studies, using 24 hour recalls, food records, or indirect methods may be needed to obtain information on food items, frequency of consumption, and portion sizes in the target population. Since food frequency questionnaires are usually developed for use in specific target populations, a food frequency questionnaire developed for use in one population may not be appropriate for use with another population with different food intake patterns. It is also extremely important that the questionnaire be tested for repeatability and validity in the target population before being used, even if it has been tested in a different population.

Table 10.3 Extract from a food frequency questionnaire using open ended response options (MacIntyre, 1998)

Food	Description	Amount	Times eaten				Office use only	
			Per day	Per week	Per month	Seldom	Code	Amount/day
Maize meal porridge	Stiff porridge						4256	
	Soft porridge						4255	
	Sour porridge						9999	
Do you pour milk on your porridge? YES NO **If NO, go to next question on sugar.** **If YES,** what type of milk: fresh, sour, milk powder (Nespray), skim milk powder (name)?								
If yes, how much milk?								
Do you pour sugar on your porridge/cereal? YES NO **If no, go to 'samp'**								
If yes, how much sugar?							9012	
Samp (only)							4043	
Samp and beans							A014	
Tshidzimba (samp, beans, and peanuts)							9816	
Rice							4040	
Macaroni/spaghetti							A018	
Bread								
White bread							4001	
Brown bread							4002	
Fat cakes							4057	
Other types of bread								
Do you spread anything on the bread? YES NO **If no, go to next section (chicken, meat, fish)** **IF YES,** What do you spread and how much?								
Margarine	Hard Soft						6508 6521	
Peanut butter							6509	
Other types of spread								

Detailed reviews of the design and evaluation of food frequency methods for use in epidemiological studies are given by Willett (1998) and Cade *et al.* (2002).

Diet history

The principal objective of the diet history is to obtain detailed information on the habitual intake of an individual. As first proposed by Burke in the 1940s, the method had several components (Burke 1947):

- an interview to obtain usual diet
- a cross-check of this information by food group
- a 3 day record of food consumed in household measures.

The 3 day record component is now seldom used as a regular component of a diet history. Its purpose originally was as a way of checking the data obtained from the diet history interview. A diet history is usually obtained by an experienced nutritionist by means of an open interview followed by some kind of cross-check using a standard list of commonly consumed foods. The interview usually begins with a review of the food that was eaten in a specific time-frame (e.g., yesterday) or on a typical day, and then moves on to explore the variations in food intake that occur for each meal over a given period. Information on the usual size of food portions is obtained with the aid of food models or photographs in the same way as for a 24 hour recall. The time-frame for a diet history can range from the previous month to the previous year.

In practical terms it is easier for respondents to reconstruct the immediate past, but the past year is often used to capture seasonal variation. Whatever the time-frame used, it is important for it to be clearly specified. In the literature the term "diet history" is sometimes used loosely to describe any form of diet recall, including the 24 hour recall and self-administered food frequency questionnaires, as well as interviewer-administered recalls of habitual or longer term intake. This broader use can be confusing and is best avoided. The dependence of the diet history on both respondent and interviewer skills may make the results obtained less comparable between individuals than those obtained from other methods, and for this reason it is often considered more appropriate to categorize diet history data (e.g., as high, medium, low) rather than to treat them as intakes expressed in terms of absolute units per day.

The diet history is favored in Scandinavia and the Netherlands, where a structured interview may be used. The structured interview is more standardized but may miss elements specific to the individual or bore the respondents with irrelevant questions. The open-ended interview allows for tailoring to the individual, but risks missing important items.

10.4 Sources of error in dietary studies

The major sources of error in dietary studies have been reviewed in detail by Bingham (1987). Four possible sources of error occur to some degree with all dietary methods, but can be minimized by careful study design and execution:

- sampling bias
- response bias
- inappropriate coding of foods
- use of food composition tables in place of chemical analysis.

In contrast, the errors that are associated with specific methods are generally much more dependent on the nature of the method and the abilities of the respondents, and therefore less easy to control. Errors of this type include:

- estimation of portion size
- recall or memory error
- day-to-day variation in intake
- effect of survey method on food intake.

Figure 10.6 illustrates the points in the dietary assessment process at which different kinds of error operate.

Sampling bias

Sampling bias arises when the sample studied is not truly representative of the population of interest. The importance of minimizing sampling bias depends on the purpose of the dietary study. Except in methodological studies, volunteers are not generally appropriate respondents because frequently the objective is to study a representative sample of a particular group in order to extrapolate the results to the population group from which the sample was drawn. For this purpose it is clearly important that as many as possible of the sample group originally selected participate in the study.

The proportion of the sample that agrees to participate in the study can vary considerably even with the same method. It depends not only on the group being studied but also on the circumstances of the study. In general, response rates tend to be greater in studies that use methods such as the 24 hour recall and food frequency questionnaires (which make fewer demands on respondents) and lower in studies such as 7 day weighed records (which require much more cooperation, effort, and time from the respondents). It is always important to try to maximize response rates, for example by increasing respondent motivation, providing specific assistance if required, and by allowing respondents as much flexibility as possible in participation within the context of the study objectives.

Response bias

Response bias arises when respondents provide incomplete or inappropriate responses. The extent of this problem is not easy to assess, but can be investigated by making measurements that are independent

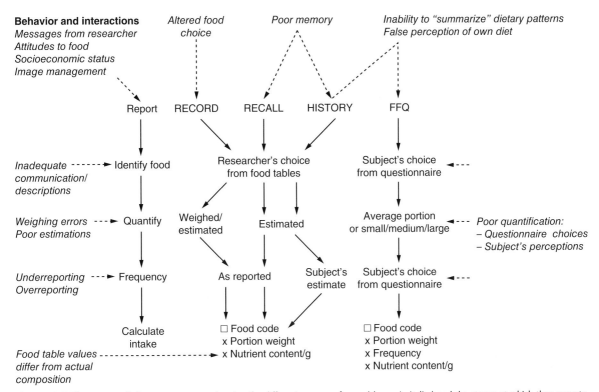

Figure 10.6 The process of dietary assessment showing the different sources of error (shown in italics) and the stages at which they operate in different dietary methods. FFQ, food frequency questionnaire.

of dietary intake, both during and after dietary study periods. Measurements suitable for this purpose will be discussed further in the context of validity. Response bias can probably best be minimized by providing the respondents with clear and well-presented instructions, adequate support, and appropriate incentives. Such incentives may include relevant dietary feedback where this is appropriate or monetary or other rewards provided that these are within ethical principles.

In dietary studies that involve more than one interviewer, the training of interviewers and the use of standard procedures for interviewing is one way of reducing unnecessary random variation (error) that might otherwise arise because different interviewers conduct interviews in different ways. The use of standard procedures, however, can also introduce systematic error; for example, if one interviewer is assigned to interview all respondents in areas of low socioeconomic status and another to interview all respondents in areas of high socioeconomic status. It is important to recognize also that standard interview procedures do not necessarily "standardize" respondent response. To date, relatively little work has focused on the respondent response aspect of dietary assessment.

Since all dietary methods engage the cognitive processes of respondents, an appreciation of the properties of human cognition and its limitations is fundamental to improving the accuracy of dietary assessments. Recently, research into the cognitive aspects of dietary assessment has been undertaken in an attempt to increase the understanding of how respondents process dietary intake data (Domel, 1997; Thompson *et al.*, 2002; Vuckovic *et al.*, 2002; Matt *et al.*, 2006).

Some of the important issues in this area that are relevant to improving the quality of dietary data include identification of:

- factors that improve communication between respondent and investigator
- the most effective cues for recall over different periods

- factors that influence retention of dietary information over time
- the ways in which individuals conceptualize foods and food quantities.

Coding

Coding refers to the allocation of a specific code to each food item. Since the nutritional content of a food varies with different processing and preparation methods, it is vital that the correct codes be assigned to each food item. Coding errors arise when the food that has been consumed is not described in sufficient detail to enable unambiguous allocation, by the investigator, to a food category in a food composition table or database. Food frequency questionnaires are often precoded to reduce the time needed for coding and the possibility of coding errors (see Table 10.3). Making it easy for respondents to describe foods with the level of detail required is therefore an important consideration in study design. This is increasingly difficult, particularly in industrialized countries where the food supply now consists of thousands of different manufactured foods, the names of which are often no longer a good guide to their nutrient content.

Coding errors are also likely to arise when more than one person is involved in coding and there is no agreed procedure and/or comprehensive coding manual. Coding errors arising exclusively from inadequate description of foods have resulted in coefficients of variation ranging from 3% to 17% for different nutrients. Note that a standard procedure for coding foods, while minimizing differences between coders (random error), can also introduce bias if the coding decisions that are made are not based on up-to-date knowledge of the local food supply and food preparation methods. Gross errors associated with weights of foods can be checked, before analysis, by means of computer routines that identify values outside a prescribed range and by using data-checking techniques such as duplicate data entry.

Use of food composition tables

Most dietary studies use food composition tables or databases rather than chemical analysis to derive the nutrient content of the foods consumed. Chapter 2 describes in detail the way in which data on food composition are derived and compiled. The purpose of this section is simply to review briefly the kinds of error that can arise as a consequence of using food composition tables to calculate nutrient intake, compared with chemical analysis of the diet, and which can lead to both random and systematic errors.

Systematic error can result from:

- the way in which results are calculated or expressed
- the analytical method used
- the processing and preparation methods in common use.

Food composition tables for different countries often use different ways of expressing results and different analytical methods. The ways in which food items are processed or prepared are also likely to differ and for these reasons different sources will not necessarily provide comparable data for the same foods. Systematic differences, which may not necessarily be errors (e.g., when foods are prepared differently in different countries), often only become evident when different food composition tables are used to evaluate the same diets.

Random error arises from the fact that most foods vary in their composition as a result of changes in composition associated with the conditions of production, processing, storage preparation, and consumption. The random error associated with the use of food composition databases generally decreases as the size of the sample group increases. This may not be true, however, in institutional settings where everyone is likely to be consuming food from the same source.

To compare calculated and analyzed data without the complication of other sources of error it is necessary that the diets are analyzed by collecting a duplicate of what has been eaten at the same time as the diet record. At group level it has been observed that mean intakes calculated from the food tables are generally within approximately 10% of the mean analyzed value for energy and macronutrients, but not for micronutrients. However, a large proportion of individuals have values that fall outside this range.

In general, calculated and analyzed values for nutrients agree more closely:

- for groups than for individuals
- for macronutrients than for micronutrients
- when data for locally analyzed foods are used.

Estimation of portion size

Estimation of portion size has long been recognized as an important source of error in dietary studies (Young *et al.*, 1953) with coefficients of variation of the differences between estimates and weights of food portions regularly reported to be around 50% for foods and 20% for nutrients (Nelson and Bingham, 1997). However, despite the fact that individuals are known to vary widely in their ability to estimate portion size, relatively few studies have attempted to quantify the size of this error or to "calibrate" their respondents in this respect. The influence of some factors on the determination of portion size is summarized in Box 10.4.

In attempts to assist respondents to describe portion sizes, a number of visual aids, known as portion size measurement aids (PSMAs), have been developed. These include:

- weighed portions of actual foods
- allowing respondents to serve out portions of food and direct weighing or measuring of the serving

---

Box 10.4

Food characteristics
- No consistent associations observed with type of food, although foods of indeterminate shape are more often associated with larger and liquid foods with smaller errors.
- Large portion sizes appear to be more difficult to estimate accurately than small portion sizes.

Visual aids
- Household measures may be associated with considerable errors.
- Food models produce more reliable results than household measures, but because only one size is usually available they may "bias" respondents to report portion sizes similar to those shown.
- Graduated food models and two-dimensional pictures may be as helpful as three-dimensional models for estimating portion size.
- The range of reference portion sizes available may influence the estimates.
- The use of multiple photographs results in more accurate estimates.

Respondents
- Respondents of all ages have been reported to have difficulty with portion size estimates.
- Women have sometimes, but not invariably, been reported to be better able to estimate portion size than men, but this may simply reflect the fact that they tend to handle food more often than men.

- commercial or home-made food models:
  - food pictures or drawings of different portion sizes
  - photographs of foods in different portion sizes
  - abstract shapes of cardboard, wooden or plastic blocks, wedges, circles, balls, and mounds in various sizes
  - household utensils and containers such as cups, spoons, jugs, glasses, bowls, and plates in various sizes
  - containers and packets of bought foods, e.g., sweet wrappers, potato crisp packets, cold drink cans and bottles, yoghurt and ice cream cups, milk cartons.

Each PSMA has advantages and disadvantages. The type of PSMA chosen will depend, among others, on the type of study, the target population, whether interviewers go from house to house or respondents go to a research centre, available resources, and the availability of appropriate PSMAs. Probably the most effective method is a combination of PSMAs such as food photographs and household utensils. Irrespective of the type of PSMA used, it is essential that respondents are able to identify and relate to the PSMA, that PSMAs be tested in the target population prior to their use, and that PSMAs are used consistently throughout the study.

Recall errors

Factors that have been studied in relation to the accuracy of dietary recall include food consumption patterns, weight status, gender, and age. Many other characteristics, such as intelligence, mood, attention, and salience of the information, however, have also been demonstrated to influence performance tests of general recall, but have not been studied in the context of dietary recall.

Short-term memory

Like the ability to estimate portion size, the ability to remember what was eaten varies with the individual. Studies that have compared the abilities of different groups to remember what they have eaten conclude that women are generally better than men and that younger adults are better than older adults. In short-term recalls of intake (e.g., 24 hour recalls) individuals more often tend to omit an item or items that they have consumed than to include ones that they have not consumed. For this reason, 24 hour recall studies often provide estimates of food intake that are lower than food records obtained over the same period. The size of the error incurred by the omission of one or more food items clearly depends on what is omitted and not only on the proportion of food omitted. For example, the effect, on 24 hour energy intake, of omitting a cup of black coffee, a glass of milk, or a bar of chocolate is quite different.

The omission of food items in 24 hour recall studies can be reduced by appropriate probing by the interviewer in relation to meals, between-meal snacks, and other activities on the previous day, but even when respondents have previously weighed their food the average energy intake may still be underestimated by as much as 20%.

Long-term memory

The diet history and most food frequency questionnaires set out to measure the habitual intake of an individual over a period of weeks or months. Individuals are not asked to recall their food intake on specific days, but to construct a picture of their "usual" food consumption pattern over a specified reference period. To provide reliable information individuals thus need to be able to remember the range of foods that they usually consume, to judge the frequency of consumption on a long-term basis, and to be able to estimate correctly the average amount that is usually consumed. These are complex cognitive tasks.

As in the case of 24 hour recalls, no attempt is usually made to assess how well individuals are able to perform these various tasks. From the limited amount of data available from comparative studies between diet histories and long-term diet records, it appears that the two methods do not give concordant results in individuals. Food frequency questionnaires are subject to the same difficulties, and have the added problem that estimates of portion size are based on standard measures or, in the case of mailed questionnaires, are made in the absence of visual aids such as food models or photographs.

When respondents are asked to report their intake over a period of weeks they rely largely on generic knowledge of their diet and tend to report items that they are likely to have eaten or items that they routinely eat, rather than items that they specifically remember having eaten during the reference period. This tendency increases with the time interval between the recall and the reference period. The accuracy of frequency estimates also deteriorates with time. While individuals appear to report more frequently eaten foods with greater frequency than less frequently eaten foods, there are differences between individuals in the way that they report the same frequency of consumption. Ranking of individuals on the basis of the usual frequency of intake is thus likely to lead to misclassification unless the extent of the differences between individuals is known and can be taken into account. It is difficult to see how such misclassification can be reduced unless it is possible to classify individuals, in some way, in terms of their ability to provide reliable information on habitual long-term intake.

Day-to-day variation in intake

We have already seen that individuals vary considerably in their intake of nutrients from day to day (see Figure 10.2). In addition, the extent of day-to-day variation differs between nutrients. The implication of the first observation is that short-term intake data (e.g., 24 hour recall data) are unlikely to provide a reliable estimate of habitual intake for most individuals. The implication of the second observation is that the length of time for which dietary data need to be collected, in order to estimate habitual intake with any given level of confidence, varies with the nutrient of interest.

Table 10.4 expresses the impact of this variation in terms of the number of days of dietary information needed to classify 80% of individuals into the correct third of the distribution. It is clear from this table that not only 24 hour recalls but also 7 day records are likely to be inadequate to classify 80% of individuals correctly into the appropriate third of the distribution for most micronutrients. This is an important reason, although not the only reason, why short-term records are only rarely used for epidemiological studies, in preference to food frequency questionnaires, despite the loss of detail and precision inevitably associated with the use of the latter.

Effect on usual diet

Recall methods clearly cannot change what has already been eaten, but what has been eaten can be misreported either consciously or unconsciously. When individuals are asked to keep records, however, they may also alter their normal habits as a consequence of the recording process. One obvious reason for

Table 10.4 Number of days of records required to enable 80% of men to be assigned into their correct third of the intake distribution

Nutrient	British civil servants	Random sample of British men	Random sample of Swedish men
Energy	7	5	7
Protein	6	5	7
Fat	9	9	7
Carbohydrate	4	3	3
Sugar	2	2	–
Dietary fiber	6	10	–
P:S ratio	11	–	–
Cholesterol	18	–	–
Alcohol	4	–	14
Vitamin C	–	6	14
Thiamin	–	6	15
Riboflavin	–	10	–
Calcium	–	4	5
Iron	–	12	9

P:S ratio, ratio of polyunsaturated to saturated fatty acids in the diet. (Reproduced from Margetts BM, Nelson M. *Design Concepts in Nutritional Epidemiology*. Oxford: Oxford University Press, 1991, with permission from Oxford University Press.)

doing so would be to simplify the process of recording. Other reasons may include a desire to eat less in order to lose weight or to be seen to conform with dietary recommendations. If this is what happens in practice, then what is measured in short-term dietary records may be actual intake or desired intake, but not usual intake.

Many studies have now demonstrated that there is a tendency, in most population subgroups, for short-term dietary records to provide estimates of energy intake that are on average around 16% lower than would be expected on the basis of measured and/or estimated levels of energy expenditure.

These studies will be discussed further in the section on precision and validity. The fact that for some groups measurements of energy intake and energy expenditure agree quite closely indicates that it is possible to achieve recording without a concomitant change in diet when there is full cooperation from respondents, and highlights the importance of efforts to achieve such cooperation.

10.5 Choosing a dietary assessment method

It is not possible to decide which dietary method to use until the purpose of the study has been clearly

defined, since this will determine the kind of information and the length of time for which it needs to be collected from each individual. Often, the purpose of the study also determines the level of precision that is required to meet the study objectives and therefore the sample size. These two considerations are the most important ones in determining the method to be used, because both the method and the size of the sample have implications for the human and financial resources needed for the study.

Purpose of the study

When dietary data are collected to describe the diet of a group for comparison with that of another group or groups, it is possible to use either a short-term method such as a 24 hour recall or record, or a longer-term method such as food records obtained over several days, a diet history, or a questionnaire about habitual intake. The final choice will depend on factors such as the importance of a representative study sample, the resources available, and the level of precision required. Usually, the most efficient approach is to measure the diet of as many individuals as possible for 1 day.

However, if the purpose of the dietary study is to determine the proportion of individuals in the group who are at risk of dietary inadequacy or excess, relative to some standard of reference, then a single day of information on each individual is no longer adequate because it is necessary to have a reliable estimate of the distribution of habitual intake in the group. As Figure 10.2 shows, a single day of intake is generally not a reliable measure of an individual's habitual intake.

To determine the distribution of habitual food intake in a group, at least 2 days (preferably not consecutive) of information from each individual or a representative subsample of individuals from the group of interest are needed. If several days of intake are available they can be used to derive a mean intake for each individual and from this the distribution of average intakes for the group. Alternatively, statistical techniques can be used to adjust 1 day intake data, for the day-to-day variation that occurs in individuals, to provide a better estimate of the underlying distribution of habitual intake for the group than is given by the 1 day data (Dodd *et al.*, 2006). While the use of appropriate statistical techniques can improve estimates of the proportion of individuals at risk of deficiency by adjusting for within-person variation, they do not enable at-risk individuals to be identified.

When the purpose of the study is to assess the diet of specific individuals it is necessary to obtain dietary information over at least a week and preferably longer. This is best done by obtaining either multiple 24 hour recalls or 24 hour food records over an extended period. The minimum number of days needed to obtain an estimate of nutrient intake with a specified level of confidence differs for different nutrients. Information on energy intake, which tends to show less day-to-day variation than other nutrients, can be obtained over a shorter period (days) than information on a nutrient for which day-to-day intake is much more variable, such as vitamin A (weeks).

Precision

In studies of groups, precision is primarily a function of sample size, while in studies of individuals it is a function of the number of days of information available. Precision increases with sample size and with the number of days for which information is collected, but so does the cost of the study. Precision therefore needs to be defined in relation to the purpose of the study.

Usually, what is required of the nutritionist is to be able to provide the statistician with an estimate of the level of difference that it is important to be able to detect (in nutritional, not statistical terms) and an estimate of the variance or standard deviation for the measurement(s) in question. For example, when looking for differences in energy intake between two groups, would a difference of 500 kJ or 1500 kJ be regarded as biologically significant?

Since the variance of a dietary measurement depends not only on the real variation within or between respondents but also on the error of the measurement, the precision of a dietary estimate can be improved not only by increasing sample size but also by reducing measurement error.

Resources

It is inevitable that the resources available, both financial and human, also influence the choice of method. They should not, however, be the primary consideration. The method used should be determined by the question to be answered. If the method or methods needed to answer the question are beyond the

resources available it is better either to abandon the study or to redefine the question than to collect inadequate data.

10.6 Repeatability and validity

This section looks at ways in which it is possible to assess the repeatability and validity of dietary methods.

Repeatability

Assessing the repeatability (also referred to as the reproducibility) of a laboratory method is relatively straightforward because, with care, it is possible to reproduce both what is measured and the conditions of measurement. This is almost always impossible in the case of a dietary intake measurement. Individuals do not eat exactly the same quantities or the same foods on different days or weeks.

All measures of repeatability obtained by applying the same method to the same individuals on more than one occasion include not only measurement error but also real day-to-day or week-to-week variability in intake.

While at first sight it might appear easier to measure the repeatability of recall methods such as the 24 hour recall and diet histories, this process also introduces additional sources of variation since the interviews have to be conducted at different times and possibly by different interviewers. Measures of repeatability for all dietary methods will thus tend to give an overestimate of the extent of measurement error because they will always include an element of variation due to real differences in what is being measured and in the conditions under which it is being measured.

Usually, the repeatability of a dietary method is determined by repeating the same method on the same individuals on two separate occasions, that is, by a test–retest study. The interval between tests depends on the time-frame of the dietary method being assessed, but should generally be short enough to avoid the effects of seasonal or other changes in food habits and long enough to avoid the possibility of the first interview or recording period influencing the second one.

The difference between the results obtained on the two occasions can be expressed in a number of different ways. Table 10.5, which was compiled from data reported in the literature, shows various mea-

Table 10.5 Measures of repeatability for energy intake obtained for a 3 day food record, a dietary history, and a food frequency questionnaire (FFQ)

Measure of repeatability	3 day food record	Dietary history	FFQ
Mean difference (kJ/day)	156	105	954
Mean difference (% of overall mean intake)	1.6	1.1	12.5
Coefficient of variation of the differences within individuals (%)	16.5	18.6	28.5
Coefficient of repeatability (kJ)	±3266	±1819	±4294
Correlation coefficient	–	0.86[a]	0.70[a]
Individuals classified in the same quartile or tertile* on both occasions (%)	56	–	60*

[a] Intraclass correlation.

sures of repeatability for energy intake obtained with different dietary methods repeated after an interval of time.

The different measures of repeatability provide different information. The correlation coefficient is widely quoted but is not a good measure of repeatability since a good correlation may be obtained even if one set of measurements has been systematically biased and has a different mean from the other set. The mean difference is not a good measure of repeatability in individuals since it depends primarily on whether the differences are random or systematic. Measures that reflect the differences between repeated measurements within individuals are to be preferred. The coefficient of variation of the differences within individuals and the coefficient of repeatability (which is simply twice the standard deviation of the differences and represents the 95% confidence limits of agreement) give much better measures of their magnitude. They are also more readily interpreted in practical terms than either a correlation coefficient or the percentage of individuals classified in the same quintile, quartile, or tertile. If the standard deviation of the difference within individuals is of the order of 20–30% of mean intake, one is unlikely to describe the method as precise or repeatable even if the mean difference at group level is only 1%.

Validity

Demonstrating that a dietary method measures what it is intended to measure is even more difficult than demonstrating that a method is repeatable, because in effect it "requires that the truth be known."

This is almost always impossible unless it is possible to observe, surreptitiously, what is consumed over short periods such as 24 hours or at most a few days. Observation is usually only feasible in institutional settings or in situations specially set up to allow unobtrusive observation of what people eat.

For methods that are designed to obtain information on habitual longer-term intake, such as the diet history or food frequency questionnaires, unobtrusive observation is impossible. This is a problem that has been faced by all investigators of dietary assessment methods and until relatively recently was usually "solved" by assessing one dietary method in relation to another dietary method, usually a 7 day weighed dietary record, which was considered to be the best available or criterion measure. Comparison with another dietary method provides at best only a relative form of validity and at worst information that is unrelated to validity but reflects either real differences or similar errors between the methods. For example, comparison of data from a single 24 hour recall or a diet history with data from a 7 day weighed record for the same individuals does not compare the same information because the time periods are not concurrent. However, because of the lack of a suitable external standard against which true validity could be judged before the 1980s it was usually assumed that most dietary intake data, and weighed records in particular, provided valid data. Usually, a method was judged acceptable if the mean intake, as measured by both methods, did not differ significantly and if correlations for nutrient intake in individuals exceeded 0.5. The magnitude of the coefficient of variation of the differences within individuals was generally ignored.

Table 10.6 shows data from three studies that provide additional information on agreement. All three studies compared data from a food frequency questionnaire with multiple days of food intake records. When different methods are compared the mean differences tend to be higher (there is greater bias) than those found in repeatability studies. However, the range of values obtained for other

Table 10.6 Measures of relative validity for energy intake obtained from a food frequency questionnaire (FFQ) compared with multiple days of records in three different studies

Measure of validity	7 days of weighed records	12 days of weighed records	15 days of records in household measures
Mean difference (kJ/day) (FFQ – record)	800	926	351
Mean difference (% of overall mean intake)	6	11	4
Coefficient of variation of the differences within individuals (%)	32.7	26.6	16.9
Coefficient of repeatability (kJ)	±8248	±4542	±2950
Correlation coefficient	–	0.69	0.71
Individuals classified in the same quintile or tertile* on both occasions (%)	43*	42	44

measures of agreement is generally similar to that obtained in repeatability studies. Agreement at the individual level is also not high, with coefficients of variation for differences in individuals ranging from 17% to 33% in these studies and less than 50% of respondents classified in the same quintile of intake. Note that even good agreement between two dietary methods does not necessarily indicate validity, but may merely indicate similar errors.

Biological measures to validate energy and nutrient intake

It is now clearly recognized that to assess the validity of any dietary method, including weighed records, it is necessary to compare the dietary data with one or more objective measures that reflect but are independent of food intake. At the group level such measures include food supply or food expenditure data, and at the individual level biochemical or physiological measures that reflect energy and nutrient intake. The latter are often referred to as biological or biochemical markers and include energy expenditure, urinary breakdown products of protein, sodium, and potassium, plasma levels of vitamins, tissue levels of minerals, and the fatty acid composition of subcutaneous adipose tissue.

> Biological marker – any biochemical index in an easily accessible biological sample that in health gives a predictive response to a given dietary component.
>
> (Bingham, 1987).

Biological markers are assumed to be objective, i.e., they do not rely on memory, or the respondents' ability to express themselves, and are free of biases introduced by the presence of the interviewers. These measures are also subject to errors of measurement and classification, but these errors are not related to the errors inherent in dietary intake assessment methodologies.

The three most widely used measures to assess the validity of dietary intake data are urinary nitrogen to validate protein intake, energy expenditure as measured by the doubly labeled water (DLW) method to validate energy intake in weight-stable individuals, and the ratio of energy intake to basal metabolic rate to identify "plausible" records of food intake.

Urinary nitrogen

One of the first to suggest an external measure as a means of validating dietary intake data was Isaakson (1980), who proposed urinary nitrogen as an independent measure of protein intake according to the equation:

$$\text{Reported protein intake (g)} = \\ (24 \text{ hour urinary N} + 2) \times 6.25 \text{ (g)}$$

Like the 24 hour recall, a single 24 hour urine collection does not necessarily reflect what is "usual." However, it appears that urinary nitrogen excretion is less variable from day to day than dietary protein intake, and that while 16 days of food intake are needed to assess habitual protein intake only eight 24 hour urine collections are needed to assess nitrogen excretion with the same level of confidence.

Although fewer 24 hour urine collections may be needed they are, in general, no more acceptable to respondents than 24 hour food records and also require access to laboratory facilities. Nevertheless, they can provide a practical independent assessment, not only of protein but also of potassium and sodium intake.

Very few validation studies have attempted to evaluate how well the different methods rank individuals. It has been observed that the correlation between urinary nitrogen and dietary nitrogen measured by diet records was better (0.65 and 0.79) than between urinary nitrogen and dietary nitrogen measured by food frequency questionnaires (0.15 and 0.24).

Doubly labeled water method

The DLW technique allows the measurement of energy expenditure in free-living respondents over several days with minimal inconvenience to the respondent and with a high level of accuracy and precision. Under controlled conditions the DLW method gives a small overestimate of 2–3% compared with whole body calorimetry, and under field conditions bias is not expected to exceed 5%.

The DLW method requires that the respondent drinks a small measured dose of water enriched with naturally occurring stable isotopes of deuterium and ^{18}O. The two isotopes disperse throughout the body, and are metabolized and then gradually lost from the body. Since the deuterium labels the body water pool, and the ^{18}O labels both the water and the bicarbonate pools, the difference between the disappearance rates of deuterium and ^{18}O can be used to calculate carbon dioxide production. The level of both isotopes is determined, using mass spectrometry, in a small sample of urine collected each day for between 5 and 28 days. Energy expenditure is calculated from carbon dioxide production using calorimetric equations. Further details of the DLW technique and the main factors influencing its accuracy and precision are provided in Chapter 3.

Using the DLW technique several investigators have compared self-reported dietary energy intake with energy expenditure based on the equation:

$$\text{Energy expenditure (EE)} = \text{Energy intake (EI)} \pm \text{Change in the body energy store}$$

Differences between measured energy intake and expenditure varied from −44% to +28% depending on the population subgroup studied. This finding confirms the need to include one or more independent measures of validity in all dietary studies to ascertain the level applicable to the particular group under study, since it is not readily predicted on the basis of gender, age, or body mass index (BMI).

The main advantage of the DLW method is that it makes minimal demands on the respondents and does not in any way interfere with their normal daily activities and therefore their habitual level of energy expenditure. Its main disadvantage is that the cost of the DLW required for each estimate is exceedingly high and the method also requires access to sophisticated laboratory equipment for mass spectrometric analysis. It is, therefore, not available for use on a routine basis for the validation of dietary intake data.

Ratio of energy intake to basal metabolic rate

Because of the limitations of the DLW method, another approach that is used compares the energy intake (EI) reported from published studies with the presumed requirements for energy expenditure, both intake and expenditure being expressed as multiples of the basal metabolic rate (BMR). The relevant equation is:

$$\text{EI:BMR} = \text{EE:BMR (PAL)}$$

where PAL is the physical activity level. To determine whether reported energy intake is a "plausible" measure of actual diet during the measurement period (i.e., represents either the habitual diet or is a low/high energy intake obtained simply by chance) an equation was developed by Goldberg and colleagues (1991) to calculate the 95% confidence limits of agreement between EI:BMR and PAL. This equation allowed for variation in EI, BMR, and PAL and also for the length of the dietary assessment period and study sample size.

For a group, if mean reported EI:BMR is below the lower 95% confidence limit (cut-off) for the given study period and sample size, then there is definitely bias to the underestimation of energy intake.

However, the identification of individual under-reporters is much more difficult, since reported EI can deviate quite markedly from energy expenditure (EE) before it falls outside the limitations of the methods. Figures 10.7 and 10.8 illustrate the limitations of both techniques. Figure 10.7 shows the energy intake and DLW EE of 264 women. The solid lines indicate EI:EE of 0.76 and 1.24. These are the 95% confidence limits of agreement between EI and EE, allowing for day-to-day variation in food intake and within-subject variation on repeat DLW measurements. Only women with an EI:EE ratio above 1.24 can be confidently

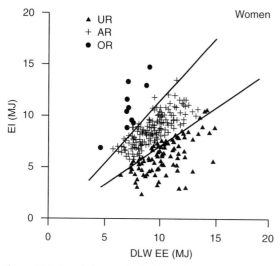

Figure 10.7 Reported energy intake (EI) against energy expenditure (EE) measured by doubly labeled water (DLW) in 264 women aged 18–90 years. The solid lines represent the 95% confidence limits of the expected agreement between EI and EE (±24%). UR, underreporters; AR, acceptable reporters; OR, overreporters (after Black, 2000, reproduced with permission).

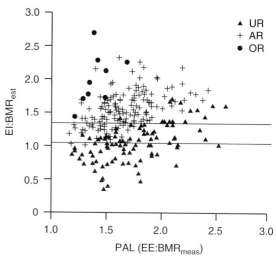

Figure 10.8 Energy intake–estimated basal metabolic rate (EI:BMR$_{est}$) against physical activity level [PAL; energy expenditure–measured BMR (EE:BMR$_{meas}$)]. Respondents are designated as acceptable reporters (AR), overreporters (OR), or underreporters (UR) by the direct comparison of EI:EE. The horizontal lines indicate the lower Goldberg cut-off for PAL = 1.55 and 1.95, 7 day records, and $n = 1$ (after Black, 2000, reproduced with permission).

identified as overreporters, and those below 0.76 as underreporters. In Figure 10.8, the same data are expressed as EI:BMR and EE:BMR, and each respondent is represented by the same symbol as in Figure 10.7. The line at EI:BMR = 1.05 indicates the Goldberg cut-off for $n = 1$ and PAL = 1.55, which has been widely used to identify low energy reporters (LERs). These data demonstrate that only about 50% of underreporters (as defined by EI:EE = 0.76) are identified as LERs. The second line at EI:BMR of 1.35 is the Goldberg cut-off for $n = 1$ and PAL = 1.95. This cut-off identifies more of the underreporters, but also includes some of the acceptable reporters. To improve on identification of underreporters it is necessary to have information on physical activity to enable respondents to be classified into different levels of activity and to calculate cut-offs appropriate for each activity level.

While the ability to separate the food and nutrient intake data of those with and without plausible energy intakes is a very important step in the evaluation of dietary intake data, it does have limitations.

- The equations for the estimation of BMR have been derived for Western populations and their

application to other populations must be done with caution.
- The ratio does not take differences in physical activity into account (Black, 2000).
- Using a single cut-off point to identify underreporters has been found to have poor sensitivity for underreporting (fails to identify underreporters), especially at high levels of energy intake (Black, 2000).
- Cut-off values differ among studies. Thus it is difficult to select an appropriate value and to compare studies.
- Cut-off values apply only to individuals in energy balance. They cannot be applied to growing children or to adults trying to lose weight (Gibson, 2005).

Characteristics of low energy reporters

A number of studies have examined the characteristics of low energy reporters (LERs). Associations between low energy reporting and a large number of factors including high body weight, high BMI, obesity, dieting, and awareness of body image were found in every study that looked at these measures. Associations with other sociodemographic factors of the type normally included in nutrition studies, such as gender, age, education, socioeconomic status, and smoking, were inconsistent.

10.7 Evaluation of food intake data

Recognizing the impact of underreporting

As indicated in Section 10.5, dietary studies are often conducted in order to compare food and nutrient intake between different groups in the population, to determine the proportion of individuals at risk of dietary inadequacy or excess, or to determine the habitual intake of individuals.

In each case it is important first to assess the validity of the data. For most investigators the use of the Goldberg cut-offs is currently the most practical option to indicate whether, and to what extent, the results are likely to be biased. However, to use the Goldberg cutoffs effectively dietary studies need to include:

- measurements of weight and height, to be able to estimate BMR from equations
- questions on activity level to provide guidance on suitable PALs for evaluation of both mean and individual data.

While the characteristics of "true" underreporters (as opposed to LERs identified by a single EI:BMR cut-off) remain to be confirmed, the associations consistently observed between high BMI, weight consciousness, and low energy reporting suggest that, in addition, questions on self-perception of body shape, dieting, and dietary restraint may also help in identifying true underreporters.

It cannot be overemphasized that it is always important to examine all dietary intake data critically because false conclusions generate false hypotheses that may take years to be disproved.

A classic case was the *luxus konsumption* hypothesis, namely that lean individuals are energy prodigal and obese individuals energy efficient. This hypothesis was generated by studies apparently showing that obese persons did not consume more energy than their lean controls. Subsequently, DLW studies demonstrated beyond doubt that obese persons recruited for studies of obesity grossly underreported their food intake.

Allowing for the effects of underreporting

Although techniques for handling biased dietary data have been developed, most are complex However, the following suggestions serve to promote critical examination of data and wariness in drawing conclusions.

If the proportion of individuals who report implausibly low intakes of energy differs between population subgroups of interest, then any comparisons between them that do not take this into account will be biased. One way to draw attention to the possibility of bias between groups is to report not only the mean or median energy intake of the groups being compared but also the EI:BMR ratio. If differences are evident then the groups should be compared both with and without LERs included. One problem that arises is that by subdividing the groups the sample size is reduced and imprecision increased, so that a difference of biological significance may be missed, not because it does not exist but because the sample size is too small to detect it statistically.

When dietary inadequacy or excess is the question of interest, it is again important to consider LERs separately. Energy intake is highly correlated with the intake of many nutrients and, consequently, intake of nutrients is also likely to be underestimated in underreporters and more likely to indicate inadequacy relative to recommendations for nutrient intake. An alternative approach is to compare nutrient intake per unit energy for both groups. If this differs between LERs and the rest of the population it provides evidence that the reporting of food intake is also likely to be selective. The nutrients for which significant differences are observed can also provide clues as to the types of food likely to be involved.

Studies that have examined macronutrient intake between respondents above and below a given value of EI:BMR have generally found that the percentage of energy derived from protein was higher and that from fat lower in LERs than in non-LERs. Results for carbohydrate have been more variable, but, when separated into starch and sugars, energy from starch tended to be higher and energy from sugars lower in LERs. Nutrient density also tends to be higher for most nutrients in LERs than in non-LERs, providing further indication of differences in food patterns between the two groups.

Table 10.7 Nutrient intakes in low energy reporting (LER) and non-LER adults in the 1995 Australian National Nutrition Survey

Nutrient	LER (n = 1291)	Non-LER (n = 9451)	Total (n = 10 851)
Energy (MJ)	4.62	10.19	9.24
Protein (g/MJ)	11.0	9.8	9.9
Fat (g/MJ)	8.1	9.0	9.0
Starch (g/MJ)	15.9	14.9	15.0
Sugars (g/MJ)	12.9	12.4	12.4
Vitamin (µg/MJ)	159	122	127
Riboflavin (mg/MJ)	0.26	0.22	0.23
Folate (µg/MJ)	37	28	29
Vitamin C (mg/MJ)	19	13	13
Calcium (mg/MJ)	106	90	92
Iron (mg/MJ)	1.8	1.5	1.5

Data used from the Australian Bureau of Statistics (abs.gov.au) (ABS, 1998).

Table 10.7 illustrates these general trends with data from the 1995 Australian National Nutrition Survey. Twelve per cent of men and 21% of women in this survey were identified as LERs. The median energy intake in non-LERs was approximately 6% higher in men and 10% higher in women than for all men and women, and vitamin and mineral intake approximately 5–10% higher in non-LER men and 6–15% higher in non-LER women. Differences of this order of magnitude are important in the context of the assessment of dietary adequacy.

Relatively few studies have reported on differences in foods eaten, but there appears to be a general tendency for LERs to report more foods such as meat, fish, vegetables, salads, and fruit, and fewer cakes, biscuits, sugar, confectionery, and fats.

10.8 Assessment of dietary adequacy

Methods for evaluating dietary adequacy are described in Chapter 7. This section simply draws attention to the limitations of these methods.

The first limitation is that the evaluation of nutrient intake can provide only an estimate of the risk of nutrient inadequacy for a population or an individual. None of the methods can identify the specific individuals who have a nutrient deficiency. Individuals with a nutrient deficiency or excess can be identified only on the basis of biochemical or clinical measures of nutritional status.

The second limitation is that all estimates of dietary adequacy/inadequacy obtained by comparison with reference values for nutrient requirements depend on how the estimate is derived (see Chapter 7).

However, irrespective of the approach that is used to assess dietary adequacy, unless the extent of under-reporting is known and taken into account, the proportion of individuals at risk of inadequacy will be overestimated. While it may become possible to distinguish more reliably in population-based studies valid from invalid reports of dietary intake, this still does not enable population-based estimates of inadequacy to be made unless those who provide valid intakes are also representative of the population as a whole. All the evidence available to date suggests that this is highly unlikely.

When the principal objective of a dietary survey is to identify the proportion of the population who may have inadequate intakes of energy and nutrients, it is essential that the dietary intake information is interpreted in the light of appropriate biological measures of nutritional status.

10.9 Assessing food intake

Nutritionists usually analyze dietary intake data by converting the information on food intake into nutrient intake using relevant food composition databases. This approach simplifies the process of analysis and enables the resulting data to be compared with energy and nutrient requirements (see Chapter 7). Describing food intake in terms of foods rather than nutrients presents two practical difficulties that do not exist when food intake is analyzed in terms of nutrients. First, the variety of foods consumed is much greater than the range of nutrients for which food composition data are available. Second, while essentially all individuals in a group contribute to nutrient intake data, not all individuals contribute food data for all foods, i.e., not all individuals are "consumers" of the same foods.

There are, however, several uses for which information on food intake is more relevant or for which information on food intake is needed in conjunction with data on nutrient intake. For example, food regulatory authorities and agencies concerned with food safety and nutritional surveillance require data on the availability and intake of foods in addition to information on nutrient intake. Similarly, nutritional epidemiologists are also interested in the relationship of different foods and dietary patterns with specific health outcomes. The use of dietary data in the context of epidemiological studies is covered in the textbook *Public Health Nutrition* (Gibney *et al.* 2004).

The analysis and presentation of food intake data depends on the objectives of the study. When the purpose is to examine intakes of specific foods, intakes of foods may be expressed as means, medians, or frequency distributions of intakes, as the number or percentage of respondents consuming specific foods, or as the percentage contribution of food items to the total food intake, energy intake, or intake of nutrients of interest. Since not all members of a sample consume a given food, it is always important to indicate whether the total sample size or only the number of respondents consuming the food has been used in statistical calculations.

Although intakes of individual food items may be reported, food intake data are usually reduced to more manageable proportions by grouping foods into appropriate categories. While this can be done in different ways, for example in terms of composition, biological origin, or cultural use, the process is relatively straightforward within a given culture or country. It is more difficult, however, to develop a classification that can be used consistently across different countries or food cultures. National food classification systems tend to differ not only because the type and range of foods differs but also because the same foods are used in different ways. For the purpose of comparing food intake patterns between countries or regions, it is, therefore, necessary to develop a food classification or coding system that allows food data from individual regions or countries to be assigned in a consistent way.

The United Nations University Food and Nutrition Program for an International Network of Food Data Systems (INFOODS) was developed for the purpose of supporting work on the classification and naming conventions for individual foods and food groups (see Chapter 2).

Indirect information on food consumption, such as that provided by FAO food balance sheets and by data from household budget and similar surveys, is usually presented in terms of foods or food groups,

but may also be converted to nutrients to provide information on the nutrient contribution of individual foods or groups of foods.

Tracking changes in the food sources of nutrients and nonnutrients is particularly important in the context of technological developments in food production and manufacture that result in the addition of nutrients to foods, in the development of foods for specific functional purposes, and in the genetic modification of foods. A specific example of the need for individual food, rather than nutrient, intake data is provided by exposure assessments to dietary nonnutrients such as food additives, pesticide residues, and other possible food contaminants.

10.10 Food safety assessments

Safety assessments for food additives are expressed in terms of the acceptable daily intake (ADI) estimated on the basis of lifetime exposure. While it is clearly not possible to collect food consumption data over the lifetimes of individuals, it is important that the dietary data used for the purpose of estimating acceptable levels of intake over a lifetime reflect, as far as is possible, the habitual level of intake of the foods being assessed.

For the purpose of food safety assessments only the intake of "consumers" is of interest. It follows, therefore, that the dietary data need to be adequate to obtain both an accurate estimate of the proportion of the population who are consumers and of the average habitual intake of consumers. Because the frequency of consumption varies between foods (some foods are eaten by most people on most days, but many other foods are eaten less frequently), the duration of the dietary recording period influences both the estimate of the proportion of consumers and the average intake of consumers. Intake data for 1 day will inevitably underestimate the true number of consumers for most foods and overestimate the average habitual intake of those consumers because not all foods are eaten every day. However, it appears that 75% or more of household menu items are normally consumed within a 14 day period and that a 14 day diary provides a good estimate of the habitual intake of most foods by consumers.

Most studies of the food intake of individuals, however, do not last for 14 days because of the increased cost and nonresponse associated with such a long study period. For the purpose of food safety assessment an approach that combines a 3 day food intake record with a food frequency questionnaire has the potential to give estimates for the intake of consumers that are similar to those obtained from 14 day records.

10.11 Perspectives on the future

It is unlikely that either the measurement or the evaluation of food intake will become less complex in future. If anything, the reverse is likely to be true given the increasing diversity in the food supply and the increasing recognition of the need to be able to assess accurately not only the intake of foods and nutrients but also the intake of nonnutrient constituents of foods and dietary supplements. While the existence of errors in association with measurements of food intake is now widely appreciated, much work still remains to be done in this area.

Other aspects of food intake measurement that also require further development in the immediate future are likely to include the following.

As all direct methods of food intake measurement involve interaction between investigators and individuals and our understanding of the cognitive aspects of these interactions is still limited, more work is needed to improve the communications aspect of dietary assessment.

As the food supply becomes more complex individuals will no longer be able to describe the foods they have eaten in adequate detail unless technological developments such as the use of barcodes and similar systems of food identification become an integral part of dietary assessment.

As the number of food constituents of interest, in relation to health, increases it is important that appropriate physiological and biochemical markers are also developed for these constituents, as well as for the nutrient constituents of foods.

Finally, since food intake data serve no useful purpose unless they can be appropriately evaluated it is essential that dietary studies include sufficient ancillary information to allow this to occur. This means routinely collecting information not only on age, gender, body size, and physiological status, but also on key aspects of lifestyle such as physical activity and the consumption of nonfood items such as

supplements (both nutrient and nonnutrient) and drugs (both social and medicinal).

Acknowledgment

This chapter has been revised and updated by Una E MacIntyre based on the original chapter by Ingrid HE Rutishauser and Alison E Black.

References

Australian Bureau of Statistics. *Australian National Nutrition Survey*. ABS, Canberra, 1998.

Bingham SA. The dietary assessment of individuals; methods, accuracy, new techniques and recommendations. *Nutr Abstr Rev (Series A)* 1987; **57**: 705–742.

Black AE. The sensitivity and specificity of the Goldberg cut-off for EI:BMR for identifying dietary reports of poor validity. *Eur J Clin Nutr* 2000; **54**: 395–404.

Burke BS. The dietary history as a tool in research. *J Am Diet Assoc* 1947; **23**: 1041–1046.

Cade J, Thompson R, Burley V, Warm D. Development, validation and utilisation of food-frequency questionnaires: a review. *Publ Health Nutr* 2002; **5**: 567–587.

Conway JM, Ingwersen LA, Vinyard BT, Moshfegh AJ. Effectiveness of the US Department of Agriculture 5-step multiple-pass method in assessing food intake in obese and nonobese women. *Am J Clin Nutr* 2003; **77**: 1171–1178.

Dodd KW, Guenther PM, Freedman LS, *et al.* Statistical methods for estimating usual intake of nutrients and foods: a review of the theory. *J Am Diet Assoc* 2006; **106**: 1640–1650.

Domel SB. Self-reports of diet: how children remember what they have eaten. *Am J Clin Nutr* 1997: **65** (suppl): 1148S–1152S.

Gibney MJ, Margetts BM, Kearney JM, Arab L. *Public Health Nutrition*. Blackwell Publishing, Oxford, 2004; 67–75.

Gibson RS. *Principles of Nutritional Assessment*, 2nd edn. Oxford University Press, Oxford, 2005.

Goldberg GR, Black AE, Jebb SA *et al.* Critical evaluation of energy intake data using fundamental principles of energy physiology. I. Derivation of cur-off limits to identify under-recording. *Eur J Clin Nutr* 1991; **41**: 569–581.

Isaksson B. Urinary nitrogen output as a validity test in dietary surveys. *Am J Clin Nutr* 1980; **33**: 4–5.

Kruger R. The determinants of overweight among 10–15 year old school children in the North West Province. University of Potchefstroom for CHE. Unpublished PhD Thesis, 2003.

MacIntyre UE. Dietary intakes of Africans in transition in the North West Province. University of Potchefstroom for CHE. Unpublished PhD thesis, 1998.

Matt GE, Rock CL, Johnson-Kozlov M. Using recall cues to improve measurement of dietary intakes with a food frequency questionnaire in an ethnically diverse population: an exploratory study. *J Am Diet Assoc* 2006; **106**: 1209–1217.

Nelson M, Bingham SA. Assessment of food consumption and nutrient intake. In: Margetts BM, Nelson M, eds. *Design Concepts in Nutritional Epidemiology*, 2nd edn Oxford University Press, Oxford, 1997.

Thompson FE, Subar AF, Brown CC, *et al.* Cognitive research enhances accuracy of food frequency questionnaire reports:

results of an experimental validation study. *J Am Diet Assoc* 2002; **102**: 212–218, 223–225.

Vuckovic N, Ritenbaugh C, Taren DL, Tobar M. A qualitative study of participants' experiences with dietary assessment. *J Am Diet Assoc* 2002; **100**: 1023–1028.

Willett W. Food-frequency methods. In: Willett W, ed. *Nutritional Epidemiology*, 2nd edn. Monographs in Epidemiology and Biostatistics. Oxford University Press, New York, 1998: 74.

Young CM, Chalmers FW, Church HN, Murphy GC, Tucker RE. Subjects' estimation of food intake and calculated nutritive value of the diet. *J Am Diet Assoc* 1953; **29**: 1216–1220.

Further reading

Black AE. Critical evaluation of energy intake using the Goldberg cut-off for EI:BMR. A practical guide to its calculation, use and limitations. *Int J Obes* 2000; **24**: 1119–1130.

Cypel YS, Guenther PM, Petot GP. Validity of portion-size measurement aids: a review. *J Am Dielet Assoc* 1997; **97**: 289–292.

Food and Agriculture Organization. *Food Balance Sheets: Application and Uses*. Available online at http://fao.org (accessed 18 July 2007).

Food and Agriculture Organization. *Food Balance Sheets and Food Consumption Surveys: Comparison*. Available online at http://fao.org (accessed 18 July 2007).

Thomson FE, Byers T. Dietary intake resource manual. *J Nutr* 1994; **124** (Suppl): 2245S–2316S.

Venter CS, MacIntyre UE, Vorster HH. The development and testing of a food portion photograph book for use in an African population. *J Hum Nutr Dietet* 2000; **13**: 205–218.

11
Food Composition

Hettie C Schönfeldt and Joanne M Holden

Key messages

- Reliable good-quality composition data of foods for human consumption are critical resources for a variety of applications.
- These data are required for a spectrum of users ranging from international to national, regional, household, and individual levels.
- In general, data obtained on food intake by individuals, or groups of individuals, are used to estimate the consumption of nutrients and to establish nutritional requirements and health guidelines.
- The determination of the consumption of nutrients can be achieved either by analyzing the foods consumed directly (by far the most accurate, but also the most costly method) or by using food composition tables/databases.
- The food described in the food composition table should be recognizably similar to that being consumed by the individual or group.

- Factors such as sampling, variability and analytical methods involved must be considered when developing such tables.
- Inadequacies of food composition tables can be minimized by calculating nutrient losses and gains during food processing and preparation.
- New activities in food composition include:
  - future composition tables could include bioavailability and the glycemic index
  - harmonizing food composition tables regionally
  - focusing on biodiversity within species
  - investigation of the composition of specific traditional and ethnic foods
  - bioactives in foods and their effect on health and well-being
  - food composition data and their role in nutrition and health claims.

11.1 Introduction

Although the amount, quality and availability of food composition data vary among countries and regions, in general most developing countries still do not have adequate and reliable data. This is despite the fact that the components of specific foods have been published for over 150 years. Over time food composition data have assumed more scientific, academic, and political importance owing to their utility. Refer to Table 11.1 for practical examples of the uses of food composition data. It was only in 1961 that a regional food composition table was developed and published for Latin America, followed by a food composition table for Africa (1968), the Near East (1970), and Asia (1972). The data in these tables were based on a very limited number of samples, a limited number of nutrients and, in today's terms, outdated analytical methodologies. However, these tables are still being used today as there are limited up-to-date tables available. Worldwide there are currently over 150 food composition tables or nutrient databases, or their electronic/magnetic equivalents, in use. Many tables are based on the data from the United States Department of Agriculture's (USDA) National Nutrient Database for Standard Reference, SR, available on the Nutrient Data Laboratory's web site: www.ars.usda.gov/nutrientdata. A comprehensive list of the food composition tables available can be obtained from the Food and Agriculture Organization of the United Nations (FAO) homepage on the World Wide Web (http://www.fao.org/infoods/directory). EuroFIR, the European Food Information Resource Consortium, is a partnership between 40 universities, research institutes, and small to-medium-sized enterprises from 25 countries in Europe. EuroFIR aims to develop and integrate a comprehensive cohort and validated network of databanks of food composition

Table 11.1 Examples of the uses of food composition data

Level	Examples
International	Role of food in the provision of nutrients and/or the estimation of adequacy of the dietary intake of population groups
	Investigation of relationships between diet, health, and nutritional status, e.g., epidemiologists correlate patterns of disease with dietary components
	Evaluation of nutrition education programs
	Nutrition intervention and food fortification programs such as in food assistance programs; foods are distributed or enriched to address the specific nutritional needs of populations, e.g., iodine or vitamin A
	In food trade nutritional labeling
National	Monitoring at governmental level, the availability of foods produced and estimating the individual intake for specific dietary requirements, e.g., protein and energy
	Food balance sheet data are used to provide data on food available nationally for the whole population and are useful in monitoring trends in food consumption over time
	Researchers work to improve the food supply by selecting or developing new strains or cultivars, improving cultivation, harvesting, preservation, and preparation
	Estimation of adequacy of the dietary intake of groups within populations
	Investigation of relationships between diet, health, and nutritional status
	Evaluation of nutrition education programs
	Food and nutrition training
	Nutrition education and health promotion
	Nutrition intervention and food fortification programs
	Food and nutrition regulation and food safety
	Nutrition labeling of foods
Regional (influenced by meal patterns and food preferences)	Institutions such as hospitals, schools, dormitories, and troops/armies (ration scale) formulate nutritionally balanced diets to the individuals in their care
	Food industries regulate the quality of their foods by routinely analyzing the components in their products
	Food industries change and improve their products to appeal to new customers by improving nutrient content or sensory appeal through the change in ingredients
	Product development
Household	Household food surveys provide data on household food consumption
	Household budget surveys
	Household food economics
Individual	Dietary intake of the individual is assessed to understand present health and to monitor changes in dietary intake
	Impact of interpretation of choice and preference via data composition
	Individual energy expenditure is the only true measurement of energy need, e.g., in the management of a sportsman's diet or in obesity
	Personal dietary needs and goals with associated likes and dislikes can be assessed on an individual basis
	Individual nutritional balance studies
	Therapeutic or restricting diets with specific nutrient contents, e.g., management of diabetes and hypertension, can only be described on an individual basis
	Individual shoppers scan the ingredient list and nutrient content on the labels of packaged foods
	Sports nutrition

data for Europe. This network, although comprehensive, has at present limited access to the broader nutrition society.

There is still a continued need to carry out food analyses as the number of foods consumed all over the world, especially unique foods, is still several times greater than the number for which analytical data exist. The recent (2008) Cross Cutting Initiative on Biodiversity for Food and Nutrition led by the FAO and Biodiversity International focused on genetic diversity within species and of underutilized, uncultivated, and indigenous foods. The investigation has highlighted the need for composition data of foods, not only at species level, but also at subspecies level. The limited amount of composition data for underutilized, uncultivated, and indigenous foods playing important roles in the consumption patterns in under-developed and developing countries increases this need for food composition analysis. Food analyses are also needed under the following circumstances:

- when the data in existing tables are based on a single or very limited number of samples
- when the content of a nutrient or other food component is not available in an existing food table
- when there is no information available on which foods are important sources of a nutrient or another food component of interest
- when there is no information on the loss or gain of nutrients in foods during preparation by the methods being used by the population under investigation
- when it is necessary to check the comparability of the various food composition tables being used in a multicenter study
- when the method available to determine a particular nutrient is considerably improved
- when scientific evidence is found correlating newly recognized food components to health
- when new foods are produced or existing foods are reformulated.

11.2 Foods

Food composition tables normally consist of a list of selected foods with data on the content of selected nutrients in each food. For a food composition table to be of value in estimating nutrient content, a significant portion of the foods consumed by the group or individual being studied, as well as the nutrients of interest, should be present in the table. To a large extent this relationship is critical in determining the quality of the information obtained by using the tables, assuming that the data in the tables are of a desirable quality.

Criteria for inclusion in tables

The identification of potential contributions of foods to the diet of the population group being studied is unquestionably the first step in identifying and selecting which foods should and should not be included in the production of a database. However, common sense dictates that it is unreasonable to expect that all foods consumed by all individuals at all times be included in a specific food composition table at any one time. Therefore, most tables aim to include all

foods that form a major part of the food supply and that are major contributors to the diet in the forms most commonly obtained or consumed, and as many as possible of the less frequently consumed foods. For instance, in the USA the number of foods contributing to quartiles of critical nutrient intakes was identified as the following: 9 foods contribute to 25% of food intake, 34 foods to 50%, 104 to 75%, and 454 to approximately 100%.

Databases can be compiled directly, where the compiler initiates sampling and analyses to obtain the data, or indirectly by drawing on the following sources of data, in order of preference:

- original analytical values
- imputed values derived from analytical values from a similar food, e.g., values for "boiled" used for "steamed"
- calculated values derived from recipes, calculated from the ingredients and corrected for preparation factors
- borrowed values (refers to using data originally generated or gathered by someone else) from other tables and databases.

Today, database compilers normally draw on a combination of the direct and indirect methods.

Description of foods

The food described in the food composition table should be recognizably similar to that being consumed by the individual or group. The precise description of foods is a difficult task and much is required to ensure that foods are described adequately. The introductory material (description and explanation) in a printed table may be almost as important as the data values. By using several words to describe a food, called an extended or multifaceted description, the chance of misinterpreting the data is reduced. As internationalization of food composition data continues, linguistic aspects of defining foods, with one definition meaning different things in different cultures and even from place to place within countries, are highlighted. For instance, sorbet or sherbet is made by beating whisked egg whites into the partly frozen mixture such as in apple sorbet and lemon sorbet. However, the term sorbet is preferred to sherbet, since the latter can also refer to a flavored, sweet, sparkling powder or drink, or a drink of sweet diluted fruit juice. The name tortilla is also applied to a variety of foods in Latin America. In Africa morogo is a collective term used for a variety of indigenous green leafy vegetables harvested from the veld. Using scientific names for food items is not necessarily a solution, since the relationship between common name and scientific name is neither consistent nor universally unique, for example the German tables group pears and apples in the same genus, while the British and US tables separate them.

Many structured food description systems have been proposed. These systems should be adapted to the specific purpose (e.g., nutrient content, pesticide regulation) for which they are intended. For example, the FAO Committee report, INFOODS Guidelines for Describing Foods: A Systematic Approach to Describing Foods to Facilitate International Exchange of Food Composition Data, published in 1991, was designed to facilitate interchange of food composition data between nations and cultures. The system is a broad, multifaceted, and open-ended description mechanism using a string of descriptors for foods. The International Food Data System Project (INFOODS) Nomenclature and Terminology Committee has developed guidelines for describing foods to facilitate international exchange of food composition data. INFOODS is a comprehensive effort, begun within the United Nations University Food and Nutrition Program to improve data on the nutrient composition of food from all parts of the world. In line with the FAO's lead role in classification of agricultural activities and products, and to facilitate international data comparability and exchange, FAOSTAT has developed and standardized the Harmonized Commodity Description and Coding System in 1996. The coding system has developed multipurpose goods' nomenclature used as the basis for trade statistical nomenclatures all over the world.

In 1975 the Food and Drug Administration (FDA) of the USA developed a controlled vocabulary for food description, based on the principle of a faceted thesaurus, where each food indexed is described by a set of standard terms grouped in facets, characteristic of the product type of a food source and process applied to food ingredients. Examples are the biological origin, the methods of cooking and conservation, and technological treatments. It is an automated method for describing, capturing, and retrieving data about food, adapted to computerized national and international food composition and consumption

databanks, and is therefore language independent. In Table 11.2 an example of the application of LanguaL is presented. More information can be obtained from the LanguaL (Langua aLimentaria or "language of food") homepage (www.langual.org). LanguaL is an international framework for food description, which the European LanguaL Technical Committee has administered since 1996. The thesaurus is organized into 14 facets of the nutritional and/or hygienic quality of foods. These include the biological origin, the methods of preparation or conservation. The European LanguaL Technical Committee has linked LanguaL to other international food categorizing and coding systems including the CIAA Food Catgorizing System, Codex Classifications, and E-numbers used for additive identifications.

Classification of foods

Most food composition tables are organized according to the classification of foods into food groups, with food items listed alphabetically within each food group. For example, the fruit group could start with apples and end with tangerines. A simple coding system could supplement the alphabetically listed foods (used in the British tables), but it presents a problem when a new food is introduced and all the codes have to change. Although food groups of different countries and organizations are never completely identical, they are usually recognizably similar. However, problems normally arise with the description of cooked mixed dishes where a dish can be equally well described by one or more food group. In some tables, particularly those for educational purposes, there are subgroups based on the content of specific nutrients such as high-fat and low-fat dairy products. Table 11.3 provides an example of major food groups that are used by the FAO for their food balance sheets and regional food composition tables.

Sampling of foods for inclusion in tables

Food sampling concerns the selection of the individual units of foods, food products, or bulk foodstuffs from the food supply or source, whether it be the marketplace, manufacturing outlet, field or the homes of the members of the study population. (Sampling also concerns the selection of the representative aliquot from the individual unit or homogenized mixture in the laboratory just before analysis.) In-

Table 11.2 Example of the international use of LanguaL

Facet	Code	English term	French term	Danish term	Hungarian term
Product type	A0178	Bread	Pain	Brød	Kenyér
Food source	B1418	Hard wheat	Blé de force (*Triticum aestivum*)	Hård hvede (*Triticum aestivum*)	Kemény búza (*Triticum aestivum*)
Part of plant or animal	C0208	Seed or kernel, skin removed, germ removed (endosperm)	Graine ou grain sans enveloppe et sans germe	Frø eller kerne, skaldele (pericarp/caryopse) fjernet, kim fjernet (endosperm)	Szénhidrát vagy hasonló vegyület
Physical state, shape, or form	E0105	Whole, shape achieved by forming, thickness 1.5–7 cm	Entier façonné épais de 1,5 à 7 cm	Hel, facon dannet ved formning, tykkelse 1.5–7 cm	Egész, formázott, 1.5–7 cm közötti vastagság
Extent of heat treatment	F0014	Fully heat treated	Transformation thermique complète	Fuldt varmebehandlet	Teljesen hőkezelt
Cooking method	G0005	Baked or roasted	Cuit au four	Bagt eller ovnstegt	Sütött vagy pirított
Treatment applied	H0256	Carbohydrate fermented	Fermenté au niveau des glucides	Kulhydratfermenteret	Szénhidrátos fermentált
Preservation method	J0003	No preservation method used	Sans traitement de conservation	Igen konservering	Tartósítási eljárást nem alkalmaztak
Packing medium	K0003	No packing medium used	Sans milieu de conditionnement	Intet pakningsmedium anvendt	Csomagoló eszközt nem alkalmaztak
Consumer group/dietary use/label claim	P0024	Human food, no age specification	Alimentation humaine courante	Levnedamiddel uden aldersspecifikation	Emberi fogyasztásra szánt élelmiszer, kormeghatározás nélkül

Table 11.3 Major food groups that are utilized by the Food and Agriculture Organization

Cereals and grain products
Starchy roots, tubers and fruits
Grain legumes and legume products
Nuts and seeds
Vegetables and vegetable products
Fruits
Sugars and syrups
Meat, poultry, and insects
Eggs
Fish and shellfish
Milk and milk products
Oils and fats
Beverages
Miscellaneous

context sampling can be defined as the selection and collection of items of food defined in number, size, and nature to represent the food under consideration. The objectives for sampling will, in the large part, determine the type and nature of the sampling plan.

One of the major objectives of food sampling is to provide representative mean values for individual components in foods. The sampling process is described in detail in Table 11.4.

Food sampling is a critical step in any food composition program. For any research project, personnel and financial resources are always limited. The selection, procurement, shipping, and storage of sample units require a significant portion of available resources. Therefore, sampling must follow a specific and detailed statement of the objectives and procedures to ensure that the selection of units is sufficient in number and weight and representative of the foods of interest. If sampling or sample preparation is done incorrectly then all subsequent analyses are a waste of time and money, as a mistake in sampling can only be corrected by repurchasing and repreparing of a new sample. Pilot studies, conducted by the investigator(s) or published in the scientific literature, can be used as the basis of sampling decisions for the current study.

Table 11.4 Sampling process of foods for food composition data

1 *Prioritizing foods for inclusion*
May be based on:
- type
- frequency and
- amount of specific foods or products consumed
- quality and quantity of existing data
- appropriateness of prior analytical methods or
- perceived benefit/risk of particular foods as sources of components of interest

May be affected by:
- changes in the forms of foods or
- levels of components, including reformulation or fortification
Levels of available resources will impact on the process of setting priorities

2 *Defining prioritized foods*
Within the context of the objective, define the specific characteristics of the food that may contribute to the variability of the estimate:
- uncooked or raw foodstuffs versus cooked forms of the food
- composition of prepared or multicomponent foods (i.e. mixed dishes)
- individual brands or cultivars or generic value

3 *Definition of sampling unit*
Collection of units (packages, bunches, or items) representative of the total population of food units:
- sample units must be taken from the available types and forms of the food for which the composition estimates are being determined. Production, consumption or sales statistics may be used. The population of items may be supplied to or distributed through an entire nation or region or be only typical of a particular subpopulation (e.g. ethnic group or tribe)
- select sample units from all the various types of food and geographical or manufacturing locations of food consumed by the population of interest. The units may be selected according to the relative importance (e.g., frequency of consumption) for given types
- sample units that are collected can be analyzed as individual units or may be combined together or composited and analyzed. The analysis of composite samples reduces the costs associated with the analysis of individual samples, but information about the variability of the component in that food will be lost

4 *Definition of sampling size*
Amount of material required:
- objective of analyses
- analyses of individual samples or composite samples of the food
- number of components to be measured; determine the number and weight of aliquots needed as required by the chemical methods
- policy for saving reserve or archive aliquots

5 *Protocol for sample collection*
Foods should be typical of the usual preparation and consumption practices
Correct units of foods should be selected
Protocols should be tested for the adequacy of food storage and transportation facilities, sample unit documentation and labeling, and packaging and short-term preservation requirements
Policies for the substitution of units should be in place in the event of unavailable sample units
Sampling among ethnic or native populations may impose additional restrictions owing to cultural or religious customs
Samples should be clearly coded for identification. Documentation should start from the planning stage, throughout purchasing, transporting, preparation and the combining of samples, to analyses including storage condition, use of reference samples, recording of data obtained (duplicate or triplicate values), as well as manipulation of the data, e.g. expression of the data on a wet (as eaten) basis, as opposed to the content of a freeze-dried sample. Correction factors applied or calculations (e.g. $N \times$ Jones factor = protein) should be recorded for each foodstuff analyzed
Documentation and handling of sample units should be under the careful control of the principal co-coordinator and all laboratory personnel should be informed before the start of the project of the reasons for handling the samples in a specific manner. The samples should preferably be marked with three-digit random codes for analysts to ensure that analyses are unbiased. Values should only be decoded as results become available, by the principal investigator. This will improve the reliability of the results if performed on a double-blind basis

Variability in foods: regional and other differences

Foods are biological materials and, as such, have a naturally variable composition. Even processed foods produced under highly controlled circumstances show some variability. Therefore, a database must be able to predict the composition of a single sample of food within the limits defined by its natural variability. Variability may be contributed by one or more of the following factors: brand, cultivars or species, season, climate, geographical location (e.g., soil type), fertilizer treatment, method of husbandry, harvesting, preservation state, stage of maturity, enrichment/fortification standards, preparation methods, food color, variation in recipes and formulations, distribution and marketing practices, and other factors. For critical components variability may affect the sufficiency, deficiency, or excess of the intake of a given component. Estimates of variability must be based on sampling and analyses specifically planned to yield such data. The intended use of the data should determine the specificity and level of precision for the estimates.

For instance, it was found that the nutrient composition of whole milk in South Africa differed among the five localities investigated between winter and summer, with the fat-soluble vitamins showing the greatest variation of all the nutrients. Vitamin A is commonly regarded as one of the micronutrients that are deficient in most developing countries and specifically in disadvantaged schoolchildren in South Africa. Considering the results of the nutrient composition of whole milk, a recommendation was made to the health authorities to fortify summer milk with retinol in the South African school-feeding intervention program, where milk is served as a mid-morning snack to 5 million primary school children.

There is a growing recognition that the composition of commodities such as meat and cereals tends to change over time. This necessitates updating food composition data every 5–10 years. In most countries this has not been possible. Changes in nutrient composition of red meat consumed are due to consumer demand for leaner cuts, changes in breeding for faster growth, and higher proportions of marketable meat as well as changes in feed to meet scientific standards or due to economic reasons.

11.3 Nutrients, nonnutrients and energy

Analytical methods

Judgment should be made on the availability of suitable methods of analyses for nutrients and whether the resources, laboratory equipment, and experience are adequate before deciding which nutrients should be included in a nutrient database. If the methods available are not well developed, one should reconsider the importance of the nutrient and whether it justifies using limited resources, in most instances and countries, to develop the method and train the staff accordingly. It will not be cost-effective to analyze food for a particular nutrient, however high in priority, if methods yield conflicting values. This implies that, as new or improved methods for measuring a nutrient emerge, foods that are important in the food supply and are known or suspected to be a good

source of that nutrient should be analyzed or re-analyzed. Food regulation sometimes limits the choice of methods.

The choice of method selected should be that which most closely reflects the nutritive content of the foodstuff analyzed. A basic understanding of the chemistry of the nutrients, the nature of the food substrate (the way in which the nutrient is distributed and held in the food matrix) to be analyzed, the effect of processing and preparation on both the food matrix and the nutrient, and the expected range of concentration of the nutrient determine the choice of method. An understanding of the role of the nutrient in the diet of individuals or populations is also a prerequisite.

The basic principle is that the method used should provide information that is nutritionally appropriate. For instance, traditionally, carbohydrate was estimated by difference, that is, by directly measuring the percentage of protein (from the nitrogen content), fat, ash, and water, and deducting these from 100 to provide the percentage of carbohydrate. This method is inadequate for all nutritional purposes as it combines in one value all of the different carbohydrate species: sugars, oligosaccharides, and polysaccharides (starch and non-starch), together with all of the errors in the other determinations, as the physiological effects of all of the components are quite different. Therefore, the sum of the individually analyzed carbohydrates is widely recommended today.

In studying the relationship between particular foods and health or disease, the biological action of related nutrients may be crucial information for particular uses of food composition data. For example, a study on the role of vitamin A and carotenoids in lung cancer requires more information than the vitamin A activity expressed in retinol equivalents. At the very least, vitamin A and provitamin A activity are required separately. Information on provitamin A could be divided into the various provitamin A carotenoids, and it may also be desirable to have information on other carotenoids present. This is also true for the vitamers of other vitamins, including vitamin B_6 (pyridoxal, pyridoxal phosphate, and pyridoxamine), folic acid (with a side-chain with one, three, or seven glutamic acid residues), vitamin D (D_2 or D_3), vitamin E (various tocopherols and tocotrienols) and vitamin K (with various numbers of saturated and unsaturated isoprene units in the side-chain).

The EuroFIR BASIS bioactives database includes critically assessed composition data on the bioactives present in edible plants and plant-based foods as well as compilation of critically assessed data on their biological effect (http://www.eurofir.net).

Criteria for inclusion in tables

As the number of nutrients is reasonably infinite, it is to some extent easier to choose and prioritize food items. Core nutrients for a nutritional database include the major proximate constituents, those that are essential, and those for which there are recommended intakes. The inclusion of micronutrients, especially trace elements, fatty acid profiles, amino acid composition and the various forms of vitamins is normally limited by the resources available. Many databases give limited coverage of the carbohydrates and carotenoids in foods, but methods are available and this limitation will probably disappear in the future.

Nutrients to be included in the food composition table will depend on the proposed use of the table. For instance, when assessing nutrient intake, two types of nutrients can often be distinguished: those nutrients that are found in small quantities in a large number of foods, such as iron and most of the B vitamins, and those that are found in large quantities in a small number of foods, such as cholesterol and vitamin A. The FAO limits the inclusion of nutrients in the table for group feeding schemes to 11 nutrients per 100 g of edible portion. The nutrients that have been selected as the most important for developing countries are energy, protein, fat, calcium, iron, vitamin A, thiamine, riboflavin, niacin, folate, and vitamin C.

Complete coverage of all nutrients in a single food database is unlikely, as priorities are set according to the importance of a food in the provision of a nutrient, resulting normally in analyses of proximates and major nutrients. However, with the growing interest in the role of biologically active compounds, residues, and toxicants in food there is increased pressure to include these in special-purpose food composition tables. Phytochemicals or phytoprotectants, often used in functional foods, are bioactive compounds found in food that may have benefits to human health.

A provisional database for food flavonoid composition has been developed and is maintained by the United States Department of Agriculture (USDA) on its National Nutrient Databank website (http://www.ars.usda.gov/nutrientdata). The database contains values for 385 food items for five subclasses of flavonoids namely flavonols, flavones, flavanones, flavan-3-ols, and anthocyanidins.

A European network established to compile and evaluate data on natural food plant toxicants, the EU AIR Concerted Action NETTOX, has previously identified 31 major compound classes called the NETTOX: a list of toxicant classes with 307 major food plants listed in Europe. This list, now known as the EuroFIR NETTOX plant list (http://www.eurofir.net) has recently been published after being updated to include additional plant parts. The list now includes 550 beneficial biological effect outputs of the bioactive compounds of 328 edible plants. This list facilitates calculations of exposure to bioactive compounds such as flavanols, phenolic compounds, phytosterols, carotenoids, isoflavones, and lignans.

For a food composition database to include all these substances will imply that there may be an over-emphasis on "nonnutrients." In general, levels of pesticides, residues, toxicants, and additives in food, with the exception of those that contribute to energy and nutrients, are often not reported in food composition tables.

Modes of expression

An increasing amount of attention is being paid to how data are presented in food composition tables. Interchange and compatibility of food composition databases are only possible if the data are uniformly expressed. To overcome ambiguities in the naming of nutrients and also to allow for the transfer of data among food composition tables, INFOODS has developed a system for identifying food components, referred to as tags. The term "tag" refers to the significant part of a generic identifier. Generic identifiers are predefined word-like strings of characters used to distinguish one element type from another. An example of a tagname and its definition is presented in Table 11.5. The latest information on this system is available on the World Wide Web via the INFOODS home page (http://www.fao.org/infoods). As already mentioned, LanguaL is a multilingual system that provides a standardized language for describing food products using faceted classification. Each food is described by a set of standard, controlled terms chosen from facets characteristic of the nutritional and/or hygienic

Table 11.5 Example of an INFOODS tagname and its definition for a food component

---

<ENERC>

Energy, total metabolizable; calculated from the energy-producing food components

Unit: kJ. The value for <ENERC> may be expressed in kilocalories instead of the default unit of kiloJoules. However, if expressed in kilocalories, kcal must be explicitly stated with the secondary tagname <Unit>

Note: It would be confusing and would imply additional information that does not exist if two <ENERC> values, i.e. one expressed in kilocalories and the other expressed in kiloJoules, were included for a single food item when one value has simply been calculated from the other using the conversion equation: 1 kcal = 4184 kJ. Consequently, one or the other should be used, but not both

Synonyms: kiloJoules; kilocalories; calories; food energy

Comments: In addition to a value for the quantity of total metabolizable energy, <ENERC> includes a description or listing of the conversion factors used to calculate this energy value from the proximate quantities. The conversion factors may be described by a keyword, or the conversion factors may be listed using secondary tagnames within <ENERC>. (More than one <ENERC> tagname may exist for a single food item if the values were calculated from the proximate components using different conversion factors.)

---

quality of a food, for example the biological origin, method of cooking and conservation, and technological treatments.

Other problems related to the method of expression of nutrients may arise from the long-standing convention of using protein values derived by applying a factor to measured total nitrogen values and from the calculation of energy values using energy conversion factors. Calculation of total carbohydrate content by difference as opposed to the sum of the individual carbohydrates is no longer the norm. The bases of expression in databases are the most commonly used units (such as g) per 100 g of edible portion. In some instances unit per 100 g of dry mass is presented, or unit per 100 ml. However, some tables list nutrient content per serving size or household measure, either as purchased or as prepared.

Quality of data

The quality of food composition data is critical for the accuracy of the estimates of compounds in food. In particular, analytical data obtained from scientific literature and laboratory reports can be evaluated for

quality. The quality of the analytical data is affected by various factors, including how the food samples were selected (sampling plan) and handled before analysis, use of appropriate analytical method and analytical quality control, and adequacy of number of samples to address variability. In addition, complete food description and identification of the components analyzed are also important.

The data quality evaluation system developed by the USDA is based on the evaluation of five categories: sampling plan, sample handling, analytical method, analytical quality control, and the number of individual samples analyzed. Detailed documentation of all the steps within each category is important for evaluating that category. Each category gets a maximum rating of 20 rating points. A quality index (QI) is generated by combining points of all the five categories and confidence codes (CCs) ranging from A to D indicating relative confidence in the data quality are assigned. These confidence codes could be released with the data and thus provide an indication of the data quality to the user of the data. Confidence code "A" indicates data of highest quality, while confidence code "D" suggests data of questionable quality. These procedures can be used to guide the planning and conducting of food analysis projects.

11.4 Information required on sources of data in tables

It is important to have information on the source of the data in a food composition table to be able to check its appropriateness for the study and to confirm its authenticity. The four major categories of sources of data are:

- primary publications, e.g., peer-reviewed articles in scientific literature
- secondary publications, e.g., reviews or published compilations with compositional data
- unpublished reports ranging from analytical records to documents prepared with limited circulation, e.g., confidential reports for clients or internal use within a company
- unpublished analytical data that can be either specifically commissioned analyses for the generation of nutrient data or analytical data that were not particularly generated for the purpose of generating food composition data.

Data in food composition tables may be original analytical values, imputed, calculated, or borrowed. Original analytical values are those taken from published literature or unpublished laboratory reports. Unpublished reports may include original calculated values, such as protein values derived by multiplying the nitrogen content by the required factor, energy values using energy conversion factors for some constituents of food, and "logical" values, such as the content of cholesterol in vegetable products, which can be assumed to be zero. Imputed values are estimates derived from analytical values for a similar food or another form of the same food. This category includes those data derived by difference, such as moisture and, in some cases, carbohydrate and values for chloride calculated from the sodium content. Calculated values are those derived from recipes by calculation from the nutrient content of the ingredients corrected by the application of preparation factors. Such factors take into account losses or gain in weight of the food or of specific nutrients during preparation of the food. Borrowed values are those derived from other tables or databases without referring to the original source. When a value for the content of a specific nutrient in a food is not included, there is a "–" or "0" value and, when a table has no values for a particular nutrient, the value is regarded as being "not included." In some tables, e.g., the National Nutrient Database for Standard Reference, SR, of the USDA, "0" value is a true zero, meaning the particular nutrient was not detected by the analytical method used; "–" indicates a missing value.

The proportion of the various types of data differs between tables and for different nutrients (Table 11.6). Details on food tables can be obtained from the Food and Agriculture Organization (http://www.fao.org/infoods). In other tables, such as those in the Netherlands, where sources of the data are given in the references, information on how the data have been obtained can also be found. However, this is not the case for all tables of food composition.

11.5 Overcoming the inadequacies of food composition tables

Nutrient losses and gains during food processing and preparation

In the absence of analytical data for all forms of foods nutrient values can be estimated by calculation using standard algorithms that have been experimentally derived. Since the content of nutrients per unit mass of food changes when foods are prepared, such losses and gains can be classified in two ways. The first can be described by a food yield factor, when the weight of the primary ingredients at the precooking stage is compared with the weight of the prepared food at the cooking stage and also with the final weight of the food as consumed at the post-cooking stage. The weight of the food can be increased due to the hydration of the dry form of a food (e.g., rice, macaroni) with cooking liquid, (e.g., water or broth) or increased due to the absorption of fat during frying of the food (e.g., potato). Alternatively, the weight of the food can decrease due to dehydration during cooking as a result of evaporative and drip losses.

The second, the nutrient retention factor, is related to changes in the amount of specific nutrients when foods are prepared. Changes in the nutrient levels can occur due to partial destruction of the nutrient as a result of the application of heat, alkalization, etc. Also, for some dietary components (e.g. β-carotene) the amount of available component may increase due to the breakdown of cell walls in the plant-based sample. Although original analytical data would be the most desirable type of data for foods at all stages of preparation, they are seldom available. Efforts are in progress in several regions to revise the nutrient losses and gain factors, including nutrient retention and yield factors, in order to compare and harmonize them and thereby improve the quality of food composition data calculated.

As food composition data are frequently lacking for cooked foods, estimates based on the use of these factors for calculating the nutrient content of

Table 11.6 Proportion of various types of data in food composition tables

Types of data	McCance and Widdowson tables, UK (developed country)	South African food composition table (developing country)
Analyses	70%	41% in 1999 (improved from 18% in 1991)
	10%	49%
Calculated	15%	10%
Estimated	5%	–

prepared foods from raw ingredients are made. Thus, the nutrient composition of a prepared or cooked food is calculated from the analytical data of uncooked food by applying suitable nutrient retention and yield factors. To obtain the nutrient content per 100 g of cooked food, the nutrient content per 100 g of raw food is multiplied by the percentage retained after cooking, and this is divided by the percentage retained after cooking, divided by the percentage yield* of the cooked product:

Nutrient content of cooked food per 100 g = [(nutrient content of raw food × retention factor)/yield of cooked food] × 100

The retention factor accounts for the loss of solids from foods that occurs during preparation and cooking. The resulting values quantify the nutrient content retained in a food after nutrient losses due to heating or other food preparations. This is called the true retention method and is calculated as follows:

% True retention = [(nutrient content per g of cooked food × g cooked food)/(nutrient content per g of raw food/g of food before cooking)] × 100

The following example uses only the yield factor to predict the nutrient content of the cooked food. The yield factors for different foods are reported in the USDA Agriculture Handbook 102 and for cooked carrots it is 92%. Selected nutrient values in SR 21 for 100 g of raw carrots are 0.93 g of protein, 33 mg of calcium and 5.9 mg of ascorbic acid. Using the yield factor the composition of 100 g of cooked carrots is calculated as 0.93 g/0.92 = 1.01 g protein, 33 mg/0.92 = 36 mg calcium and 5.9 mg/0.92 = 6.4 mg of ascorbic acid. This compares favorably to the determined values for carrots of 0.76 g of protein and 30 mg of calcium, but less so for ascorbic acid at a value of 3.6 mg, probably because it is heat sensitive; therefore, applying the nutrient retention factor for ascorbic acid (70%) would have resulted in a more accurate prediction (5.9 × 0.7/0.92 = 4.9) of 4.9 mg/100 g) (http://www.ars.usda.gov/nutrientdata).

Missing values in food composition tables

In general, original analytical data provide information of the highest quality for inclusion in a food composition table or nutrient database. However, it is seldom possible to construct a food composition table with only such data. A plan of action should be developed by the compilers of the database to deal with missing food items and values for particular nutrients. Very often, values of a biologically similar food are used. For composite or mixed dishes the composition of the dish is estimated by calculation from a standard recipe and applying appropriate nutrient retention factors and, in some cases, adjusting for changes in moisture content due to cooking loss or gain in the different cooking procedures. If a food item forms an important part of the population's diet and analysis is not possible, existing food composition databases should be searched to see whether data on the same or a similar food item could be borrowed. If a value for a nutrient is missing a similar approach can be followed, as it is more desirable to have a slightly incorrect estimated value of lower quality than no value at all. A value of "−" or "0" assigned to missing nutrient values may lead to underestimation of nutrient intakes, especially if those nutrients make a significant contribution to the diet.

Bioavailability and glycemic index

Nutrient composition information in food composition tables indicates the amount of nutrients as analyzed in that specific food sample and does not give an indication of the absorption or bioavailability of the nutrient from that food item. However, when dietary reference intakes such as recommended dietary allowances (RDAs) are drawn up, the recommendation makes provision for the amount of ingested nutrient that may not be absorbed. The concept of bioavailability has developed from observations that measurements of the amount of a nutrient consumed do not necessarily provide a good index of the amount of a nutrient that can be utilized by the body. The bioavailability of a nutrient can be defined as the proportion of that nutrient ingested from a particular food that can be absorbed and is available for utilization by the body for normal metabolic functions. This is not simply the proportion of a nutrient absorbed, and cannot be equated with solubility or diffusibility in in vitro-simulated physiological systems. Bioavailability is not a property of a food or of a diet per se, but is the result of the interaction between the nutrient in question, other components of the diet and the individual consuming the diet. Owing to the many factors

*Yield of cooked food (%) = (weight of edible portion cooked food/weight of raw food) × 100

influencing bioavailability, tables of food composition cannot give a single value for a nutrient's bioavailability. Most research until now has centered upon inorganic constituents, particularly iron, but the concept is applicable to virtually all nutrients. Iron incorporated into heme is more readily absorbed than iron in the nonheme form, and these two forms of iron are sometimes listed separately in food composition tables. Yet, such information does not take into account, for example, the effect of ascorbic acid (vitamin C) and organic acids (citric, malic, tartaric, and lactic acid) on nonheme iron absorption. Iron absorption is also increased in a state of iron deficiency and research has shown that vitamin A and iron intake has to be increased simultaneously to alleviate anemia. In the coming years, it can be expected that much more work will be carried out on bioavailability than in the past, because of its key role in relating functional nutritional status to nutrient intake.

Future research will probably also focus more on the measurement of the bioavailability of food constituents. Several vitamins and minerals, such as calcium, iron, zinc, and a number of B vitamins, are already being studied, with limited attention to carotenoid bioavailability. Inhibitors of absorption and the effects of processing and storage on the foodstuffs must be determined. As bioavailability is also influenced to a large extent by the meal in which a food constituent is consumed, this means that more information will be needed not only on daily food consumption but also on intake of other constituents at individual meals.

There is an increasing demand from users of food composition tables for information on the glycemic index (GI) of food, which is used as a tool in the selection of food in the management of diabetes, as opposed to the previous system of carbohydrate exchange. The GI is a food-specific measure of the relative tendency of carbohydrate in food to induce postprandial glycemia. The body's response to a 50 g carbohydrate dose induced by either glucose or white bread is taken as the reference and assigned a value of a 100. Responses to all other foods are rated in comparison and listed in tabular format. New datasets with complementary values, based on the GI and available carbohydrate content of food, have been proposed, of which one is a measure of the relative glycemic response to a given mass of whole food and the other is the mass of a food responsible for a given specific glycemic response. A more recently proposed identification of a food's GI value lies in indicating the specific food's category of GI as high, medium, or low. Accurate numerical values of a food's GI are difficult to obtain as various factors, including human subject variability both between and within subjects during analysis as well as response during ingestion of the food, can differ significantly.

Both bioavailability and GI are food indices that are influenced not only by the characteristics of the food, but also by the response of the individual to the food (i.e., absorption, metabolism, and excretion of the metabolites). For example, quantitative analysis of carotenoids alone could lead to a misinterpretation of vitamin A value. Therefore, the bioavailability of test foods in a single mixture may be investigated using the digestive system of nutrient-depleted rats (i.e., measuring retinol accumulation factor as a measure of total carotenoid bioavailability), or in humans using the relative dose–response test. Advances in analytical chemistry such as improvements in analytical methods, information science, computer hardware and software will assist in filling these gaps in special-purpose databases in the future.

How to calculate a recipe not included in the database

If the composition of a composite or mixed dish is not known, it can be estimated by calculation from a standard recipe and applying appropriate nutrient retention factors and, in some cases, adjusting for changes in moisture content due to cooking loss or gain during cooking. The following guidelines are suggested.

- Identify the ingredients of the recipe from the most appropriate foods available in the food composition database table.
- Quantify the ingredients in mass (g).
- Calculate the nutrient values for the specific amount of each ingredient.
- Add up the nutrient values of the individual ingredients.
- Calculate the nutrient composition for 100 g of the recipe.
- Apply suitable retention factors to the mineral and vitamin nutrient values if the recipe food is cooked. Note that if individual ingredients are in a cooked form this step is not necessary.

- Compare the moisture content of the calculated recipe with a similar cooked composite dish. If the moisture content differs by more than 1%, adjust the moisture content of the recipe food. All of the nutrients of the recipe food must be adjusted (concentrated or diluted) according to either the decrease or increase in moisture content.
- Assign to a suitable food group and list.

This is only an estimation of the make-up of a composite or mixed dish of unknown composition. Refer to Table 11.7 for an example of the calculation of the composition of a dish from a recipe. However, if this dish is a very important part of the diet of an individual or group and the information is crucial in assessing the adequacy of the diet, analysis should be considered.

Accurate estimation of portion size

Food composition tables and databases are mainly used in nutritional epidemiology to estimate the composition of foods consumed by individuals. All subjects have difficulties in estimating the exact portion sizes of food consumed. This issue is further complicated by the difference between the weight of a product as purchased and that of the actual item consumed (e.g., in meat after cooking there is at least a 25% cooking loss, without bone and with or without visible fat). Standardized portion sizes for individual foods within countries may help, but a set of standard food models (small, medium, and large) for use in dietary assessment may be of more value.

11.6 Description of food composition tables and databases and how to retrieve data

A food composition table or database is easier to use if the format allows easy access to the data available. Advances in information technology have led to more and more food composition tables being available in electronic form, progressively replacing the printed format. Printed food composition tables, although limited by physical proportions such as the size of both the written text and the printed table, continue to be popular in developing and underdeveloped countries. The printed word is seen as authoritative and only a limited level of literacy or knowledge on nutrition is necessary to be able to access the data.

Table 11.7 Calculation of the composition of a dish from a recipe

Recipe for scrambled eggs with onions
2 large eggs
$^1/_6$ cup whole milk
$^1/_8$ teaspoon salt
$^1/_4$ cup chopped raw onions
2 teaspoons oil
Add milk and salt to eggs and beat with a fork. Fry onions in the oil. Pour egg mixture into frying pan with the onions, and stir mixture with a fork while cooking until it solidifies. Makes one serving.

Calculation of nutrient content of scrambled eggs from nutrient values for raw ingredients
Step 1: Add nutrient levels for the specified quantities of ingredients
The nutrients in the raw eggs, whole milk, salt, raw onions and oil are added together
Step 2: Readjust quantities of those nutrients in the raw ingredients that are lost during cooking due to evaporation or heat

Nutrient loss on cooking	Eggs	Milk	Onions
Thiamin (%)	15	10	15
Riboflavin (%)	5		
Niacin (%)	5		
Ascorbic acid (%)		25	20
Folacin (%)			30

Step 3: Determine weight of the recipe before cooking
1 large egg = 57 g; 57 g × 2 eggs = 114 g; refuse factor to calculate weight without shell of 11%;
1 14 g × 0.89 = 101.46 g
1 cup whole milk = 244 g × $^1/_6$ = 40.66 g
1 teaspoon salt = 5.5 g × $^1/_8$ = 0.69 g
1 cup chopped raw onions = 170 g × 0.25 = 42.5 g
1 teaspoon oil = 4.53 g × 2 = 9.06 g
Total weight = 194.37 g
Step 4: Determine weight of recipe after cooking
Weight loss during cooking due to evaporation is estimated to be 8%
Weight of recipe after cooking = 194.37 g × 0.92 = 179 g
Step 5: Determine the nutrient levels of the recipe per 100 g and per serving
Divide the nutrient levels by 1.79 to determine the nutrient content of 100 g scrambled eggs
The calculated nutrient levels represent the nutrient content of one serving

Electronic data and access to them are more limited in remote areas in these countries, and a higher level of computer literacy and equipment is necessary, which is generally seen as a luxury and not a necessity.

However, electronic databases have many advantages over printed tables, including virtually unlimited capacity to store information, rapid access to individual data items, and easy sorting and manipulation of data for use in a wide range of calculations. However, the ease of accessing data in an electronic or a computerized database is dependent on the database access software and not only on the way in which data are stored. The development of relational databases has led to the opening up of possibilities to link different databases in regions and countries with each other. This has led to the identification of new challenges such as food identification, compatibility of data, data interchange and data quality.

11.7 Converting foods to nutrients

Entering data

Before the computer age, the conversion of food consumption into nutrient intake had to be done manually, which was a laborious and time-consuming task. Later, much of the work, especially for larger surveys, was done on mainframe computers, and has since passed on to microcomputers, because of their ready accessibility and ease of use. Data on food and nutrient intakes were often subsequently transferred to a mainframe computer, where they were combined with other survey data for further analysis. Today, there is little that cannot be done on a microcomputer, including data manipulation such as sorting and calculations.

Before proceeding to calculate nutrient intake from data on food consumption, it is necessary to ensure that mistakes that have crept into the data set during acquiring, coding, merging, transcription, and storage are reduced to an acceptable level. Regardless of the method used for the collection of data on food consumption, consideration should be given to how the data will be entered into the computer. Suitable forms should be designed for the collection of data. These can be on paper or in a personal computer-based program that can save time and eliminate errors associated with the transcription of data from paper to the computer. The use of carefully prepared forms, with information to guide those collecting the data, can reduce the chance of error during the collection of data and, if a separate process, during entry into the computer. The collection and entry of data are subject to human and computer error; therefore, procedures must be developed to ensure that the quality of data is as high as possible. Editing and error-

checking routines should be incorporated in the data entry process and subsets of data entered into the computer should be compared with the original written records. Where mistakes are found, the extent of the error should be determined, because it could involve data for the previous (or next) subject or day, or those previously (or subsequently) entered by the operator involved. In addition to such checks, frequency distributions of all amounts of food and food codes should be carried out. The Food Surveys Research Group of the Agricultural Research Service of the USDA has developed an automated method for collecting and processing dietary intake data. The three computer systems, Automated Multiple Pass Method (AMPM), Post-Interview Processing System (PIPS) and Survey Net collect, process, code, review, and analyze data for nutrient intakes. The system has been used for the National Health and Nutrition Examination survey since 2002.

Converting data in food intake to nutrient intake

A crucial aspect of food composition research is the transmission of information from those working in food composition and analysis to those working in food monitoring, to scientists trying to improve the food supply, to workers in epidemiological, training and nutrition programs, and to regulators. Yet there is little discussion in the scientific literature of the issues relating directly to the compilation of food composition databases, which are the primary means of transmission of food composition data to most professionals in the field. If good food statistics are available in a country, as well as access to food intake and food composition databases, estimates of a higher quality can be made regarding the nutrient intake of the individual or population as a whole. However, few data on food composition exist for the 790 million people in developing countries who are chronically undernourished and where malnutrition in the form of deficiencies of iron, iodine, and vitamin A is rife.

11.8 Perspectives on the future

No universal food database system has been developed that fulfills all of the needs of compilers and users of food databases, despite the fact that it would represent the primary scientific resource from which all other nutritional studies flow. However, recent international collaboration has considerably improved the development and compatibility of food composition data. It is essential for the development of nutritional sciences that this resource be maintained and improved to serve at both national and international levels. The quest for continued improvement in quality of representative food composition data are at the core of most food composition programs.

Recent advances in food composition

Harmonizing of regional food composition tables

High-quality, comprehensive food composition data for foods commonly consumed is important across an ever increasing list of applications, e.g., in epidemiological research studying the effect of specific foods on health and well-being. Integrated, comprehensive, and validated food composition databanks from individual countries within a region will contribute immeasurably towards shifting the barriers of current scientific understanding. Towards this end

Europe has moved much closer to obtaining this goal, preceded by the ASEAN Food Composition Tables (2000) (www.fao.org/infoods/tables_asia_en.stm).

Focusing on biodiversity within species

The FAO has begun a study on the development of baseline data for the Nutritional Indicator for Biodiversity – 1. food composition. The aim is to collect food composition data at the inter- and intraspecies level for regions and countries. The process includes obtaining information on food composition data at the interspecies level (variety, cultivar, breed) and on underutilized and wild foods at the species level, as well as reviewing all available food composition data at national, regional, and international levels. The data collected are reported in a template, naming the country and the INFOODS regional data centre. Table 11.8 gives an example of the format of reporting at the national level. For the baseline reporting, at the beginning of 2008 data from 254 publications from 49 countries were included.

Table 11.8 Template for reporting on the nutritional indicator of biodiversity in the food composition literature

Publication	Material examined	References	\multicolumn{4}{c}{Number of foods on subspecies level with following number of components}
			1	2–9	10–30	>30
1. Food composition databases (FCDB)						
Reference database of national FCDB						
User database of national FCDB						
Other national FCDB						
2. Literature						
National peer-reviewed journals	Indicate journals and years					
National laboratory reports	Indicate laboratories and years					
Reports from national research institutes	Indicate research institutes and years					
National conference presentations (incl. posters)	Indicate conferences and years					
Theses	Indicate universities and years					
Other (specify)	Indicate publication and years					
Material examined						
Letter	Material examined					
A						
B						
References						
Number	Full reference					DOI, CiteXplore ID[1], other international publication code

Investigating specific traditional and ethnic foods

Traditional and ethnic foods reflect cultural inheritance and in many cases form key components in the dietary patterns in many countries. In many instances traditional foods include underutilized vegetable species and in the current evolved world there are still many of these species and subspecies of which the nutrient information is lacking. Traditional and ethnic foods contribute considerably to the diet of many populations, and may have significant health contributions. Research and analysis on these foods has slowly emerged as a matter of great interest, but with financial constraint on such type of research, much is still to be done.

Ethnic minority populations have become significant parts of the population in many countries, and similarly in many developing countries traditional foods form a major component of these populations' diet. Inequalities in health status are observed in these subpopulations compared with the general population. These inequalities, which could be due to socioeconomic status, have highlighted the need for the expansion of nutrient data on ethnic and traditional foods. A limited budget is mostly all that is available for the analysis of these foods, which is one of the main reasons why there are limited data available. Often composition data for ethnic foods are derived or borrowed from other food composition tables or derived from recipes. Variation and modification in recipes and cooking practices between individuals are also some of the complications to consider when the composition of ethnic and traditional foods is investigated.

Bioactives in foods and their effect on health and well-being

Dietary constituents commonly found in foods with health-promoting or beneficial effects when ingested are part of the emerging evidence that drives consumers, researchers, and the food industry in their quest for validated information. It is generally recognized that a diet high in plant foods is associated with decreased incidence of certain diseases such as cancers and cardiovascular disease. One of the several plausible reasons for this decrease in incidence of disease is the antioxidant properties of plant-derived foods, which may prevent some of the processes involved in the development of cancer (protecting DNA from oxidative damage) and cardiovascular disease (inhibiting oxidative damage to low-density lipoprotein cholesterol). Apart from containing antioxidants, plant foods contain other compounds, not classified as traditional essential nutrients, but as bioactives. These bioactives, backed up with substantial evidence, may play a role in health promotion.

Thousands of plant bioactives have been identified and the major classes of plant bioactives are flavonoids and other phenolic compounds, carotenoids, plant sterols, glucosinolates, and other sulfur-containing compounds (http://www.eurofir.net). The USDA has prepared several Special Interest databases on flavonoids, proanthocyanidins, isoflavones, and ORAC (antioxidant powers assayed by oxygen radical absorption capacity assay). The ORAC database contains values for total phenols also.

Nutrition and health claims

Focusing on the relationship between diet and health, consumers are demanding more information on the food they purchase and consume. Not only has there been an increase in demand for nutrition information, but the increased prevalence of noncommunicable diseases such as cardiovascular disease and diabetes mellitus, as a consequence of obesity, has led to increase in the need for nutrition communication and guidance in making healthy food choices. Food labeling has become an important communicator to the consumer, with the provision that it is based on the truth and not misleading. The Codex Alimentarius Commission (http://www.codexalimentarius.net) aims to strengthen local and regional efforts towards harmonizing and simplifying the process of making a nutritional or health claim.

Towards this end they proposed the following areas for further development:

- labeling to allow consumers to be better informed about the benefits and content of foods
- measures to minimize the impact of marketing on unhealthy dietary patterns
- more detailed information about healthy consumption patterns including steps to increase the consumption of fruits and vegetables
- production and processing standards regarding the nutritional quality and safety of products.

Nutrition and health claims are used to present products as having an additional nutritional or health benefit. In most cases, consumers perceive products carrying certain claims to be better for their health and well-being. Nutrient profiling is the first step towards a possible health claim. At present, different systems for the setting of nutrient profiling range from a simple algorithm to a scientifically complicated approach. It is difficult to develop a single system that reflects both the nutrition contribution of a food or food group to the diet and the effect of the matrix on nutrient bioavailability. This discussion is continuing.

Further reading

Brussard JH, Löwik MRH, Steingrímsdóttir L, Møller A, Kearney J, De Henauw S, Becker W. A European food consumption survey method – conclusions and recommendations. *European Journal of Clinical Nutrition* 2002; **56** (Suppl. 2): S89–S94.

Food and Agriculture Organization of the United Nations. *Expert Consultation on Nutrition Indicators for Biodiversity 1. Food Composition*. Rome, 2008.

Greenfield H, Southgate DAT. *Food Composition Data. Production. Management and Use*. Food and Agriculture Organization of the United Nations, Rome, 2003

Greenfield H. 1990. Uses and abuses of food composition data. *Food Australia* **42** (8) (Suppl.).

Gry S, Holden J. Sampling strategies to assure representative values in food composition data. *Food, Nutrition and Agriculture* 1994; **12**: 12–20.

Klensin JC. *INFOODS Food Composition Data Interchange Handbook*. United Nations University Press, Tokyo, 1992.

Ireland J, Van Erp-Baart AMJ, Charrondière UR, Møller A, Smithers G, Trichopoulou A. Selection of food classification system and food composition database for future food consumption surveys. *European Journal of Clinical Nutrition* 2002; **56** (Suppl. 2): S33–S45.

Rand WM, Pennington JAT, Murphy SP, Klensin JC. *Compiling Data for Food Composition Data Bases*. United Nations University Press, Tokyo, 1991.

Southgate DAT. Food composition tables and nutritional databases. In: Garrow JS, James WPT, Ralph A, eds. *Human Nutrition and Dietetics*, 10th edn, Churchill Livingstone, Edinburgh, 2000: 303–310.

Truswell AS, Bateson DJ, Madafiglio KC, Pennington JA, Rand WM, Klensin IC. (1991) INFOODS guidelines for describing foods: a systematic approach to describing foods to facilitate international exchange of food composition data. *Journal of Food Composition and Analysis* 1991; **4**: 18–38.

Verger Ph, Ireland J, Møller A, Abravicius JA, Den Henauw S, Naska A. Improvement of the comparability of dietary intake assessments using currently available individual food consumption surveys. *European Journal of Clinical Nutrition* **56** (Suppl. 2): S18–S24, 2002.

Websites

Codex Alimentarius Commission: http://www.codexalimentarius.net

Eurocode2: http://www.eurofir.org/eurocode

EuroFIR: http://www.eurofir.net

Food and Agriculture Organization of the United Nations: http://www.fao.org

INFOODS: United Nations University of International Food Data Systems Project: http://www.fao.org/infoods/directory

LanguaL: http://www.langual.org

United States Department of Agriculture National Nutrient Databank: http://www.ars.usda.gov/nutrientdata

12
Food and Nutrition: Policy and Regulatory Issues

Michael J Gibney and Aideen McKevitt

Key messages

- The human food supply is highly regulated and while in the past there was an emphasis on food safety, there is now a rapidly expanding regulatory base covering nutrition.
- Any policy decision in the nutrition regulatory framework needs to be informed by up-to-date and relevant data on prevailing food and nutrient intake patterns. These metrics are compared with agreed standards for optimal food and nutrient intake and on the basis of any discrepancy, public health nutrition programs encompassing regulatory issues are initiated.
- Public health nutrition programs can be supply driven or demand driven. In the supply-driven option, the government takes the decision centrally to alter some properties of foods the most common approach being mandatory food fortification. In

demand-driven approaches, efforts are made to create a demand for a new food-purchasing pattern through a nutrition communication process.
- A nutrition communication process should always be built on actual studies of consumers attitudes and beliefs, and a number of tools are commonly used to communicate nutrition and health messages including nutritional labeling and nutrition claims.
- Globalization of the food supply has been accompanied by evolving governance issues that have produced a regulatory environment at national and global level led by large national, international agencies in order to facilitate trade and to establish and retain the confidence of consumers in the food supply chain.

12.1 Introduction

Few areas of our lives are more regulated than that of the food supply and within that regulatory framework, three distinct divisions are evident: food chemicals, food microbial hazards, and nutrition. In the past, the chemistry and microbiology aspects of food regulation tended to dominate but in recent times, the regulatory environment for nutrition has begun to receive increasing attention given that (a) the role of diet in noncommunicable chronic disease has been so extensively accepted and woven into policy and (b) food producers have made efforts to develop innovative products to help reduce the burden of disease risk. The present chapter is intended to provide new students of nutrition with a brief insight into the present direction of food regulation as it relates to dietary choices.

12.2 Reference points in human nutrition

Chapter 10 in this textbook outlines the many options that are available for measuring food intake and converting those data into nutrient intakes. Such data are fundamental to the development of nutrition-related regulatory policy. The more detailed the level at which data are collected, the more useful they are for advising and informing policy. Prevailing dietary habits, as measured through dietary surveys, represent the first reference point for nutrition policy. The second set of reference points are those targets set out by expert committees that will move populations toward everhealthier diets. Chapter 7 of this textbook describes the basic principles involved in setting out target values for the assessment of dietary intakes, primarily for micronutrients. These are defined using variable terms across the globe but, generally, all definitions employ the term "reference" and hence they can be classified as reference nutritional data. Such data were historically developed to ensure the adequacy of the human diet from the point of view of micronutrients. However, as our knowledge of diet and chronic disease has evolved, a second set of reference nutrition values had to be developed, this time to minimize the risk of chronic disease. Table 12.1 shows a non-exhaustive list of these nutrients and the risk factor or chronic disease they are associated with.

In addition to these data, recommendations are made for ideal body weight and there are specific sets of dietary guidelines for such life stages as lactation, pregnancy, aging, etc. However, the regulatory environment in nutrition is dominated by the above nutrients and also the micronutrients.

The whole purpose of devising these two sets of metrics – nutrient intakes and nutrient reference values – is to first measure where we are in relation to our nutritional well-being and second to set targets to move the population toward a healthier diet. There is however, a very slight antagonism between the establishment of an ideal pattern of nutrient intake and developing public health nutrition programs to achieve that goal. The reason is that the former does so in isolation from the real world of everyday eating. Its focus is on experimental studies that, for example, help delineate the optimal balance of dietary fatty acids to minimize plasma cholesterol. That optimal may be very significantly different from prevailing dietary habits and to attempt to bridge the gap too fast might produce a public health nutrition program that is unrealistic. Thus nutritionists can look at prevailing intakes against ideal intakes and then set out

interim attainable targets in realistic public health nutrition programs that can be implemented over a defined and reasonable period of time. In summary, it is not possible to develop a meaningful nutrition regulatory framework without access to both nutrient intake data and dietary reference data.

12.3 Exploration of dietary patterns

With a given set of population nutrient intake data and a given set of nutritional reference values, it is possible to divide the population into those closest to some nutritional ideal and those furthest from such an achievement. These two contrasting groups can now be laid against one another and a wide range of data, listed in Box 12.1, can be examined.

Based on these comparisons and using appropriate statistical techniques, it is possible to begin to discern the reasons why one group are near achieving some nutritional ideal and why another are set far off the mark. These reasons now feed into policy advice and begin to form the nucleus of a nutrition regulatory structure that may help the population improve their diet. Given that the focus of this text is nutrition, it would be worthwhile to single out food patterns for a more critical analysis. The following is a hypothetical finding in relation to three foods that appear to be important in determining the nutritional adequacy of "achievers" and "non-achievers" of some nutrient goal.

Look at Table 12.2. At first glance C seems unimportant and A and B seem to be important and going in opposite directions. These are very typical data that emerge from such analyses and they hide two very important statistics that should always be sought in studies of this nature. The first missing statistic is "% consumers" and the second is the "intake among

Table 12.1 Nutrients and associated risks

Nutrient	Effects
Saturated fatty acids	Blood cholesterol
Monounsaturated fatty acids	Blood cholesterol
n-6 polyunsaturated fatty acids	Blood cholesterol
Trans unsaturated fats	Blood cholesterol
n-3 polyunsaturated fatty acids	Blood cholesterol
Total fat	Obesity
Sodium	Blood pressure
Sugar	Dental caries
Fiber	Digestive disorders
Folic acid	Neural tube defects
Fruits and vegetables	Certain cancers

Box 12.1

Nutrients
Foods
Eating habits
Anthropometry
Socioeconomic data
Physical activity
Education
Others

consumers only." Now reconsider the above data with these additional statistics and look at Table 12.3.

Now everything has changed with the five consumers converting population average intakes into consumer-only intakes. For any program in public health nutrition, three important strategies which are often lost are (a) strategies to increase or decrease the five people eating a target food, (b) strategies to alter the frequency with which a target food is consumed, and (c) the portion size when the food is eaten. Thus were we to look solely at population averages, food C was of no interest. Now it is of interest if not intriguing: "achievers" universally eat this food while only 30% of "non-achievers" partake of it and, among the small group of "non-achievers" who do eat the food, they eat it at a much higher level (which might be the same amount more frequently or a higher amount less frequently).

12.4 Options to change food and nutrient intakes

Once the above analysis is complete and peer reviewed, definite directions in the consumption of nutrients and foods become apparent. In this section we focus on some of the options but the reader should always bear in mind that all options are possible and none is exclusive. Broadly speaking we can think of two contrasting options: "supply-driven" nutrition policy and "demand-driven" nutrition policy.

Supply-driven nutrition policy takes the food supply and in some way modifies it so that individuals consuming a habitual diet will have their nutrient intake altered without having to make any major changes in food choice. Mandatory fortification of foods with micronutrients is by far the best example of supply-driven food nutrition policy. There are certain essential prerequisites to the development of a successful supply-driven fortification program. These are shown in Box 12.2.

Let us now consider these factors for a typical fortification process, the mandatory addition of folic acid to flour in the USA to reduce the incidence of the neural tube birth defect, spina bifida (Box 12.3).

Let us contrast the data in Box 12.3 with the evidence linking saturated fatty acids (SFAs) to plasma cholesterol shown in Box 12.4.

Box 12.2

a There is unequivocal evidence that the lack of a particular nutrient very strongly predisposes to some serious condition
b The evidence is based on properly conducted human nutrition intervention trials
c The effect of the nutrient in question on the problem to be solved is not dependent on other conditions being met
d There are no adverse effects from the fortification strategy
e The scale of the problem is a true public health issue

Box 12.3

a+b There is certainly unambiguous evidence from randomized controlled trials involving high-risk women who had a previous spina bifida baby that folic acid significantly reduces the risk of a second event
c The effect is independent of any other factor from age, smoking, weight, and ethnicity, and so on
d There is some concern that fortifying with folic acid might cause some B_{12} deficiency to go undiagnosed but the scale of that problem is not enough to halt the fortification program
e This problem is a truly important public health issue

Table 12.2 Achievers and non-achievers of nutrient goals

	Achievers	Non-achievers
	(g/day population average)	
Food A	100	40
Food B	20	60
Food C	50	50

Table 12.3 Achievers and non-achievers of nutrient goals with consumer-only intakes

	Achievers	Non-achievers	Achievers	Non-achievers	Achievers	Non-achievers
	g/day population average		% consumers		Consumer-only intake	
Food A	100	40	20	80	500	50
Food B	20	60	50	50	40	120
Food C	50	50	100	30	50	150

Box 12.4

a+b There is certainly strong evidence that elevated levels of SFAs can raise plasma LDL cholesterol. However, within the category SFAs, some individual fatty acids are more potent than others and these are not uniquely found in one single dietary source of fat

c The effect of SFAs is to some extent also dependent on the simultaneous intakes of *trans* unsaturated fatty acids and different forms of unsaturated fatty acids

d+e There are no adverse effects known and the problem is not truly important

---

From the data in Boxes 12.3 and 12.4 it is easy to defend the folic acid option but less easy to defend the SFA option for supply-driven policy. It should be borne in mind that a supply-driven policy effectively takes away from the individual the right to choose in this regard and thus there are always social and sometimes ethical dimensions to this approach.

Demand-driven nutrition policy is based on educating the consumer to demand newer and healthier types of foods from the food supply. This is a chicken-and-egg situation. Consumers may want something that is not within the scope of industry to produce either for economic or technical reasons. Equally many companies have developed food products with very obvious health benefits which were market failures because the consumer saw no benefit. The success of this area is thus very market driven. Industry made spreadable fats low in SFAs, which consumers liked. They developed immune-boosting probiotics, cholesterol-lowering phytosterols, high-fiber ready-to-eat cereals and cereal bars, juices with various antioxidants, low-fat milks, n-3 PUFA-enriched eggs, and so on. For demand-driven food supply to work, we need to invoke a major new area of public health nutrition – communication.

12.5 Nutrition communication

One of the great attractions of the science of human nutrition is the breadth of topics to be covered from molecular biology, through population science to communication. The greatest mistake a nutrition regulatory policy initiative can make is for scientists to think they know the consumer and his or her beliefs. The only way that this can be understood is to study what consumers feel and believe before we can expect them (a) to listen to our communication, (b) believe it, (c) understand it, or (d) care about it. The present section assumes that is a given. In terms of nutrition communication, there are three very important areas to consider: nutrition labeling, nutrition claims, and nutrition profiling.

Nutrition labeling

In most countries, packaged foods bear a label listing particular nutrients in particular ways. The number of nutrients listed can vary either because of the prevailing food policy or because it suits a manufacturer to have more or less nutritional information imparted to the consumer. The standard format is to express the target nutrients per 100 g of the food or per some specified portion of the food. Generally, nutrition labeling was a "back of pack" issue, generally considered less important. Today, it is becoming increasingly a "front of the pack" issue, with visuals to immediately let the consumer see what a typical serving supplies in terms of target nutrients and then to express these as a percentage of some reference intake. Often colors are used where a serving greatly exceeds some nutritional standard (red) or green if it is well below.

Nutrition labels fulfill a very important role in nutrition communication – helping the consumer see the nutrient content of the food. However, there are aspects that are not so obvious which we need to bear in mind. Comparisons of the nutritional composition of different foods are often difficult to interpret. For example, in choosing a packaged sandwich, the consumer can unite their gastronome preferences with nutritional data to make a choice. On the other hand, if the choice was a carton of ready-to-eat soup versus a sandwich, the comparison is much more difficult; when it comes to making a decision on any two foods versus another set of two foods, then the decision process is exceeded for almost everybody. Another limitation of nutritional labeling is that fresh foods are often not packaged and thus are not labeled for nutritional content. The same is true for meals, snacks outside the home, in bars, restaurants, canteens, delicatessens, and the like. Notwithstanding the shortcomings, nutrition labeling is a very positive step in helping consumers make informed choices.

Nutrition claims

In general, claims in the field of food and health can be divided in several ways in matrix form. The first division is into claims which are "generic" (any manufacturer can use it if they meet the criteria) and claims which are "unique," that is specific to a brand which has some unique attribute on which a claim can be made. In the USA, the Food and Drug Administration (FDA) has favored generic claims such as "saturated fats raise cholesterol" or "calcium helps bone health." The FDA accepts petitions in this area where industry groupings put forward a scientific case as to why such a generic claim might be used. If accepted, the regulator can now decide what the conditions for making a claim are. For example, a typical serving of the food would have to achieve a minimum percentage of some reference value before a claim could be made. A product where a serving size gave 1% of the requirement for calcium would surely not be allowed to make any claim on bone health.

   The other type of claim can be classified into three levels (Table 12.4)

   At the time of writing, there are developments in different parts of the world as to how such claims can be handled. As one goes up from level 1 to level 3, the scientific rigor must increase exponentially. Quite probably, level 2 and level 3 will need to be accompanied by significant supportive evidence from human dietary intervention studies. Again, such claims will require that certain specified attributes of the food be met before a claim can be made, and different parts of the globe are taking various approaches to these issues. As with many aspects of labeling communication, some reflection will help reveal the complexity of the task. If companies are to innovate and develop new foods with enhanced nutritional properties or functions, they need to invest in research and development. If their research, industry supporting human intervention studies, shows clear evidence of an effect

in lowering the risk of a disease or condition, they need to be able to make that claim and to prevent others who have not done this research from simply adopting that claim. In that way, they stand a chance of developing a market leader and of recouping their research investment. This approach is perfectly understandable but it does cause problems for smaller companies and for industrial sectors in less developed countries for which such high stakes are unthinkable. The terms and conditions for the use of such claims has led to a third area in nutrition communication – nutrition profiling.

Nutrition profiling

This is by far the newest area and without doubt the most controversial. In the EU, the law now requires that for a food to make a claim, it must meet certain nutritional standards. This is often referred to as the Jelly Bean Rule – that is, if you added zinc to jelly beans, would one support the promotion of jelly bean consumption on the grounds that increased zinc intake may assist in minimizing poor immune function. The idea is that if the food supply needs zinc to be added, then a more suitable vehicle needs to be found. In principle this is not complex. In the real world it is an intellectual minefield. In terms of developing nutrient profiles for whatever reason, there are two approaches in operation. One seeks to take a single set of criteria and apply that universally to all foods. This has been the approach of what is called the UK Traffic Light System. All foods are classified into three types, which can be described as good (green), bad (red), or neither (orange). Inevitably, the application of such a simple system to something as complex as the human food chain leads to exceptions. Walnuts might get a red color because of their high fat content, and yet walnuts have been shown along with other nuts to be protective against heart disease. Maybe walnuts are now exceptionally excluded from a red sign. But the process goes on to exceptionally include or exclude and the objectivity of the simple approach becomes gradually replaced with the subjectivity of exceptions.

   The second nutrient-profiling approach is to take each food category separately and devise nutritional standards for each category. An example of this is the Swedish Keyhole Method. For breads, certain standards are set and breads that meet these standards carry the keyhole symbol, which consumers recognize

Table 12.4 Nutrition claims

Level 1. Nutrition content	This product is a rich source of some omega-3 fats
Level 2. Function claim	This product is rich in omega-3 fats, which promote heart health
Level 3. Disease reduction claim	This product is rich in omega-3 fats, which reduce the risk of cognitive impairment in older people

as a mark of nutritional quality. The huge advantage of this system is that the standards are not universal. One is judging packet soups against packet soups as an example but not against mayonnaise or chocolate or breakfast cereals. At present, the area of nutrition profiling is very much at the development stage and it remains to be seen how exactly this progresses. Besides the use of nutrient profiling for permitting claims, there is interest in its use in deciding significant nutrition policy issues about individual foods. Advertising of foods is one critically important area where this approach may be applied.

12.6 Global players in food and nutrition regulation

Food and nutrition regulation spans the entire food chain – from processing of seeds, to planting seeds, to tilling crops, storage and harvest of crops, and sale of crops. Animal and fish farming are equally complex. Where these primary products enter the realm of the food processor, another range of regulations apply, for example what is permitted to be added to the food, what must be in a food (nutrition), what must not be in a food (pesticides), the physical and biological environment in which the food is processed, in addition to packaging, labeling, transport, storage, sales, and advertising.

Globalization is one of the driving forces shaping the world economy and the pace of globalization of the food trade has accelerated in the past decades. New methods and technologies in food production and processing have contributed to this acceleration. Productivity of animals and crops has risen to unprecedented levels. Globalization of the food trade benefits consumers in terms of quality, affordability, and guaranteed supply. It also offers diversity of products, which can contribute to improved nutrition and health. Globalization has been accompanied by evolving governance issues that have produced regulation at a national and global level in an attempt not only to facilitate trade but also to establish and retain the confidence of the consumer in the food supply chain. The distances that food and feed are now transported potentially create conditions more conducive to contamination of the supply chain, where even a single source can have serious consequences.

Modern food and nutrition regulation must deal with this range of activity on a global scale and must

be reviewed continuously to take account of issues such as food sources from new areas with differing climates, growing and harvesting techniques, and public health infrastructure. In addition, there are very many national approaches to food regulation reflecting different perceptions about the value of new technology, different degrees of protection given by governments to food producers, and even different interpretations of the science involved in the regulatory process. The implication of globalization for food regulation therefore requires both international cooperation among national food regulators and the effective balancing of gains from trade with regulatory differences.

UN and UN agencies

Globally, a range of agencies plays a role in food and nutrition regulation. The UN was established in 1945 as was the Food and Agriculture Organization (FAO), which was established as a specialized UN agency. The principal role of the FAO is the provision of food security for all. Coupled with this is its mandate to raise nutrition levels and agricultural productivity in order to raise the standard of living for rural communities and thereby contribute to the growth of the global economy.

The World Health Organization (WHO) is another agency of the UN and is a sister organization of the FAO. Established in 1948, its objective is the attainment by all peoples of the highest possible levels of health. The WHO is the directing and coordinating authority for health within the UN system. The WHO is governed by its member states through the World Health Assembly (WHA), which is composed of representatives from each member state. The WHO considers that freedom from hunger and malnutrition is a basic human right and alleviation of these global problems is fundamental for human and national development. While the WHO has traditionally focused on nutritional deficiency and associated morbidity and mortality, the issue of malnutrition characterized by obesity and the long-term implications of unbalanced dietary and lifestyle practices that result in chronic diseases such as cardiovascular disease, cancer, and diabetes has assumed increasing importance in recent years. Countries, particularly developing countries where both under- and overnutrition coexist, are of particular concern. In light of these challenges and trends the WHO aims to build and implement a science-based, comprehensive, integrated, and action/policy-oriented "Nutrition Agenda" at the global, regional and country levels that addresses the whole spectrum of nutrition problems towards attaining the Millennium Development Goals (MDGs) and other nutrition-related international commitments, including the prevention of the diet-related chronic diseases. The Millennium Declaration (later restated as MDGs with specific measurable targets that should be met by 2015) was signed by 147 heads of state in 2000 and passed unanimously by the members of the UN General Assembly. The MDGs seek to eliminate hunger, poverty, maternal and child malnutrition with particular emphasis on maternal and fetal undernutrition and malnutrition, and micronutrient malnutrition. The UN Children's Fund (UNICEF) was established by the UN General Assembly in 1946. UNICEF provides long-term humanitarian and developmental assistance to children and mothers in developing countries with special emphasis on pregnancy, breastfeeding and the first 3 years of life.

FAO/WHO and Codex Alimentarius

In the 1950s food regulators, traders, consumers, and experts were looking increasingly to the FAO and WHO for leadership about the plethora of food regulations that were impeding trade and that for the most part were not providing adequate protection for consumers. As a result, the Joint FAO/WHO Expert Committee on Food Additives (JECFA) was established in 1956. Its remit now covers the evaluation of contaminants, naturally occurring toxicants and residues of veterinary drugs in food. In the early 1960s a Joint FAO/WHO Meeting on Pesticide Residues (JMPR) was set up to provide independent scientific advice to the FAO and WHO with recommendations from panels of independent experts on the use of pesticides in agriculture and safe levels of residues in foods. The Joint FAO/WHO Meeting on Microbiological Risk Assessment (JEMRA) began in 2000. The aim of JEMRA is to optimize the use of microbiological risk assessment as the scientific basis for risk management decisions that address microbiological hazards in foods. Other examples of *ad hoc* joint expert consultations on new or emerging food and nutrition problems are the Joint FAO/WHO Expert Consultation on Acrylamide or the *ad hoc* Committee on Foods derived from Biotechnology.

The FAO also recognized the need for international agreement on food standards, labeling requirements, methods of analysis, etc. In 1963, the Sixteenth World Health Assembly approved the establishment of the Joint FAO/WHO Food Standards Program and adopted the statutes of the Codex Alimentarius Commission (CAC).

The CAC is the pre-eminent global food standards organization and has had an important impact on food producers, processors, and consumers. The principal aims of Codex are to protect consumers' health, ensure fair practices in the food trade by the development of science-based food quality and safety standards, guidelines, and recommendations, and promote coordination of all food standards work undertaken by governmental and international organizations. The harmonization of food standards facilitates trade between countries and underpins it with a guarantee that food that is traded will be safe and of the same quality as the same product made elsewhere. Membership of CAC is open to all member nations and associate members of the FAO and/or WHO. By 2007, some 174 countries and one Member Organization (European Community) were members. CAC meetings are held yearly and alternately at the FAO headquarters in Rome and the WHO headquarters in Geneva. At these meetings draft and final standards, guidelines, and codes of practice are adopted. Each member of the Commission has one vote. Decisions of the Commission are taken by a majority of votes cast. Representation is on a country basis. National delegations are led by senior officials appointed by their governments. Delegations may include representatives of industry, consumers' organizations, and academic institutions. Countries not members of the Commission sometimes attend in an observer capacity. A number of international governmental organizations and international NGOs also attend in an observer capacity. These organizations may put forward their points of view at every stage except in the final decision, which is taken by member governments. The Commission and member governments have established country Codex Contact Points and many member countries have National Codex Committees to coordinate activities nationally.

Codex Alimentarius is the Latin name for food law or food code. The main aim of Codex is to define international standards, codes of practice, and other guidelines and recommendations. The main work on standard setting is carried out in more than 20 Codex Committees and Task Forces. These include committees dealing with "vertical" and "horizontal" standards, task forces dedicated to a particular task of limited duration and regional coordinating committees. In addition, the experts' meetings organized and supported by the FAO and the WHO, JMPR, JEMRA, and JECFA provide the scientific basis (risk assessment) for the work of the CAC. At the beginning the CAC concentrated on commodity standards called "vertical standards," for example standards for cereals; fats and oils; fish and fish products; fresh fruits and vegetables; processed and quick frozen fruits and vegetables; fruit juices; meat and meat products; milk and milk products; sugars, cocoa products, and chocolate. In the 1980s it was generally agreed that diversification of food products was occurring so rapidly that the setting of detailed standards was in fact hindering trade. Thus a move toward "horizontal" standards began. "Horizontal standards" are general standards that have application across a wide range of foods, for example general principles: food additives and contaminants; food labeling; food hygiene, methods of analysis and sampling; pesticide residues, residues of veterinary drugs in foods; food import and export inspection and certification systems; nutrition and foods for special dietary uses. These standards are then published in one of the Codex's 13 volumes. Codex standards pass through various stages of ratification by members – the eight-step process – the final one being that of acceptance. When members accept a Codex standard they are committed to allowing products conforming to that standard on to their market.

A major concern of national governments is that food imported from other countries should be safe and not jeopardize the health of consumers or pose a threat to health and safety of their animal and plant populations. So governments of importing countries introduce laws and regulations to reduce or eliminate such threats. In the food area these measures could become disguised barriers to trade as well as being discriminatory. One of the main principles of the Codex Alimentarius is that harmonization of food laws and adoption of internationally agreed standards would result in fewer barriers to trade and freer movement of food products among countries.

WTO: Sanitary and phytosanitary measures and technical barriers to trade

The General Agreement on Tariffs and Trade (GATT) began in 1948. Countries subsequently agreed to lengthy "rounds" of negotiations to develop rules for "non-tariff barriers" to trade. The completion of the Uruguay Round of Multilateral Trade Negotiations 1986–1994 led to the formation of the World Trade Organization (WTO) on 1 January 1995. The Uruguay Round Agreements (which began at Punta del Este, Uruguay) for the first time incorporated agriculture and food under its rules. Two of the Uruguay Round Agreements relevant to international food regulation are the Agreement on the Application of Sanitary and Phytosanitary Measures (SPS) and the Agreement on Technical Barriers to Trade (TBT). The SPS Agreement allows governments to take scientifically justified sanitary and phytosanitary measures to protect human health. The agreement commits members to base these measures on internationally established guidelines and risk assessment procedures. The SPS Agreement has chosen the standards guidelines and recommendations established by the CAC for food additives, veterinary drug and pesticide residues, contaminants, methods of analysis and sampling, and codes and guidelines of hygienic practice. A national standard that provides a greater level of protection than Codex is considered to be a trade barrier unless the WTO decides that the stricter national standard is based on a risk assessment that demonstrates that the Codex standard, guideline, or recommendation provides insufficient protection or that the country maintaining the stricter standard has other scientific justification. The TBT agreement seeks to ensure that technical regulations and product standards including packaging, marking and labeling requirements, and analytical procedures for assessing conformity with technical regulations and standards do not create unnecessary obstacles to trade. The importance of Codex standards is also stated in the Technical Regulations and Standards provisions contained in Article 2 of the TBT Agreement. So, although CAC standards are not enshrined in international law, WTO endorsement of these standards through the SPS and TBT agreements has effectively made them mandatory, and Codex standards are the benchmarks standards against which national measures and regulations are evaluated. Both the SPS and TBT

Agreements call on the WTO member countries to seek harmonization of regulations based on the work of the CAC, and foods which meet CAC Codex standards, recommendations and guidelines should be traded freely in international trade.

Adherence to Codex standards has become critical as they are used as guidelines for the resolution of disputes under the enhanced WTO dispute settlement procedure. Annex 2 of the WTO covers all disputes arising from the GATT and WTO agreements. A dispute is triggered when a WTO member complains that another member(s) has failed to live up to the obligations of the GATT or WTO agreements, i.e., a benefit guaranteed under one or other of these agreements has been "nullified or impaired" by another member(s). The dispute settlement procedure encourages the governments involved to discuss their problems and settle the dispute by themselves. The first stage is therefore consultations between the governments concerned. If the governments cannot resolve their dispute they can ask the WTO director-general to mediate or try to help. If consultations fail, the complaining country can ask for a panel to be appointed. If the panel decides that the disputed trade measure does break a WTO agreement or an obligation, it recommends that the measure be made to conform with WTO rules. The panel may suggest how this could be done. Either side can appeal a panel's ruling. Appeals are limited to points of law and legal interpretation — they cannot re-examine existing evidence or examine new issues. The appeal can uphold, modify, or reverse the panel's legal findings and conclusions. If a member does not comply with WTO recommendations on bringing its practice in line with WTO rules, then trade compensation or sanctions, for example in the form of duty increases or suspension of WTO obligations, may follow. An interesting case that illustrates the working of the Dispute Settlement Understanding is the long-running dispute between the EU and the USA and Canada concerning the EU ban on the use of growth-promoting hormones in beef and the import of meat treated with hormones (http://www.wto.org/english/tratop_e/dispu_e/cases_e/ds320_e.htm).

Setting international food standards requires the participation of all countries. In recent years there has been a significant increase in the membership of the Codex. Developing countries now constitute a significant proportion of total membership. However, many countries are still faced with resource constraints to effective participation in Codex activities. The FAO and WHO technical assistance programs support the efforts of developing countries to strengthen their national food safety systems to protect local consumers and to take advantage of international food trade opportunities. In addition, the FAO/WHO Codex Trust Fund supports the participation of countries in Codex technical committee meetings, and countries have been funded to attend sessions of the CAC.

Europe

Having considered the global agencies and institutions that impact on food and nutrition regulation, the EU will be considered as an example of evolution toward a modern system of food and nutrition regulation.

The EU is an association of 27 Member States that have agreed to integrate and coordinate much of their economic policy and some other policy areas. The original European Economic Community (EEC) was formed following the signing of the Treaty of Rome in 1957 and consisted of six Member States, increasing over time to 9, 12, 15, 25, and 27 Member States in 2007 following the accession of Romania and Bulgaria. The emphasis in the early years was to concentrate on the free movement of foodstuffs through the common market. EU food regulation developed in an uncoordinated fashion over a period of more than 40 years and resulted in a fragmented framework characterized by different national traditions of member states as well as different policy areas such as trade and agriculture to which they were linked.

From a consumer health point of view, the dominant areas were related to food safety, in particular toxicology and microbiology. Nutrition issues in EU policy were dominated by compositional standards for infant foods and clinical foods. The Community may not act in a policy area unless given the power to do so by Treaty and the Treaty of Rome did not explicitly mention consumer protection or public health. These goals were added to the Single European Act and the Maastricht Treaty.

Three institutions, the European Commission, the Council of the European Union, and the European Parliament – the interinstitutional triangle – take decisions in the legislative field. The main differences in the decision-making process are related to whether the Council decides by qualified majority or unanimity and the degree to which the European Parliament is involved in the process. In legislative initiatives, the Commission has sole right of initiating policy. The legislative process usually starts with the expectation that the Community should act in a particular policy area. The prompt for action often comes from external pressure perhaps in response to pressure from a particular Member State, the Council of Ministers, the European Parliament, trade associations, research on risks and hazards, technical developments, etc. These influences build up pressure for action.

In 1974, a Scientific Committee for Food (SCF) was established by the European Commission "to advise the Commission on any problem relating to the protection of the health and safety of persons arising or likely to arise from the consumption of food, in particular on nutritional, hygienic and toxicological issues." The SCF was located in the Directorate General Industry (DG111). At various times, scientific committees were criticized on a number of grounds by the European Parliament and by industry and consumer NGOs. Following the bovine spongiform encephalopathy (BSE) crisis in the UK, there was a further decrease in confidence in the scientific committees and, with the new powers in public health granted by the Maastricht Treaty, the European Parliament forced the Commission to totally revise the structures of the scientific committees. Indeed, the Santer Commission in its very first year almost collapsed under pressure from the European Parliament to speed up the reform and to restore consumer confidence in the issuing of scientific advice to the Commission. A major reorganization of the Commission's services ensued. The responsibility for monitoring the implementation of food safety legislation and for providing scientific advice, hitherto jointly share by the Commissioners for Agriculture and Industry, was transferred to the Commissioner for Consumer Affairs. The rationale at the time was that it was necessary to separate monitoring, compliance with and enforcement of the law from the law-making function itself. This latter function remained for a time with the Agriculture and Industry Commissioners. Two years later, however, the legislation function on food safety was transferred to the Health and Consumer Protection Commissioner. The Commission also announced that the way in which scientific advice on food safety was provided at European level would be reorganized and strengthened. A Scientific Steering Committee to oversee the work of

the eight regrouped scientific committees was created. The Green Paper on the general principles of food law was published in 1997 to launch a debate on the future development of EU food law. Its aim was to provide the Commission with a solid background for a major program of new or amending legislation it would later propose in the 2000 White Paper on food safety. In January 2002 Regulation (EC) No. 178/2002 laying down general principles and requirements of food law, establishing the European Food Safety Authority and laying down procedures in matters of food safety was adopted. The Regulation sets out the general principles of EU food law, establishes a European Food Safety Authority, and establishes a rapid alert system for the notification of direct or indirect risks to human health deriving from feed or food, and sets down clear procedures for the handling by the Commission and the Member States of food safety emergencies and crises. The main principles of EU food law contained in the Regulation includes all food and feed at all stages of production, processing, and distribution; food law must be based on a system of risk analysis founded on risk assessment, risk management, and risk communication; the precautionary principle will be applied in the case of a potential risk to human health where there is scientific uncertainty as to what measures to take; public authorities at all levels will apply the principle of transparency in consulting with and informing the public on actual or potential risks and the actions that are taken or proposed to deal with them. The Regulation provides for a system to allow the traceability of all food and feed at all stages of the food and feed chain; food operators are responsible at all stages of the food chain for ensuring that the food they produce complies with the requirements of food law and must verify that the requirements are met; food business operators have an obligation, when they have reason to believe that food that has been imported, produced, processed, manufactured, or distributed is not in compliance with requirements, to withdraw the product from the marketplace, to inform the responsible public authorities, and to inform consumers of the reasons for withdrawal; food imports and exports must meet the requirements of EU food law.

European Food Safety Authority

The primary responsibility of the European Food Safety Authority (EFSA) is to provide independent scientific advice on all matters with a direct or indirect impact on food safety. The Authority has been given a wide brief, so that it can cover all stages of food production and supply, from primary production to the safety of animal feed, right through to the supply of food to consumers. It gathers information from all parts of the globe, keeping an eye on new developments in science. It shares its findings and listens to the views of others through a network (advisory forum) that will be developed over time, as well as interacting with experts and decision-makers on many levels. Although the Authority's main "customer" is the Commission, it is open to respond to scientific questions from the European Parliament and the Member States and it can also initiate risk assessments on its own behalf. The Authority carries out assessments of risks to the food chain and indeed can carry out scientific assessment on any matter that may have a direct or indirect effect on the safety of the food supply, including matters relating to animal health, animal welfare, and plant health. The Authority also gives scientific advice on non-food and feed, genetically modified organisms (GMOs), and on nutrition in relation to Community legislation.

EU nutrition and public health

With regard to public health, the Community's role is to complement national policies, to encourage cooperation between the Member States and to lend support to their action when it comes to improving public health, preventing human disease, and reducing risks to human health. In keeping with the principle of subsidiarity, Community action in the field of public health is designed to fully respect the responsibilities of the Member States for the organization and delivery of health services and medical care.

In 2000 the European Commission adopted a Communication on the Health Strategy of the European Community. This described how the Commission was working to achieve a coherent and effective approach to health issues across all the different policy areas and emphasized that health services must meet the population's needs and concerns, in a context characterized by the challenge of aging and the growth of new medical techniques, as well as the more international dimension of health care (contagious diseases, environmental health, increased mobility of persons, services and goods). A new Health Strategy for the EU 2008–2013 was adopted in 2007. The Strat-

egy encompasses work not only in the health sector but across all policy areas. In the nutrition arena, the scientific community has estimated that an unhealthy diet and a sedentary lifestyle might be responsible for up to one-third of the cases of cancers, and for approximately one-third of premature deaths due to cardiovascular disease in Europe. Nutrition and physical activity are key determinants for the prevalence of obesity, which continues to rise in the EU among children and adults.

In terms of nutrition the two main objectives are to collect quality information and make it accessible to people, professionals, and policy-makers, and to establish a network of Member State expert institutes to improve dietary habits and physical activity habits in Europe. The long-term objective is to work toward the establishment of a coherent and comprehensive community strategy on diet, physical activity, and health, which will be built progressively. It will include the mainstreaming of nutrition and physical activity into all relevant policies at local, regional, national, and European levels and the creation of the necessary supporting environments. At Community level, such a strategy would cut across a number of Community policies and needs to be actively supported by them. It would also need to actively engage all relevant stakeholders, including the food industry, civil society, and the media. Finally, it would need to be based on sound scientific evidence showing relations between certain dietary patterns and risk factors for certain chronic diseases. The European Network on Nutrition and Physical Activity, which the Commission established, will give advice during the process. The Community approach is inspired by the WHO's Global Strategy on Diet Physical Activity and Health, which was adopted unanimously by the World Health Assembly.

In 2005, the Commission launched a new forum, called "Diet, Physical Activity and Health – a European Platform for Action." The platform brought together all relevant players active at European level that were willing to enter into binding and verifiable commitments that could help to halt and reverse current obesity trends. This included retailers, food processors, the catering industry, the advertising business, consumer and health NGOs, the medical professions, and the EU presidency. It enables all individual obesity-related initiatives to be more promptly shared among potential partners and across the EU as a whole. In December 2005 the Commission published a Green Paper called "Promoting healthy diets and physical activity: a European dimension for the prevention of overweight, obesity and chronic diseases." This was followed in May 2007 by the Commission's white paper outlining strategies/initiatives in the area of diet, physical activity, and health aimed at promoting good health and quality of life and reducing risks of disease. Nutrition is clearly recognized as having a key role in public health and, together with lifestyle, has a central position within the strategy and actions of the Community in public health.

12.7 Perspectives on the future

The food we eat is an area of everyday life that is very heavily regulated from the food safety point of view, including chemical and microbial hazards, but increasingly from the nutritional point of view. The bedrock of sensible nutrition regulation planning is the availability of good data and the intelligent use of that data to both inform and challenge the policy-makers. Globalization of the food supply has been accompanied by evolving governance issues that have produced a regulatory environment at the national and global level led by large national, and international agencies in order to facilitate trade and to establish and retain the confidence of consumers in the food supply chain.

Further reading

Websites

BEUC European Consumers Organisation: http://www.beuc.org/Content
CIAA: http://www.ciaa.be/asp/index.asp/
DG-SANCO: www.europa.eu.int/comm/dg24
EUROPA: http://europa.eu
European Commission: http://ec.europa.eu/index_en.htm
European Court of Justice: http://curia.europa.eu/en/index.htm
European Food Safety Authority: http://www.efsa.europa.eu
EUROPA Food and Feed Safety: http://ec.europa.eu/food/index_en.htm
European Food Information Council: http://www.eufic.org
Eur-Lex The portal to European Union Law: http://eur-lex.europa.eu/en/index.htm

European Parliament: http://www.europarl.europa.eu
International Life Sciences Institute: http://www.ilsi.org
Institute of Food Science and Technology (IFST): http://www.ifst.org
Food Standards Agency (FSA): http://www.foodstandards.gov.uk
European Food Information Council: http://www.eufic.org
European Union: http://.europa.eu

EU food agencies

France – L'Agence Française de Sécurité Sanitaire des Aliments: http://www.afssa.fr
Ireland – Food Safety Authority of Ireland: http://www.fsai.ie
Sweden – National Food Administration: http://www.slv.se
UK – Food Standards Agency: http://www.foodstandards.gov.uk

US sites

Arbor Nutrition Guide: http://www.arborcom.com/
Centre for Disease Control and Prevention, Atlanta (CDC): http://www.cdc.gov
Centre for Food Safety and Applied Nutrition: http://www.cfsan.fda.gov/list.html
Centre for Nutrition Policy and Promotion: http://www.usda.gov/cnpp
Environmental Protection Agency (EPA): http://www.epa.gov
Food and Drug Administration (FDA): http://www.fda.gov/default.htm
Food and Nutrition Information Center, USDA: http://www.nal.usda.gov/fnic
Food and Safety Inspection Service (FSIS): http://www.fsis.usda.gov
Iowa State University Extension, including a Food Safety Project: http://www.extension.iastate.edu/foodsafety
Institute of Food Technologists – a non-profit scientific society: http://www.ift.org
United States Department of Health and Human Services: http://www.os.dhhs.gov
United States Department of Agriculture (USDA): http://www.usda.gov

Worldwide

Codex Alimentarius: http://www.codexalimentarius.net
Consumers International: http://www.consumersinternational.org
Dept. of Plant Agriculture, University of Guelph, Ontario, Canada: http://www.plant.uoguelph.ca/safefood
Food and Agriculture Organization of the United Nations (FAO): http://www.fao.org
Food Standards Australia New Zealand: http://www.foodstandards.gov.au
International Food Information Council (IFIC): http://www.ific.org
International Standards Organization (ISO): http://www.iso.ch
World Health Organization (WHO): http://www.who.int
World Trade Organization: http://www.wto.org

13
Nutrition Research Methodology

J Alfredo Martínez and Miguel A Martínez-González

Key messages

- This chapter identifies critical aspects and factors involved in nutritionally orientated investigations as well as the measurement qualities concerning research procedures.
- It describes how to select methods and techniques as well as animal models to assess nutrient utilization and functions.

- It defines indicators and markers of dietary intake and metabolism in human studies.
- It helps to choose methods to investigate the causal relationships between diet and disease.

13.1 Introduction

Research is a meticulous process to discover new, or collate old, facts by the scientific study of a subject or through a critical investigation. In this context, nutrition research involves advances in knowledge concerning not only nutrient functions and the short- or long-term influences of food and nutrient consumption on health, but also studies on food composition, dietary intake, and food and nutrient utilization by the organism.

The design of any investigation involves the selection of the research topic accompanied by the formulation of both the hypotheses and the aims, the preparation of a research protocol with appropriate and detailed methods and, eventually, the execution of the study under controlled conditions and the analysis of the findings leading to a further hypothesis. These stages of a typical research program are commonly followed by the interpretation of the results and subsequent theory formulation. Other important aspects concerning the study design are the selection of statistical analyses as well as the definition of the ethical commitments.

This chapter begins with a review of some of the important issues in statistical analysis and experimental design. The ensuing sections look at *in vitro* techniques, animal models, and finally human studies.

The primary purpose is to provide a primer in nutrition research methods early in a student's career to allow a more critical review of the many studies that, from time to time, a student will need to consider in the course of their study.

13.2 Statistical analysis and experimental design

In all areas of research, statistical analysis of results and data plays a pivotal role. This section is intended to give students some of the very basic concepts of statistics as it relates to research methodology.

Validity

Validity describes the degree to which the inference drawn from a study is warranted when account is taken of the study methods, the representativeness of the study sample and the nature of its source population. Validity can be divided into internal validity and external validity. Internal validity refers to the subjects actually sampled. External validity refers to the extension of the findings from the sample to a target population.

Accuracy

Accuracy is a term used to describe the extent to which a measurement is close to the true value, and

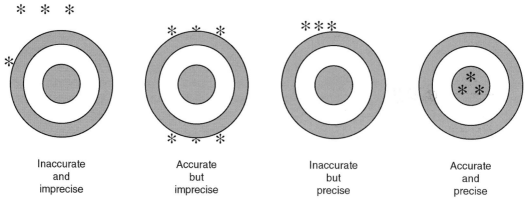

Figure 13.1 Accuracy and precision.

it is commonly estimated as the difference between the reported result and the actual value (Figure 13.1).

Reliability

Reliability or reproducibility refers to the consistency or repeatability of a measure. Reliability does not imply validity. A reliable measure is measuring something consistently, but not necessarily estimating its true value. If a measurement error occurs in two separate measurements with exactly the same magnitude and direction, this measurement may be fully reliable but invalid. The kappa inter-rate agreement statistic (for categorical variables) and the intraclass correlation coefficient are frequently used to assess reliability.

Precision

Precision is described as the quality of being sharply defined or stated; thus, sometimes precision is indicated by the number of significant digits in the measurement.

In a more restricted statistical sense, precision refers to the reduction in random error. It can be improved either by increasing the size of a study or by using a design with higher efficiency. For example, a better balance in the allocation of exposed and unexposed subjects, or a closer matching in a case–control study usually obtains a higher precision without increasing the size of the study.

Sensitivity and specificity

Measures of sensitivity and specificity relate to the validity of a value. Sensitivity is the proportion of

Table 13.1 Estimation of sensitivity and specificity

	True condition or outcome present	True condition or outcome absent
Test +	A	B
Test −	C	D

$$\text{Sensitivity} = \frac{A}{A+C} \quad \text{Specificity} = \frac{D}{B+D}$$

subjects with the condition who are correctly classified as having the condition. Specificity is the proportion of persons without the condition who are correctly classified as being free of the condition by the test or criteria. Sensitivity reflects the proportion of affected individuals who test positive, while specificity refers to the proportion of nonaffected individuals who test negative (Table 13.1).

Data description

Statistics may have either a descriptive or an inferential role in nutrition research. Descriptive statistical methods are a powerful tool to summarize large amounts of data. These descriptive purposes are served either by calculating statistical indices, such as the mean, median, and standard deviation, or by using graphical procedures, such as histograms, box plots, and scatter plots. Some errors in the data collection are most easily detected graphically with the histogram plot or with the box-plot chart (box-and-whisker plot). These two graphs are useful for describing the distribution of a quantitative variable. Nominal variables, such as gender, and ordinal variables, such as educational level, can be presented simply tabulated as proportions within categories or ranks. Continuous variables, such as age and weight, are customarily presented by summary statistics describing the frequency distribution. These summary statistics include measures of central tendency (mean, median) and measures of spread (variance, standard deviation, coefficient of variation). The standard deviation describes the "spread" or variation around the sample mean.

Hypothesis testing

The first step in hypothesis testing is formulating a hypothesis called the null hypothesis. This null hypothesis can often be stated as the negation of the research hypothesis that the investigator is looking for. For example, if we are interested in showing that, in the European adult population, a lower amount and intensity of physical activity during leisure time has contributed to a higher prevalence of overweight and obesity, the research hypothesis might be that there is a difference between sedentary and active adults with respect to their body mass index (BMI). The negation of this research hypothesis is called the null hypothesis. This null hypothesis simply maintains that the difference in BMI between sedentary and active individuals is zero. In a second step, we calculate the probability that the result could have been obtained if the null hypothesis were true in the population from which the sample has been extracted. This probability is usually called the p-value. Its maximum value is 1 and the minimum is 0. The p-value is a conditional probability:

$$p\text{-Value} = \text{prob}(\text{differences} \geq \text{differences found} \mid \text{null hypothesis (H}_0) \text{ were true})$$

where the vertical bar (|) means "conditional to." In a more concise mathematical expression:

$$p\text{-Value} = \text{prob}(\text{difference} \geq \text{data} \mid H_0)$$

The above condition is that the null hypothesis was true in the population that gave origin to the sample. The p-value by no means expresses the probability that the null hypothesis is true. This is a frequent and unfortunate mistake in the interpretation of p-values.

An example of hypothesis testing is shown in Box 13.1. Hypothesis testing helps in deciding whether or not the null hypothesis can be rejected. A low p-value indicates that the data are not likely to be com-

---

Box 13.1 Example of hypothesis testing

Among a representative sample of 7097 European men, the authors found that each 10 unit increase in the leisure-time physical activity was associated with -0.074 kg/m^2 in BMI. Physical activity was measured in units of MET-hours/week (1 MET-hour is the energy expenditure during 1 resting hour).

What is the probability of finding, in such a sample, a BMI 0.074 kg/m^2 lower (or still lower) for those whose energy expenditure is 10 MET-hours higher, if the actual difference in the whole European population were 0? This probability is the p-value; the smaller it is, the stronger is the evidence to reject the null hypothesis.

In this example, the p-value was 0.001, i.e., chance would explain a finding like this, or even more extreme, in only 1 out of 1000 replications of the study. The conclusion is that we reject the null hypothesis (population difference in BMI = 0) and (provisionally) accept the hypothesis that states that lower physical activity during leisure time is associated with a higher BMI. We call this the alternative hypothesis.

Table 13.2 Right and wrong decisions in hypothesis testing

	Truth (population)	
Decision	Null hypothesis	Alternative hypothesis
Null hypothesis	Right decision (probability = $1 - \alpha$)	Type II error (probability = β)
Alternative hypothesis	Type I error (probability = α)	Right decision (power = $1 - \beta$)

---

patible with the null hypothesis. A large p-value indicates that the data are compatible with the null hypothesis. Many authors accept that a p-value lower than 0.05 provides enough evidence to reject the null hypothesis. The use of such a cut-off for p leads to treating the analysis as a decision-making process. Two possible errors can be made when making such a decision (Table 13.2).

A type I error consists of rejecting the null hypothesis, when the null hypothesis is in fact true. Conversely, a type II error occurs if the null hypothesis is accepted when the null hypothesis is in fact not true. The probabilities of type I and type II errors are called alpha (α) and beta (β), respectively.

Power calculations

The power of a study is the probability of obtaining a statistically significant result when a true effect of a specified size exists. The power of a study is not a single value, but a range of values, depending on the assumption about the size of the effect. The plot of power against size of effect is called a power curve. The calculations of sample size are based in the principles of hypothesis testing. Thus, the power of a study to detect an effect of a specified size is the complementary of beta $(1 - \beta)$. The smaller a study is, the lower is its power. Calculation of the optimum sample size is often viewed as a rather difficult task, but it is an important issue because a reasonable certainty that the study will be large enough to provide a precise answer is needed before starting the process of data collection (Box 13.2).

The necessary sample size for a study can be estimated taking into account at least three inputs:

Box 13.2 Example of sample size calculation

Let us suppose that we want to compare the proportion of subjects who develop a given outcome depending on whether they have been assigned to diet A or diet B. We expect that 5% of subjects in the group assigned to diet A and 25% of those assigned to diet B will develop the outcome of interest. We are willing to accept a type I error with a 5% probability and a type II error with a 10% probability. A simplified equation* for sample size (n) calculation would be:

$$n = \frac{(z_{\alpha/2} + z_\beta)^2 \, 2pq}{(p_A - p_B)^2}$$

$$n = \frac{(1.96 + 1.28)^2 \, 2 \times 0.15 \times 0.85}{(0.05 - 0.25)^2}$$

$$n = 65$$

where $z_{\alpha/2}$ and z_β are the values of the normal distribution corresponding to alpha 0.05 ($z_{\alpha/2} = 1.96$) and beta 0.10 ($z_\beta = 1.28$), P_A and P_B are the expected proportions, p is the average of both proportions $(0.05 + 0.25/2 = 0.15)$ and $q = 1 - p$. Therefore, in this example:

$$z_{\alpha/2} = {}_{0.05 \text{ (two tailed)}} = 1.96$$
$$z_\beta = {}_{0.10 \text{ (one tailed)}} = 1.28$$
$$p_A = 0.05 \ (q_1 = 0.95)$$
$$p_B = 0.25 \ (q_2 = 0.75)$$

These values are substituted in the equation and thus the required sample size for each group is obtained **(65). Therefore, we shall need 130 participants, 65 in each group.**
*When the outcome is a quantitative variable, sample means (x_A and x_B) replace proportions in the denominator, while the product terms $p_A q_A$ and $p_B q_B$ are replaced by the respective variances (s^2) of the two groups in the numerator:

$$n = \frac{(z_{\alpha/2} + z_\beta)^2 \left[S_A^2 + S_B^2 \right]}{(\bar{x}_A - \bar{x}_B)^2}$$

- the expected proportion in each group and, consequently, the expected magnitude of the true effect
- the beta error (or alternatively, the power) that is required
- the alpha error.

The p-value has been the subject of much criticism because a p-value of 0.05 has been frequently and arbitrarily misused to distinguish a true effect from lack of effect. Until the 1970s most applications of statistics in nutrition and nutritional epidemiology focused on classical significance testing, involving a decision on whether or not chance could explain the observed association. But more important than the simple decision is the estimation of the magnitude of the association. This estimation includes an assessment about the range of credible values for the association. This is more meaningfully presented as a confidence interval, which expresses, with a certain degree of confidence, usually 95%, the range from the smallest to the largest value that is plausible for the true population value, assuming that only random variation has created discrepancies between the true value in the population and the value observed in the sample of analyzed data.

Options for statistical approaches to data analysis

Different statistical procedures are used for describing or analyzing data in nutritional epidemiology (Table 13.3). The criteria for selecting the appropriate procedure are based on the nature of the variable considered as the outcome or dependent variable. Three main types of dependent variable can be considered: quantitative (normal), qualitative (very often dichotomous), and survival or time-to-event variables.

Within bivariate comparisons, some modalities deserve further insights (Table 13.4).

The validity of most standard tests depends on the assumptions that:

- the data are from a normal distribution
- the variability within groups (if these are compared) is similar.

Tests of this type are termed parametric and are to some degree sensitive to violations of these assumptions. Alternatively, nonparametric or distribution-free tests, which do not depend on the normal

Table 13.3 Common statistical methods used in nutritional epidemiology

Dependent variable ("outcome")	Univariate description	Bivariate comparisons	Multivariable analysis (Katz, 2006)
 Quantitative (normal)	Mean, standard deviation	*t*-Tests (two groups) Analysis of variance (more than two groups) Regression and correlation (two quantitative variables)	Multiple regression
 Qualitative (dichotomous)	Proportion, odds	Chi-squared McNemar paired test Fisher's exact test Cross-tables Odds ratio Relative risk	Multiple logistic regression Conditional logistic regression (matched data)
 Survival	Kaplan–Meier (product-limit) estimates and plots	Log-rank test (Mantel–Haenszel)	Proportional hazards model (Cox regression)

Table 13.4 Common statistical methods for comparison of means

	Two samples		More than two samples	
	Parametric	Nonparametric	Parametric	Nonparametric
Independent samples Paired or related samples	Student's *t*-test Welch test (unequal variances) Satterthwaite test (unequal variances) Paired *t*-test	Mann–Whitney U-test Wilcoxon test	Analysis of variance Bonferroni, Scheffé, Tamhane, Dunnet, Sidak, or Tukey post-hoc tests Analysis of variance for repeated measurements General linear models ANCOVA (analysis of covariance)	Kruskal–Wallis test Friedman's test

distribution, can be used. Nonparametric tests are also useful for data collected as ordinal variables because they are based on ranking the values. Relative to their parametric counterparts, nonparametric tests have the advantage of ease, but the disadvantage of less statistical power if a normal distribution should be assumed. Another additional disadvantage is that they do not permit confidence intervals for the difference between means to be estimated.

A common problem in nutrition literature is multiple significance testing. Some methods to consider in these instances are analysis of variance together with multiple-comparison methods specially designed to make several pairwise comparisons, such as the least significant difference method, the Bonferroni and Scheffé procedures, and the Duncan test. Analysis of variance can also be used for replicate measurements of a continuous variable.

Correlation is the statistical method to use when studying the association between two continuous variables. The degree of association is ordinarily measured by Pearson's correlation coefficient. This calculation leads to a quantity that can take any value from −1 to +1. The correlation coefficient is positive if higher values of one variable are related to higher values of the other and it is negative when one variable tends to be lower while the other tends to be higher. The correlation coefficient is a measure of the scatter of the points when the two variables are plotted. The greater the spread of the points, the lower the correlation coefficient. Correlation involves an estimate of the symmetry between the two quantitative variables and does not attempt to describe their relationship. The nonparametric counterpart of Pearson's correlation coefficient is the Spearman rank correlation. It is the only nonparametric method that allows confidence intervals to be estimated.

To describe the relationship between two continuous variables, the mathematical model most often used is the straight line. This simplest model is known as simple linear regression analysis. Regression analysis is commonly used not only to quantify the association between two variables, but also to make predictions based on the linear relationship. Nowadays, nutritional epidemiologists frequently use the statistical methods of multivariable analysis (Table 13.3). These methods usually provide a more accurate view of the relationship between dietary and nondietary exposures and the occurrence of a disease or other outcome, while adjusting simultaneously for many variables and smoothing out the irregularities that very small subgroups can introduce into alternative adjustment procedures such as stratified analysis (Katz, 2006).

Most multivariate methods are based on the concept of simple linear regression. An explanation of the variation in a quantitative dependent variable (outcome) by several independent variables (exposures or predictors) is the basis of a multiple-regression model. However, in many studies the dependent variable or outcome is quite often dichotomous (diseased/nondiseased) instead of quantitative and can also be explained by several independent factors (dietary and nondietary exposures). In this case, the statistical multivariate method that must be applied is multiple logistic regression. In follow-up studies, the time to the occurrence of disease is also taken into account. More weight can be given to earlier cases than to later cases. The multivariate method most appropriate in this setting is the proportional hazards model (Cox regression) using a time-to-event variable as the outcome (Table 13.3).

13.3 *In vitro* studies

Scientific research involves studies across a reductionist spectrum. As studies become more reductionist, more and more confounding factors are stripped away. *In vitro* studies represent part of the reductionist approach in nutrition research. The range of techniques used is large.

- Chemical analysis studies provide data on nutrient and nonnutrient content of foods.
- Digestibility techniques, in which a substrate is exposed to enzymes capable of digesting the substrate, help to refine the gross chemical analytical data to predict nutritional potential.
- Intact organs such as the liver of experimental animals can be used in studies such as perfused organ studies. In such studies, the investigator can control the composition of material entering an isolated organ and examine the output. Sections of organs can also be used, such as the everted gut sac technique. A small section of the intestine is turned inside out and placed in a solution containing some test material. Uptake of the test material into the gut can be readily measured.
- Another approach is the construction of mechanical models that mimic an organ, usually the gut (in nutrition research). Many of these models successfully predict what is observed *in vivo* and have advantages such as cost and flexibility in altering the experimental conditions with great precision. System biology is a recently launched platform to integrate metabolic pathways using computational biology.

The application of molecular biology techniques to tissue and cell culture systems has provided researchers with powerful strategies to evaluate and establish metabolic pathways and regulatory roles of nutrient and nonnutrient components of food. Thus, Northern, Southern and Western blotting techniques to quantitate specific RNA, DNA, and proteins in tissues in response to nutrients are common tools in the nutrition laboratory. The influence of some nutrients or nutritional conditions on ribosomal dynamics as well as on cell hyperplasia or hypertrophy processes has been estimated through RNA, DNA, or protein/DNA values, respectively.

Furthermore, molecular biological approaches have allowed numerous *in vitro* discoveries that have aided our understanding of the genetic basis of nutrient functions and metabolic states *in vivo*. The polymerase chain reaction (PCR) can be used for DNA and/or messenger RNA (mRNA) amplification to determine the genetic background and/or gene expression in very small cellular samples. Transfection studies allow the insertion of DNA into cells to examine nutrient function. Thus, cell lines that usually lack the expression of a particular gene can be transfected with DNA containing the gene promoter, as well as all or part of the transfected gene of interest, to study the interactions of various nutrients with the expression of a particular gene. Conversely, knockout cell lines allow us to investigate the consequences of losing a specific gene. In either case, nutrient function at the cell level and the cell–gene level may be studied and provide definitive results. Gene regulation by nutrients has been assessed in different isolated cells and tissues using appropriate indicators and markers of gene expression RNA levels.

The integration of biochemical and molecular technologies into nutrition research allows the potential for an integrated systems biology perspective examining the interactions among DNA, RNA protein, and metabolites. Following the completion of the human genome sequence, new findings about individual genes functions and their involvement in body homeostasis is emerging. Thus, technologies to achieve a simultaneous assessment of thousands of gene polymorphisms, the quantitation of mRNA levels of a large number of genes (transcriptomics) as well as proteins (proteomics), or metabolites (metabolomics) is rapidly progressing. Advances in DNA and RNA microarray-based tools as well in the application of classic two-dimensional gel electrophoresis, various Liquid chromatography-mass spectrometry (LC-MS) techniques, image scanning, or antibody arrays is contributing to unraveling the intimate mechanisms involved in nutritional processes. Epigenetics studies constitute a rising methodology to be applied in nutritional research.

13.4 Animal models in nutrition research

Whole animal systems have been used in measuring the utilization, function, and fate of nutrients. Thus,

a part of our knowledge regarding nutrition concepts stems from animal experiments, which are often extrapolated to humans and referred to as animal models. There are many reasons for choosing an animal study over a human study. We can and do subject animals to experimental conditions that we would ethically not be allowed to apply to humans. For example, to study the manner in which a nutrient influences the scale and histopathology of atherosclerosis, animal studies are needed. Just as studies with humans are governed by the rules of ethics committees, so too are studies with animals. These rules involve the regulation of facilities, accommodation and animal care, competence, alternatives to animal experimentation, anesthesia and euthanasia procedures, registration, supply of animals, and the involvement of an ethical committee.

In general, the use of animals as models for human nutrition research can be examined from three aspects:

- the animal model
- the experimental diet and its delivery
- the experimental techniques available.

The animal model

Many species have been used in the study of nutrition. Many are pure-bred strains such as the Wistar rat, the Charles River mouse, or the New Zealand white rabbit. Some animal models have been specially selected to exhibit particular traits, making them very useful models for research. The Wattanable rabbit has defective low-density lipoprotein (LDL) receptor function, making this animal model very useful for studying the role of diet in influencing LDL receptor-mediated arterial disease. The ob/ob mouse develops gross obesity because of an alteration in a genetic profile (leptin synthesis). In recent times there has been a rise in the use of transgenic animal models that have been produced through advanced molecular genetic techniques. In such models, specific genes can be inserted or deleted to fulfill specific functions. For example, the peroxisome proliferator-activated receptor-alpha (PPAR-α) is not expressed in one knockout mouse model, giving rise to fat accumulation. Another example of a transgenic mouse presents an overexpression of the Cu/Zn-superoxide dismutase enzyme.

The experimental diet and its delivery

The nature of the diet and its mode of delivery are centrally important in understanding the role of animal models in human nutrition issues. There are several types of diets offered to laboratory animals.

Commercially available diets made to internationally accepted nutritional norms are often referred to as chow diets or laboratory chow. For the vast majority of laboratory animals in studies where nutrient intake is not the central area of interest, such chow diets are used. However, when nutrition is the area of research, special diets will almost always have to be formulated. The type of diet that needs to be formulated will depend on the nature of the research question.

Terms such as semipurified, purified, and chemically defined diets are often used but frequently it is difficult to know exactly which type of term fits different formulations. The least refined experimental diet uses ingredients such as barley, soybean, and wheat. An example is given in Table 13.5, taken from a study of rapeseed glucosinolates on the iodine status of piglets.

The purpose of the study was to assess the effects of glucosinolate derived from ground rapeseed. A direct comparison between the ground rapeseed and the control is not possible because the ground rapeseed contains twice as much fat as the controls. Thus, the rapeseed oil diet is included because it contains no glucosinolate, but the same amount of fat as the control diet. The ingredients used in these diets, in general, contain several nutrients. Thus, the main ingredient, barley, contains protein, carbohydrate, and fat as well as fiber and micronutrients. That can

create problems when there is a need to examine the effects of specific nutrients, such as fatty acids. The fatty acids naturally present in barley cannot be ignored. In the case of the rapeseed oil diet in Table 13.5, 40 g of the 56 g of fat per kilogram of diet comes from the rapeseed oil, but 16 g (or 28.6%) comes from barley lipid.

To deal with this, more refined diets are used. An example of such a diet is given in Table 13.6. In this instance, the authors were examining how different dietary fats influence blood cholesterol in normal mice and in transgenic mice not expressing the gene for the cholesteryl ester transfer protein (CETP), which is a key protein in lipid metabolism. In this instance, the ingredients are almost all pure. Thus, casein is pure protein and nothing else. Similarly, sucrose is pure carbohydrate and cellulose is pure fiber. The diets differ only in the source of fat. The high-fat diet obviously has more fat and thus more energy per kilogram of diet. It is thus critically important to note that as the energy density goes up, most other things must also go up to ensure a common concentration, not on a weight-for-weight basis but on a weight-for-energy basis. A simple illustration is the level of the mineral mix used: 2.5 g/100 g in the control diet, 3.2 g/100 g in the low-fat diet and 4.2 g/100 g in the high-fat diet. But when considered on a weight-for-energy basis, all five diets contain 2.0 g/MJ. The only changes are in fat and in maize starch, which always vary in opposite directions.

Variations in diet composition are often the key for the design of nutrition experiments. In this context, different feeding regimens can be applied to laboratory animals depending on scientific criteria. In *ad libitum* feeding the animals have free access to food; in controlled feeding animals are offered a limited amount of food (restricted feeding) or receive as much food as can be fed to them (forced feeding). A specific form of restricted feeding is pair feeding, which involves the measurement of food consumed by some animals to match or equalize the intake of a test group on the following day. There are many reasons why pair feeding is critically important. An experiment may seek to examine how a new protein source, rich in some nutrient of interest, influences some aspect of metabolism. Let us consider a compound in the protein source that may reduce blood LDL cholesterol. A control diet is constructed based on casein. In the experimental diets, this casein is

Table 13.5 An example of less refined experimental diets to test the effects of rapeseed-derived glucosinolate

	Control (g/kg)	Rapeseed oil (g/kg)	Ground rapeseed (g/kg)
Soybean meal[a]	220	240	195
Rapeseed oil	5	40	–
Ground rapeseed	–	–	100
Barley	755	700	685
Mineral/vitamin	20	20	20
Total	1000	1000	1000
Energy (MJ/kg)[b]	12.6	13.3	13.0
Protein (g/kg)	183	177	182
Fat (g/kg)	29	56	58
Glucosinolate (mmol/kg)	0	0	1.9

[a]Solvent-extracted soybean meal.
[b]Metabolizable energy.
From Schone *et al.* (2001). Reproduced with permission.

Table 13.6 An example of more refined experimental diets to examine the cholesterolemic effects of fats in transgenic CETP mice

	Control diet		Low-fat diet		High-fat diet	
	(g/100 g)	(g/MJ)	(g/100 g)	(g/MJ)	(g/100 g)	(g/MJ)
Casein	20	12	19	12	24	12
L-Cystine	0.03	0.18	0.28	0.18	0.36	0.18
Maize starch	40	24	48	31	13	6
Dextrinized starch	13	8	12	8	16	8
Sucrose	10	6	9	6	12	6
Cellulose	5	3	5	3	6	3
Soybean oil	7	4	0	0	0	0
Safflower oil	0	0	2	1.2	2.4	1.2
Experimental oil[a]	0	0	0	0	22	11
Mineral mix	3.5	2.1	3.3	2.1	4.2	2.1
Vitamin mix	1	0.6	0.9	0.6	1.2	0.6
Energy (%)						
Total fat	16.9		5.7		48.6	
Sugar	10.1		10.9		10.5	
Starch	54.1		22.3		22.1	
Protein	20.2		20.9		20.7	
MJ/kg	16.7		15.9		20.1	

[a] Three different experimental oils were used (butter, safflower, high oleic safflower) for three different high-fat diets varying in types of fatty acids.
From Chang and Snook (2001). Reproduced with permission.

replaced on an isonitrogenous basis with the test protein source. Otherwise the diets are identical. After several weeks of *ad libitum* feeding a blood sample is taken and the results show that blood cholesterol rose with the experimental diet. Then the researcher begins to look at other data and observes that growth rates in the control rats were far higher than in the experimental group because the latter had a much lower food intake. Quite simply, the new protein source was unpalatable. The experiment will now have to be carried out as a pair-fed study. The food intake of rats given the experimental diet will be measured each day. On the following day the control rats will be rationed to that amount. Food intakes and probably growth rates are identical. Only the protein source differs. Now the researcher can truly reach conclusions as to the effect of the new protein source on LDL cholesterol metabolism. The intake or supply of nutrients may be administered orally, intravenously, intraperitoneally, or by means of some specific tools (gavage, stereotaxis, etc.).

The experimental techniques available

The outcome or variables of interest to be assessed condition the experimental techniques to be applied, which may include growth curves, nutrient and energy balance, nutrient utilization and signalling, etc., using cellular, molecular or other strategies.

Another approach to investigate nutritional processes is to overexpress, inactivate, or manipulate specific genes playing a role in body metabolism (Campión *et al.* 2004). These new technologies allow the study of the regulation and function of different genes. The current standard methods for manipulating genes in nutrition research depend on the method of introducing/blocking genes. Thus, genetic manipulation can be sustained for generations by creating germline transmission. In this way, there are examples of transgenic animals, overexpressing or knocking out genes, but still controlling this gene manipulation in a spatial or temporal manner. However, when the aim is not to transfer genetic information to subsequent generations, the most usual method is gene transfer to somatic cells. Different viral and nonviral vectors are used for the *in vivo* gene transfer, allowing a transient or permanent overexpression of the gene of interest. The RNAi (interference) approach allows the creation of new *in vivo* models by transient ablation of gene expression by degrading target mRNA. Moreover, by inserting RNAi encoding sequences in the genome, permanent silencing of the target gene can be obtained. Undoubtedly, new models of investigation will be developed, combining the different genetic manipulation techniques to achieve the creation of new models to understand the function and the regulation of metabolism, nutritional, and disease-related genes. Indeed, research concerning inhibiting/activating the expression of different genes (transgenic/knockout animals), gene transfer, and RNAi application is allowing us to specifically investigate functions and metabolism of regulatory processes.

13.5 Human studies

In human nutrition, man is the ultimate court in which hypotheses are both generated and tested. Nutritional epidemiology, through its observational studies, demonstrates possible links between diet, physical activity, and disease (Willett, 1998). It is not the only way in which such possible links are generated but it is a critically important one in modern nutrition. Experimental human nutrition takes the hypothesis and through several experiments tries to understand the nature of the link between nutrients and the metabolic basis of the disease. Once there is a reasonable body of evidence that particular nutritional conditions are related to the risk of disease, experimental nutritional epidemiology examines how population level intervention actually influences the incidence of disease (see Section 13.6). In effect, experimental human nutrition and experimental nutrition epidemiology both involve hypothesis testing. However, the former is more often intended to understand mechanisms and generally involves small numbers. The latter, in contrast, uses very large numbers to examine the public health impact of a nutrition intervention that, under the controlled conditions of the laboratory, showed promise.

Human nutrition experimentation

The use of experimental animals for human nutrition research offers many possible solutions to experimental problems. However, the definitive experiments, where possible, should be carried out in humans. Studies involving humans are more difficult to conduct for two major reasons. First, humans vary enormously compared with laboratory animals. They vary genetically and they also vary greatly in their lifestyle, background diet, health, physical activity, literacy, and in many other ways. Second, it is far more difficult to manipulate human diets since we do not eat purified or semi-purified diets.

Experimental diets in human nutrition intervention studies

In the 1950s, an epidemiological study across seven countries presented data to suggest that the main determinant of plasma cholesterol was the balance of saturated, monounsaturated, and polyunsaturated fatty acids (MUFAs and PUFAs). To test this hypothesis, a series of studies was carried out on human volunteers using "formula diets." Dried skimmed milk powder, the test oil, and water were blended to form a test milk with specific fatty acid compositions. The volunteers lived almost exclusively on these formulae. Although this type of study is simple to conduct, it does not represent the true conditions under which normal humans live. At the other end of the spectrum of options for manipulating human diets is that of issuing advice that the subjects verify by way of a food record. It is difficult to prove that subjects actually ate what they say they have eaten. Sometimes, adherence to dietary advice can be ascertained using tissue samples (blood, saliva, hair, fat) and biomarkers. For example, adherence to advice to increase oily fish intake can be monitored using platelet phospholipid fatty acids.

In between these two extremes of formula feeds and dietary advice lies an array of options in which convenience is generally negatively correlated with scientific exactitude. In the case of minerals and vitamins, it is possible simply to give out pills for the volunteers to take and measure compliance by counting unconsumed pills and perhaps using biomarkers. When it comes to macronutrients this is not generally possible. Whereas asking someone to take a mineral supplement should not alter their eating habits, asking someone to consume a liter of milk a day or a bowl of rice bran per day will alter other aspects of the diets of the volunteers. It will not then be possible to attribute definitively an event to the intervention (1 l/day of milk or 1 bowl/day of rice bran). The event could have been caused by possible displacement of some other foods by the intervention. The only option in human intervention experiments is to prepare foods for volunteers to eat, which differ only in the test nutrient. If the objective is to examine the effect of MUFAs relative to saturated fatty acids (SFAs) on blood lipids, then fat-containing foods can be prepared that are identical except for the source of fat.

The more foods and dishes that can be prepared in this way, the more successful the experiment will be.

The final dilemma is where the test foods will be consumed. A volunteer may share the test foods, which are almost always supplied free of charge, with friends or family. To be sure of consumption, volunteers may be asked to consume the test meal in some supervised space, usually a metabolic suite. This, however, is a very costly option. Nutritional intervention studies with different macronutrient distribution of food content within energy-restricted diets are typical in nutrition research (Abete *et al.* 2006).

Study designs in human nutrition

The randomized clinical trial is the most powerful design to demonstrate cause–effect relationships. It is unique in representing a completely experimental approach in humans. The major strength of randomized trials is that they are able to control most biases and confounding even when confounding factors cannot be measured. The CONSORT statement has established the CONsolidated Standards Of Reporting Trials (http://www.consort-statement.org/). The CONSORT guidelines comprise a checklist and a flow diagram offering a standard way for reporting the research and assessing its quality. The major methodological issues to be considered and reported in a randomized trial include the following aspects: enrolment, allocation, follow-up, and inclusion in analysis of participants, sample size, proceedings for the randomization, blinding of the allocation, blinded assessment of the outcome, comparability of groups regarding major prognostic variables, ascertainment and measurement of end-points, statistical analyses, subgroup analyses, results description, ancillary analyses, adverse events, interpretations, generalizability, and overall quality of the reported evidence.

As the researcher designs the options for altering the intake of nutrient under investigation, so too the design of the study requires careful thought. The metabolic effect of the nutrient in question may be influenced by age, gender, and other variables, such as high levels of alcohol intake or physical activity, smoking, health status, prescribed drug use, and family history. On an experiment-by-experiment basis, the researcher must decide which attributes will exclude a volunteer (exclusion criteria).

The volunteers recruited can now be assigned to the various treatments. When the numbers are small, randomly assigning subjects to the treatments may lead to imbalances that could confound conclusions. For example, if one has 45 volunteers for three treatments, it could be that the 15 assigned to treatment A include the five heaviest subjects and the five lightest subjects. Another treatment may be predominantly one gender. In such instances, a minimization scheme can be used. Minimization is a technique in which individuals are allocated to treatment groups, ensuring a balance by minimizing the differences between groups in the distribution of important characteristics (age, weight, physical activity). To apply minimization, during the recruitment process the investigators must keep an ongoing analysis of differences between groups in the major variables that may affect the result and allocate new individuals to the group that leads to a more balanced distribution of these characteristics. Another option is stratified randomization in which strata are identified and subjects are randomly allocated within each stratum. While stratification and minimization are potentially very useful, it is impractical to stratify individuals for many variables at the same time or to try to minimize every conceivable variable that may affect the result. To a considerable extent, the need to balance groups becomes less important when all subjects are rotated through all treatments (crossover designs). For this to happen, the number of experimental periods must equal the number of treatments. For any given period, all treatments must be represented. An important factor to consider in this type of design is whether or not a washout period is needed between treatments, and its duration.

Consider the situation above if the study was to examine the effect of fish oil (treatment A) versus olive oil (treatment B) on lymphocyte function. If it is deemed necessary that 20 days are needed to alter the membrane phospholipids of lymphocytes, then it is likely that 30 days will be needed to return to baseline. If it is necessary that each treatment should commence at baseline, then a washout period, where volunteers resume their normal routine, is needed.

A final consideration is the occasion when it is not possible to balance all confounding factors. Take as an example a study to examine the effect of supplemental calcium on bone mineral density in premenopausal women. The treatment group will receive a supplement of 1000 mg of calcium as a tablet and the control will receive a placebo tablet. What factors might one wish to balance in such a study? Among the possibilities are age, parity, use of oral contraceptives, intake of coffee, smoking, and physical activity. To balance these factors adequately is impossible. However, if they are recorded, then, when the data are being evaluated on a statistical basis, they can be included to ascertain their effect on the measured outcome, bone mineral density. To accomplish this aim, multivariate methods such as multiple regression or logistic regression should be used (see Section 13.2).

13.6 Epidemiological designs

Epidemiology is a health-related science dealing with the distribution and determinants of health and illness in populations. Nutritional epidemiology integrates the knowledge derived from nutrition research, to examine diet–disease relationships at the level of free-living populations. Nutritional epidemiology provides scientific evidence to understand the role of nutrition in the cause and prevention of disease.

The comparison and choice of different epidemiological study designs depends on exposure measures, outcome measures, costs, and expected length of follow-up. The selection of a study method is often influenced by pragmatic issues such as feasibility, as well as by ethical questions.

Epidemiological studies can be divided into two broad categories (Figure 13.2): experimental and nonexperimental (observational) studies. Observational studies can be further divided into descriptive and analytical studies. In a wide sense, an experiment is a set of observations, conducted under controlled

circumstances, in which the scientist manipulates the conditions to ascertain the effect of such manipulation on the observations.

Experimental studies in nutritional epidemiology

It is necessary to consider that in biological experimentation, it is not possible for the scientist to control completely all of the relevant circumstances, and the manipulation will consist of increasing at most the degree of variation in the factor that the scientist is investigating. The ideal will be to obtain two almost identical sets of circumstances where all factors are the same. If a strong variation is then introduced in only one of these factors, all of the observed differences between the two sets that occurred thereafter would be causally attributed to the single factor that the investigator had manipulated.

Experimental epidemiological designs are those in which the investigator assigns the exposure to each subject. In these studies, the treatment (or exposure) is assigned with the aim of attaining maximum comparability between treated and untreated groups regarding all other characteristics of the subjects apart from the treatment or exposure of interest. In epidemiological research, the best way to achieve identical sets of circumstances is to assign subjects randomly to exposure (treatment) or control groups. This process is called randomization. All randomized studies are experimental designs.

Exposure, from an epidemiological point of view, describes lifestyle or environmental factors that may be relevant to health. Outcome is another generic term used to describe the health-related events or variables that are being studied in relation to the effect of an exposure. In nutritional epidemiology, the primary exposure of interest is dietary intake, whereas outcome measures usually involve disease occurrence or nutritional status indicators (anthropometry, clinical signs of disease/health status, biological or physiological measures or dietary habits).

It is also possible to design experimental studies assigning whole population groups to different exposures. These studies are called community trials. For example, if a whole town is assigned to receive an educational program about healthy eating and another neighboring town is assigned to control (no educational program), this would be a community trial; when randomization is used, it is termed "cluster-

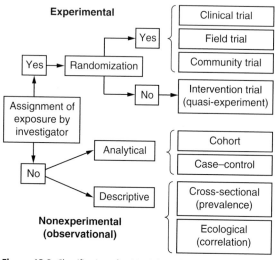

Figure 13.2 Classification of epidemiological designs.

randomization." However, when the number of randomized units is scarce, even though each unit may be large, there would be no guarantee that the groups to be compared would be identical. Conversely, if the randomization has been done on an individual basis and the whole sample is large enough, a random scheme will usually accomplish its objective of distributing the participants in groups that are essentially homogeneous in all measured and unmeasured factors. This balance makes groups directly comparable and ensures the validity of causal inferences extracted from a randomized design (individual randomization).

In general, experimental studies with individual randomization provide the strongest evidence for the effect of an exposure on an outcome. Experimental studies are the inferentially strongest designs to demonstrate causality, but they may raise substantial ethical problems because the scheme of random assignment is used to help not the subject, but the experiment. Subjects are exposed only to meet the needs of the protocol of the study and not the individual needs of the participant. Therefore, randomized experiments with humans can only be conducted under strict ethical conditions (see Boxes 13.3 and 13.4). It is not permissible to carry out experimental studies where the exposure is potentially harmful. Therefore, under these conditions, nonexperimental (observational) study designs must be applied. The design options in nutritional epidemiology must take into account the setting, uses, advantages, and limitations (Table 13.7).

Experimental designs in epidemiology

Experimental epidemiologists try to conduct controlled studies, and in these studies it is the investigator who assigns the exposure. Human studies, however, unlike animal studies, involve aspects that the investigator cannot control. This is particularly so when they are carried out on a free-living population. Two study designs dominate this area of epidemiology: randomized controlled trials and crossover studies. In these studies, subjects are randomly assigned to

---

Box 13.3 Sample ethics form for completion prior to research

The proposal respects the fundamental ethical principles including human rights and will deal only with individuals adequately informed and willing to participate. Also, all research data partners will obtain national authorization from an ethical committee or equivalent body before any intervention with subjects. The study does not involve any genetic manipulation.

- Requested specifications:
  - Human embryos or fetus   No   Yes
  - Use of human embryonic or fetal tissue   No   Yes
  - Use of other human tissue   No   Yes
  - Research on persons   No   Yes
  - If yes, further specify if it involves:
    - children   No   Yes
    - persons unable to consent   No   Yes
    - pregnant women   No   Yes
    - healthy volunteers   No   Yes
  - Use of nonhuman primates   No   Yes
  - Use of transgenic animals   No   Yes
  - Use of other animals   No   Yes
  - Genetic modification of animals   No   Yes
  - Genetic modification of plants   No   Yes
- Other specifications:
  - The regulations, concerning human and medical research, will be respected with precise reference to the recommendations of the Helsinki (1964), Tokyo (1975), Venice (1983) and Hong Kong (1989) committees, as well as other EU regulations RD 561/1993, 65/65 CEE, 75/318 CEE, Directive 91/507 and 89/843 EN-C (ISBN 92-825-9612-2).

Box 13.4 Sample of an informed consent form

This form will cover the following aspects:

I .... (name)

I have read the volunteer's information

I have felt free to make questions concerning the study

I have received enough information

I have talked to the following personnel responsible (names . . .)

I understand that my participation is on a voluntary basis

I understand that I can withdraw from the study:

  1. If I wish

  2. Without further explanations

Therefore, I freely confirm my availability to be involved in the trial

Date

Signature

In addition, all the partners agree with the following statement

  In implementing the proposed research I shall adhere most strictly to all national and international ethical and safety provisions applicable in the countries where the research is carried out.

  I shall conform in particular to the relevant safety regulations concerning the deliberate release into the environment of genetically modified organisms.

Table 13.7 Design options in nutritional epidemiology

Design	Setting	Uses	Advantages	Limitations
Clinical trial	Secondary prevention (diseased participants)	Treatment–outcome association	Strongest evidence for causality Highest internal validity Very low potential for bias	Low external validity Ethical problems High cost
Field trial	Primary prevention (healthy participants)	Exposure–onset of disease association	Strong evidence for causality High internal validity Low potential for bias	Very large sample and long follow-up Low external validity Can assess only single-nutrient effects Highest costs
Community trial	Group randomization (towns, work-sites, schools)	Evaluation of community interventions or educational activities	If multiple, and small groups are randomized, it has the advantages of an experimental design	Low internal validity if the number of randomized units is low
Quasi-experiment	Intervention study (not randomized)	Evaluation of community interventions or educational activities	High feasibility More applicable Investigator controls exposure	Difficulties in finding comparable groups High potential for bias Underlying trends may alter results
Cohort	Participants are initially classified as exposed or nonexposed and followed up in time to monitor the incidence of the outcome. Retrospective or historical cohort studies are conducted using previously collected information (files)	The most powerful observational tool in nutritional epidemiology to study diet–health associations	Very low potential for bias Ability to study rare exposures, complex dietary patterns and multiple outcomes of a single exposure Allows direct estimation of risks and rates Minimal ethical problems	Large sample and very long follow-up No ability to study rare outcomes Bias by low follow-up (attrition) Requires collaborative participants High costs
Case–control	Exposure is compared between subjects with and without the outcome. Nested case–control studies are conducted within an ongoing cohort using the data of cohort members who develop the disease (cases) and a sample of nondiseased members (controls)	Practical analytical tool in nutritional epidemiology to study diet–health associations	Ability to study rare outcomes Ability to study multiple potential causes of a single outcome No problems with losses to follow-up Minimal ethical problems Low cost	Potential for biased recall of exposure and biased participation of controls Inability to study rare exposures and multiple outcomes of a single exposure Inability to estimate risks and rates
Cross-sectional	Past exposure and outcome are simultaneously assessed in a representative sample of the population	Estimation of the prevalence of a disease or an exposure Population assessment in health planning Monitoring trends if it is periodically repeated	Highest external validity Relatively low costs Minimal ethical problems A wide spectrum of information about diet and health can be collected	Difficult to assess the temporal sequence: very low ability for causal inference Potential for biased participation and response bias
Ecological	The unit of analysis is not the individual but a community. Exposure and/or disease are not measured at the individual level	Generation of new hypothesis and contextual or multilevel analysis	Ability for assessing exposures at the community level Relatively low costs Minimal ethical problems	Very low internal validity ("ecological fallacy")

either an exposed or a nonexposed group, commonly referred to as the treatment and the placebo group. The placebo is a substance that is indistinguishable from the treatment and enables both subjects and investigators to be blinded to the treatment. Changes in indicators of health or disease status are compared between the two groups at the end of the experiment to identify the effect of the exposure.

Crossover designs in epidemiology operate on the same principles as the repeated-measures designs common to basic science research. All study subjects receive the treatment and the placebo for equal periods, with a washout period in between, and the order of treatment or placebo administration is selected at random for each study subject. Crossover designs are appropriate only for studies of treatments that have no lasting effects, a feature that limits their utility in nutritional epidemiology.

In general, experimental epidemiological study designs are well suited to the identification of causal relationships between specific exposures and indicators of health or disease status. Application of these methods is limited, however, by the difficulty in controlling exposures and by the enormous expense associated with population-based intervention trials aimed at modifying risk or chronic diseases. It is perhaps more feasible to apply experimental study designs to contrast the effects of pharmacological doses of specific nutrients or food components the exposures of which can be more easily controlled. This approach has been increasingly selected from the 1990s to assess the effects of specific micronutrients (β-carotene, α-tocopherol, folic acid, and other minerals and vitamins) using large-scale randomized trials.

When only one micronutrient is compared with a placebo, the study is called a single trial, whereas multiple or factorial trials involve designs where several micronutrients are compared with a placebo. In a 2×2 factorial design, two treatments are evaluated simultaneously by forming four groups (treatment A, treatment B, both treatments, and placebo).

Experimental studies keep the highest internal validity among epidemiological designs. However, they may lack generalization (i.e., they may have low external validity) and their applicability to free-living populations may be poor insofar as the dietary intake patterns do not correspond to isolated nutrients but to the combination of more complex food items.

Moreover, the induction time needed to appraise the effect of a postulated cause may last longer than the observation period of a randomized trial, thus precluding the ability of the trial to ascertain the causal relationship.

Quasi-experimental studies are those in which the assignment of exposure is controlled by the investigator, but subjects are not randomly allocated. They are sometimes called intervention trials (Figure 13.2).

Some randomized trials are referred to as primary prevention trials and others as secondary prevention trials. Primary prevention trials are those conducted among healthy individuals with the aim of preventing the onset of disease. For example, in the Women's Health Initiative (Howard et al., 2006) more than 48 000 healthy postmenopausal women were randomly assigned to receive either a low-fat diet or placebo to prevent the onset of cardiovascular disease (CVD). All participants were free of this disease at the start of the study and they were followed up for several years to assess the incidence of fatal and nonfatal coronary heart disease, fatal and nonfatal stroke, and CVD (composite of both). This is an example of a primary prevention trial. Primary prevention trials are also called field trials.

Secondary prevention trials are conducted among patients who already suffer from a particular disease and they are randomly assigned to treatment or placebo groups to prevent adverse outcomes. For example, to study the benefits of a Mediterranean-style diet, in the Lyon Diet Heart Study, patients were randomized to two different dietary patterns after suffering a myocardial infarction (de Lorgeril et al., 1999). The outcome was not the onset of disease but the incidence of reinfarction or cardiac death during the follow-up period.

Nonexperimental (observational) epidemiological studies

When experiments are not feasible or are unethical, other nonexperimental designs are used. In nonexperimental (observational) studies the investigator has no control over the exposure, because the participants freely assign themselves or not to the exposure. In nonexperimental studies the investigator may take advantage of "natural experiments," where exposure only appears in some defined groups. An example of this would be an "experiment" where dietary intake is culturally determined, such as in Indonesia, where the rice consumed is white rather than brown, and beriberi is common as a result of vitamin B_1 deficiency.

Nonexperimental (observational) designs can be further classified into four main subtypes:

- cross-sectional studies
- case–control studies
- cohort studies
- ecological studies.

Among observational studies, the main differences between study designs relate to the time when exposure and outcome are measured. The initiative "STrengthening the Reporting of OBservational studies in Epidemiology (STROBE), http://www.strobe-statement.org" provides a check-list to assess the methodological quality of the three major epidemiological designs: cohort studies, case–control studies, and cross-sectional studies (Von Elm and Egger 2004).

Cross-sectional (prevalence) studies

Cross-sectional or prevalence studies measure both exposure and outcome in the present and at the same point in time. Cross-sectional surveys provide a snapshot of descriptive epidemiological data on nutrition, identifying nutritional needs in the population and forming a basis for health promotion and disease prevention programs at a single point in time. Several countries conduct regular cross-sectional surveys on representative samples of their populations focusing on dietary habits and frequencies of illness. Dietary factors can then be correlated with prevalence of illness, which may be helpful for national nutrition policy.

Case–control studies

In case–control studies, outcome is measured in the present, and past exposure is ascertained. Usually the dietary and lifestyle patterns of patients with a disease (cases) are compared with those of age- and gender-matched people without disease (controls).

Subjects are identified and recruited on the basis of the presence or absence of the disease or the health outcome variable of interest. Ideally, the controls are randomly selected from the same study base as the cases, and identical inclusion and exclusion criteria are applied to each group. The presence of specific dietary exposures or other factors of etiological interest in subjects is generally established using interviews, questionnaires, or medical record reviews. Within the general framework for case–control studies, there are several options for study design and control selection.

For example, controls may be matched with cases at an individual level on the basis of age, gender, or other variables believed to affect disease risk. Matching eliminates variability between cases and controls with respect to the matching variables and thus leads to a higher efficiency in the analysis. Nevertheless, matching does not control for the confounding effects of these risk factors on the observed relationship. Case–control studies are by far the most logistically feasible of the analytical study designs in epidemiology, but their application to questions of interest to nutritionists is limited by the particular nature of diet–disease relationships.

The insight to be gained from a comparison of dietary exposures between cases and controls is limited by the possibility that the dietary patterns of subjects have changed since the time when diet was most important to the disease initiation process. Retrospective case–control studies attempt to overcome this limitation by measuring past diet using food frequency or diet history methods. One concern is that recall of past diet by cases may be influenced by their present disease status. For example, patients who have had a heart attack may attach an unfair level of importance to their intake of specific foods, based on misinformation.

A primary factor in choosing between a case–control design and a cohort design is whether the exposure or the outcome is rare. If the outcome is rare, case–control studies are preferable, because a cohort would need a very large sample to observe a sufficient number of events. If the exposure is rare, cohort studies are preferable.

A nested case–control design consists of selecting as cases only those members of a previously defined cohort who develop the disease during their follow-up period. A random sample or a matched sample of non-cases is also selected from the cohort to make up the control series as the comparison group.

Cohort studies

In cohort studies exposure is evaluated in the present and outcome ascertained in the future.

Cohort studies are most commonly longitudinal or prospective, with subjects being followed forward in time over some predefined period to assess disease onset. They may also be retrospective (historical cohorts), with groups identified on the basis of exposure sometime in the past and then followed from that time to the present to establish presence or absence of the outcome. The feasibility of retrospective cohorts depends on the availability of good-quality data from pre-existing files. The research costs associated with cohort study designs mean that such studies are less common than other approaches. Nevertheless, a substantial effort to develop large cohort studies in nutritional epidemiology has been made since the early 1980s. Cohort studies can assess multiple outcomes, whereas case–control studies are restricted to assessing one outcome, but may be able to assess many different exposures. If an absolute measure of the effect of the exposure on the outcome is required, the only design that is appropriate is a cohort study, as case–control studies cannot be used to estimate incidence.

For example, to ascertain the relationship between olive oil consumption and coronary heart disease, a case–control study would compare the previous consumption of olive oil between cases of myocardial infarction and healthy controls. A cohort study would start with a roster of healthy individuals whose baseline diet would be recorded. They would then be followed up over several years to compare the occurrence of new cases of myocardial infarction between those consuming different levels of olive oil as recorded when they were healthy at baseline.

Ecological studies

Epidemiological studies can be classified according to whether measurements of exposure and outcome are made on populations or individuals. Observational investigations in which the unit of observation and analysis is not the individual but a whole community or population are called ecological studies. In ecological studies, measures of exposure routinely collected and aggregated at the household, local, district, regional, national, or international level are compared with outcome measures aggregated at the same level. An example of an ecological study would be plotting the mortality rates for colon cancer in several countries against the average intakes of saturated fat in these same countries and calculating the correlation between the two variables.

Studies considering the individual (instead of the population) as the unit of observation are always preferable because in an individually based study it is possible to relate exposure and outcome measures more directly, preventing many flaws that are likely to invalidate the findings of ecological studies. One of these flaws is known as the "ecological fallacy" and it is the bias resulting because an association observed between variables on an aggregated level does not necessarily represent the association that exists at an individual level. A major advantage of individually based studies over aggregated studies is that they allow the direct estimation of the risk of disease in relation to exposure.

Ecological studies measure diet less accurately because they use the average population intake as the exposure value for all individuals in the groups that are compared, leading to a high potential for biased ascertainment of diet–disease associations. Ecological studies, also termed correlation studies, may compare indicators of diet and health or disease within a single population over time to look for secular trends, or to compare the disease incidence rates and dietary intake patterns of migrant groups with those of comparable populations in the original and new country. Ecological comparisons have been important in hypothesizing diet and disease associations. Nevertheless, they are not able to establish causal relationships.

Definition of outcomes and end-points

Epidemiological outcomes must be clearly defined at the outset of a study. For example, a study of diet and CVD may specify that the outcome (CVD) is verified by specific clinical tests such as cardiac enzyme level or electrocardiographic changes. Taking the word of the patient or the doctor is not sufficient. Two main measures of the frequency for an outcome are used in epidemiology: prevalence and incidence.

Prevalence

The prevalence of an outcome is the proportion of subjects in a population who have that outcome at a given point in time. The numerator of prevalence is the number of existing cases and the denominator is the whole population:

$$\text{Prevalence} = \frac{\text{Existing cases}}{\text{Total population}}$$

Incidence

The incidence of an outcome is the proportion of new cases that occur in a population during a period of observation. The numerator of incidence is the number of new cases developing during the follow-up period, while the denominator is the total population at risk at the beginning of the follow-up time:

$$\text{Incidence} = \frac{\text{New cases}}{\text{Population inititally at risk}}$$

When calculated in this fashion, incidence is a proportion. However, incidence can also be expressed as a rate (velocity or density), when the time during which each person is observed (i.e., person-time of observation) is included in the denominator. Then it is called incidence rate or incidence density and it is expressed as the number of new cases per person-time of observation.

Other epidemiological methods

Epidemiological studies have also been conducted to assess: consumer attitudes to and beliefs about food, nutrition, physical activity patterns, and health to provide policy-makers, researchers and the food industry with data to promote health messages concerning the relation between food or nutrient intake and chronic diseases. These surveys seek information about influences on food choice, health determinants, criteria about perceptions of healthy eating, regular sources of nutritional information, expected benefits and barriers to healthy diet implementation, in order to identify consumers' knowledge, attitudes, and beliefs concerning food and health interactions and to promote more focused nutrition education messages.

Meta-analysis and pooled analysis

The role of meta-analysis for systematically combining the results of published randomized trials has become routine, but its place in observational epidemiology has been controversial despite widespread use in social sciences. Some have argued that the combining of data from randomized trials is appropriate because statistical power is increased without concern for validity since the comparison groups have been randomized, but that in observational epidemiology the issue of validity is determined largely by confounding and bias rather than limitations of statistical power. Thus, the greater statistical precision obtained

by the combination of data may be misleading because the findings may still be invalid. An alternative to combining published epidemiological data is to pool and analyze the primary data from all available studies on a topic that meets specified criteria. Ideally, this should involve the active collaboration of the original investigators, who are fully familiar with the data and its limitations. This kind of study conducted with a combination of the original data from several studies, is the basis of pooled analysis or pooling projects. In a pooled analysis, the range of dietary factors that can be addressed may be considerably greater than in the separate analyses because any one study will have few subjects in the extremes of intake and, sometimes, the studies will vary in distribution of dietary factors. The advantages of pooled analyses in nutritional epidemiology are so substantial that they are becoming common practice for important issues, such as alcoholic intake and breast cancer, body size and breast cancer, or alcohol beverages and coronary heart disease.

Analysis of epidemiological data requires careful consideration of the criteria for acceptable data quality, but also of the presentation of categorized or continuous independent variables and the application of empirical scores. The study of subgroup analysis and interactions and error correction are other issues of interest. Other limitations are the requirement of sample to be considered as representative, compliance, inaccuracies of information in retrospective studies, and confounding effects by factors that are simultaneously associated with both the exposure and the outcome.

13.7 Perspectives on the future

Future nutrition research will develop new methods for studying those processes whereby cells, tissues and the whole body obtain and utilize substances contained in the diet to maintain their structure and function in a healthy manner. Particular emphasis will be paid to molecular and cellular based strategies devised to understand better the genetic basis of nutritional outcomes.

It can also be anticipated that many ongoing large cohort studies with tens of thousands of participants will provide valuable information on the role of nutrition in disease prevention, and also on nutritional management of a large number of diseases by dietary means, and gene–nutrient and gene–environment interactions. Moreover, pooling of data from several cohort studies may provide a very powerful tool to assess the benefits of a healthy diet. An increasing interest in a dietary pattern approach instead of a single nutrient approach will be seen in nutritional epidemiology in the forthcoming decades. In addition, large primary prevention trials using the approach of assessing the effect of an overall dietary pattern (Estruch *et al.*, 2006; Howard *et al.*, 2006) are growing nowadays and their results will be on the rise during the next decade (Martinez-Gonzalez, 2004).

Nutritional epidemiology will also adopt a wider, multidisciplinary approach, with more studies concerning the impact of factors affecting social determinants of eating patterns, food supplies, and nutrient utilization on health to facilitate the decisions of policy-makers, food industry managers, investigators, and consumers.

References

Abete I, Parra MD, Zulet MD, Martinez JA. Different dietary strategies of weight loss in obesity: role of energy and macronutrient content. *Nutr Res Rev* 2006; **19**: 5–12.

Campión J, Milagro FI, Martinez JA. Genetic manipulation in nutrition, metabolism, and obesity research. *Nutr Rev* 2004; **62**(8): 321–330. Review.

Chang CK, Snook JT. The cholesterolaemic effects of dietary fats in cholesteryl ester transfer protein transgenic mice. *British Journal of Nutrition* 2001; **85**: 643–648.

Estruch R, Martínez-González MA, Corella D, Salas-Salvadó J, Ruiz-Gutiérrez V, Covas MI, Fiol M, *et al.* Effects of a mediterranean-style diet on cardiovascular risk factors: a randomized trial. *Annals of Internal Medicine* 2006; **145**: 1–11.

Howard BV, Van Horn L, Hsia J, Manson JE, Stefanick ML, Wassertheil-Smoller S, Kuller LH, *et al.* Low-fat dietary pattern and risk of cardiovascular disease. *JAMA* 2006; 295: 655–666.

Katz MH. *Multivariable Analysis: a Practical Guide for Clinicians*, 2nd edn. Cambridge University Press, Cambridge: 2006.

Lorgeril de M, Salen P, Martin JL, Monjaud I, Delaye J, Mamelle N. Mediterranean diet, traditional risk factors, and the rate of cardiovascular complications after myocardial infarction: final report of the Lyon Diet Heart Study. *Circulation* 1999; **99**: 779–785.

Martínez-González MA, Estruch R. Mediterranean diet, antioxidants, and cancer: the need for randomised trials. *European Journal of Cancer Prevention* 2004; **13**: 327–335.

Schone F, Leiterer M, Hartung H, Jahreis G, Tischendorf F. Rapeseed glucosinolates and iodine in sows affect the milk iodine concentration and the iodine status of piglets. *British Journal of Nutrition* 2001; **85**: 659–670.

Von Elm M, Egger M. The scandal of poor epidemiological research. *BMJ* 2004; **329**: 868–869.

Further reading

Altman DG. *Practical Statistics for Medical Research.* Chapman & Hall, London, 1991.

Armitage P, Colton T. *Encyclopaedia of Biostatistics*, 2nd ed. John Wiley and Sons, New York: 2007.

Breslow NE. *Statistics. Epidemiologic Reviews* 2000; **22**: 126–130.

Corthésy-Theulaz I, den Dunnen, JT, Ferre P, Geurts JMW, Müller M, van Belzen, N, van Ommen B. Nutrigenomics: the impact of biomics technology on nutrition research. *Annals of Nutrition & Metabolism* 2005; **49**: 355–365.

Fernandez-Jarne J, Martínez E, Prado M, *et al.* Risk of non-fatal myocardial infarction negatively associated with olive oil consumption: a case-control study in Spain. *International Journal of Epidemiology* 2002; **31**: 474–480.

Kumanyika SK. Epidemiology of what to eat in the 21st century. *Epidemiology Reviews* 2000; 22: 87–94.

Kussmann M, Raymond F, Affolter M. OMICS – driven biomarker discovery in nutrition and health. *Journal of Biotechnology* 2006; **124**: 758–787.

Leedy PD. *Practical Research: Planning and Designs*, Vol. 2. Macmillan, New York, 1980.

Moreno-Aliaga MJ, Marti A, García-Foncillas J, Martínez JA. DNA hybridization arrays: a powerful technology for nutritional and obesity research. *British Journal of Nutrition* 2001; **86**: 119–122.

Scheweigert FJ. Nutritional proteomics: methods and concepts for research in nutritional science. *Annals of Nutrition & Metabolism* 2007; **51**: 99–107.

Willett W. *Nutritional Epidemiology.* Oxford University Press, London, 1998.

14
Food Safety: A Public Health Issue of Growing Importance

Alan Reilly, Christina Tlustos, Judith O'Connor, and Lisa O'Connor

Key messages

After reading this chapter the student should have an understanding of:
- the reasons for increased concern about the safety of food
- chronic effects of food-borne illness
- vulnerable groups
- economic consequences of food-borne illness
- emerging food-borne pathogens

- types and sources of bacterial contamination in foods
- bacteria
- food-borne viruses
- parasites
- transmissible spongiform encephalopathies and food
- chemical contamination and food
- food safety control programs.

14.1 Introduction

In recent years the reported incidence of food-borne diseases has continued to increase worldwide, with a number of extremely serious outbreaks occurring on virtually every continent (Kaferstein, 2003). In addition, various high-profile food safety issues, including bovine spongiform encephalopathy (BSE), dioxins, acrylamide, *Escherichia coli* O157 and Sudan Red 1 have presented themselves to consumers, industry and regulators alike.

In a nutritional context, food-borne illness is often associated with malnutrition. In recent times food safety issues have been perceived by the public and governments as posing a greater potential risk to consumer health than nutritional aspects of the diet. To convey positive public health nutritional messages, nutritionists must understand the scientific basis of "food scares" that affect attitudes to food, nutrition, and health. This chapter aims to highlight the reasons for concern about the safety of food, the types and sources of biological and chemical contaminants in foods, and possible control and prevention strategies.

14.2 Factors contributing to food safety concerns

Although it is difficult to determine the global incidence of food-borne disease, the World Health Organization (WHO) estimates that in 2005 alone, 1.8 million people died from diarrheal diseases, and in industrialized countries around 30% of the population is estimated to suffer from food-borne diseases each year (WHO, 2007). In the USA, for example, an estimated 76 million cases of food-borne diseases, resulting in 325 000 hospitalizations and 5000 deaths occur each year (Mead *et al.*, 1999).

Changing food supply system

The increasing incidence of food-borne diseases is due to a number of factors, including changes in food production on the farm, new systems of food processing, longer distribution chains, and new food preparation and storage methods. Changing lifestyles have led to a far greater reliance on convenience foods that are prepared outside the home, and which may have a longer preparation to consumption time. In addition, the food chain has become longer and more complex, giving increased opportunities for food contamination. International trade in foods has expanded dramatically, and today the Food and Agriculture Organization of the United Nations (FAO) estimates over 500 million tonnes of food, valued around US$400–500 billion, move in international trade annually. Globalization of the food trade presents a major challenge to food safety control authorities, in that food can become contaminated in one country and cause outbreaks of food-borne illness in another. It is not unusual for an average meal to contain ingredients from many countries that have been produced and processed under different standards of food safety.

Chronic effects of food-borne illness

Food-borne diseases are classified as either infections or intoxications. Food-borne infections are caused when viable microorganisms are ingested and these can then multiply in the human body. Intoxications are caused when microbial or naturally occurring toxins are consumed in contaminated foods. Illnesses that relate to the consumption of foods that are contaminated with chemical toxins or microorganisms are collectively referred to as food poisoning.

The health consequences of food-borne illness are varied and depend on such factors as the individual's susceptibility, the virulence of the pathogen, and the type of disease. Symptoms are often mild and self-limiting in healthy individuals and people recover within a few days from acute health effects. Acute symptoms include diarrhea, stomach pain and cramps, vomiting, fever, and jaundice. However, in some cases microorganisms or their products are directly or indirectly associated with long-term health effects such as reactive arthritis and rheumatoid syndromes, endocarditis, Reiter syndrome, Guillain–Barré syndrome, renal disease, cardiac and neurological disorders, and nutritional and other malabsorptive disorders. It is generally accepted that chronic, secondary after-effect illnesses may occur in 2–3% of cases of food-borne infections and that the long-term consequences to human health may be greater than the acute disease. In one salmonellosis outbreak, associated with drinking contaminated milk, about 2% of patients developed reactive arthritis. It is estimated that up to 10% of patients with hemorrhagic colitis develop hemolytic uremic syndrome (HUS), a life-threatening complication of *Escherichia coli* O157:H7 infection characterized by acute renal failure, hemolytic anemia, and thrombocytopenia.

Vulnerable groups

Vulnerable groups tend to be more susceptible to food-borne infections and generally suffer more severe illness because their immune systems are in some way impaired. The immune system of infants and young children is immature. In pregnant women, increased levels of progesterone lead to the downregulation of cell-mediated immunity, increasing the susceptibility of both mother and fetus to infection by intracellular pathogens (Smith, 1999). In older people, a general decline in the body's immune response occurs with age, as does a decrease in stomach acid production. Immune responses in older people are also adversely affected if that person is malnourished through poor diet. Furthermore, age-related loss of sensory abilities, such as sight and taste, can lead to difficulties in choosing and preparing food. An aging population is one factor influencing the increase in the prevalence of food-borne disease. In 1999, 20% of Europe's population was older than 60 years of age, but this is predicted to rise to 35% by 2050 (Kaferstein, 2003). Other groups in which the immune system may be suppressed, making them more susceptible to food-borne infection, include cancer patients, transplant patients receiving immunosuppressant drugs, and patients with acquired immunodeficiency syndrome (AIDS). In nonindustrialized countries, political unrest, war, and famine lead to increased malnutrition and can expose poorer populations to increased risk of food-borne disease.

Improved surveillance

Improved surveillance systems lead to an increase in the reported incidence of food-borne disease. Using information technology, many countries have developed enhanced surveillance systems to gain a better picture of the true incidence of food-borne disease. International outbreaks are more readily detectable with the use of electronic databases for sharing molecular typing data (such as PulseNet in the USA and EnterNet in Europe) and rapid alert systems, websites, or list servers. However, even with this enhanced surveillance, it is unlikely that statistics reflect the true incidence of food-borne disease worldwide.

Economic consequences of food-borne illness

As well as morbidity and mortality associated with food-borne diseases, there are direct economic costs incurred, including the cost of medical treatment and industry losses. WHO estimates that in the USA diseases caused by the major food-borne pathogens have an annual cost of up to US$35 billion. The annual cost for illness due to E. coli O157 infections in the USA has been estimated at US$405 million, which includes costs for medical care (US$30 million), lost productivity (US$5 million) and premature deaths (US$370 million); however, this estimate does not include costs due to pain and suffering, and expenditure on outbreak investigations (Frenzen *et al.*, 2005). The cost of salmonellosis in England and Wales in 1992 was estimated at between US$560 million and US$800 million. Over 70% of costs were directly associated with treatment and investigation of cases, and costs to the economy of sickness related to absence from work. In 2006, Cadbury Schweppes, the world's largest confectionary company, were forced to recall seven Cadbury-branded products in the UK and two in Ireland due to *Salmonella* contamination. The estimated cost of the product recall was £30 million, including a £5 million marketing campaign to rebuild consumer confidence. In addition, Cadbury Ltd in the UK was fined £1 million and ordered to pay costs totaling £152 000 for distributing the contaminated chocolate products which led to illness in 42 people being reported, three of whom were hospitalized (Cadbury press release, 2007).

Bearing these figures in mind, the true estimates of food-borne disease and the likely economic costs are unknown. In industrialized countries only a small proportion of cases of food-borne diseases is reported, and even fewer are investigated. Very few non-industrialized countries have established food-borne disease reporting systems, and in those that have, only a small fraction of cases is reported.

Emerging food safety issues

The emergence of new food-borne pathogens is one factor leading to increased concern about food safety. During the twentieth century improvements in sewage treatment, milk pasteurization, and water treatments, and better controls on animal disease have led to the control of food-borne and water-borne diseases such as typhoid, tuberculosis, and brucellosis. However, new food-borne pathogens have emerged. Food-borne organisms such as E. coli O157, *Campylobacter jejuni*, and *Salmonella* Enteritidis phage type 4 were virtually unknown in the 1970s, but have come to prominence as virulent pathogens associated with foods of animal origin. *Cyclospora cayetanensis* emerged as a food-borne pathogen in 1995, when it was associated with outbreaks of illness traced to raspberries imported into the USA from Guatemala. *Cryptosporidium parvum* emerged as a pathogen of worldwide significance during the 1990s and has been linked to contaminated drinking water and to a range of foods including salads, unpasteurized milk, and apple juice. Some known pathogens such as *Listeria. monocytogenes* have only recently been shown to be predominantly food-borne and, since they can grow at refrigeration temperatures, have increased in importance with the expansion of the cold chain for food distribution. *Enterobacter sakazakii* has recently been implicated in outbreaks of infection associated with powdered infant formula. Many of these emerging pathogens are of animal origin and do not usually cause serious illness in the animal host.

Another concern is that a proportion of food-borne illness is caused by pathogens that have not yet been identified, and therefore cannot be diagnosed. In the USA, it is estimated that unknown food-borne agents caused 65% of the estimated 5200 annual deaths from food-borne disease (Mead, 1999; Frenzen, 2004). This is of concern since many of today's commonly recognized food-borne pathogens were not recognized as causes of food-borne illness 30 years ago. In this regard, *Mycobacterium avium* subspecies *paratuberculosis* (Map) is an organism of potential concern. Map is the causative agent of Johne's disease in cattle, but it has been proposed that Map is also the causative agent of Crohn's disease in humans, and that it may be transmitted via milk (including pasteurized milk) and possibly other foods.

During the 1980s and 1990s, antibiotic-resistant food-borne pathogens emerged that are associated with the inappropriate use of antibiotics in animal husbandry. For example, *Salmonella typhimurium* DT 104 routinely shows resistance to five different antibiotics. Strains of *Salmonella* and *Campylobacter* are showing resistance to fluoroquinolones since these compounds were introduced for use in animals.

In recent years a new range of foods has been implicated with food-borne disease. For instance, the internal contents of an egg were always presumed to be safe to eat raw, and uncooked eggs have been traditionally used in many different food products. This situation has changed with the emergence of *S. Enteritidis* infection in egg-laying flocks, resulting in contamination in shell eggs and a major increase in food-borne illness worldwide associated with uncooked eggs. Animal products are no longer the only focus for food safety controls, as fresh produce is emerging as an important vehicle for food-borne disease (McCabe-Sellers and Beattie, 2004). Between 1990 and 2003, 12% of food-borne outbreaks in the USA were linked to produce and produce dishes; the most common produce foods being salads and alfalfa sprouts. Of the produce-associated outbreaks, 40% were due to norovirus or hepatitis A, and 30% were caused by bacteria commonly associated with an animal reservoir, such as *Campylobacter*, *E. coli* O157 and *Salmonella* (Dewaal *et al.*, 2006).

Finally, chemical risks to food, such as pesticide residues, acrylamide, and the use of food additives, continue to concern consumers.

14.3 Food-borne bacteria

The major cause of food-borne diseases is the consumption of microbiologically contaminated foods. There are many types of food-borne pathogens, including bacteria, viruses, and parasites. The characteristics of food-borne bacterial intoxications and infections are summarized in Tables 14.1 and 14.2, respectively. Food-borne pathogens are covered in more detail by Doyle *et al.* (2001).

14.4 Food-borne viruses

It is only in recent years that the role of viruses as etiological agents of food-borne illness have emerged. Difficulties in attributing viral illness to food have mainly been due to the diagnostic difficulties in detecting viruses in an implicated food and under-reporting owing to the mild nature of illness in many cases. A report from the US Centers for Disease Control (CDC) in 2000, on surveillance of food-borne disease outbreaks from 1993 to 1997, revealed

that viruses accounted for 6% of all food-borne outbreaks and 8% of cases. Hepatitis A accounted for the majority of these, followed by norovirus. Data published by the European Food Safety Authority (EFSA) revealed that viruses accounted for 10.2% of all food-borne outbreaks reported during 2006. Caliciviruses (including norovirus) accounted for the majority (61.7%) of these food-borne viral outbreaks.

Food-borne viruses are generally enteric, being transmitted by the fecal–oral route. However, transmission by person-to-person contact and via contaminated water is common. Hepatitis A and norovirus are more commonly transmitted via foods than other food-borne viruses. The most important food-borne viruses are hepatitis A, norovirus, astrovirus, and rotavirus. These are discussed in detail below.

Hepatitis A virus

Hepatitis A is one of the more severe food-borne diseases. The illness results from immune destruction of infected liver cells, and a few weeks of debility are common (Table 14.3). It is a member of the picornaviruses.

Infections are more likely to be asymptomatic or mild in young children than in adolescents or adults. The virus can be shed in feces for up to 14 days before the onset of illness. It is therefore possible for an infected food handler with poor personal hygiene (hand-washing, in particular) to contaminate food during this period. The virus may be shed in the feces for 1–2 weeks after onset of symptoms.

Food becomes contaminated with this virus via infected persons or via fecally contaminated water, as is usual with shellfish. Examples of other foods implicated in hepatitis A outbreaks are oysters, raw mussels, drinking water, bakery products and caviar. Hepatitis A has been shown to be more heat resistant than most enteric viruses and is also quite resistant to drying. The virus is susceptible to chlorination treatment, however, and water-borne hepatitis A outbreaks have been linked to untreated water.

Noroviruses

Norovirus was the first enteric virus reported to be food-borne. It was formerly known as Norwalk-like virus (NLV) or small round structured virus (SRSV) and has recently been classified as a member of the calicivirus family. Noroviruses are difficult to detect, especially from foods.

Table 14.1 Characteristics of food-borne bacterial intoxications

Bacteria	Comment	Food-borne illness (a) Onset (b) Duration	Food-borne illness (a) Symptoms (b) Infectious dose	(a) Min. temp (b) Opt. temp (c) Min. pH[a] (d) Min. A_w[b]	Forms spores	Heat resistance	(a) Gram stain (b) Aerobic/anaerobic	(a) Source (b) Associated foods[b]
Bacillus cereus (Emetic)	Vegetative cells are inactivated by normal cooking temperatures; however, spores are quite heat resistant. Emetic illness is caused by consumption of heat-stable emetic toxin produced by cells growing to high numbers in food. This is most likely to happen when cooked foods are not served while hot or not cooled rapidly	(a) 1–5 h (b) 6–24 h	(a) Nausea and vomiting (b) >10^5 cells (12–32 µg toxin/kg)	(a) 10°C (b) 30–35°C (c) 4.3 (d) 0.95	Yes	Heat-sensitive, but can form heat-resistant spores (D_{121} = 0.03–2.35 min) Emetic toxin: extremely heat resistant (can withstand 121°C for 90 min)	(a) Gram positive (b) Facultative anaerobe	(a) Soil, dust and vegetation (b) Cooked rice, cereals and cereal-based products, herbs and spices
Clostridium botulinum Group I (proteolytic) Group II (nonproteolytic)	Food-borne botulism is caused when food becomes contaminated with spores from the environment, which are not destroyed by initial cooking or processing. If the food is packaged anaerobically and provides a suitable environment for growth, spores will germinate, leading to toxin production. The toxin is heat sensitive, so further heat treatment of the food would prevent illness. The so called "botulinum cook" (heat treatment to 121°C for 3 min or equivalent) is used for low acid canned food products to destroy these spores	(a) 12–36 h, but may be as long as 8 days (b) Variable (from days to months)	(a) Blurred and/or double vision, dryness of the mouth followed by difficulties swallowing and finally breathing. Vomiting and mild diarrhea may occur in the early stages (b) 0.005–0.5 µg toxin	Group I (a) 10°C (b) 30–40°C (c) 4.6 (d) 0.94 Group II (a) 3.3°C (b) 25–37°C (c) 5.0 (d) 0.97	Yes	Toxin: destroyed by 5 min at 85°C Group I Spores: D_{100} = 25 min D_{121} = <0.001 min 0.1–0.2 min Group II Spores: D_{100} < 0.1 min D_{121} = <0.001 min	(a) Gram positive (b) Obligate anaerobe	(a) Soil, sediment, intestinal tract of fish and mammals (b) Canned foods, smoked and salted fish, honey

| Staphylococcus aureus | Food handlers play a major role in transmission. S. aureus is carried in nose/throat of ~40% of healthy individuals and can be easily transferred to food via the hands. Most implicated foods have been ready-to-eat foods that have been contaminated by poor handling practices and stored at incorrect temperatures, allowing S. aureus to grow to levels (>10⁵ cells/g) that will produce sufficient heat-stable staphylococcal toxin | (a) 1–6 h
(b) 1–2 days | (a) Nausea, vomiting, abdominal pain and diarrhea
(b) <1.0 μg toxin (>10^5 cells/g) needed to produce sufficient toxin) | (a) 7°C
(b) 35–37°C
(c) 4.5
(d) 0.83 | No | Toxin: heat resistant (able to withstand boiling for up to 30 min) | (a) Gram positive
(b) Facultative anaerobe | (a) Exposed skin lesions, nose, throat and hands
(b) Generally foods of animal origin that have been physically handled and have not received a subsequent bactericidal treatment |

[a] Under otherwise optimal conditions; limits will vary according to strain, temperature, type of acid (in the case of pH), solute (in the case of A_w), and other factors.

[b] Not an exhaustive list.

Min., minimum; Opt., optimal; A_w, water activity.

Table 14.2 Characteristics of food-borne bacterial infections

Bacteria	Comment	Food-borne illness		(a) Min. temp (b) Opt. temp (c) Min. pH[a] (d) Min. A$_w$[b]	Heat resistance	(a) Gram stain (b) Aerobic/ anaerobic	(a) Source (b) Associated foods[b]
		(a) Onset (b) Duration	(a) Symptoms (b) Infectious dose				
Bacillus cereus (diarrheal)	Vegetative cells are inactivated by normal cooking temperatures; however, spores are quite heat resistant. The diarrheal enterotoxin is produced when spores germinate in the small intestine after consumption of contaminated food	(a) 8–16 h (b) 12–14 h	(a) Abdominal pain and diarrhea (b) >10^5 cells	(a) 10°C (b) 30–35°C (c) 4.3 (d) 0.95	Heat-sensitive, but forms heat-resistant spores (D$_{121}$ = 0.03–2.35 min)	(a) Gram positive (b) Facultative anaerobe	(a) Soil and dust (b) Meat, milk, vegetables, fish and soups
Clostridium perfringens	Illness results from consumption of food containing high numbers of cells (>10^6/g) followed by enterotoxin production in the large intestine. When contaminated food is cooked, sporulation is induced. As the food cools, the spores germinate and vegetative cells continue to multiply, unless the food is cooled quickly and stored under refrigerated conditions	(a) 12–18 h (can be 8–22 h) (b) 24 h	(a) Diarrhea and severe abdominal pain (b) >10^6 cells/g	(a) 15°C (b) 43–45°C (c) 5.0 (d) 0.95	Heat-sensitive, but forms heat-resistant spores (D$_{95}$ = 1.3–2.8 min)	(a) Gram positive (b) Obligate anaerobe	(a) Soil and animal feces (b) Meat, poultry, gravy, dried and precooked foods

Organism	Description	Incubation	Symptoms / Infective dose	Growth parameters	Heat	Characteristics	Sources
Campylobacter	*C. jejuni* is one of the most common causes of bacterial food poisoning in many industrialized countries. Although campylobacters are fragile organisms, and do not survive or multiply very well on foods, the low infectious dose means that a small level of contamination may result in illness. Compared with other food-borne bacteria with low infectious doses, relatively few outbreaks have been identified	(a) 2–5 days (b) 1–7 days	(a) Moderate to severe diarrhea, sometimes bloody diarrhea. Severe abdominal pain. Vomiting is rare. Complications are uncommon, but include bacteremia, reactive arthritis and Guillain–Barré syndrome (b) 500 cells	(a) 32°C (b) 42–43°C (c) 4.9 (d) 0.98	Heat-sensitive	(a) Gram negative (b) Fastidious microaerophile	(a) Chickens, birds, cattle, flies, and water (b) Undercooked chicken, raw milk, beef, pork, lamb, shellfish, and water
Verotoxigenic *Escherichia coli* (VTEC)	VTEC is of considerable concern due to the severity of illness. The organism is easily killed by cooking, but the low infective dose means that foods must be cooked thoroughly and protected from cross-contamination	(a) 1–6 days (b) 4–6 days	(a) Diarrhea and severe abdominal cramps, bloody diarrhea (hemorrhagic colitis), approx. 5% (mostly children) develop hemolytic uremic syndrome (HUS) (b) 10–100 cells	(a) 7°C (b) 37°C (c) 4.5 (d) 0.97	Heat-sensitive	(a) Gram negative (b) Facultative anaerobe	(a) Cattle, sheep, pigs, deer (b) Undercooked beef burgers, raw milk, salad vegetables, and unpasteurized apple juice
Listeria monocytogenes	*L. monocytogenes* causes serious illness in individuals with impaired cell-mediated immunity. Highly susceptible individuals include pregnant women, neonates, older people and immunocompromised individuals. The organism is also reported to cause febrile gastroenteritis (FG) in healthy persons. Foods associated with transmission tend to be processed, ready-to-eat foods, with long shelf-lives (>5 days) stored at refrigeration temperatures	(a) Up to 10 weeks (FG: 20–27 h) (b) Days to weeks (FG: self-limiting, usually 1–3 days)	(a) Flu-like symptoms, meningitis and/or septicemia. While pregnant women may experience a mild flu-like illness, infection may result in miscarriage, stillbirth or birth of a severely ill infant. (FG: fever, watery diarrhea, nausea, headache and pains in joints and muscles) (b) Unknown	(a) 0°C (b) 30–37°C (c) 4.3 (d) 0.90	Heat-sensitive	(a) Gram positive (b) Facultative anaerobe	(a) Soil, improperly made silage (b) Fresh soft cheeses, raw milk, deli meats, pâté, hot dogs, raw vegetables, ice cream, and seafood

Table 14.2 *Continued*

Bacteria	Comment	Food-borne illness (a) Onset (b) Duration	(a) Symptoms (b) Infectious dose	(a) Min. temp (b) Opt. temp (c) Min. pH[a] (d) Min. A_w[b]	Heat resistance	(a) Gram stain (b) Aerobic/anaerobic	(a) Source (b) Associated foods[b]
Salmonella	Although there are approx. 2400 different *Salmonella* serotypes only a small number account for most human infections, with S. Typhimurium and S. Enteritidis predominating. Undercooked food from infected food animals is most commonly implicated. Egg-associated salmonellosis is an important public health problem	(a) Usually 12–36 h, but may be 6–72 h (b) 2–5 days	(a) Fever, abdominal pain, diarrhea, nausea and sometimes vomiting. Can be fatal in older people or those with weakened immune system (b) ~10^6 cells	(a) 7°C (b) 35–37°C (c) 4.0 (d) 0.93	Heat-sensitive	(a) Gram negative (b) Facultative anaerobe	(a) Water, soil, animal feces, raw poultry, raw meats, and raw seafood (b) Raw meats, poultry, eggs, raw milk and other dairy products, raw fruits and vegetables (e.g., alfalfa sprouts and melons)
Vibrio cholerae serogroup non-O1	*Vibrio cholerae* non-O1 is related to V. cholerae O1 (the organism that causes Asiatic or epidemic cholera), but causes a disease reported to be less severe than cholera. It has been generally believed that water was the main vehicle for transmission, but an increasing number of cases have been associated with food	(a) 1–3 days (b) Diarrhea lasts 6–7 days	(a) Diarrhea, abdominal cramps, fever, some vomiting, and nausea (b) >10^6 cells	(a) 10°C (b) 37°C (c) 5.0 (d) 0.97	Heat-sensitive	(a) Gram negative (b) Facultative anaerobe	(a) Costal waters, raw oysters (b) Shellfish
Vibrio parahaemolyticus	V. parahaemolyticus can be considered to be the leading cause of seafood-borne bacterial gastroenteritis. It is frequently isolated from fish from both marine and brackish-water environments	(a) 12–24 h (b) <7 days	(a) Diarrhea, abdominal cramps, nausea, vomiting, headache, fever, chills (b) >10^6 cells	(a) 5°C (b) 37°C (c) 4.8 (d) 0.94	Heat-sensitive	(a) Gram negative (b) Facultative anaerobe	(a) Costal and estuarine waters, raw shellfish (b) Fish and raw shellfish

Organism	Characteristics	Onset/duration	Symptoms/infective dose	Growth parameters	Heat	Gram/oxygen	Sources
Vibrio vulnificus	*V. vulnificus* is considered to be one of the most invasive and rapidly lethal of human pathogens. Infection starts with a gastrointestinal illness, and rapidly progresses to a septicemic condition. It is mostly associated with the consumption of raw oysters. Human infections are rare, but those at most risk either have underlying illnesses or are immunocompromised	(a) 16 h (b) Days to weeks	(a) Wound infections, gastroenteritis, primarily septicemia (b) Unknown in healthy individuals but in predisposed <100 cells	(a) 8°C (b) 37°C (c) 5 (d) 0.96	Heat-sensitive	(a) Gram negative (b) Facultative anaerobe	(a) Coastal waters, sediment, plankton, shellfish (b) Oysters, clams, crabs
Yersinia enterocolitica	*Y. enterocolitica* is psychrotrophic and known to be quite resistant to freezing, surviving in frozen food for extended periods. The organism is present in a wide range of animals, especially pigs. Milk and pork have been implicated in outbreaks, especially in countries where pork is eaten raw or undercooked	(a) 3–7 days (b) 1–3 weeks	(a) Diarrhea, abdominal pain and fever. Intestinal pain, especially in young adults, may be confused with appendicitis (b) Unknown	(a) −1.3°C (b) 25–37°C (c) 4.1 (d) 0.96	Heat-sensitive	(a) Gram negative (b) Facultative anaerobe	(a) Wide range of animals (e.g., pigs, dogs, cats) and water (b) Undercooked pork, raw milk and water

[a] Under otherwise optimal conditions; limits will vary according to strain, temperature, type of acid (in the case of pH), solute (in the case of A_w) and other factors.
[b] Not an exhaustive list.
Heat-sensitive: cells destroyed by typical cooking temperatures; Min.: minimum; Opt.: optimal; A_w: water activity.

Table 14.3 Characteristics of the illnesses caused by hepatitis A and norovirus

	Hepatitis A (picornavirus)	Norovirus (calicivirus)
Properties	Particles are featureless spheres 28 nm in diameter, single-stranded RNA coated with protein	Particles are spheres 25–35 nm in diameter, single-stranded RNA coated with protein that has characteristic cupped surface depressions
Infection	Infection via intestine to liver, incubation period 15–20 days (mean 28 days)	Infection of intestinal lining, incubation period 24–48 h
Illness	Illness from immune destruction of infected liver cells: fever, malaise, anorexia, nausea, abdominal discomfort, often followed by jaundice; severity tends to increase with age: ranges from unapparent infection to weeks of debility, occasionally with permanent sequelae	Nausea, vomiting, diarrhea, etc., lasting for 24–48 h
Shedding	Shedding of virus peaks during the second half of the incubation period (10–14 days), usually ends by 7 days after onset of jaundice	During illness (in vomitus and feces), possibly 7 days after onset
Diagnosis	Based on detection of IgM class antibody. Hepatitis A virus in the patient's blood serum (kits available)	Detection of virus in stool ELISA or PCR or of antibody against the virus in patient's blood serum; no standard methods, reagents not readily available for most agents
Immunity	Immunity is durable (possibly lifelong) after infection	Apparently transient

ELISA, enzyme-linked immunosorbent assay; IgM, immunoglobulin M; PCR, polymerase chain reaction.

Exposure is by contact with infected individuals or fecally contaminated water or other materials. Shellfish (bivalve molluscs) have been the predominant food vehicle. Shellfish beds may frequently become contaminated with human feces from sewage discharges. Aerosolization of vomitus-containing virus particles has been proposed as another mode of transmission of the virus and may also be a source of food contamination. Sensitive detection assays have now revealed that shedding of the virus in feces may continue for up to a week after the illness subsides.

Astroviruses

Under the electron microscope, astroviruses appear as small, round viruses that have surface projections resembling a five- or six-pointed star (Greek *astron*, star). The illness differs from the norovirus in that the incubation period is longer (3–4 days), the duration of illness is longer (often lasting for 7–14 days), and vomiting is less common, with diarrhea being the predominant symptom. In addition, the very young (<1 year) appear to be the most susceptible group, whereas norovirus affects all age groups. Astrovirus outbreaks have been reported to occur in crèches, schools, hospital wards, and nursing homes, but in many cases there was no well-defined mode of transmission. One large outbreak linked to contaminated food from a common supplier occurred in Osaka, Japan, in 1991, affecting 4700 teachers and pupils from 14 schools in the city.

Rotaviruses

Serogroup A rotaviruses are the single most important cause of infantile gastroenteritis worldwide, affecting an estimated 130 million infants and causing 873 000 deaths every year. The rotavirus genome consists of 11 segments of double-stranded RNA surrounded by a double-shelled viral capsid. When examined by electron microscopy, the double-shelled particles resemble a wheel-like structure morphologically (Latin *rota*, wheel). The incubation period of the illness is 1–3 days, and the illness is characterized by fever, vomiting, and diarrhea. Although the majority of rotavirus infections involve infants, outbreaks of food-borne, and water-borne disease affecting all age groups have been reported, albeit infrequently.

Other viruses

Picornaviruses other than hepatitis A can also be transmitted by the food-borne route. Polioviruses are transmitted by food but virulent strains of this agent are now extremely rare. Coxsackie virus and echovirus have been associated with food-borne outbreaks, but data are limited. Hepatitis E has been linked to a number of water-borne outbreaks but there has been no association with food. One food-borne outbreak of parvovirus linked to consumption of cockles has been reported.

14.5 Food-borne parasites

Food-borne parasitic diseases are a major public health problem affecting millions of people, predominantly in nonindustrialized countries. The incidence of parasitic disease associated with the consumption of foods of animal origin has declined in industrialized countries in recent years, where improvements in animal husbandry and meat inspection have led to considerable safety and quality gains. The situation in nonindustrialized countries is very different, in that these diseases are associated with poor standards of sanitation and hygiene, low educational standards, and extreme poverty.

Parasites are organisms that live off other living organisms, known as hosts. They may be transmitted from animals to humans, from humans to humans, or from humans to animals. Food-borne parasitic disease occurs when the infective stages of parasites are eaten in raw or partially cooked protein foods, or in raw vegetables and fruits that are inadequately washed before consumption. These organisms then live and reproduce within the tissues and organs of infected human and animal hosts, and are often excreted in feces. The parasites involved in food-borne disease usually have complex life cycles involving one or two intermediate hosts (Figure 14.1). The food-borne parasites known to cause disease in humans are broadly classified as helminths (multicellular worms) and protozoa (single-celled microscopic organisms). These include the major helminthic groups of trematodes, nematodes, and cestodes, and some of the emerging protozoan pathogens, such as cryptosporidia and cyclospora. The illnesses they can cause range from mild discomfort to debilitating illness and possibly death.

These infections occur endemically in some 20 countries, where it is estimated that over 40 million people worldwide, mainly in eastern and southern Asia, are affected. Of major concern are the fish-borne trematode infections. The trematode species concerned all have similar life cycles involving two intermediate hosts. The definitive host is man and other mammals. Food-borne infection takes place through

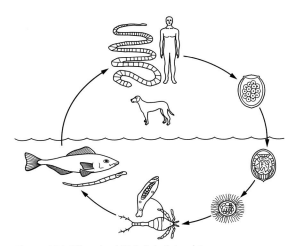

Figure 14.1 Life cycle of *Diphyllobothrium latum*.

the consumption of raw, undercooked, or otherwise underprocessed freshwater fish or crustaceans containing the infective stages (metacercariae) of these parasites. Table 14.4 summarizes the distribution, the principal reservoirs, and freshwater fish or crustaceans involved in the transmission of these parasites in the food chain. The most important parasites with respect to the numbers of people affected are species of the genera *Clonorchis*, *Opisthorchis*, and *Paragonimus*. The diseases caused by food-borne trematodes include cholangiocarcinoma, gallstones, severe liver disease, and gastrointestinal problems.

Nematodes

The food-borne roundworms of primary importance in humans belong to the phylum Nematoda and are known as nematodes. Undercooked or raw fishery products and pork meat are the usual foods involved.

Where fishery products are the food vector, the definitive hosts of roundworms causing disease in humans are piscivorous marine mammals such as seals. Marine invertebrates and fish are the two intermediate hosts and humans are infected when they consume raw or minimally processed products. Fish are the secondary hosts and are infected when they consume the invertebrate primary host or fish that are already infected. There are many species of nematodes and a very large number of species of fish, worldwide, that are known to act as intermediate hosts. The most common species of nematode causing disease in humans is *Anisakis simplex*, sometimes referred to as

Table 14.4 Food-borne trematode infections

Parasite	Distribution	Principal reservoirs (other than humans)	Food involved in transmission to humans	Disease
Liver flukes				
Clonorchis sinensis	Widespread in China, Taiwan, Macao, Japan, Korea and Vietnam. Migrants to other countries found to be infected; cases in Hawaii attributed to consumption of fish imported from China	Dogs, cats, and many other species of fish-eating mammals	Many species (c. 110) of freshwater fish, mainly Cyprinidae, e.g., carp, roach and dace, most important being Pseudorasbora parva. Metacercariae in fish muscles	The liver flukes, Opisthorchis viverrini, O. felineus and Clonorchis sinensis, are biologically similar, food-borne trematodes that chronically infect the bile ducts and, more rarely, the pancreatic duct and gallbladder of humans and other mammals
Opisthorchis felineus	Commonwealth of Independent States (CIS), eastern and central Europe	Cats, dogs, and other mammals that eat fish or fish waste	Freshwater fish of family Cyprinidae. Metacercariae in muscle and subcutaneous tissue	
Opisthorchis viverrini	Laos and north-eastern Thailand (Mekong River basin)	Dogs, cats, fishing cats (Felis viverrina), and other mammals that feed on fish and fish waste	Some 10 species of freshwater fish including Puntius orphoides and Hampala dispar Metacercariae in fish muscles	
Faciola hepatica	Europe, the Middle East, the Far East, Africa, Australia, USA	Sheep, cattle		Inflammation of the bile ducts which eventually leads to fibrosis
Intestinal flukes				
Heterophyes heterophyes	Mediterranean basin, especially Egypt and eastern Asia	Dogs, cats, jackals, foxes, pelicans, hawks, and black kite	Brackish water and freshwater fish, especially mullet (Mugil spp.), Tilapia, and others. In Japan, species of fish genera Acanthogobius and Glossogobius also involved. Metacercariae in muscle and skin	The parasite can irritate the lining of the small intestine, resulting in diarrhea and abdominal pain. In some instances the lining of the small intestine breaks down, and the eggs produced by the parasite enter the bloodstream. Once in the bloodstream the eggs can be carried to other organs where they can cause significant pathology, especially in the liver, heart, and brain
Metagonimus yokogawai and related species	Eastern and southern Asia	Dogs, cats, pigs, and fish-eating birds	Freshwater fish, e.g., sweetfish (Plecoglossus altivelis), dace (Tribolodon hakonensis), trout, and whitebait. Metacercariae in gills, fin, or tail	Similar to Heterophyes heterophyes

Nanophyetus spp.	Eastern Siberia (mountain tributaries of Amur River) and parts of Sakhalin peninsula, north-western USA	Dogs, cats, rats (?), and badgers	Salmonid and other fish. Metacercariae in muscles, fins, and kidneys	Nanophyetiasis Diarrhea, usually accompanied by increased numbers of circulating eosinophils, abdominal discomfort and nausea. Sometimes asymptomatic
Spelotrema brevicaeca	Philippines	Sea birds	Crustaceans, amphipods, isopods, and brachyures	
Haplorchis spp.	Eastern and southern Asia	Cats, dogs, and fish-eating birds	Fish, frogs, and toads. Metacercariae in muscle	Most infections are light and asymptomatic. Heavy infections show symptoms of diarrhea, abdominal pain, fever, ascites, anasarca, and intestinal obstruction
Fasciolopsis buski	Oriental countries	Pigs	Uncooked contaminated water plants such as water cress	
Lung fluke *Paragonimus westermani* and related species in Asia, Africa and the Americas	Siberia, west Africa (Nigeria, Cameroon), the Americas (Ecuador to USA), Japan, Korea, Thailand, Laos, China	Domestic and wild carnivora that feed on crustaceans	Freshwater and brackish water crabs (*Eriocheir, Potamon, Parathelphusa*), crayfish and shrimps. Metacercariae in muscles, gills, liver (hepatopancreas), and cardia region. Wild boar meat suspected as a source of infection	Paragonimiasis

Based on data from *Food Control*, **6**, Abdussalam *et al*., Food safety measures for the control of food-borne trematode infections, page 9, copyright 1995 with permission from Elsevier.

the herringworm. The other species involved in anisa-kiasis in North America, Europe, and Japan is *Pseudo-terranova decipiens* (the codworm or sealworm).

Nematodes are commonly present in fish caught in the wild, most frequently in the liver and belly cavity, but can also occur in the flesh. Anisakiasis is an uncommon disease because the parasite is killed by heating (55°C for 1 min), and by freezing (−20°C for 24 h). There is a risk of illness from fishery products consumed raw, for example sushi, or after only mild processing, such as salting at low concentrations or smoking. Many countries now require that fish used for these mildly processed products be frozen before processing or before sale.

Trichinella spiralis is the cause of trichinosis in humans. This most commonly results from the consumption of contaminated raw or undercooked pork or pork products. Since the mid-1980s outbreaks have been associated with raw and undercooked horse-meat. Isolated cases have been reported from the consumption of bear meat and ground beef in the USA. The incidence of trichinosis can be controlled by avoiding feeding infected waste foods to pigs or by fully cooking pig swill. Freezing pork products (−15°C for 20 days) or thorough cooking (78°C at the thermal center) before human consumption will destroy trichina larvae.

Cestodes

Cestodes are tapeworms and the species of major concern associated with consumption of fish is the fish tapeworm, *Diphyllobothrium latum*. Humans are one of the definitive hosts, along with other fish-eating mammals. Freshwater copepods and fish are the intermediate hosts. The plerocercoid is present in the flesh of the fish and infects humans following the consumption of raw or minimally processed fish. The recorded epidemiology of *D. latum* shows it to be prevalent in many countries worldwide. The incidence is relatively high in Scandinavia and the Baltic region of Europe. Diphyllobothriasis in humans can be prevented by cooking or freezing fish before consumption. Infections with tapeworms are also associated with eating undercooked or raw pork and beef.

Taenia saginata (the beef tapeworm) and *Taenia solium* (the pork tapeworm) are unique among parasites in that they have no vascular, respiratory, or digestive systems. Humans are their definitive hosts and they rely solely on the human body for all of their nourishment. Infections can be prevented by sanitary disposal and treatment of human waste and by thorough cooking and freezing of contaminated pork and beef.

Protozoa

The protozoal human parasites are unicellular organisms that colonize the intestinal epithelium and form cysts. These are excreted and may survive for long periods in the environment. There are five genera of concern in foods: *Giardia*, *Entamoeba*, *Toxoplasma*, *Cyclospora*, and *Cryptosporidium*.

Table 14.5 summarizes the distribution, principal reservoirs and route of transmission of these parasites in the food chain.

14.6 Transmissible spongiform encephalopathies and food

Transmissible spongiform encephalopathies (TSEs) are fatal degenerative brain diseases which include BSE in cattle; scrapie in sheep; kuru, Creutzfeldt–Jakob disease (CJD), and new variant CJD (vCJD) in humans. They are characterized by the appearance in the brain of vacuoles – clear holes that give the brain a sponge-like appearance – from which the conditions derive their name.

Several theories have been proposed to explain the nature of the agents that cause TSE. Prusiner was awarded the Nobel Prize in 1997 for the prion theory, which postulates that the agent is a proteinaceous infectious particle (PrP) that is capable of replication without the need of an agent-specific nucleic acid. The disease-associated prion (PrP^{Sc}) has been shown to have a different helical shape to normal cellular prion protein (PrP^{C}) found on neuronal cells and some other cells, for example lymphoid cells. However, while it is widely acknowledged that PrP^{Sc} is very closely associated with the causative agent, there is a reluctance by some to accept PrP^{Sc} as the sole agent responsible for transmission. Another hypothesis suggests the agent is an unconventional virus, while a third suggests that it is a virion that has similar properties to a virus but uses host proteins to coat its nucleic acid.

Bovine spongiform encephalopathy

BSE, sometimes referred to as "mad cow disease," was first identified in the UK in 1986. The disease is fatal

Table 14.5 Food-borne protozoa

Occurrence	Transmission	Definitive host	Incubation	Infective dose	Pathogenesis
Giardia intestinalis worldwide	Food-borne, water-borne, person–person	Humans, domestic, and wild animals	3–25 days	Low (~10 cysts)	Chronic diarrhea, malabsorption, weight loss
Entamoeba histolytica worldwide	Food-borne, water-borne, person–person (food handlers)	Humans	2–4 weeks	Very low (~1 cyst)	Amebiasis, abdominal pain, fever, diarrhea, ulceration of the colon (severe cases)
Toxoplasma gondii worldwide	Food-borne (raw or inadequately cooked infected meat), water-borne, fecal–oral (infected cats)	Humans, cats, several mammals	5–23 days	~1–30 cysts	Mostly asymptomatic. In severe cases: hepatitis, pneumonia, blindness, severe neurological disorders. Can also be transmitted transplacentally resulting in a spontaneous abortion, a stillborn, or mental/physical retardation
Cyclospora cayetanensis worldwide	Food-borne, water-borne	Humans	Several days to weeks	Not known, probably very low	Often asymptomatic. Abdominal cramps, vomiting, weight loss, diarrhea
Cryptosporidium parvum worldwide	Food-borne, water-borne, animal–person, fecal–oral	Humans, domestic, and wild animals	Difficult to define, in most cases 3–7 days, occasionally longer	Very low (~1 cyst)	Often asymptomatic. Abdominal cramps, vomiting, weight loss, diarrhea

to cattle within weeks to months of its onset. The incubation period is between 2 and 10 years. Affected animals may display changes in temperament, such as nervousness or aggression, abnormal posture, lack of coordination, and difficulty in standing, decreased milk production, or loss of body weight despite continued appetite. Most cattle with BSE show a gradual development of symptoms over a period of several weeks or even months, although some can deteriorate very rapidly. While the original source of the agent responsible for BSE remains unknown, currently the most plausible explanation is that a novel TSE appeared in the UK cattle population in the 1970s and subsequently spread through contaminated meat and bone meal fed to cattle. The International Office for Epizootic Diseases (OIE) reports cases on its website (www.oie.int).

Creutzfeldt–Jakob disease and new variant CJD

CJD is a fatal disease of humans, first described in the 1920s and found worldwide. CJD is predominantly a sporadic disease, but about 14% of cases are familial

(inherited) and associated with genetic mutations. Less than 1% are iatrogenic (i.e., accidentally transmitted from person to person as a result of medical or surgical procedures). Classically, sporadic CJD occurs in those over 65 years of age and presents as a rapidly progressive dementia with myoclonus (shock-like contractions of isolated muscles), usually fatal within 6 months. Surveillance of CJD, a human neurological disease, was reinstituted in the UK in 1990 to evaluate any changes in the pattern of the disease that might be attributable to BSE. The overall incidence of CJD rose in the UK in the 1990s, although a portion of this increase was due to improved ascertainment of CJD in older people as a result of the reinstitution of surveillance.

New variant CJD, also referred to as variant CJD (vCJD), is a newly recognized disease in humans, which was first diagnosed in the UK in the mid-1990s. In contrast to the traditional forms of CJD, vCJD has affected younger patients (average age 29 years) and has a longer duration of illness (approximately 14 months). Early in the illness, patients usually experience behavioral changes, which most commonly take the form of depression or, less often, a schizophrenia-like disorder. Neurological signs such as unsteadiness, difficulty walking, and involuntary movements develop as the illness progresses and, by the time of death, patients become completely immobile and mute.

The link between BSE and vCJD

A geographical association exists whereby the majority of BSE cases occurred in the UK and the majority of vCJD cases were also reported there. The emergence of BSE preceded vCJD, indicating a temporal association. Studies of stored human brain tissue internationally have not identified the histopathological changes characteristic of vCJD before the current BSE epidemic. Incubation period and pathological lesion studies in mice and molecular typing studies demonstrate that vCJD is similar to BSE but different from other TSEs. It is now widely accepted that vCJD was transmitted to humans through the consumption of contaminated food.

Estimates of future prevalence of vCJD vary widely as too little is known about the disease, especially regarding the incubation period between exposure to the infective agent and the emergence of symptoms.

14.7 Chemicals affecting food safety

Chemicals may be present in food owing to their natural occurrence in soil (e.g., cadmium, lead) or from fungal contamination (e.g., aflatoxins, ochratoxin), from algal contamination [e.g., amnesic shellfish poisoning (ASP), diarrhetic shellfish poisoning (DSP), azaspiracid shellfish poisoning (AZP), paralytic shellfish poisoning (PSP)], from industrial or other pollution [e.g., lead, mercury, polychlorinated biphenyls (PCBs), dioxins], from agricultural and veterinary practices (e.g., pesticides, fertilizers, veterinary drugs) or from food processing and packaging techniques [e.g. acrylamide, polycyclic aromatic hydrocarbons (PAHs), 3-monochloropropane-1,2-diol (3-MCPD), bisphenol A diglycidyl ether (BADGE)] (Box 14.1).

Toxicological assessment of these substances is largely carried out on an international basis by expert groups such as the Joint Expert Committee on

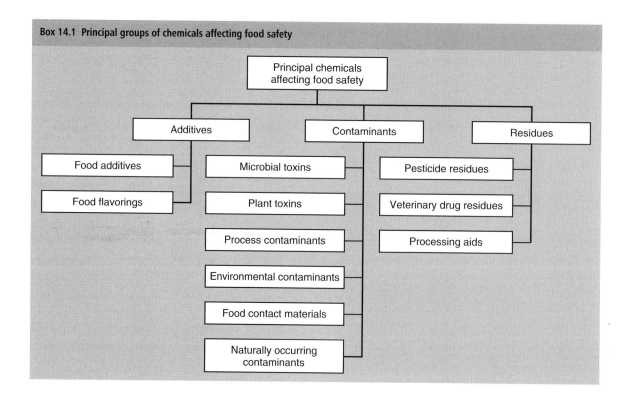

Box 14.1 Principal groups of chemicals affecting food safety

Food Additives and Contaminants (JECFA) or Joint Meeting on Pesticide Residues (JMPR), both jointly organized by the WHO and FAO. These expert groups advise on acceptable or tolerable levels of intake of these substances.

Acceptable and tolerable levels of intake

The acceptable daily intake (ADI) level of a chemical is the daily intake that, during a lifetime, would pose no appreciable risk to the consumer, on the basis of all facts known at the time. It is expressed in mg/kg of body weight (Box 14.2).

The tolerable weekly intake (TWI) represents permissible human weekly exposure to those contaminants unavoidably associated with the consumption of otherwise wholesome and nutritious foods. The term tolerable signifies permissibility rather than acceptability for the intake of contaminants that have no necessary function in food, in contrast to those of permitted pesticides or food additives. For cumulative toxicants, such as lead, cadmium, and mercury, the tolerable intakes are expressed on a weekly basis to allow for daily variations in intake levels, the real concern being long-term exposure to the contaminant.

The maximum tolerable daily intake (MTDI) has been established for food contaminants that are not known to accumulate in the body, such as tin, arsenic, and styrene. The value assigned to the provisional MTDI represents permissible human exposure as a result of the natural occurrence of the substance in food and drinking water.

One of the most difficult issues in food safety is to advise on the potential risks to human health for substances found in food which are both genotoxic (damaging DNA, the genetic material of cells) and carcinogenic (leading to cancer). For these substances, it is generally assumed that even a small dose can have an effect. JECFA addressed this issue in 1978 and introduced the concept of an "irreducible level," which it defined as "that concentration of a substance which cannot be eliminated from a food without involving the discarding of that food altogether, severely compromising the ultimate availability of major food supplies" (FAO/WHO, 1978).

Until now the risk assessors have advised to keep the exposure to such substances at the lowest possible level. This approach is known as the ALARA principle ("as low as reasonably achievable"). A disadvantage of this approach is that it cannot be used to compare risks posed by different substances. Furthermore, the application of the ALARA principle does not take into account the effectiveness of a substance and the actual (sometimes extremely low) level of occurrence in food.

A different approach, "the margin of exposure" (MoE) approach, which can be used to assess the risks to human health of exposure to a substance in the absence of a tolerable daily intake or similar guidance value, has recently been endorsed by the EFSA Scientific Committee (EFSA, 2005) and the WHO/FAO Joint Expert Committee on Food Additives (WHO/FAO, 2005). The margin of exposure is defined as the reference point on the dose–response curve (usually based on animal experiments in the absence of human data) divided by the estimated intake by humans. It enables the comparison of the risks posed by different genotoxic and carcinogenic substances. Differences in potency of the substances concerned and consumption patterns in the population are taken into account when applying the MoE approach.

Setting the acceptable daily intake

JECFA generally sets the ADI of a substance on the basis of the highest no-observed-effect level in animal studies. In calculating the ADI, a "safety factor" is applied to the no-observed-effect level to provide a conservative margin of safety on account of the inher-

Box 14.2 Levels of intake of a chemical	
No observed effect level (NOEL) ↓	Greatest concentration or amount of an agent, found by study or observation, that causes no detectable, usually adverse, alteration of morphology, functional capacity, growth, development, or lifespan of the target
/Safety factor ↓	Uncertainty factor for extrapolating animal data to humans
/Safety factor ↓	Human interspecies variation
Acceptable daily intake (ADI)	Daily intake that, during a lifetime, would pose no appreciable risk to the consumer, on the basis of all facts known at the time. It is expressed in mg/kg of body weight

ent uncertainties in extrapolating animal toxicity data to potential effects in humans and for variation within the human species. JECFA traditionally uses a safety factor of 100 (10×10) in setting ADI values based on long-term animal studies. It is intended to provide an adequate margin of safety for the consumer by assuming that the human being is 10 times more sensitive than the test animal and that the difference in sensitivity within the human population is in a 10-fold range. However, different safety factors apply depending on the substance and test species in question.

Maximum levels for food commodities

These levels are calculated taking the above-mentioned levels into consideration. Depending on the substance, different principles apply. Residues such as pesticides and residues of veterinary drugs in foodstuffs are limited by setting a maximum residue limit (MRL). Additives are regulated by setting maximum limits or by applying the "quantum satis" principle (the least amount required to exert the desired technological function).

For contaminants, maximum levels/limits are established for those foods that provide a significant contribution to the total dietary exposure. However, as a general principle the levels in all foods should always be kept as low as reasonably achievable (the ALARA principle).

In Europe, additives, pesticides, veterinary residues, and a wide range of contaminants are regulated by EU legislation in the form of directives or regulations that are transposed into national legislation by each member state.

Pesticide residues

Pesticides are chemicals or biological products used to control harmful or undesired organisms and plants, or to regulate the growth of plants as crop protection agents. They are classified into the groups shown in Box 14.3.

Most pesticides are toxic substances that are highly selective, especially those developed since the early 1980s, and only have an effect on those pests or plants to which they are applied. Unlike other environmental contaminants, pesticides are applied under controlled conditions that should conform to "good agricultural practice" (GAP). This defines the effective use of pesticides, up to the maximum allowable dose, applied in a manner that ensures the smallest amount of residue in the foodstuff.

Pesticides can also be toxic to humans since certain biochemical pathways are relatively conserved across species, as are some enzymes and hormones. In the context of food safety, exposure to pesticides is classified as acute or chronic. An acute intoxication usually has an immediate effect on the body, whereas a chronic effect may reveal itself over the lifespan. The severity depends on the dose and the toxicity of the pesticide compound or breakdown product. Toxic effects that have been identified include enzyme inhibition, endocrine disruption, and carcinogenic action, depending on the compound in question.

In Europe the control of pesticides is based on Council Directive 91/414/EEC. Under this legislation, pesticides must be evaluated for safety based on dossiers prepared by their manufacturers. If a pesticide is accepted it is placed on a positive list with an MRL assigned to it.

In the case of a limited number of highly toxic pesticides, for which the ADI is necessarily based on acute toxicity rather than chronic toxicity, the level of exposure is considered in relation to the acute reference dose (ARfD). ARfD values are measures of the maximum level of intake at one meal, or consump-

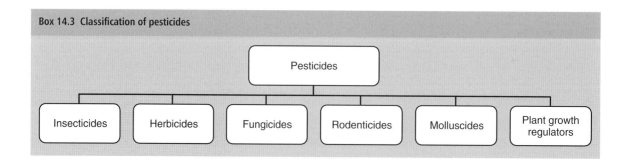

Box 14.3 Classification of pesticides

Pesticides
- Insecticides
- Herbicides
- Fungicides
- Rodenticides
- Molluscides
- Plant growth regulators

tion over a day. This is the maximum intake level, which is judged to result in no adverse toxicological effect following such exposure. The ARfD value includes a safety factor to ensure that older people, infants and children, and those under stress due to illness are protected.

Veterinary drug residues

Veterinary drugs include antibacterial compounds, hormones, and nonsteroidal anti-inflammatory preparations. As animal husbandry practices have intensified over the past few decades, antibacterial substances have been increasingly used as growth promoters to increase feed conversion efficiency, and for prophylaxis and therapy to prevent outbreaks and treat disease. Similarly, hormones are administered to increase growth rate and meat yield. Table 14.6 shows the main types of antibacterial and hormonal compounds.

Veterinary drugs are metabolized in the animal and are excreted in the urine and feces over time as the detoxification process continues. Hence, residue traces of drugs or their metabolites can be found in major organs, muscles, and body fluids. In general, antibacterial drugs are found in greatest concentration in the kidney, lesser concentrations in the liver and lowest concentrations in the muscle tissue, whereas hormones tend to concentrate in the liver.

The excessive use of antibacterial compounds in animal husbandry has raised concerns about the development of resistant bacteria and the effect that this may have on the usefulness of antibiotics in human medicine. There have also been concerns about the risk of allergic reactions in humans to antibacterial residues in food of animal origin. The use of hormones has raised issues surrounding the effects of hormone residues in foods of animal origin on human metabolism.

Environmental and industrial contaminants

These contaminants are of environmental origin or are by-products of industrial processes.

Polyhalogenated hydrocarbons (PHHs) are a category of environmental contaminants that includes toxaphene, dioxins, and polychlorinated biphenyls (PCBs). Certain polyhalogenated hydrocarbons are manufactured for use in plastics, paints, transformers, and herbicides; although their use is now either banned or severely restricted. In most industrialized nations the compounds have become ubiquitous in the environment. Hence, contamination of the food chain is inevitable and it has been estimated that in Western industrialized countries 90% of human exposure is through ingestion of contaminated foods such as fish and milk.

Foods that are rich sources of fats and oils tend to accumulate PHHs because the compounds are lipophilic and bioaccumulate in lipid-rich tissues and fluids. Oily fish from areas such as the Baltic Sea, where levels of PHHs in the water are high, may contain elevated levels of these contaminants. Similarly, cows that graze on polluted pasture can accumulate unacceptable concentrations of PHHs in their milk. A recent incident in Belgium introduced PCBs and dioxins into the food chain via contaminated animal feed resulting from the accidental incorporation of industrial oil into the feed ration. The biological half-life of PHHs can range from a matter of months to 20 years in human adipose tissue. Hence, they are persistent and accumulate in the body. Exposure to PHHs can result in a variety of toxic effects that can be carcinogenic, including dermal toxicity, immunotoxicity, reproductive effects, and endocrine disruption.

Metals, metalloids, and their compounds have long been associated with food poisoning, with lead and mercury probably the best documented hazards. Metals are released into the environment as a result of natural geological action and also as a result of man-made pollution from industrial processes.

Metals have an affinity for biological tissue and organic compounds, and hence they are often easily absorbed into the body and can often accumulate in organs and fat deposits. Table 14.7 shows some of the main metals linked with food-borne toxicity.

Table 14.6 Main types of veterinary drugs

Antibacterial compounds	Hormones
Aminoglycosides	β-Agonists
β-Lactams	Resorcylic lactones
Fluoroquinolones	Steroids
Macrolides	Stilbenes
Sulfonamides	Thyrostat
Tetracyclines	
Quinolones	

Table 14.7 Metals in the food chain

Metal	Main food sources
Lead	Shellfish, finfish, kidney, liver
Cadmium	Shellfish, kidney, cereals, vegetables
Mercury	Finfish
Arsenic	Meat, vegetables, seafood

Lead toxicity has many symptoms, but the main issue relates to its effects on the nervous system of children. Here, lead interferes with the transmission of nervous signals around the body. This can manifest itself in a reduced intelligence quotient (IQ) and coordination problems. In adults, exposure to lead can result in hypertension and other blood effects such as anemia. Cadmium is most often accumulated from occupational exposure or smoking and is known to affect the respiratory system. However, food exposure tends to be at a low level over longer periods. In this regard, cadmium bioaccumulates in the kidney and can cause renal damage. Mercury and its compounds also bioaccumulate in the body, where they are most frequently associated with neural effects and renal damage. In particular, methylmercury is highly toxic particularly to the nervous system, and the developing brain is thought to be the most sensitive target organ for methylmercury toxicity.

Arsenic is most often an occupational hazard, but it can also be ingested with food and is responsible for acute and chronic poisoning. The toxicity of arsenic depends on its oxidation state and the type of complex that it forms with organic molecules in the body. Chronic effects include gastroenteritis, nephritis, and liver damage. Arsenic is also considered to be a carcinogen. Other metals are also known contaminants and their toxic effects are diverse. Although this is not an exhaustive list, these metals include aluminum, copper, tin, zinc, and chromium.

Process contaminants

These types of contaminant occur during the processing and production of foods, and include acrylamide, PAHs, chloropropanols, and nitrosamines.

Acrylamide is a reactive unsaturated amide that has found several industrial uses. In 2002, it was discovered to occur in a variety of fried and baked foods, in particular carbohydrate-rich foods that had been subjected to high-temperature cooking/processing.

Acrylamide has been shown to be neurotoxic in humans. It has been shown to induce tumors in laboratory rats and has been classified as a probable human carcinogen, and as such several international bodies have concluded that dietary exposure should be as low as reasonably achievable. The most significant pathway of formation of acrylamide in foods has been shown to arise from the reaction of reducing sugars with asparagines via the Maillard reaction at temperatures above c. 120°C. Acrylamide has been found in a wide range of heat-treated foods; it is found in both foods processed by manufacturers and foods that are cooked in the home. Acrylamide has been found to be most prevalent in fried potato products (such as French fries and potato chips), cereals, bakery wares, and coffee.

PAHs are a group of over 100 different chemicals that are formed during certain technological processes and are common environmental contaminants. They are formed during incomplete combustion of coal and oil. They are also formed during barbecuing or grilling meat. Human exposure usually results from air pollution and from cigarette smoke. Foods most likely to be contaminated by PAHs are grilled or charred meats. PAHs are toxins that have been documented by the WHO as genotoxic, immunotoxic, and carcinogenic. Long-term exposure to foods containing PAHs can lead to serious health risks. In a recent Europe-wide incident, PAHs were found in pomace olive oil, which resulted in a major product recall.

3-Monochloro-propane-1,2-diol (3-MCPD) is a member of a group of contaminants known as chloropropanols, which includes known genotoxic animal carcinogens such as 1,3-dichloropropan-2-ol. 3-MCPD is a by-product in soy sauce and in hydrolyzed vegetable protein produced through acid hydrolysis. It can also be present as a contaminant in some food additives, and in epichlorhydrin/amine copolymers, used as flocculants or coagulant aids in water treatment, and may be present in drinking water (opinion of the European Scientific Committee on Food, adopted on 30 May 2001).

Microbial toxins

Food poisoning can occur as a result of the ingestion of food containing preformed toxins that originate from bacterial growth, fungal growth, or algal growth. In the case of bacteria the toxin is absorbed into the bloodstream via the intestine and therefore illness results from intoxication rather than infection. In the case of fungi, several species are involved in the production of toxic substances during growth on foodstuffs. These toxins are known as mycotoxins. Algal toxins are usually associated with seafood, most notably molluscan shellfish.

Bacterial toxins

Three bacteria are most commonly associated with preformed toxin production: *Clostridium botulinum*, *Staphylococcus aureus* and *Bacillus cereus* (see Table 14.1).

Fungal toxins (mycotoxins)

Mycotoxins are secondary metabolites of molds that can induce acute and chronic symptoms, such as carcinogenic, mutagenic, and estrogenic effects in humans and animals. Acute toxicity due to mycotoxins is associated with liver and kidney damage. Chronic toxicity resulting from the exposure of low levels of mycotoxins in the human diet is a major food safety concern. In nonindustrialized countries mycotoxins have been reported to be responsible for increased morbidity and mortality in children owing

to suppression of their immune systems and greater susceptibility to disease.

The principal fungi that are associated with mycotoxin production are the genera *Aspergillus*, *Penicillium*, and *Fusarium*. *Aspergillus* and *Penicillium* are sometimes referred to as storage fungi as they can grow at low water activity levels and are associated with the post-harvest spoilage of stored food commodities such as cereals, nuts, and spices. *Fusarium* species are plant pathogens and can infect plants in the field and produce mycotoxins preharvest. Table 14.8 provides an overview of the most important mycotoxins.

Seafood toxins

Fish and fishery products are nutritious foods and are desirable components of a healthy diet. Food-borne illnesses resulting from the consumption of seafood are associated with both finfish and molluscan shellfish. The major risk of acute illness is associated with the consumption of raw shellfish, particularly bivalve molluscs. The consumption of these toxic shellfish by humans can cause illness, with symptoms ranging from mild diarrhea and vomiting to memory loss, paralysis, and death. Toxins associated with phyto-

Table 14.8 Mycotoxins in the food supply

Mycotoxin	Producing fungi	Main foods affected	Toxicity
Aflatoxins	*Aspergillus flavus* and *A. parasiticus*	Nuts, cereals, dried fruit, herbs and spices, milk (aflatoxin M1)	Carcinogenic, hepatotoxic
Ochratoxin A	*Aspergillus ochraceus*, *Penicillium verrucosum*, and other *Aspergillus* and *Penicillium* spp.	Coffee, dried fruit, cereals, beans, pulses, wine, beer, grape juice; kidney, liver and blood from animals fed with contaminated feed	Nephrotoxic, immunotoxic
Patulin	*Aspergillus clavatus*, also several species of *Penicillium*, *Aspergillus*, and *Byssochlamys*	Fruits and grains, predominantly apples and apple products	Cytotoxic
Trichothecenes (nivalenol, deoxynivalenol, T2-toxin, etc.)	*Fusarium* spp.	Wheat, maize, barley, oats, rye, malt, beer, bread	Dermotoxic, enterotoxic, hemotoxic, immunotoxic
Fumonisins	*Fusarium* spp.	Cereals, mainly corn	Carcinogenic, cytotoxic, hepatotoxic
Sterigmatocystin	*Aspergillus versicolor*, *A. nidulans*, and other *Aspergillus* spp.	Cereals, green coffee, herbs and spices, raw meat products	Hepatotoxic and nephrotoxic, carcinogenic
Citrinin	*Penicillium* spp., *Aspergillus* spp.	Cereals	Nephrotoxic
Zearalenone	*Fusarium graminearum*	Maize, barley, oats, wheat, rice, sorghum, bread	Estrogenic effects, feed refusal, vomiting
Moniliformin	*Fusarium* spp.	Cereals, maize	Nephrotoxic, causes necrosis of the heart muscle

plankton are known as phycotoxins. These toxins have been responsible for incidents of wide-scale death of sea-life and are increasingly responsible for human intoxication.

Various seafood poisoning syndromes are associated with toxic marine algae and these include paralytic shellfish poisoning (PSP), amnesic shellfish poisoning (ASP), diarrhetic shellfish poisoning (DSP), neurotoxic shellfish poisoning, and azaspiracid shellfish poisoning (AZP). There are also different types of food poisoning associated with finfish and these include ciguatera poisoning, scombroid or histamine poisoning, and puffer fish poisoning. Consumption of raw molluscan shellfish poses well-known risks of food poisoning, but intoxication from finfish is not so well known. Most of the algal toxins associated with seafood poisoning are heat stable and are not inactivated by cooking. It is also not possible visually to distinguish toxic from nontoxic fish. Many countries rely on biotoxin monitoring programs to protect public health and close harvesting areas when toxin algal blooms or toxic shellfish are detected. In nonindustrialized countries, particularly in rural areas, monitoring for harmful algal blooms does not routinely occur and deaths due to red-tide toxins commonly occur. Table 14.9 provides an overview of the most important types of fish poisoning.

Naturally occurring plant toxins

Certain plants contain naturally occurring compounds that are toxic to humans or that reduce the bioavailability of nutrients in foods. Examples of naturally occurring toxins are listed in Table 14.10. Some species of mushroom also contain toxic compounds, for instance agaritine. Some cereal-based diets have restricted bioavailability of nutrients as a result of the presence of antinutritional factors such as phytate and tannins or polyphenols.

Food processing methods have evolved that reduce human exposure to both natural toxins and antinutritional compounds. For instance, cassava is a staple food of over 500 million people worldwide. Certain bitter varieties of cassava contain high levels of linamarin, a cyanogenic glycoside. The consumption of these varieties has been associated with health defects such as goiter and paralysis of the legs. Traditional processing of cassava in Africa that involves grating, soaking roots in water, and lactic acid fermentation completely removes the cyanide.

Adequate cooking of legume seeds such as kidney beans and disposal of the cooking water will remove the natural toxins present in these food products.

Antinutritional factors are those components of plants that interfere with metabolic processes and can lead to deficiencies of key nutrients in the diet. These are generally classified as enzyme inhibitors and mineral binding agents. Enzyme inhibitors are polypeptides and proteins that inhibit the activities of digestive enzymes, and most are thermolabile and are reduced by cooking. For example, trypsin inhibitors may cause poor protein digestion and a shortage of sulfur-containing amino acids in the diet. Lectins are proteins that occur in beans that alter the absorption of nutrients in the intestinal wall. Cooking beans will inactivate lectins. Tannins (polyphenols) occur in cereals, specifically in the seed coat. These form complexes with proteins and inhibition of digestive enzymes. Phytate is a natural component in plants and on digestion forms insoluble complexes with metal ions in the body. The result is reduced bioavailability of essential minerals such as iron. In addition, a range of natural plant toxins can cause allergic reactions in humans, but there is a general lack of knowledge about their properties and modes of action.

Food additives

Food additives are added to foods for a specific technological purpose during manufacture or storage and become an integral part of that foodstuff. Additives can be natural or synthetic and are usually categorized by their function (Table 14.11). For example, preservatives prevent the growth of bacteria, gelling agents maintain the structure of some foods during storage, and emulsifiers maintain the stability of fat structures. Without additives it would not be possible to manufacture many of the foods available today, especially convenience foods and low-fat foods.

Safety considerations involving additives have centered on allergic reactions and food intolerances. Additives have also been blamed for inducing hyperactivity in children. Studies have been conducted into allergies and they often find that the actual prevalence rate is much lower than the perceived prevalence rate.

At the international level, additives are controlled by means of safety evaluation and the development of a positive list. To ensure transparency and choice, all additives that are used in prepackaged food should be labeled with their function and their name or

Table 14.9 Types of fish poisoning

Poisoning	Implicated foods	Associated toxin	Symptoms	Occurrence
Paralytic shellfish poisoning	Mussels, oysters, clams or scallops that have fed on toxigenic dinoflagellates (*Gonyaulax* spp.)	Saxitoxins	Neurotoxic; symptoms include numbness, tingling and burning of the lips, staggering, drowsiness, and in severe cases respiratory paralysis	Worldwide
Amnesic shellfish poisoning	Mussels and clams that have recently fed on a marine diatom *Nitzchia pungens*, viscera of crabs and anchovies	Domoic acid	Vomiting, cramps, diarrhea, disorientation, and difficulty in breathing	USA, Canada, and Europe
Diarrhetic shellfish poisoning	Toxic mussels, clams, and scallops that have fed on marine dinoflagellates (*Dinophysis* spp.)	Okadaic acid and associated toxins	Abdominal pain, nausea, vomiting, and severe diarrhea	Europe, Japan, Chile, New Zealand, and Canada
Neurotoxic shellfish poisoning	Shellfish that have fed on the dinoflagellate *Gymnodinidum breve*	Brevitoxins	Nausea, diarrhea, tingling and burning of the lips, tongue, and throat	Florida coast and Gulf of Mexico
Azaspiracid shellfish poisoning	Mussels, oysters, clams, scallops, and razor fish	Azaspiracid	Nausea, vomiting, severe diarrhea, and stomach cramps	Ireland, suspected cases in Norway, the Netherlands, Scotland, and Japan
Ciguatera fish poisoning	Flesh of toxic reef fish from tropical areas feeding on dinoflagellates (*Gambierdiscus toxicus*) and their toxins. Common species are amberjack, barracuda, moray eel, groupers, trevally, Spanish mackerel, and snapper	Ciguatera	Gastrointestinal (diarrhea, vomiting, abdominal pain, nausea); neurological (paresthesia of the extremities, circumoral paresthesia, temperature reversal, ataxia, arthralgia, malign headache, severe pruritus, vertigo, and stiffness, convulsions, delirium, hallucinations, photophobia, transient blindness, salivation, perspiration, watery eyes, metallic taste in mouth, blurred vision, hiccups, exacerbation of acne, dysuria); cardiovascular (dyspnea, bradycardia, hypotension, tachycardia)	Tropical reef waters, particularly in the island states of the South Pacific
Scombroid or histamine poisoning	Consumption of scombroid and scombroid-like marine fish species that have not been chilled immediately after capture. Commonly involved are members of the Scombridae family, e.g., tuna and mackerel, and a few nonscombrid relatives, e.g., bluefish, dolphin fish, and amberjack	Scombroid or histamine.	Initial symptoms are that of an allergic response with facial flushing and sweating, burning–peppery taste sensations around the mouth and throat, dizziness, nausea, and headache. A facial rash can develop as well as mild diarrhea and abdominal cramps. Severe cases may blur vision and cause respiratory stress and swelling of the tongue. Symptoms usually last for approximately 4–6 h and rarely exceed 1–2 days	Worldwide
Puffer fish poisoning	Consumption of fish species belonging to the Tetraodontidea family, particularly those species caught in waters of the Indo-Pacific Ocean regions	Tetrodotoxin	Symptoms of puffer fish poisoning are similar to paralytic shellfish poisoning as the actions of both toxins are similar. Mild poisoning results in tingling and numbness of the lips, tongue, and fingers, and in severe cases death by asphyxiation due to respiratory paralysis	Most frequent in Japan, where puffer fish (called fugu in Japan) are eaten as a delicacy, Indo-Pacific Ocean region

Table 14.10 Naturally occurring plant toxins

Compound	Food species	Common name
Glycosides:		
Linamarin	*Manihot escaleatum*	Cassava
Dhurrin	*Sorghum* spp.	Sorghum
Prunasin	*Prunus* spp.	Cherries
Glycoalkaloids:		
Solanin	*Solanium tuberosiem*	Potatoes
Pyrrolizidine alkaloids:		
Acetyllycopsaimine	*Symphytum* spp.	Comfrey
Senecionine	*Senccio jacobata*	Ragwort
Glucosinolates:		
Sinigrin	*Brassica* spp.	Cabbage
		Broccoli
		Brussels
		sprouts

Table 14.11 Categories of food additives according to function

Acid	Flour treatment agent
Acidity regulator[a]	Gelling agent
Anticaking agent	Glazing agent[c]
Antifoaming agent	Humectant
Antioxidant	Modified starch
Bulking agent	Preservative
Color	Propellant gas and packaging gas
Emulsifier	
Emulsifying salt	Raising agent
Enzyme[b]	Sequestrant[d]
Firming agent	Stabilizer[e]
Flavoring	Sweetener
Flavor enhancer	Thickener

[a] These can act as two-way acidity regulators.
[b] Only those used as additives.
[c] These substances include lubricants intended for the final consumer.
[d] Inclusion of these terms in this list is without prejudice to any future decision or mention thereof in the labeling of foodstuffs.
[e] This category also comprises foam stabilizers.
Source: European Union Directive 89/107/EEC, http://eur-lex.europa.eu/. © European Communities.

approval number (E number). However, there are some exemptions specifically applying to additives that are in a foodstuff as a result of carry-over from an ingredient.

14.8 Food safety control programs

Each nation has a responsibility to ensure that its citizens enjoy safe and wholesome food. Governments aim to identify major food safety issues that can then

be controlled through the development and implementation of targeted food safety control programs. This can be achieved either through legislation, or the use of standards or codes of practice. At the international level, the WHO and the FAO have worked since the 1960s on developing food standards that aim to protect the health of consumers and facilitate international trade of foods and animal feeding stuffs. This work is carried out by the Codex Alimentarius Commission (CAC), an intergovernmental body managed by the FAO and WHO. Food safety standards developed by the CAC serve as the baseline for harmonization of global food standards, codes of practice, guidelines, and recommendations. Harmonization of standards and recognition that different national food safety controls are equivalent are enshrined in the international agreements of the World Trade Organization (WTO).

The purpose of food safety legislation is to protect consumers' health and interests by providing controls throughout the food chain. A recent overhaul of EU food safety legislation now places the primary responsibility for food safety with the food business operator. It also recognizes that food safety must start at primary production (i.e., the farmer) and places increased importance on the safety of animal feed. This concept of food safety control from "farm-to-fork" or "gate-to-plate" has been endorsed internationally, but implemented differently in different countries.

The traditional "inspection and detection" aspects of food safety control are now being replaced with strategies for prevention of hazards occurring in the first place. In many countries, food businesses are now legally obliged to adopt the principles of HACCP (hazard analysis and critical control point) in order to predict what biological, chemical or physical hazards are likely to occur in their process, so that they can implement control measures to prevent them happening.

14.9 Perspectives on the future

As our society changes, so do the bacteria involved in food-borne disease. Changes in food production systems and the globalization of the food supply, as well as changes in the food we are eating, and where this food is prepared, expose us to an ever-changing spectrum of contamination. The global nature of our food supply poses greater risks to consumer health from the mass production and distribution of foods and increased risk for food contamination. New food development has led to changing vectors for the spread of disease. Inappropriate use of antibiotics in animal husbandry can lead to the emergence of antibiotic-resistant food-borne pathogens such as *S. typhimurium* DT 104.

Food safety and nutrition are inextricably linked because food-borne infections are one of the most important underlying factors of malnutrition, especially in poorer countries. Repeated episodes of food-borne infections can, over a period of time, lead to malnutrition, with serious health consequences. A safe food supply is essential for proper nutrition, basic health and well-being.

Maintaining a safe food supply is not difficult; however, it requires attention to detail at all stages of the food chain from agricultural inputs through farms, processing, the distribution network to retailers and catering outlets to consumers. There can be no gaps in the continuum from farm to fork if consumer protection is to be optimum. To ensure consumer protection, food standards have to be based on sound science and the principles of risk analysis. At the national level, food safety controls must be well coordinated and based on proportionate food legislation. The food industry must also recognize its primary responsibility for producing safe food and for ensuring that foods placed on the market meet the highest standards of food safety and hygiene. A multisectoral effort on the part of regulatory authorities, food industries. and consumers alike is required to prevent food-borne diseases.

Acknowledgment

This chapter has been revised and updated by Alan Reilly, Christina Tlustos, Judith O'Connor, and Lisa O'Connor based on the original chapter by Alan Reilly, Christina Tlustos, Wayne Anderson, Lisa O'Connor, Barbara Foley, and Patrick Wall.

References

Abdussalam M, Käferstein FK, Mott K. Food safety measures for the control of food borne trematode infections. *Food Control* 1995; **6**: 71–79.

Cadbury Schweppes. *Press Release* 2007. Available at: http://www.cadbury.com/media/press/Pages/2006fullyearresults.aspx

CDC. Surveillance for Foodborne Disease Outbreaks – United States, 1993–1997. *Morbidity and Mortality Weekly Report* 2000; **49**: (SS01)1–51.

Dewaal CS, Hicks G, Barlow K, Aldterton L, Vegosen L. Foods associated with food-borne illness outbreaks from 1990 through 2003. *Food Protection Trends* 2006; **26**: 466–473.

Doyle MP, Beuchat LR, Montville TJ, eds. *Food microbiology: fundamentals and frontiers, 2nd ed.* American Society for Microbiology, Washington DC, 2001.

EFSA. Opinion of the Scientific Committee on a request from EFSA related to a harmonised approach for risk assessment of substances which are both genotoxic and carcinogenic. *EFSA Journal* 2005; **282**: 1–31.

EFSA. The community summary report on trends and sources of zoonoses, zoonotic agents, antimicrobial resistance and food-borne outbreaks in the European Union in 2006. Available at: http://www.efsa.europa.eu/cs/BlobServer/DocumentSet/Zoon_report_2006_en,0.pdf?ssbinary=true

European Commission. Opinion of the Scientific Committee on Food on 3-monochloro-propane-1,2-diol (3-MCPD) updating the SCF opinion of 1994 adopted on 30 May 2001. Available at: http://ec.europa.eu/food/fs/sc/scf/out91_en.pdf

FAO/WHO. *Evaluation of certain food additives and contaminants. 22nd Report of the Joint FAO/WHO Expert Committee on Food Additives.* WHO Technical Report Series No. 631. WHO, Geneva, 1978: 14–15.

Frenzen PD. Deaths due to unknown foodborne agents. *Emerging Infectious Diseases* 2004; **10**: 1536–1543.

Frenzen PD, Drake A, Angulo FJ, the Emerging Infections Program Foodnet Working Group. Economic cost of illness due to *Escherichia coli* O157 infections in the United States. *Journal of Food Protection* 2005; **68**: 2623–2630.

Käferstein, FK. Actions to reverse the upward curve of foodborne illness. *Food Control* 2003; **14**: 101–109.

McCabe-Sellers BJ, Beattie SE. Food safety: emerging trends in foodborne illness surveillance and prevention. *Journal of the American Dietetic Association* 2004; **104**: 1708–1717.

Mead PS, Slutsker L, Dietz V, McCaig LF, Bresee JS, Shapiro C, Griffin PM, Tauxe RV. Food-related illness and death in the United Sates. *Emerging Infectious Diseases* 1999; **5**: 607–625.

Smith JL. Foodborne infections during pregnancy. *Journal of Food Protection* 1999; **62**: 818–829.

WHO. Food safety and foodborne illness. *Fact sheet No. 237.* Available at: http://www.who.int/mediacentre/factsheets/fs237/en/

WHO/FAO. Joint FAO/WHO expert committee on food additives sixty-fourth meeting, Rome, 8--17 February 2005. Available at: ftp://ftp.fao.org/es/esn/jecfa/jecfa64_call.pdf

15
Food and Nutrition-Related Diseases: The Global Challenge

Hester H Vorster and Michael J Gibney

Key messages

- This chapter deals with the current situation, trends and types of nutrition-related diseases in developed and developing countries.
- It shows that in developed countries excessive intakes of macronutrients (overnutrition) and suboptimal intakes of micronutrients (hidden hunger), mainly because of low fruit and vegetable consumption, lead to obesity and related noncommunicable diseases (NCDs).
- The chapter also shows that developing countries are suffering from a double burden of disease because of the persistence of

undernutrition and related deficiency and infectious diseases (including human immunodeficiency virus/acquired immunodeficiency syndrome HIV/AIDS), and the emergence of NCDs as a result of the nutrition transition. It explains the vicious cycle of poverty and undernutrition and how this is related to underdevelopment and increased risk of NCDs in the developing world.
- Current global challenges for food and nutrition interventions on different levels are highlighted.

15.1 Introduction

The relationship between nutrition and health was summarized in Figure 1.2, illustrating that the nutritional quality and quantity of foods eaten, and therefore nutritional status, are major modifiable factors in promoting health and well-being, in preventing disease, and in treating some diseases. It is now accepted that our nutritional status influences our health and risk of both infectious and noncommunicable diseases.

But it is also accepted that billions of people in both developed and developing countries suffer from one or more forms of malnutrition, contributing to the global burden of disease. Mankind has an inherent preference for palatable, sugary, salty, fatty and smooth (finely textured, refined) foods. These foods are mostly energy-dense and low in micronutrients. Food production, processing, manufacturing, marketing

and promotion have responded to this preference by making high energy-dense foods available at increasingly affordable prices. This has led to changes in food consumption patterns which unfortunately coincided with more sedentary, less active lifestyles. The resultant overnutrition of especially macronutrients is the major cause of obesity and also, together with obesity, a risk factor for many of the noncommunicable disease (NCDs) such as type 2 diabetes, coronary heart disease, stroke, hypertension, dental disease, osteoporosis, and some forms of cancer.

These changes from traditional low-energy dense, high-fiber diets to the dietary pattern described above are collectively known as the nutrition transition (NT). The NT has proceeded gradually over centuries in the developed world and accelerated during the industrial revolution with a resultant gradual and then accelerated emergence of the NCDs. However, globalization characterized by urbanization, acculturation, global trade, and information exchange has led to a very rapid NT in developing countries. The consequence is that, different from developed countries, obesity and the NCDs emerged before the problems of undernutrition and specific nutritional deficiencies have been solved. Developing countries now suffer from a double burden of nutrition-related diseases because of the coexistence of under- and overnutrition. This dual burden is further exacerbated by the HIV/AIDS and TB pandemics in these countries.

The purpose of this chapter is to describe the major nutrition-related diseases in the developed and developing world, to show the interrelationships between the causes and consequences of under- and overnutrition, and to identify the global challenges in addressing the heavy burden of malnutrition that contribute to underdevelopment, disability, and premature death.

15.2 Nutrition-related diseases in developed countries

The current situation

Economic development, education, food security, and access to health care and immunization programs in developed countries have resulted in dramatic decreases in undernutrition-related diseases. Unfortunately, many of these factors have also led to unhealthy behaviors, inappropriate diets, and lack of physical activity, which has exacerbated the development of chronic diseases, also known as noncommunicable diseases (NCDs). These NCDs are now the main contributors to the health burden in developed countries (these are countries with established market economies).

In 2002, 28.2 million global deaths (58.6%) were from NCDs. In the same year the predicted mortality for 2020 was 49.6 million (72.6% of all deaths). This is an increase from 448 to 548 deaths per 100,000, despite an overall downward trend in mortality rates. Although the burden will fall increasingly on developing countries (see 15.3) NCDs remain the major cause of death in developed countries.

Definition, terminology and characteristics

The NCDs that are related to diet and nutrient intakes are obesity, hypertension, atherosclerosis, ischemic heart disease, myocardial infarction, cerebrovascular

disease, stroke, diabetes mellitus (type 2), osteoporosis, liver cirrhosis, dental caries, and nutrition-induced cancers of the breast, colon, and stomach. They develop over time in genetically susceptible individuals because of exposure to interrelated societal, behavioral, and biological risk factors. Together with tobacco use, alcohol abuse, and physical inactivity, an unhealthy or inappropriate diet is an important modifiable risk factor for NCDs. Diet, therefore, plays a major role in prevention and treatment of NCDs. NCDs are sometimes called "chronic diseases," but some infectious diseases such as HIV/AIDS and tuberculosis are also chronic. They have also been called "diseases of affluence," which is a misnomer because in developed, affluent countries, they are more common in lower socioeconomic groups. Some scientists have a problem with the term "noncommunicable" because lifestyles, including diets, are transferable between populations. The term "noncommunicable" should therefore be seen as no transfer of an infectious agent from one organism to another. Because of its first emergence in "Westernized" societies and associations with Western lifestyles, it is often called "Western" diseases, also a misnomer. It is becoming more prevalent in developing countries in other parts of the world. Another misconception is that it is a group of diseases affecting only older people. The risk factors for NCDs accumulate throughout the life course – from infancy to adulthood, and manifest after decades of exposure. The increase in childhood obesity is especially of concern because it has long-term implications for NCDs in the developed world.

Risk factors for NCDs

Table 15.1 lists the risk factors for NCDs. The factors are interrelated and form a chain of events starting with societal factors such as socioeconomic status and environments that influence behavior, leading to the development of biological risk factors that cause the NCDs. The biological risk factors often cluster together. For example, obesity (abnormal body composition) is associated with insulin resistance, hyperlipidemia, and hypertension, which all contribute to the development of both cardiovascular disease and diabetes. Cardiovascular disease is furthermore one of the complications of untreated diabetes. The mechanisms through which these risk factors contribute to the development of NCDs are discussed in detail in

Table 15.1 Risk factors for nutition-related noncommunicable diseases (NCDS)

Societal	Behavioral	Biological	NCDs
Socioeconomic status	Smoking	Tobacco addiction	Lung disease
Cultural habits	Alcohol abuse	Alcohol addiction	*Cardiovascular disease*
Environmental factors	Lack of physical activity	Dyslipidemia	Atherosclerosis
	Inappropriate diets:	Hyperlipidemia	Cerebrovascular disease
	inadequate	Insulin resistance	Stroke
	fiber	Hypertension	Ischemic heart disease
	micronutrients	Obesity (body composition)	Myocardial infarction
	excess		Diabetes
	total fat		Osteoporosis
	saturated fat		Dental caries
	trans fat		Cirrhosis
	cholesterol		Diet-induced cancers
	salt (NaCl)		
	energy		

appropriate chapters and sections of this series of textbooks.

The role of nutrition

The evidence that diets and specific nutrient deficiencies and excesses influence the development of NCDs and may therefore be used in prevention and treatment is solid. It comes from extensive research which collectively gave convincing evidence of the relationships between nutrition and NCDs: first, from ecological studies which compared different populations, the effects of migration of populations, food availability during economic development, and differences in dietary and nutrient intakes. Second, numerous epidemiological studies have established the associations between diet and biological risk factors of NCDs. Third, interventions with specific nutrients and foods in placebo-controlled trials using both healthy and diseased subjects confirmed the relationships seen in epidemiological studies. And last, molecular and genetic research has elucidated many mechanisms through which diet and nutrients affect genetic mutation and expression, adding to our knowledge of how nutrition influences NCD development. This body of knowledge has led to several sets of international dietary recommendations and guidelines to reduce the burden of nutrition-related NCDs. An example of one such set of guidelines from the World Health Organization (WHO) is shown in Box 15.1. These generic recommendations could be used as the basis for the development of country-specific strategies and food-based guidelines for dietary prevention of NCDs.

Box 15.1 The WHO population nutrient intake goals for prevention of death and disability from NCDs[a]

Dietary factor (food or nutrient)	Recommended goal (range)
Total fat	15–30% of total energy
Saturated fatty acids	<10% of total energy
Polyunsaturated fatty acids (PUFAs)	6–10% of total energy
n-6 PUFAs	5–8% of total energy
n-3 PUFAs	1–2% of total energy
Trans fatty acids	<1% of total energy
Monounsaturated fatty acids (MUFAs)	By difference[b]
Total carbohydrate	55–75% of total energy[c]
Free sugars[d]	<10% of total energy
Protein	10–15% of total energy
Cholesterol	<300 mg per day
Sodium chloride (sodium)	<5 g per day (<2 g per day)
Fruits and vegetables	≥400 g per day
Total dietary fiber	>25 g per day
Non-starch polysaccharides	>20 g per day

[a] WHO Technical Support Series No. 916.
[b] MUFAs are calculated as total fat minus saturated plus polyunsaturated plus trans fatty acids).
[c] Energy from carbohydrate is the percentage energy available after taking into account that consumed as fat and protein.
[d] Free sugars refers to all monosaccharides and disaccharides added to foods by the manufacturer, cook, or consumer, plus sugars naturally present in honey, syrups, and fruit juices. It does not include sugars present in milk, fruit and vegetables.

Prevention of NCDs in developed countries

The complex chain of events where behavioral and lifestyle factors influence the development of the biological risk factors for NCDs, emphasizes the need for a multisectoral approach in which all factors in the chain are targeted throughout the life course. In addition to the medical treatment of some biological risk factors (such as pharmacological treatment of hypercholesterolemia) and of the NCD itself (such as blood glucose control in diabetes) there is convincing evidence that primary prevention is possible, cost-effective, affordable, and sustainable. In the developed world, early screening and diagnosis, and access to health care make primary prevention more feasible than in many developing countries. However, overcoming the barriers to increase physical activity and changing dietary behavior towards more prudent, low-fat, high-fiber diets may be more difficult. The strategies and programs to prevent NCDs would be similar in developed and developing countries, although the context and specific focus of different interventions may vary. Because the future burden of NCDs will be determined by the accumulation of risks over a lifetime, the life course approach is recommended. This will include optimizing the nutritional status of pregnant women (see Box 15.3), breastfeeding of infants, ensuring optimal nutrition status and growth of children, preventing childhood obesity and promoting "prudent" diets for adolescents, adults, and older people. Addressing childhood obesity in developed countries is one of the biggest nutritional challenges these countries is facing today. Increases in the prevalence of childhood obesity have been documented for most developed countries. In the USA, the National Health and Nutrition Examination Surveys (NHANES) showed substantial increases over the last two decades in overweight and obese children aged 2–19 years. More than 15% of American children are currently considered obese. The International Obesity Task Force estimates that at least 22 million of the world's children under 5 years of age are overweight or obese. Overweight and obesity have dire consequences in children. These children already display many of the other biological risk factors of NCDs. There are also immediate health consequences such as risks to develop gallstones, hepatitis, sleep apnea, and others. Moreover, these children have a lack of self-esteem, are often stigmatized

and have difficulties with body image and mobility. Overweight and obese children often become overweight or obese adults and carry the long-term risk of premature morbidity and mortality from NCDs. Children in the developed world are exposed to a food environment in which high energy-dense and micronutrient-poor foods, beverages, and snacks are available, affordable, and aggressively marketed. This illustrates that to address the problem of childhood obesity, active and responsible partnerships and common agendas should be formed between all stakeholders (for example between governments, NGOs and the food industry). There are indications that dialogue with the food industry is not sufficient, and that many countries are now considering or already implementing legislation to create a more healthy food environment for children. The problems of childhood overweight and obesity and consequent increases in NCDs are not only seen in developed countries. They are emerging in developing countries and in some the total number of children affected exceeds those in developed countries. Timely interventions are needed to prevent the escalation experienced in developed countries.

15.3 Nutrition-related diseases in developing countries

The poverty–malnutrition cycle

Malnutrition in developing countries affects individuals throughout the life course: from birth to infancy and childhood, through adolescence into adulthood, and into old age. Malnutrition affects, therefore, critical periods of growth and mental development, maturation, active reproductive as well as economical productive phases.

The health of populations in developing countries is largely determined by their environment. "Environmental" factors include social and economic conditions depending on and influencing availability and distribution of resources, agricultural and food systems, availability and access to nutritious food and safe drinking water, implementation of immunization programs, exposure to unhygienic surroundings and toxins, women's status and education, as well as the "political" milieu including dictatorships, conflict, and war, which often determine the availability of health services. There is a close, interrelated association between undernutrition and poverty in developing countries.

Figure 15.1 illustrates this relationship, also showing some of the mechanisms responsible for perpetuating the relationship over generations.

Approximately 243 million adults in developing countries are severely undernourished, with a body mass index less than 17 kg/m². This means that high proportions of especially Asian and African pregnant women are undernourished. Intrauterine (fetal) growth retardation is common in these women, leading to low birthweight babies (weight at full term less than 2500 g). Almost a quarter of newborns in the developing world (30 million of the 126 million babies born each year) have low birth weights compared with only 2% in the developed world. These babies, especially when exposed to inappropriate breastfeeding and weaning practices, leading to further nutritional insults, have growth impairment and mental underdevelopment. In addition, because of undernutrition, their immune systems are compromised. The result is stunted children that cannot benefit optimally from education and with an increased risk of infectious disease. In 2000, more than 150 million preschool children in the developing world were underweight, while approximately 200 million were stunted.

Figure 15.1 also shows that these physically and mentally underdeveloped children eventually develop into adults with "decreased human capital" and decreased competence. These adults are often not able to create enabling environments for themselves or their children to escape poverty and undernutrition in the next generation. But moreover, these "underdeveloped" adults are at increased risk of obesity and other NCDs because of early programming (possibly through epigenetic or DNA methylation changes) in the undernourished fetus. It is especially when these adults are exposed to low micronutrient quality and high energy-dense diets that they rapidly become overweight and obese. This phenomenon explains to a certain extent the coexistence of under- and overnutrition in the same household with undernourished, wasted, and stunted children being cared for by an overweight or obese mother or care-giver.

Obesity and noncommunicable diseases in developing countries

Obesity and other NCDs are increasingly becoming major public health problems in the developing world. The WHO estimates that almost 80% of all deaths worldwide that are attributable to NCDs are already occurring in developing countries. A disturbing observation is that they often occur at younger ages than in the developed world. Obesity and other NCDs have similar biological risk factors in developed and developing countries (and will not be discussed in detail here). However, the context in which they develop may differ, being linked with fetal and infant undernutrition. Also, underdevelopment and a lack of resources in developing countries limit the availability of diagnostic and therapeutic care of people suffering from NCDs, leading to increased morbidity and mortality.

The other two groups of nutrition-related diseases in developing countries are nutrient deficiency diseases and infectious diseases, which will now be briefly discussed.

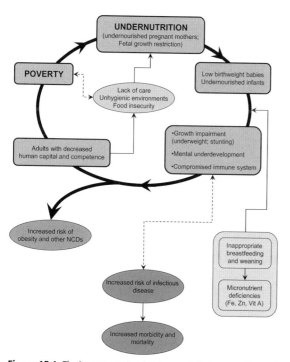

Figure 15.1 The intergenerational vicious cycle between undernutrition and poverty.

Major nutrient deficiency diseases in developing countries

It is estimated that nearly 30% of humanity suffer from one or more forms of malnutrition. About 60%

of the approximately 11 million deaths each year of children aged under 5 years in the developing world are associated with malnutrition. In addition to the undernutrition related to poverty, hunger, and food insecurity, leading to stunted physical and mental development, specific nutrient deficiencies are causes of specific diseases (as discussed in Chapters 4, 5, 8, and 9 of this textbook). The major nutrient deficiency diseases prevalent in developing countries are briefly summarized in Box 15.2, to illustrate the scope of the problem and to identify the nutrition challenges in the developing world for the twenty-first century.

Nutrition-related infectious disease in developing countries

Nutrition is a major determinant of the human body's defense against infectious diseases. Optimal nutrition is necessary for the integrity of the physical barriers (skin, epithelium) against pathogens. Specific nutrients furthermore play important roles in defining acquired immune function (both humoral and cell-mediated responses) and to influence, modulate, or mediate inflammatory processes, the virulence of the infectious agent, and the response of cells and tissues to hypoxic and toxic damage.

The immune system and the influence of malnutrition on its functions are discussed in detail in the clinical nutrition textbook of the series. Given the high prevalence of malnutrition (undernutrition) in developing countries, it is not surprising that infectious diseases are still dominating mortality statistics in these countries. In children under 5 years of age these are diarrhea and common childhood illnesses in which malnutrition could lead to premature childhood deaths. In some developing countries, children die of AIDS-related diseases. HIV/AIDS is an infectious disease that has pandemic proportions in developing countries. It will be discussed in more detail here to illustrate the complex role of nutrition in this tragic situation.

15.4 HIV/AIDS

Introduction

Infection with HIV and the consequent development of AIDS is a global pandemic already responsible for more than half of total deaths in some developing countries. It is estimated that since the early 1980s when the syndrome was described and the virus identified, this infectious disease has already killed more than 25 million people, including at least half a million children. A third of these deaths occurred in sub-Saharan Africa, where more than half of the 33.4–46 million people currently infected with HIV live. The pandemic has a devastating and tragic social, economic and demographic impact on previous development and health gains in developing countries. It affects mostly young, sexually active adults in their reproductive years as well as babies born from infected mothers. To understand the nutritional challenges of HIV/AIDS it is necessary to understand how the virus is transmitted and to follow the clinical course of the infection. The virus characteristics, its binding to cell surface receptors, its entry into cells of the immune system, its replication and transcription, as well as its genetic variability, and different classes of the virus have been intensively researched and described,

Box 15.2 Nutrient deficiency diseases in developing countries: prevalence (scope)		
Nutrient	Consequence: disease	Estimated: 1995–2006
Iron	Anemia; poor brain development in infancy	Maternal anemia pandemic: more than 80% in some countries; globally, more than 2000 million people
Protein, energy	Kwashiorkor, marasmus marasmic kwashiorkor, wasting	Millions of children are at risk
Vitamin A	Blindness; increased mortality from infectious diseases (children under 5 years especially vulnerable)	140–250 million children suffer from subclinical deficiency
Iodine	Goiter, cretinism (infants) with severe brain damage and mental retardation	In 1999, 700 million people in developing countries; remarkable progress made with universal salt iodization
Zinc	Its role in stunting and life-threatening childhood illnesses is only now becoming clear	Thought to be common in children and during pregnancy

forming the basis for the development of antiretroviral drugs to treat HIV/AIDS. More about this can be found in the clinical nutrition textbook of this series or at http://en.wikipedia.org/wiki/HIV.

Transmission of HIV

Because there is still no vaccine against HIV and no cure available, the emphasis is on prevention of transmission of the virus. It is transmitted from person to person via certain body fluids: blood (and blood products), semen, pre-seminal fluid, vaginal secretions, and breast milk.

The majority of HIV infections are acquired through unprotected sexual contact when sexual secretions of one partner come into contact with genital, oral, or rectal mucous membranes of another. The estimated infection risk per 10 000 exposures (without a condom) to an infected source varies from 0.5 to 50, depending on the type of exposure.

The blood transmission route is responsible for infections in intravenous drug users when they share needles with contaminated persons. Although blood and blood products are these days mostly checked for HIV, unhygienic practices in some developing countries, needle prick injuries of nurses and doctors, as well as procedures such as tattoos, piercings, and scarification rituals pose some risk for infection.

Transmission of the virus from an infected mother to her child can occur *in utero* during pregnancy, during childbirth (intrapartum), or during breastfeeding. The transmission rate between untreated infected mothers and children is approximately 25%. This risk can be reduced to 1% with combination antiretroviral treatment of the mother and cesarean section. The overall risk of a breastfeeding mother to child is between 20% and 45%. Recent studies have shown that this risk can be reduced three- to fourfold by exclusive breastfeeding for up to 6 months. Exclusive breastfeeding for 6 months is therefore the present recommendation from the WHO for infected mothers in developing countries "unless replacement feeding is acceptable, feasible, affordable, sustainable and safe for them and their infants before that time."

The clinical course of HIV infection: progression to AIDS

The different stages of HIV infection dictate different types of nutritional intervention. Even before infection, the vicious cycle of undernutrition and poverty in developing countries may increase vulnerability to infection: the hopelessness and despair of poverty could lead to alcohol abuse, violence, rape, and irresponsible sexual behaviors, increasing exposure to the virus. In addition, malnutrition could compromise the integrity of the immune system, increasing vulnerability to infection. Breaking this cycle by appropriate public health nutrition interventions in poverty alleviation programs may indirectly also impact on HIV transmission.

- Stage 1: Incubation period
  There are no symptoms during this stage and its duration is usually 2–4 weeks.
- Stage 2: Acute infection (seroconversion)
  There is rapid viral replication during this stage. It may last from a week to several months with a mean duration of 28 days. The symptoms in this stage include fever, lymphadenopathy, pharyngitis, rash, myalgia, malaise, headache, and mouth and esophageal sores.
- Stage 3: Asymptomatic or latency stage
  This stage may last from a few weeks up to 10 or 20 years, depending on the nutritional status and drug treatment of the individual. It is characterized by none or only a few symptoms, which may include subclinical weight loss, vitamin B_{12} deficiency, changes in blood lipids and liver enzymes, and an increased susceptibility to pathogens in food and water.
- Stage 4: Symptomatic HIV infection
  CD4+ cell counts (the immune cells containing the CD4 receptor, which binds the virus and which is destroyed during viral replication) have decreased from normal values of 1200, to between 200 and 500 cells/μl. Wasting is a characteristic symptom and is defined as an involuntary loss of more than 10% of baseline body weight. Other symptoms include loss of appetite, white plaques in the mouth, skin lesions, fever, night sweats, TB, shingles, and other infections. Nutrition interventions may help to preserve lean body mass, "strengthen" the immune system and slow progression to stage 5.
- Stage 5: AIDS
  The CD4+ counts are now below 200 cells/μL. The immunosuppression is severe and leads to many possible opportunistic or secondary infections with fungi, protozoa, bacteria and/or other viruses.

Malignant diseases and dementia may develop. This is the final stage, and if not treated by antiretroviral drugs and specific drugs for the secondary infections it invariably leads to death.

Nutrition and HIV/AIDS

The role of nutrition in HIV/AIDS is complex. As mentioned above, malnutrition could contribute to increased vulnerability to infection in developing countries. The virus probably increases nutritional needs, while its effects on the nervous and digestive system lead to decreased appetite and intakes, impaired digestion, and malabsorption. The consequent loss of lean body mass gave the infection its original African name of "thin disease." There are indications that improved nutrition may slow the progression of HIV infection to AIDS. There is evidence that nutritional support can help in the tolerance of antiretroviral drugs and their side-effects and assist in the management of some of the secondary infections of AIDS.

The optimal diet for people living with HIV/AIDS is not known. At least one study (the THUSA study in South Africa) indicated that asymptomatic infected subjects who regularly included animal-derived foods in their diets had better health outcomes than those on plant-based diets and with high omega-6 polyunsaturated fat intakes. The nutritional recommendations for people living with HIV/AIDS are therefore evidence informed and not totally evidence based at this stage. Global recommendations have recently been evaluated by the Academy of Science of South Africa, and some of their conclusions are summarized in Box 15.3.

The transmission of the virus and the different stages in the progression of infection to AIDS indicate that different levels of nutrition intervention and support are needed, as illustrated in Box 15.4. Specific nutrient requirements during HIV infection are discussed in the clinical nutrition textbook of this series.

15.5 The global challenge to address malnutrition

Background

The nutritional problems and diseases facing mankind at the beginning of the twenty-first century have been

---

Box 15.3 Nutritional recommendations for HIV/AIDS

1 Nutrition recommendations should do no harm
2 Optimum nutrition at population level is necessary as part of a set of general measures to reduce the spread of HIV and TB
3 The focus should be on diversified diets including available, affordable and traditional foods. However, fortified foods as well as macro- and micronutrient supplements at safe levels (not more than twice daily recommended level) may be helpful
4 Ready-to-use therapeutic food supplements are effective in reversing poor nutritional status found in severely affected individuals
5 Because micronutrient deficiencies may hasten disease progression and facilitate mother-to-child transmission of HIV, multivitamin, zinc and selenium supplementations are indicated, but vitamin A supplementation may increase mother-to-child transmission and zinc supplementation may be harmful in pregnant women
6 HIV-infected pregnant women, lactating mothers and their babies need special advice and care to ensure best possible outcomes
7 Established, well-described steps and protocols should be followed in public health nutrition interventions and in the therapeutic (medical) nutritional support of patients

General Principles from ASSAf (2007).

Box 15.4 Types of nutrition interventions needed

Stage	Nutrition intervention needed
Poverty/malnutrition cycle	Public Health Nutrition (PHN) programs as part of other programs to alleviate poverty and improve socioeconomic development
Increased vulnerability	Targeted nutrition (TN) programs for vulnerable groups including advice to pregnant mothers
Decreased immunocompetence	TN programs for PLWH, including food assistance; food-based dietary guidelines plus advice on safe foods and drinking water
Transmission High risk behavior Asymptomatic HIV People living with HIV (PLWH) AIDS	Individual therapeutic or medical nutrition (IMN) programs: i Facility based IMN programs with defined algorithms ii Home-based care IMN programs with practical advice Food and supplement assistance

identified and briefly discussed in this chapter. In developed countries these are mainly childhood and adult obesity and the NCDs related to a combination of overnutrition, lack of activity, smoking, alcohol abuse, and stressful lifestyles. In developing countries the magnitude of undernutrition is staggering. Moreover, obesity and NCDs have emerged in these countries and are increasingly becoming major causes of mortality. This double burden is further exacerbated by the HIV/AIDS pandemic.

Dietary patterns responsible for the problems

The dietary patterns and nutrient intakes responsible and contributing to these problems have been intensively researched in epidemiological, clinical, and basic molecular studies. There is a huge body of scientific evidence available to identify the immediate deficiencies and excesses in intakes, as well as all the environmental factors associated with suboptimal dietary patterns that lead to the nutrition-related diseases highlighted in this chapter. Broadly, these dietary problems can be summarized as:

- hunger and food insecurity in developing countries, with infants, pregnant women, and older people being the most vulnerable
- "hidden hunger" or micronutrient deficiencies in both developed and developing countries, especially of iron, vitamin A, zinc, iodine, and all dietary antioxidants
- overconsumption of unfortified and refined staple foods in "low-quality diets"
- availability and intake of too many high-fat, sugary, and refined convenience and fast foods, increasing total fat, saturated fat, trans fat, omega-6 fatty acid, sugars, and salt intake
- not enough fish and other sources of omega-3 fatty acids in the diet
- not enough vegetables and fruit and their products in the diet
- not enough dietary fiber-rich foods in the diet;
- too little dietary variety
- over-reliance on dietary supplements in the developed world.

Suggestions to meet the challenge

In an ideal world, every human being would be able to exercise their right (often constitutionally defined) to regularly access, at affordable prices, adequate (enough, sufficient), safe (uncontaminated), and nutritious food to prevent undernutrition and to ensure optimal nutritional status for health, well-being, a quality life, ability to actively and productively work and play, and moreover to reach their mental and physical development potential. This is often defined as being food and nutrient "secure."

The above situation would be possible if all stakeholders in the global community (UN agencies, governments, NGOs, food industries, academics, civil society, and others) worked together in partnerships to create a food and nutrition environment in which healthy food choices were available, acceptable, and affordable and where consumers were educated, informed, and motivated to make the right choices.

But we do not live in an ideal world, as the high prevalences of nutrition problems indicate. So the questions that need to be answered are what should be done and by whom to rectify the situation?

Clearly, the time for individual, separate programs to address undernutrition in one way and overnutrition and NCDs in another is past. What is needed is a holistic, integrated approach that will promote and make optimum nutrition possible. Several UN agencies, separately or in combination have developed "strategic directions" and described policy principles, strategies to introduce this on different levels in different settings, as well as actions to promote healthy diets. The challenge is huge, for there are many barriers to overcome: from war, to uncommitted political agendas, to "unhealthy" food preferences of individuals. The lessons learned from the failure of many developing countries to be on-track in reaching the Millennium Development Goals by 2015 plead for a new approach and global leadership. This could be possible in partnerships in which there is recognition and respect for different agendas, but where partners are willing to develop a common nutrition agenda and agree on steps to reach common goals. But there are also many success stories. For example great strides have been made in the past few decades to reduce child undernutrition in some developing regions. A global database on child growth and malnutrition covers 95% of the world's under-5 population (http://www.who.int/nutgrowthdb). Much is being done by several UN agencies and international donors and NGOs to improve the global nutrition situation, assisting countries in nutrition surveillance

Box 15.5 UN Agencies: Intersectorial nutrition policies and strategies to address the double burden of nutrition problems throughout the life course

1 Nutrition surveillance
2 Combating micronutrient deficiencies
   • Fortification
   • Salt iodization
3 Nutrition advocacy
4 Developing national food-based dietary guidelines
5 Addressing nutrition and HIV/AIDS
6 Addressing obesity and other diet-related diseases
7 Improving maternal, infant and young child nutrition cycle
   Improving nutrition of school-age children and adolescents (integrated school-based program, nutrition friendly schools, health promoting schools)
   • Ensuring appropriate fetal development
   • Implementation of new growth reference
   • Improving infant and young child nutrition (breastfeeding, complementary feeding, baby-friendly hospitals, global strategy on infant and young child feeding).

and implementation of targeted programs. In Box 15.5 one such an example is given, namely the topics of the WHO's integrated and intersectorial food policies and strategies to address the double burden of nutrition problems throughout the life course.

There is agreement that policies and programs should be implemented at all "levels" – from global macrolevels to individual microlevels. These programs will include a variety of actions – from food assistance of displaced people to educating consumers how to choose healthy diets. The development of food-based dietary guidelines in both the developed and developing world to assist people to choose an adequate but prudent diet for optimal nutrition is an example of the latter. There is total agreement in the body of literature on the nutrition challenges of the twenty-first century that the focus should be on prevention of nutrition-related diseases to minimize their serious economic and social consequences.

Further reading

ASSAf. *HIV/AIDS, TB and Nutrition*. Scientific inquiry into nutritional influences on human immunity with special reference to HIV infection and active TB in South Africa. Pretoria, Academy of Science of South Africa, 2007: 1–283 (www.assaf.org.za).

Murray CJ, Lopez AD, eds. *The Global Burden of Disease. A Comprehensive Assessment of Mortality and Disability from Diseases, Injuries, and Risk Factors in 1999 and Projected to 2020*. Geneva, Harvard University Press and WHO, 1996: 1–989.

Standing Committee on Nutrition (SCN). Working together to end child hunger and undernutrition. *SCN News* 2007; 34: 1–80.

United Nations Administrative Committee on Coordination, Sub-Committee on Nutrition (ACC/SCN), in collaboration with the International Food Policy Research Institute (IFPRI). *4th Report of the World Nutrition Situation: Nutrition Throughout the Life Cycle*. Geneva, IFPR, 2000.

World Cancer Research Fund and American Institute for Cancer Research. Food, Nutrition, Physical Activity and the Prevention of Cancer: A Global Perspective. Washington DC, AICR, 2007.

World Health Organization. *Global Strategy on Diet, Physical Activity and Health. Diet, Nutrition and the Prevention of Chronic Diseases*. WHO. Technical Report Series, no 916. Geneva, WHO 2007: 1–149 (http://www.who.int/dietphysicalactivity/publications/trs916/en/).

Index

Note: page references in italics refer to information in figures or tables.

abdominal girth 25
acetyl-CoA 105–7, 178–9
acidity regulators *348*
acrylamide 344
additives *10*, 346–7, *348*
　regulation 299–300
　sodium-containing *200*
adipose tissue *15*
　component lipids 104
　　and dietary fat intake 106
　endocrine control 103
aflatoxins *345*
agricultural residues *10*
AIDS/HIV 355–7
　nutrition needs 61, 357
alanine 51, *52*
albumin *214*
aluminium 233–4, *236*
Alzheimer's disease 215
amino acids
　biochemical roles and functions 50, *51*, 63
　　discovery and history 50–1
　　homeostasis and turnover 58–61, 78
　　metabolic needs 58–64
　　metabolites and derivatives 53–4
　biochemical structures 51–4
　body requirements 66–7
　　by species *62*
　　estimation and determination 65–7
　　in catabolic states 62, 72
　　influencing factors 58, 71–2
　　meeting needs 67–9
　classification 54–8
　sources 56–7
　　digestibility 68–9
ammonia 56–7, 61–2
amylopectin 80
amylose 80
anemia
　iron-deficiency 207
　megoblastic 175
　pernicious 168, 169
　and folate 175
　and scurvy 183
　and vitamin B12 168, 169
animal meat
　dietary fats 91–2
　drug residues 343
animal studies 311–14
anthropometry 22–3
antioxidants 291
　intracellular 61
　mode of action *222*
apoproteins 97, 99

impact on cholesterol 119–20
　properties *98*
appetite 33–4
　hormonal regulation 35
　metabolic factors 35
　neurophysiological factors 34–5
arachidonic acid cascade 109–11, *110*
arginine 51, *52*, 60
arginine—nitric oxide pathways 54
arsenic 233–4, *236*, 344
ascorbic acid *see* vitamin C
asparagine *52*
aspartate 51, *52*
aspartic acid 57
assessment of nutritional status *see* nutritional status assessments
astroviruses 334
atherogenic lipoprotein phenotype (ALP) 103
atherosclerosis
　and homocysteine levels 174
　lipid-mediated 100, 102–3
　　cholesterol-lowering drugs 91, 95
　　nutritional modifications 103–4
　　postprandial lipemia 98
　　TAG regulation hypothesis 103–4
athletes, energy requirements 43
ATP production 77
avidin 177

Bacillus cereus 328, *330*
bacterial contamination *10*, 327
　emerging pathogens 326–7
　pathogen characteristics *328–33*
　toxins 345
Bartter's syndrome 196
basal metabolic rate 37–8
　and energy intake ratios 269–70
beriberi 153–4
bias 260–3
bile acids 95
bioactives 291
bioavailability of foods, defined 286–7
biochemical markers 130
bioelectric impedance 25–6
bioflavonoids 186
biological markers 130
biotin 176–8
　deficiencies 177
　functions 177
blood clotting, and vitamin K 150–2
blood glucose, regulation mechanisms 77–9
body composition 12–30
　levels
　　atomic 13
　　cellular 14
　　molecular 13
　　relative relationships 14–15
　　whole body 14

body composition (*cont.*)
  measurement techniques 15–27
    advantages and disadvantages *27*
    anthropometry 22–3
    bioelectric impedance 25–6
    carcass analysis 15–16
    creatinine excretion 26–7
    CT imaging 21–2
    densitometry 16–18
    dilution methods 18–19
    dual-energy X-ray absorptiometry (DEXA) *18*, 19–21
    infrared interactance 25
    MRI imaging 22
    multicompartment models 20–1
    N-methyl-histidine excretion 26–7
    skinfold thickness 23–4
    total body electrical conductivity (TOBEC) 26
    ultrasound 25
    in vivo neutron activation analysis 16
    weight/height indices 22–3
  prospects for future 29–30
  use and misuse of data 27–9
body fat
  biochemical components 104
  deposition sites 104
  measures 27–9
    comparative analysis *29*
    densitometry 16–18
    skinfold thickness 23–4
  see also adipose tissue
body mass index (BMI) 22–3
  obesity measures 45
body protein mass 58
bone mass, and calcium 191–2
boron *233–4, 236*
bowel cancer
  prevention
    folate supplements 174–5
    role of butyrate 84
Boyle Gay-Lussac's law 17–18
brain
  and lipids 105, 114–15
    role of docosahexaenoate 114
bread/flour, fortified 174, 193
BSE (bovine spongiform encephalopathy) 338–9
bulking agents *348*
burning foot syndrome 179–80
butyrate 83–4

cadmium *233–4, 236*, 344
calcitriol 143–4
calcium 189–94
  absorption and transport 189–91
    influencing factors *191*
  daily requirements 193–4, *194*
  food sources 193–4, *193*
  functions 191
    deficiency conditions 191–2
  homeostatic regulation *190*
  interactions 194
  nutritional status 192–3
  tissue distribution 189–91
  toxicity 192
  and vitamin D 144, 192

Campylobacter 331
cancer
  and folate 174–5
  and selenium 219
  and vitamin B6 164
  and vitamin C 185, 219
carbohydrates 74–85
  classes 74–5
  digestive breakdown and absorption 74–6
    fermentation in the colon 82–3
    of short-chain fatty acids 83–4
  food sources *76*
  malabsorption problems 75–6
  metabolic utilization 77
  oral pH and dental caries 84–5
  types
    glycemic 76–9
    nonglycemic 79–84
    resistant starch and dietary fibre 81–2
carbon recycling 107
carcass analyis 15–16
cardiovascular disease 351–3
  and homocysteine levels 174
  and lipids
    ALP findings 102–3
    cholesterol-lowering drugs 91, 95
    homeostasis and transport 95, 100–3, 102–3
    hormonal control 103
    nutritional modifications 103–4
    postprandial regulation 98
    triacylglycerol (TAG) hypothesis 103–4
carnitine 186
carotenoids 135–7, 291
  antioxidant function 139
  see also vitamin A
case-control studies *318*, 320
cassava 346
cell membranes 90–1, 104
cell signaling mechanisms, arachidonic acid cascade 109–11, *110*
ceruloplasmin *214*
cestodes 338
chemicals affecting foods 340–6
  acceptable intake levels 341–2
  classes *340*
chemotherapy, and folate supplements 172–3
children
  energy requirements 42
  malnutrition 299
chloropropanols 344
cholecystokinin (CCK) 34, 93
cholera *332*
cholesterol 86
  biliary 95
  biosynthesis 114–15
  dietary intake 116–17
    impact on blood lipids 115–16
    role of MUFAs 116
    sources 90, 91–2, 114–15
  dietary regulation cf. drug lowering regimes 117
  functions, brain lipid membranes 105, 114–15
  homeostasis 95
    genetic factors 119–20
    hormonal control 103
    LDL receptor pathways 100–1, 102–3
    HDL reverse transport pathways 101–2, 102–3

re-esterification processes 96
  role of plant sterols 91, 116
  triacylglycerol (TAG) hypothesis 103–4
  storage, structural pools 104
cholesterol-lowering drugs 117
  effectiveness 117
  mode of action 95
  and plant sterols 91, 116
choline 186
chromium 230–2
chylomicrons 97–8, 100
  properties 98
chyme 93
clinical trials 318
Clostridium botulinum 328
Clostridium perfringens 330
cobalamins 167–70
Codex Alimentarius Commission (CAC) 299–300
coding systems 262
coenzyme A (CoA) 178–9
coenzyme Q 187
cohort studies 318, 320–1
colon
  bacteria 82–3
  carbohydrate breakdown 79–84
colorectal cancer
  prevention
    butyrate 84
    folate supplements 174–5
community nutrition, clinical roles 7
community trials 318
composite dishes, food composition calculations 287–8
congenital hyperthyroidism 224
conjugated fatty acid isomers 90
CONSORT guidelines 315
contaminants see bacterial contamination; chemicals affecting
        foods; viruses and foods
copper 212–17
  daily requirements and sources 216–17
  functions 213
    deficiency conditions 213–14
    enzyme components 181, 213, 214
  genetic diseases 215–16
  interactions 217
  metabolism and absorption 213
  nutritional status measures 216
  supplements 111
  toxicity 214–15
  transport and tissue distribution 213
corneal conditions 140
coronary heart disease, fish oil supplementation 117–18
correlation 310
coxsackie viruses 334
creatine 53
creatinine 61
  excretion 26–7
cretinism 224
Creutzfeldt-Jakob disease (CJD) 339–40
cross-sectional studies 318, 320
Cryptosporidium parvum 339
CT imaging, body composition analysis 21–2
cultural beliefs 8
cyanide 10
Cyclospora cayetanesis 339
cysteine 51, 52, 54, 61

cystic fibrosis 114
cystine 52
cytochrome C oxidase 214

daily nutrient recommendations see dietary reference
        standards
data accuracy and validity 247–8, 266–8, 305–6
data analysis 305–10
densitometry 16–18
dental caries
  and fluoride 229–30
  role of carbohydrates 84–5
depression, and food intake 35
desaturation processes 108–9
developing countries 353–5
  impact of HIV/AIDS 355–7
  infectious disease 355
  nutrient deficiencies 354–5
  obesity and NCDs 354
  poverty and malnutrition 353–4
DHA see docosahexaenoate
diabetes 78, 351–3
  and dyslipidemia 103
  and vitamin D status 144
diet history information 259–60
  see also nutritional status assessments
diet quality assessments 272
diet-induced disease see nutrition-related diseases
dietary assessment methods see nutritional status assessments
dietary data, accuracy and validity 247–8, 266–8
dietary fats 90, 92
  digestion and absorption 92–8
  nutritional and metabolic effects 112–14
  see also lipids
dietary fiber 81–3, 116
  intake levels 82
dietary patterns 294–5, 358–9
dietary reference standards 122–31
  concepts and approaches 122–3
    changes to 125
  definitions and terminology 123–5
  future studies 131
  identification methods 128–31
    animal experiments 130–4
    balance studies 129
    biochemical markers 130
    biological markers 130
    deprivation studies 128–9
    factorial methods 129–30
    radioactive tracer studies 129
    tissue nutrient level measures 130
  interpretation and uses 125–7
    for population studies 127–8
digestion
  carbohydrates 74–6
  fats 92–8
  food intake regulation 34
  proteins 68–9
dihydrofolate reductase 172–3
dioxins 343
disaccharides 80
disease
  body energy needs 44
  evolutionary perspectives on diet 114
  food-borne illnesses 325

disease (*cont.*)
    global challenges 350–9
        in developed countries 351–3
        in developing countries 353–5
        nutrient intake goals 352–3
docosahexaenoate 118
    early brain development 114
dopamine *53*
double labeled water (DLW) measures 39–40, 269
Down's syndrome 216
dual-energy X-ray absorptiometry (DEXA) *18*, 19–20
    multicompartment models 20–1
dUMP suppression test 175–6
Duncan test 309
dyslipidemia 103

echovirus 334
ecological studies *318*, 321
eicosanoids 109–11
eicosapentaenoic acid 117–18
elderly
    energy requirements 42
    height/weight measures 24
emulsification processes 92–3
emulsifiers *348*
energy availability, carbohydrate metabolism 77
energy balance
    concepts and definitions 31–2
    components 32–3
    future perspectives 47–8
    in disease and trauma states 44
    in infancy and childhood 42
    in old age 42
    in physically active individuals 43
    in pregnancy and lactation 43
    measures 268–71
energy expenditure 35–40
    concepts and definitions 32–3, 35–6
    historical aspects 36
    influencing factors
        physical activity 39
        resting metabolic rate 37–8
        thermic effects of feeding 38–9
    measurement 36–7, 268–71
        double labeled water (DLW) 39–40, 269
        urinary nitrogen measures 268–9
energy intake 32, 33–5
    dietary sources 33
    influencing factors 34–5
    regulation mechanisms 33–4
energy requirements 40–2
Entamoeba histolytica 339
enterohepatic circulation 95
environmental contaminants *10*, 343–4
epidemiological designs 316–22
    cross-sectional studies 320
    experimental studies 316–19
    non-experimental studies 319–20
error 246–7
    recall problems 263–4
    sources 260–2
essential fatty acid deficiencies 113–14
estrogen 103
ethics and nutrition studies *317*

ethnicity
    BMI and body fat analysis *23*
    food patterns 291
Europe
    food safety regulation 302–3
    public health policies 303–4
European Food Safety Authority (EFSA) 302–3
exercise, and energy balance 43
experimental diets 314–15

Fanconi's syndrome 199
fat-free mass (FFM), density calculations *17*
fats *see* dietary fats; fatty acids; lipids
fatty acids
    classification and terminology 87–90
    dietary intake
        effects on serum cholesterol 115–16, 119
        imbalances of n-3 to n-6 117–18
        trans fatty acids 113, 116
    digestion and absorption 92–3
        and colonic fermentation 83–4
    metabolism
        biosynthesis 105–6
        desaturation 108–9
        hydrogenation 109
        ketogenesis and ketosis 107
        oxidation 106–7
        peroxidation 107–8
        role of eicosanoids 109–11
    nutritional and metabolic effects 112–14
        deficiencies 113–14
        impact of *trans* fats 113
    storage 104–5
        as body fat 104
        whole body profiles *105*
    transport and circulation 95–8, 100–4
    see also lipids
fermentation processes, colonic 82–3
ferroxidase *214*
fiber
    dietary 81–3
    intake levels 82
field trials *318*
fish
    dietary fats 92, 117–18
    parasites 338
    poisoning *347*
    toxins 345–6
FIVIMS (Food Insecurity and Vulnerability Information and Mapping System) 6
flavins 155–8
flavonoids 291
flavor enhancers *348*
flukes 336–7
fluoride 228–30
    daily requirements and sources 230
    functions 229
        deficiency symptoms 229
    metabolism and absorption 228–9
    toxicity 229–30
folic acid 170–6
    daily requirements 175
    equivalents and viamers 170–1
    functions 171–5

metabolism and absorption 171
   tissue uptake 171
nutritional status assessment 175–6
food additives *10, 200,* 346–7
   regulation 299–300
Food and Agriculture Organization (FAO) 6
   food classification systems *280*
food composition data 262, 276–92
   benefits and uses *277*
   criteria for inclusion 278
      descriptions and classification of foods 278–9
      sampling methods 279–81
   data analysis methods 282–4
   data presentation 283–4
   data quality 284
   data sources 284–5
   future studies 289–92
   problems
      bioavailability 286–7
      composite recipes 287–8
      food preparation effects 285–6
      missing values 286
      portion estimates 288
   retrieval of data 288–9
      food—nutrient data conversion 289
   see also food labeling and profiling
food diaries 249–53
Food and Drug Administration (FDA) 279
food frequency questionnaires 256–9
food intake
   assessments 272–3
      of dietary adequacy 272
   measures
      choice of method 265–6
      direct 244–60
      evaluating data 271–2
      indirect 239–44
      sources of error 260–5
      underreporting 271–2
      validity and repeatability 266–71
   regulation 33–5
      appetite and satiety 33–4
      central nervous system factors 34–5
      circulatory factors 35
      digestive factors 34
      external signals 35
      peripheral signals 35
   thermic effects 38–9
food labeling and profiling 296, 297–8
food policy and regulation 293–304
   base-line dietary patterns 294–5
      making changes 295–6
   communication and policy dissemination 296–8
      nutrition claims 297
      nutrition labeling 296–8
   European agencies 301–4
   UN and UN agencies 298–9
   WHO/FAO and Codex Alimentarius 299–300
   WTO sanitary measures and trade barriers 300–1
food preparation, nutrient losses 285–6
food processing, contaminants 344
food profiling 297–8
food safety 10, 324–49
   assessments 273–4

concerns and contributing factors 324–7
   bacterial pathogens *10,* 327, *328–33*
   changing supply systems 324–5
   chemical contaminants 340–6
   emerging pathogens 326–7
   food additives 346–7
   food-borne illnesses 325–6
   parasites 335–8
   prion diseases (BSE/vCJD) 338–40
   setting safe intake levels 341–2
   toxins 344–6
   virus contaminants 327, 334–5, *334*
control programmes 348
European regulation 302–3
future studies 304, 348–9
surveillance systems 325
UN/UN agencies regulation 298–300
food sampling, for food composition tables 279–81
food supply
   system changes 324–5
   trade agreements and tariffs 300–1
food-borne illnesses 325
   bacterial contamination 327, *328–33*
   economic consequences 326
   emerging pathogens 326–7
   parasite infections 335–8
   surveillance 325
   virus contamination 327, 334–5, *334*
   vulnerable groups 325
formiminoglutamate test (FIGLU) 175
fructooligosaccharides (FOSs) 82
fructose *75,* 76–7, 79
functional foods 10, 82, 291, 296
fungal toxins 345
fungicides 342–3

galactose 75–6
gene expression regulation
   role of fatty acids 120
   role of retinol 137
genetics, blood lipid metabolism 119–20
germanium *233–4, 236*
ghrelin 35
Giardia intestinalis 339
glucose 36
   absorption 75–6
   metabolism 77
      role of biotin 178
   rate of uptake 76–7, 78
   regulation 77–9
      and diabetes 78
glucose-galactose malabsorption syndrome 76
glucosinolates 291
GLUT proteins 75–6
glutamate *51, 52,* 56–7
glutamine *50, 51, 52,* 56–7
glutathione 61
glycemic index (GI) 78–9, 186–7
glycine *51, 52,* 54, 56–7
glycoalkoids *348*
glycogen 77
glycolysis 77
glycosides *348*
goitre 224

Graves' disease 225
growth, amino acid and protein needs 55, 62–3
gum arabic 116

hazardous substances *10*
health status, and nutrition *4*
heavy metals *10*, 343–4
hemochromatosis 208
hepatitis E 334–5
hepatitis-A virus 327, *334*
herbicides 342–3
high-density lipoproteins (HDL) 98–9
    properties *98*
    reverse cholesterol transport 101–2, *102–3*
histidine *51*, 175–6
history of nutrition science 7–9
HIV/AIDS 355–7
    nutrition needs 61, 357
homocysteine *53*, 173–4
    elevated levels 174
household surveys 243–4
    expenditure data 243
    food account methods 243–4
    food inventory methods 244
    food procurement data 244
Human Genome Project 50
human nutrition science *see* nutrition studies
hunger 33–4
hydrogenation processes 90, 92, 109
    partial 92, 109, 113, 116
hydroxylases, and vitamin C 181–2
hypercalcemia 192
hypertension, and homocysteine levels 174
hyperthyroidism 225
hypocalcemia 195
hypokalemia 195
hypophosphatemia 199
hypothalamus 34–5
hypothesis testing 307
hypothyroidism 224, 225–6

in vitro studies 310–11
in vivo neutron activation analysis (IVNAA) 16
incidence, defined 322
industrial contaminants 343–5
industrial pollution *10*
infants
    energy requirements 42
    and vitamin B6 165
    and vitamin D 144–5
INFOODS (International Food Data System Project) (UN) 273, 279, 283–4, 290
informed consent *317*
infrared interactance 25
inositol 186–7
insecticides 342–3
insulin 35
    functions, lipoprotein metabolism 103, 104
intestinal flukes 336–7
iodine 223–6
    daily requirements 225
    food sources 225
    functions 223–4
        deficiency symptoms 224, *355*

    genetic diseases 225
    interactions 225–6
    metabolism and absorption 223
    nutritional status measures 225
    toxicity 224–5
    transport and tissue distribution 223
iron 205–9, *355*
    daily requirements 208–9
    food sources 208–9
    functions 206–7
        deficiency symptoms 207
    genetic diseases 208
    interactions 209
    metabolism and absorption 205–6, *207*
        role of vitamin C 184–5
    nutritional status measures 208
    toxicity 207–8
    transport and tissue distribution 205–6
isoflavones 291
isoleucine *51, 52*

JECFA (Joint FAO/WHO Expert Committee on Food Additives) 299–300
JEMRA (Joint FAO/WHO Meeting on Microbiological Risk Assessment) 299–300

Kaplan-Meier estimates *309*
Kashan-Beck disease 218–19
Kayser-Fleischer rings 215
Keshan's disease 218–19
ketogenesis 107
ketosis 107
Kruskal-Wallis test *309*
kynureninase 165–6

lactation, energy requirements 43
lactose *75*
    intolerance 75
LanguaL 279, *280*, 283–4
lead *233–4, 236*
    toxicity 344
lecithin 90
lectins 346
leptin 35
leucine *51, 52*, 53, 161
leucovorin rescue 173
leukotrienes 109–11
linoleate 104, 106, 108, 109, 113, 117, *118*
    deficiencies 114
lipemia, postprandial 97–8
lipids 86–120
    background history 86–7
    classification and types 87–91
        circulating 98–104
        fats and oils 90
        hydrogenated and conjugated fatty acid isomers 90
        long-chain saturated and monounsaturated fatty acids 89
        medium- and short-chain fatty acids 88
        milk and plasma lipids 105
        phospholipids 90–1
        polyunsaturated fatty acids (PUFAs) 89
        saturated fatty acids 87–8
        simple lipids 87
        sterols 91
        unsaturated fatty acids 87–8

dietary intake 92
dietary sources 91–2
digestion and absorption 92–4
metabolism (long-chain fatty acids) 105–11
  role of eicosanoids 109–11
solubilization 93–4
storage and deposition 96–8
  body lipid pools 104–5
  whole body fatty acid profiles *105*
structural and cell membrane functions 90–1, 104
transport 95–8, *96*
  HDL reverse cholesterol pathways 101–2, 102–3
  LDL receptor pathways 100–1, 102–3
lipolysis 93
lipoprotein lipase (LPL) 98
lipoproteins 92
  assembly and secretion 96–7
  classification and distribution *98*, 99
    VLDLs 98–103
  homeostasis 95, 100–3
  structures and metabolism *95*, 98–9
    metabolic determinants 100
  transport pathways 99–100, 102–3
Listeria monocytogenes 330
lithium 233–4, *236*
liver, cholesterol homeostasis 95, 100–3, *101, 102*
liver flukes *336*
long-chain fatty acids 89
  dietary sources *92*
  metabolism
    biosynthesis 105–6
    carbon recycling 107
    desaturation 108–9
    hydrogenation 109
    ketogenesis 107
    oxidation 106–7
    perioxidation 107–8
    role of eicosanoids 109–11
  nutritional regulation 111–12
low energy reporters (LERs) 270–1
low-density lipoproteins (LPLs)
  hormonal control 103
  influence of dietary fats 115–16
  properties *98*
  receptor pathways 100–1, 102–3
lung flukes *337*
lysine *52*

mad cow disease 338–9
magnesium 194–7
  daily requirements 196–7
  food sources *197*
  functions 195
    deficiency conditions 195–6
  genetic diseases 196
  homeostasis and absorption 194–5
  interactions 197
  nutritional status assessments 196
  tissue distribution 194–5
  toxicity 196
malabsorption syndromes 75–6
malaria, and riboflavin 157
malnutrition
  global challenges and perspectives 5–7, 298–9, 357–9
  and poverty 353–4

targets and initiatives 6, 298–300
  UN/UN agency responses 298–9
manganese 226–7
Mann-Whitney U-test *309*
meat
  dietary fats 91–2
  drug residues 343
  overcooked 344
Mediterranean diet 116, 117
medium-chain fatty acids 88–9, 112
  dietary sources *92*
megoblastic anemia 175
memory, recall errors 263–4
menadiol 149–50
menaquinone 149–50
Menkes' syndrome 215
mercury 344
meta-analysis 322
metabolic rates, at rest 37–8
methionine *51, 52*
  load test 165–6
  metabolism *172*, 173–4
methyl-folate trap 173–4
methylmalonic aciduria 170
microbial toxins 344–5
milk 193
  sunlight exposure 155
milk lipids 105
Millenium Development Goals 6, 299, 358
minerals and trace elements 188–237
  definitions 188
  future study areas 232, 236–7
  periodic table *189*
  ultratrace elements 232–6
molds and toxins 345
molybdenum 227–8
monosaccharides *75*, 80
monounsaturated fatty acids (MUFAs) 89, 113, 116, 117
motor neurone disease 216
MRI techniques, body composition analysis 22
mRNA, protein synthesis 53
MUFAs *see* monounsaturated fatty acids (MUFAs)
mycotoxins *345*

NCDs (non-communicable diseases) *see* nutrition-related diseases
nematodes 335–8
neurotransmitters, synthesis *51*
niacin 158–62
  classification and equivalents 159–60
  daily requirements 162
    availability 160
  functions 161
    deficiency conditions 161–2
  metabolism and absorption 160–1
    catabolism 160
    urinary excretion 160–1
  nutritional status assessment 162
  toxicity 162
nickel *233, 235, 236*
nicotinamide 159–60
nicotinic acid 159–60
night blindness 139

nitrogen
  biochemical precursors 60–1
  body requirements *60*, 64
  protein synthesis 56–7
  sources 56–7
nitrogen cycles *56*, 59, *59*
nitrosamines 344
  and vitamin C 185
nonglycemic carbohydrates 79–84
nonstarch polysaccharide (NSP) *see* dietary fiber
noroviruses 327, 334, *334*
novel foods *see* functional foods
nutrient recommendations *see* dietary reference standards
nutrients
  dietary reference standards 122–31
  food composition data 262, 276–92
  labeling and profiling 296–8
  see also carbohydrates; lipids; minerals and trace elements;
    proteins; vitamins
nutrition claims 297
nutrition labeling 296
nutrition studies 1–10
  approaches 2
  conceptual frameworks 2–3
  development history 7–9
  disease risk associations *294*
  global perspectives 5–7
  and health 4
  key study components 4–5
  reference points 293–4
  research areas and challenges 9–10
  research methodology 305–23
    experimental design and statistical analysis 305–
      10
    future studies 322–3
    use of animal models 311–14
    use in epidemiological studies 316–22
    use in human studies 314–16
    use of *in vitro* studies 310–11
  scientific theory vs clinical practice 7
  see also nutritional status assessments
nutrition-related diseases
  in developed countries 351–3
  in developing countries 353–5
nutritional status assessments
  considerations 238–9
  direct measures of intake 244–60
    basic concepts and definitions 246–8
    for longer periods 256–60
    for specified days 248–56
  future study areas 274
  indirect measures of intake 239–44
    approaches *240*
    commodity-level food supply data 240–2
    household surveys 243–4
    product-level food supply data 242–3
  method choice 265–71
    repeatability and validity 266–71
  safety assessments 273–4
nutritionists, roles 7

obesity 44–7
  basic metabolic principles 44–5
  definitions 45
  in developed countries 351–3

  in developing countries 354
  etiology 46
  health implications 103, 351–3
  role of physical activity 46–7
observational studies 319–20
oils 90
oleate 104, 108, 113, *118*
oligosaccharides *75*, 80, 82
omega fatty acids *see* polyunsaturated fatty acids (PUFAs)
ORAC database 291
oral contraceptives, and vitamin B6 166–7
ornithine *53–4*
osteomalacia 144–5
oxidation processes, fatty acids 106–7
oysters, pathogens *333*

PAHs 344
Paleolithic diets 114
palmitate 104, 108
pancreas, blood glucose regulation 77–8
pantothenic acid 178–80
  non-nutritional uses 180
parasites 335–8
parathyroid hormone 144
partially hydrogenated fatty acids 92, 109, 113, 116
patulin *345*
PCBs (polychlorinated biphenyls) 343
PDCAAS (protein digestibility-corrected amino acid score)
  69–70
pectin 116
pellagra 161–2
Pendred's syndrome 225
periodic table *189*
pernicious anemia 168, 169
peroxidation (auto-oxidation) 107–8
pesticide residues 342–3
pesticides *10*
phenylalanine *51*, *52*
phospholipids 90–1, 104
phosphorus 197–200
  food sources *193*, 200
  functions 198–9
    deficiency conditions 199
  genetic diseases 199
  homeostasis and absorption 197–8
  interactions 200
  nutritional status assessments 200
  tissue distribution 197–8
  toxicity 199
phylloquinone 149–50
phytate 346
phytestrogens 187
phytoceuticals 187
phytosterols 95
  food sources 92
plant proteins 70–1
plant sterols 91, 116, 291
plant toxins 346
plasma lipids
  overview 105, *118*
  see also cholesterol; triacylglycerols (TAGs)
polioviruses 334
pollutants *see* chemicals affecting foods
polyhalogenated hydrocarbons (PHHs) 343–4
polysaccharides *75*, 80

polyunsaturated fatty acids (PUFAs) 89
    basic functions 104
    deficiencies 113–14
    desaturation 108–9
    dietary intake 113
        impact on serum cholesterol 115–16, 119
        imbalances of n-3 to n-6 114, 117–18
        n-3 deficiencies 113–14
        nutrient—gene interactions 119–20
    hydrogenation 109
    nutritional and metabolic effects 113–14
        clinical importance 114
    nutritional regulation 111–12
    oxidation and peroxidation 107–8
    storage 104, 105
pooled analysis 322
pork, pathogens and parasites *333, 338*
portion size estimates 263, 288
potassium 202–5
    body composition measures 19
    daily requirements 204–5
    food sources 204–5
    functions 203–4
        deficiency symptoms 204
    homeostasis and absorption 203
    interactions 205
    toxicity 204
    transport and tissue distribution 203
poverty and malnutrition 353–4
power calculations 307–8
pregnancy
    and anticoagulants 151–2
    energy requirements 43
    and folate 174
prion diseases 338–40
processed foods, partial hydrogenation processes 92
propionate 83–4
prostaglandins 109–11
proteins 49–72
    background and discovery 50–1
    biochemical roles *51*
        amino acid functions *50*
    biochemical structures 49
    biochemical synthesis and degradation 58–62
    body requirements 58–63, 64–5
        by age and physiological groups 58, 64–5
        dietary recommendations 63–5
        during illness and trauma 72
        estimation 63–5
        influencing factors 58, 71–2
        growth needs 55, 62–3
        metabolic needs 58–64
        over supply 61–2
    classification of amino acids 54–8
    deficiencies *355*
    food sources 70–1
        and digestibility 68–9
        and nutritional quality 69–70
        worldwide availability *71, 355*
    future considerations 72
protozoa 338, *339*
public health nutrition 9–10
    role of nutritionists 7
PUFAs *see* polyunsaturated fatty acids (PUFAs)
puffer fish *347*

pyridoxines 162–4
pyruvate 77

quality of diets 272
quasi-experiments *318*
questionnaires 256–9

recipes, food composition calculations 287–8
recommendations and standards *see* dietary reference standards
records of food intake 248–53
reference values for nutrients *see* dietary reference standards
regional food differences 281–2
reliability of data 306
research methodology
    animal models 311–14
    in vitro studies 310–11
    statistical analysis 305–10
residues 342–4
resistant starch 81
response bias 260–2
resting metabolic rate (RMR) 37–8
retinol *134,* 135, 137
    see also vitamin A
retinol binding protein (RBP) 137
riboflavin *see* vitamin B2 (riboflavin)
rickets 144–5, 192
rotaviruses 334
rubidium *233, 235, 236*

salivary glands 75
Salmonella 332
salt intake trends *203*
    see also sodium and chloride
sample size calculations *308*
sampling bias 260
satiety 34
saturated fatty acids 89
    dietary sources *92*
    nutritional and metabolic effects 112, *118*
        and LDL cholesterol 119
    public health policies *296*
    see also long-chain fatty acids
SCFAs *see* short-chain fatty acids
Schilling test 170
scurvy 182–3
seafood pathogens *332, 347*
    toxins 345–6
seed oils 91
selenium 217–23
    daily requirements 220–1
    food sources 220–1
    functions 218
        deficiency conditions 218–20
    genetic diseases 220
    interactions 221–3
    metabolism and absorption 217–18
    nutritional status measures 220
    toxicity 220
    transport and tissue distribution 217–18
selenoproteins 218, *219*
serine *51, 52*
sex hormones, functions, lipoprotein metabolism 103
short-chain fatty acids (SCFAs) 83–4, 88
    absorption 83–4
    roles 83

silicon *233, 235, 236*
Siri's formula 16–17, *17*
skeletal mass, measures 24
skinfold thickness measures 23–4
sodium and chloride 200–2
    daily requirements 202
    functions 201
        deficiency symptoms 201
    genetic diseases 202
    homeostasis and absorption 200–1
    intake trends *205*
    interactions 202
    nutritional status assessments 202
    in processed foods *200*
    toxicity 201–2
    transport and tissue distribution 200–1
solanine *10*
soy beans 187
spina bifida 174
squalene 187
standards *see* Codex Alimentarius Commission (CAC); dietary
        reference standards
Staphylococcus aureus 329
starch
    digestion *75*, 80
    resistant 81
starches, modified 82
statistical analysis 305–10
stearate 104, 108
stone-age diets 114
strontium 146
studies on food intake *see* nutritional status assessments
sucrase-isomaltase deficiency 75
sugar alcohols 80
surveillance systems 325

t-tests *309*
tag names 283–4
TAGs *see* triacylglycerols
tannins 346
tapeworms 338
taurine 53, 187
teeth
    dental caries 85–6
    and fluoride 229–30
terpines 187
testosterone 103
thiamin *see* vitamin B1 (thiamin)
threonine *52*
thymidylate synthetase 172–3
thyroid hormones, and vitamin D 144
thyrotoxicosis 225
tin *233, 235, 236*
total body electrical conductivity (TOBEC) 26
total body potassium (TBK) 19
total body water (TBW) 18–19
toxins *10*, 344–6
    bacterial 345
    fungal 345
    microbial 344–5
    naturally occurring 346–7
    seafood 345–6
Toxoplasma gondii 339
trace elements *see* minerals and trace elements
trade agreements and tariffs 300–1

traffic light system food profiling 297–8
trans fatty acids 107–8, 113, 116
transmissible spongiform encephalopathy (TSE) 338–40
triacylglycerols (TAGs) 90
    dietary sources 91–2
    functions 104
    lipoprotein assembly 96–7
        impact of n-3 PUFAs 119
    postprandial lipemia 97–8
    re-esterification 96
    regulation of cholesterol deposition 103–4
        impact of n-3 PUFAs 119
    synthesis 104
trichinosis 338
triglycerides, dietary sources 91
tryptophan *51, 52*, 159–62
    load test 165
tyrosinase *214*
tyrosine *51, 52*

ubiquinone 187
ultrasound measurements 25
UNICEF (UN Children's Emergency Fund) 6, 299
United Nations (UN)
    food and nutrition regulation 298–9
    global challenges 358–9
    nutrient recommendations 124–5
    University Food and Nutrition Program INFOODS 273,
        279
unsaturated fatty acids 87–8
    partial hydrogenation 92
    types 88–9
urea cycle enzymes *61*
urea production 61–2
urinary nitrogen measures 268–9

validity
    defined 305
    of diet measures 267–71
valine *51, 52*
vanadium *233, 235, 236*
verotoxigenic *Escherichia coli* (VTEC) *331*
very low-density lipoproteins (VLDL) 98–9
    hormonal control 103
veterinary drug residues 343
Vibrio cholerae 332
Vibrio parahaemolyticus 332
Vibrio vulnificus 333
viruses and foods 327, 334–5, *334*
    astroviruses 334
    emerging pathogens 325–6
    hepatitis-A 327
    noroviruses 327, 334
    rotaviruses 334
vision
    role of vitamin A 137, *138*
    and night blindness 139
vitamins 132–87
    functions 132–3
        deficiency conditions 132–3
    future study areas 185–7
vitamin A 133–41
    classification and units 134–5
    daily reference levels 139

drug/nutrient interactions 141
functions 137–9
  deficiency conditions 139
metabolism and storage 135
status assessments 139–40
teratogenicity 140–1
toxicity 140
vitamin B1 (thiamin) 152–5
  daily requirements 154
  functions 153
    deficiency conditions 153–4
  metabolism and absorption 153
  status assessment 154–5
vitamin B2 (riboflavin) 155–8
  daily requirements 157–8
  functions 156–7
    deficiency conditions 157
  metabolism and absorption 155–6
    homeostasis 156
    and oxidative stress 157
  nutrient/drug interactions 158
  nutritional status assessments 158
  photolytic destruction 155
vitamin B6 162–7
  classification and vitamers 162–3
  daily requirements 164–5
  functions 164
    deficiency conditions 164
    non-nutritional uses 166–7
  metabolism and absorption 163–4
  nutritional status assessments 165–6
  toxicity 167
vitamin B12 167–70
  daily requirements 169
  functions 169
    deficiency conditions 169
  metabolism and absorption 168–9
    and folate 174
  nutritional status assessment 170
  structure and vitamers 167–8
vitamin C 180–5
  classification and structures 180–1
  daily requirements 183–4
    benefits of high doses 184–5
  functions 181–2
    deficiency conditions 182–3
    pro-and anti-oxidant roles 182
  metabolism and absorption 181
  nutritional status assessments 184
  pharmacological uses 185
  toxicity 185
vitamin D 141–6
  classification and units 141
  daily recommendations 145
  drug/nutrient interactions 145–6
  functions 144

deficiency conditions 144–5
metabolism and absorption 141
  to calcitriol 143
metabolites 143
regulation 143–4
synthesis (skin) 141–3
toxicity 145
vitamin E 146–9
  classification and units 146
  daily requirements 148
    high intake levels 149
  functions 146–8
    deficiency conditions 148
  metabolism and absorption 146
  nutrient interactions 149
  nutritional status assessment 148–9
vitamin K 149–52
  dietary sources 149–50
  functions 150–1
    deficiency conditions 152
  metabolism and synthesis 149–50
  toxicity and interactions 152
vitamin Q 187

waist-to-hip ratios 25
warfarin, contraindications, pregnancy 151–2
weight/height indices 22–3
Wernicke-Korsakoff syndrome 154
WHO (World Health Organization) 123–4
  food and nutrition regulation 298–300
  nutrient intake goals (disease prevention) 352
WHO/FAO (World Health Organization/Food and Agriculture
    Organization) 6, 124, 299–300
  Codex Alimentarius Commission (CAC) 299–
    300
Wilson's disease 215
WTO (World Trade Organization), trade agreements and tariffs
    301–2

X-linked hypophosphatemia 199
xerophthalmia 139

Yersinia enterocolitica 333

Zellweger's syndrome 114
zinc 209–12
  daily requirements 211–12
  food sources 211–12
  functions 210
    deficiency symptoms 210–11, 355
  genetic diseases 211
  interactions 212
  metabolism and absorption 209–10
  nutritional status measures 211
  toxicity 211
  transport and tissue distribution 209–10